CRITICAL NEEDS AND G

# PREVENTION, AMELIORATION, AND
# RESOLUTION OF LYME AND
# OTHER TICK-BORNE DISEASES

The Short-Term and Long-Term Outcomes

WORKSHOP REPORT

Committee on Lyme Disease and Other Tick-Borne Diseases:
The State of the Science

Board on Population Health and Public Health Practice

## INSTITUTE OF MEDICINE
*OF THE NATIONAL ACADEMIES*

THE NATIONAL ACADEMIES PRESS
Washington, D.C.
**www.nap.edu**

**THE NATIONAL ACADEMIES PRESS**    500 Fifth Street, N.W.    Washington, DC 20001

This project was supported by Contract No. N01-OD-4-2139 between the National Academy of Sciences and the National Institutes of Health. Any opinions, findings, conclusions, or recommendations expressed in this publication are those of the author(s) and do not necessarily reflect the view of the organizations or agencies that provided support for this project.

International Standard Book Number-13:   978-0-309-21109-3
International Standard Book Number-10:   0-309-21109-3

Additional copies of this report are available from the National Academies Press, 500 Fifth Street, N.W., Lockbox 285, Washington, DC 20055; (800) 624-6242 or (202) 334-3313 (in the Washington metropolitan area); Internet, http://www.nap.edu.

For more information about the Institute of Medicine, visit the IOM home page at **www. iom.edu.**

The serpent has been a symbol of long life, healing, and knowledge among almost all cultures and religions since the beginning of recorded history. The serpent adopted as a logotype by the Institute of Medicine is a relief carving from ancient Greece, now held by the Staatliche Museen in Berlin.

Cover images courtesy of the Centers for Disease Control and Prevention's Public Health Image Library.

IOM (Institute of Medicine). 2011. *Critical needs and gaps in understanding prevention, amelioration, and resolution of Lyme and other tick-borne diseases: The short-term and long-term outcomes: Workshop report.* Washington, DC: The National Academies Press.

*"Knowing is not enough; we must apply.
Willing is not enough; we must do."*
—Goethe

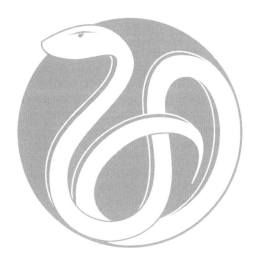

# INSTITUTE OF MEDICINE
### OF THE NATIONAL ACADEMIES

**Advising the Nation. Improving Health.**

# THE NATIONAL ACADEMIES
*Advisers to the Nation on Science, Engineering, and Medicine*

The **National Academy of Sciences** is a private, nonprofit, self-perpetuating society of distinguished scholars engaged in scientific and engineering research, dedicated to the furtherance of science and technology and to their use for the general welfare. Upon the authority of the charter granted to it by the Congress in 1863, the Academy has a mandate that requires it to advise the federal government on scientific and technical matters. Dr. Ralph J. Cicerone is president of the National Academy of Sciences.

The **National Academy of Engineering** was established in 1964, under the charter of the National Academy of Sciences, as a parallel organization of outstanding engineers. It is autonomous in its administration and in the selection of its members, sharing with the National Academy of Sciences the responsibility for advising the federal government. The National Academy of Engineering also sponsors engineering programs aimed at meeting national needs, encourages education and research, and recognizes the superior achievements of engineers. Dr. Charles M. Vest is president of the National Academy of Engineering.

The **Institute of Medicine** was established in 1970 by the National Academy of Sciences to secure the services of eminent members of appropriate professions in the examination of policy matters pertaining to the health of the public. The Institute acts under the responsibility given to the National Academy of Sciences by its congressional charter to be an adviser to the federal government and, upon its own initiative, to identify issues of medical care, research, and education. Dr. Harvey V. Fineberg is president of the Institute of Medicine.

The **National Research Council** was organized by the National Academy of Sciences in 1916 to associate the broad community of science and technology with the Academy's purposes of furthering knowledge and advising the federal government. Functioning in accordance with general policies determined by the Academy, the Council has become the principal operating agency of both the National Academy of Sciences and the National Academy of Engineering in providing services to the government, the public, and the scientific and engineering communities. The Council is administered jointly by both Academies and the Institute of Medicine. Dr. Ralph J. Cicerone and Dr. Charles M. Vest are chair and vice chair, respectively, of the National Research Council.

**www.national-academies.org**

# COMMITTEE ON LYME DISEASE AND OTHER TICK-BORNE DISEASES: THE STATE OF THE SCIENCE

# Reviewers

This report has been reviewed in draft form by persons chosen for their diverse perspectives and technical expertise, in accordance with procedures approved by the National Research Council's Report Review Committee. The purpose of this independent review is to provide candid and critical comments that will assist the institution in making its published report as sound as possible and to ensure that the report meets institutional standards for objectivity, evidence, and responsiveness to the study charge. The review comments and draft manuscript remain confidential to protect the integrity of the process. We wish to thank the following individuals for their review of this report:

**Abdu F. Azad, Pharm.D., Ph.D., M.P.H.,** Professor of Microbiology and Immunology, University of Maryland

**Stephen W. Barthold, D.V.M., Ph.D.,** Professor of Pathology and Director of the Center of Comparative Medicine, University of California at Davis

**Linda Lobes,** Director, Michigan Lyme Disease Association

**Robert Smith, M.D., M.P.H.,** Maine Medical Center Research Institute

**Ellen Stromdahl, Ph.D.,** Entomologist, US Army Public Health Command

Although the reviewers listed above have provided many constructive comments and suggestions, they did not see the final draft of the report before its release. The review of this report was overseen by **Linda McCauley, Ph.D., F.A.A.N., R.N.**, Dean, Nell Hodgson Woodruff School of Nursing, Emory University. Appointed by the National Research Council, she was responsible for making certain that an independent examination of this report was carried out in accordance with institutional procedures and that all review comments were carefully considered. Responsibility for the final content of this report rests entirely with the authoring committee and the institution.

# Contents

# Preface: A Walk in the Woods

Lyme disease and many other tick-borne diseases (TBDs) are zoonotic diseases in which a pathogen moves from an animal host to a person through ticks. Scientists now understand the complexities associated with such disease transmissions, including the role of ecosystems as it relates to the life cycle of the pathogen.

A walk in the woods in certain geographic areas of the United States constitutes a risk factor for exposure to Lyme disease or other tick-borne illness. The same phrase, a "walk in the woods," is also a metaphor for a process of conflict resolution. A "walk in the woods" is a model named for the classic 1982 saga of two Cold War nuclear arms reduction negotiators from the United States and Russia who broke an impasse in their talks by accompanying each other for a walk in the woods around Geneva, Switzerland, leading them to new insights and compromise, and ultimately a newly crafted agreement based on shared interests. This saga was later immortalized in a Broadway play symbolizing the advantage of interpersonal bargaining and interest-based negotiation.

It was obvious to participants at the workshop that a significant impasse has developed in the world of Lyme disease. There are conflicts within and among the science; policy; politics; medicine; and professional, public, and patient views pertaining to the subject, which have created significant misunderstandings, strong emotions, mistrust, and a game of blaming others who are not aligned with one's views. Lines in the sand have been drawn, sides have been taken, and frustration prevails. The "walk in the woods" process of conflict resolution or a similar process seems necessary for creating a new environment of trust and a better environment for more constructive dialogue to help focus research needs and achieve better outcomes. Such a process does not imply a compromise of the science but rather is needed to shift to a more positive and productive environment to optimize critical research and promote new collaborations.

Pamela Weintraub spoke eloquently about her personal experience and her family's challenges with Lyme disease. Ms. Weintraub also made the point that the impasses and mistrust that exist have been instrumental in impeding progress toward developing solutions by creating an environment that is unproductive and even accusatory. Thus, a "walk in the woods" seems to be in order not only in considering factors in disease transmission but also as a process by which to find common ground, align interests, and develop a national strategy to address the complex and serious issues of TBD, including Lyme disease.

The committee believes that the project will provide a snapshot of the state of the science for TBDs, but it recognizes that not all topics could be covered in as much depth during a 2-day workshop as would be satisfying to the committee or the scientific community. Furthermore, the committee was cognizant of the societal issues that could affect the scientific agenda, but we did not allow the controversy to affect the scientific discussion. During the process, the committee also noted a lack of precision in describing research. In the report, the committee has not attempted to impose uniform terminology or definitions, opting to retain those employed by the individual speakers. The committee realizes that the lack of precise, uniform terminology is hampering the reporting and the discussions of stages of Lyme disease and other tick-borne diseases. Although the committee was not charged to produce recommendations, we hope that this body of work will result in further discussions of research gaps, opportunities, and priorities.

Many individuals and organizations contributed to this report. The committee thanks the authors of the commissioned papers, who worked diligently over the summer and the early fall to produce the extensive background that contributed to discussions at the workshop. The committee also thanks the presenters at the workshop, the members of the research community, and the public who shared their perspectives before and during the meeting, as well as the many individuals who participated in other public forums, on phone calls, and by e-mail. We understand and appreciate the negative impact that some of these diseases have on the quality of peoples' lives. The convergence of science with real-life situations has highlighted both the need for more scientific knowledge and the serious societal issues and challenges that need to be addressed through scientific advancements.

The committee also extends its thanks to Sandra Hackman for providing preliminary drafts of some of the presentations; to Trevonne Walford for ensuring that the meetings and listening sessions ran smoothly and providing research and writing support; to Pam Lighter for assisting with the committee formation and background information; to Rita Deng for collecting initial data on the federal programs; to Andrea Bankoski for analyzing the federal program data; and to Carol Mason Spicer for drafting sections of the report and helping to provide critical comments. Hope Hare was instrumental in preparing the document for review and publication. We also thank Christine M. Coussens, who was the study director for the project. Together with Rose Marie Martinez, the board director, Christine helped the committee navigate the sociobiology issues. Although this was a challenging assignment, the committee welcomed the opportunity to help improve understanding of this group of diseases and, more importantly, to improve the lives of those who have been profoundly impacted by them.

# Acronyms

| | |
|---|---|
| ACA | Acrodermatitis chronica atrophicans |
| ADNI | Alzheimer's Disease Neuro-Imaging Initiative |
| AHSV | African horse sickness virus |
| ALS | Amyotrophic lateral sclerosis |
| ANA | Antinuclear antibodies |
| APC | Antigen-presenting cell |
| Arp | Arthritis-related protein |
| | |
| CALDA | California Lyme Disease Association |
| CBC | Complete blood count |
| CCHF | Crimean-Congo hemorrhagic fever |
| CCHFV | Crimean-Congo hemorrhagic fever virus |
| CDC | Centers for Disease Control and Prevention |
| CF | Complement fixation |
| CFS | Chronic fatigue syndrome |
| CME | Canine monocytic ehrlichosis |
| CRASP | Complement regulator-acquiring surface protein |
| CRF | Case report form |
| CSF | Cerebrospinal fluid |
| CSTE | Council of State and Territorial Epidemiologists |
| | |
| DbhA | DNA-binding protein HU-alpha |
| Dbp | Decorin-binding protein |
| DC | Dense-cored cell |

| DFA | Direct fluorescent antibody |
| DGGE | Denaturing gradient gel electrophoresis |
| DNA | Deoxyribonucleic acid |
| | |
| ECCMID | European Conference on Clinical Microbiology and Infectious Diseases |
| ECDC | European Centre for Disease Control |
| EEE | *Ehrlichia ewingii* ehrlichiosis |
| EIA | Enzyme immunoassay |
| ELISA | Enzyme-linked immunosorbent assay |
| EM | Erythema migrans |
| ESCMID | European Society of Clinical Microbiology and Infectious Diseases |
| EST | Expressed sequence tag |
| EUCALB | European Union Concerted Action on Lyme Borreliosis |
| | |
| FDA | Food and Drug Administration |
| FISH | Fluorescent in situ hybridization |
| | |
| GIS | Geographic Information Systems |
| | |
| HA | Human anaplasmosis |
| HBV | Hepatitis B virus |
| HCV | Hepatitis C virus |
| HE | Human granulocytic ehrlichiosis |
| HEE | Human ehrlichosis ewingii |
| HGA | Human granulocytic anaplasmosis |
| hgt | Horizontal gene transfer |
| HIV | Human immunodeficiency virus |
| HME | Human monocytic ehrlichiosis |
| HPA | Hypothalamic–pituitary–adrenal |
| Hsps | Heat-shock protein genes |
| | |
| IDSA | Infectious Diseases Society of America |
| IFA | Immunofluorescence assay |
| IFAT | Indirect immunofluorescence |
| IFN | Interferon |
| IFN- | Interferon gamma |
| IgG | Immunoglobulin G |
| IgM | Immunoglobulin M |
| IHA | Indirect hemagglutination |

| | |
|---|---|
| IL | Interleukin |
| ILADS | International Lyme and Associated Diseases Society |
| IOE | *Ixodes ovatus Ehrlichia* |
| IOM | Institute of Medicine |
| | |
| KFD | Kyasanur forest disease |
| | |
| LA | Latex agglutination |
| LD | Lyme disease |
| LFA-1 | Lymphocyte function associated antigen |
| LPS | Lipopolysaccharide |
| LTT | Lymphocyte transformation |
| | |
| MA | Microagglutination |
| MHC | Major histocompatibility complex |
| MLST | Multilocus sequence typing |
| MRI | Magnetic resonance imaging |
| MSF | Mediterranean spotted fever |
| MSP | Major surface protein |
| | |
| NatCapLyme | National Capital Lyme and Tick-borne Disease Association |
| NDVI | Normalized difference vegetation index |
| NEDSS | National Electronic Disease Surveillance System |
| NETSS | National Electronic Telecommunications System for Surveillance |
| NIAID | National Institute of Allergy and Infectious Diseases |
| NIH | National Institutes of Health |
| NIP | Nymphal infection prevalence |
| NK | Natural killer |
| NKT | Natural killer T |
| NNDSS | National Notifiable Disease Surveillance System |
| NSAIDs | Non-steroidal anti-inflammatory drugs |
| | |
| OMP | Outer membrane protein |
| Osp | Outer surface protein |
| | |
| PCR | Polymerase chain reaction |
| PFGE | Pulsed-field gel electrophoresis |
| PLS | Post-Lyme syndrome |
| POTS | Postural orthostatic tachycardia syndrome |
| | |
| RC | Reticulate cell |
| RELU | Rural Economy and Land Use |

| RMSF | Rocky Mountain spotted fever |
|---|---|
| Sca | Stem cell antigen |
| SCID | Severe combined immunodeficiency |
| SFG | Spotted fever group |
| SNP | Single-nucleotide polymorphism |
| STARI | Southern tick-associated rash illness |
| TBD | Tick-borne diseases |
| TBE | Tick-borne encephalitis |
| TFSS, T4SS | Type IV secretion system |
| TG | Typhus group |
| TIBOLA | Tick-borne lymphdenopathy |
| TLR | Toll-like receptor |
| T-RFLP | Terminal restriction fragment length polymorphisms |
| TRP | Tandem repeat protein |
| TRs | Tandemly repeated sequences |
| VBD | Vector-borne disease |
| VMP | Variable membrane protein |
| WHO | World Health Organization |
| WTD | Whitetail deer |

# Overview

Tick-borne diseases (TBDs) represent some of the world's most rap-idly expanding arthropod-borne infectious diseases, yet significant gaps remain in our understanding and knowledge about them. In the United States, many tick-borne diseases such as anaplasmosis and the borrelioses, ehrlichioses, and rickettsioses are on the rise. Reasons include shifts in the prevalence and distribution of animal reservoirs and tick vectors as well as the movement of humans into areas where the animal hosts and tick populations are abundant. From a public health standpoint, the burden of disease is of growing concern, as is the incomplete understanding of the complex interactions of ticks, hosts, pathogens, and habitats that underlie changing disease patterns and the potential for climate change to exacerbate these trends.

The Committee on Lyme Disease and Other Tick-Borne Diseases: The State of the Science was formed at the request of the National Institute of Allergy and Infectious Diseases to hold a 2-day workshop on the state of the science of Lyme disease and other TBDs. The committee was requested to be inclusive in the breadth of scientific approaches and disciplines, but to exclude treatment guidelines from the workshop. Furthermore, the work-shop was to provide a forum for broad scientific and public input and to produce a workshop report that would highlight the major themes of the workshop and commissioned papers. The committee was not constituted to develop conclusions or recommendations. The committee recognized that the limitation of a 2-day workshop meant that not all proposed topics or speakers could be accommodated; it did its best to cover a range of topics and speakers.

The presentations summarized in this document represent the views of the individual speakers and should not be interpreted as a consensus or an endorsement by the Institute of Medicine, the committee, or its sponsors. Furthermore, the committee recognizes that the language and terminology used to describe various facets and manifestations of Lyme disease and coinfecting conditions are not uniform throughout the report—this reflects differences in scientific perspective among speakers and authors. As highlighted by many presenters, a standard lexicon that is consistently applied and understood would improve and advance research efforts related to Lyme disease and other tick-borne diseases. Furthermore, addressing the major knowledge gaps identified in this report is likely to lead to standardization of terminology as the unknown becomes the known.

The following sections of the overview summarize the committee's highlights of presentations and discussions from the scientific portion of the agenda. The committee appreciates the time and efforts of the presenters and commissioned paper authors and the many participants who shared their stories to provide a context for these discussions. The interactions with patients and advocates were useful and constructive and served as an effective reminder of why scientific observations and gaps in knowledge need to be filled. Science is lagging behind as the burden of these diseases increases. The reader is directed to Chapter 3 for the rich presentation of participant views.

## EMERGING INFECTIONS, TICK BIOLOGY, AND HOST–VECTOR INTERACTIONS

The recognized number of serious diseases transmitted by ticks has increased over the past 30 years. The emergence and increased incidence of several major TBDs has been attributed to specific human activities and behaviors that disrupt ecosystems. Increases in human population and demographic shifts have brought dramatic changes in the distribution and composition of natural habitats, as people modify the land for living spaces, agriculture, or recreation. These changes mean that people and animals interact at many more interfaces, creating new opportunities for the transmission of zoonotic pathogens, including those responsible for TBDs. This session examined the natural history of ticks and their wildlife and domestic hosts; outlined the contributions of animal health experts to understanding human TBD; explored genetic diversity among pathogens, vectors, and hosts; and showed how scientists are investigating the microbial community found within the ticks themselves. During the session, the individual speakers highlighted a number of research gaps and opportunities for studying TBDs. Some of these gaps and opportunities cut across individual presentations and comments from the audience. A few of the themes discussed included

- Regional differences in the distribution of ticks and tick-borne pathogens and their contribution to human disease.
- Environmental systems and the "One Health" (i.e., the interface of human, animal, and environmental health that includes complexities of the ecosystems or the interface of biological communities and their physical or abiotic environment) approach to understanding tick-borne diseases.
- The biology and dynamic characteristics of disease vectors.
- The risk of TBDs as they relate to ecological fragmentation and reduced wildlife diversity.
- The tick microbiome and its role in transmission of pathogens to humans.

## SURVEILLANCE, SPECTRUM, AND BURDEN OF TICK-BORNE DISEASE, AND AT-RISK POPULATIONS

An understanding of the science of Lyme disease and other TBDs begins with the surveillance, spectrum, and burden of disease. This session focused on the current state of knowledge of the prevalence, incidence, patterns, and severity of key TBDs in the United States and their impact on patients. The presenters discussed efforts to track the movement of pathogens in the environment, how infection moves from animals to people, and the burden of human infection and disease, especially among vulnerable populations. Some themes discussed included

- The relative contributions of changes in surveillance, clinical recognition, and testing patterns to the rising incidence of all of the major tick-borne diseases.
- The impact of coinfection in severity of human TBDs.
- Biological understanding of persistent symptoms.

## PATHOGENESIS

Understanding pathogenesis of an infectious disease at the cellular and molecular levels is critical for discovering, developing, and implementing methods to prevent infection, and to improve patient outcomes after treatment. Scientists rely on several approaches to study the pathogenesis of tick-borne diseases. These include *in vitro* laboratory studies, *in vivo* studies of experimental and natural infections in animals, and patient studies based on clinical trials and specimens from biopsies and autopsies. While no one approach can represent the full spectrum and complexity of human disease, the ability to "reduce" or "control" the number of variables by using in vitro and in vivo models allows more rapid and less equivocal determination of key variables in disease progression—knowledge required to improve prevention, diagnosis, and treatment of tick-borne disease in patients. This session focused on the state of the science regarding the pathogenesis of tick-borne infections—specifically those caused by pathogens in the genera *Anaplasma*, *Borrelia*, *Ehrlichia*, and *Rickettsia*. Themes discussed included the following:

- Research based on animal models for the testing of hypotheses related to the clinical manifestations and severity of symptoms or disease.
- The role of the immune response to tick-borne infection and its effect on bacterial load and disease manifestations.
- New technologies in animal models that explore mechanisms of pathogen persistence following antibiotic treatment.
- Translating research findings from the animal model to clinical application.

## DIAGNOSTICS AND DIAGNOSIS

Diagnostics and diagnosis, which are essential to improve outcomes of tick-borne diseases, have different connotations. Diagnostics provide a cluster of objective measures directed toward identifying the cause of a disease. After scientists discover the causative agent of an emerging infectious disease, such as *Borrelia burgdorferi* or *Ehrlichia* chaffeensis, they develop, evaluate, and refine diagnostic tests over time. Diagnosis, in contrast, rests on a patient's history and symptoms and observed physical and laboratory findings in a particular epidemiologic context. Ultimately, accurate diagnosis requires knowledge of the epidemiology and clinical manifestations, as well as specific and sensitive diagnostic tests. In this session, the presenters explored the limitations of existing tests for Lyme borreliosis and other tick-borne diseases, and they discussed promising new approaches to diagnostics that may improve the diagnosis of these diseases, and the challenges and needs for improving initial diagnosis. Some themes discussed in this session included

- The current status of diagnostic tests and biomarkers for TBDs.
- The role of central system sensitivity and fatigue and other sequelae as possible biomarkers of TBDs.
- Measurement of qualitative symptoms reported by patients.
- Biorepositories for tick-borne diseases.
- Syndromic-based diagnostics for TBDs.

## PREVENTION

Research efforts have been focused on ameliorating the symptoms and consequences of tick-borne diseases through treatment. However, the development, deployment, and evaluation of strategies to prevent the occurrence of tick-borne diseases were also discussed as a high priority. Prevention of infection is much more preferable to treating the short- and long-term consequences of disease. In this session, the presentations addressed current and future opportunities for vaccine development, the role and effectiveness of behavior change, and vector-control strategies. A few of the themes discussed in this session included

- Research and development of safe, effective, multipathogen human and animal vaccines for tick-transmitted diseases.
- Land-use practices and public education as current tools to improve mitigation and prevention of TBDs.
- Social and behavioral considerations for TBD prevention interventions.
- Educational programs for the public.
- Assessing the impact of educational programs for patients and clinicians.

## SUMMATION

The committee invited a panel of stakeholders to listen to the presentations and discussions during the course of the 2-day workshop and to share their observations regarding the research gaps and priorities in the science of tick-borne diseases. The panel members were not asked to come to a consensus but rather to express their individual viewpoints. The panelists included a representative from a patient advocacy group, a clinician specializing in Lyme disease, a clinician–scientist specializing in *Ehrlichia* and *Anaplasma*, a clinician–scientist studying pathogenesis, and a European clinician–scientist who provided a global perspective. Following the discussion, the committee invited participants to share their thoughts. A few of the views presented during this session included perspectives on the following:

- Research funding gaps for other TBDs.
- Contribution of a national integrated research plan for advancing the science on TBDs.
- The merits of a long-term study of Lyme disease and other TBD patients.
- The role of public–private partnerships and other collaborative efforts to enhance the research on TBDs.

# 1

# Introduction

People live in a world of growing interdependency and complexity. The old English word "connexity" is an appropriate description that helps to define the combination of connectivity and complexity that is our reality. Tick-borne diseases (TBDs), including Lyme disease, are certainly embedded in our world of "connexity." This group of diseases defies simple cause and effect explanations and, while science has enabled us to uncover critical information on TBDs, we also realize that much more remains hidden.

TBDs represent some of the world's most rapidly expanding arthropod-borne diseases, yet there still are significant gaps in our understanding and an incomplete knowledge of them. While we can map the genome of *Borrelia burgdorferi*, the spirochete that causes Lyme disease, we still lack clarity in the natural history, epidemiology and true ecology of this pathogen as well as for other microbes involved with other TBDs. The state of the science is promising, but we lack a national, integrated research road map and an appreciation of the process of system thinking in considering these diseases and their human impact.

Rather than focusing on a more reductionist approach to science and research, we must fully understand parts in relationship with the whole and how they influence one another. The field of complex systems is relevant to the study of TBDs. This new field cuts across traditional disciplines of science, medicine, and the social sciences. It focuses on parts, wholes, and relationships. TBDs are problematic because causes and effects are not obviously related or are not closely associated in time and space. In addition, ecological knowledge has been grossly underused both to understand emerging infectious diseases and to reduce the burden of disease and mitigate its expression.

Vector-borne diseases, including diseases transmitted by ticks, continue to be a public health concern in the United States and abroad. Ticks are arthropods that belong to two large groups: hard (ixodid) and soft (argasid) ticks. Soft ticks undergo no more than seven molts during their life cycle while hard ticks undergo three (see Figure 1-1). The life cycle duration varies

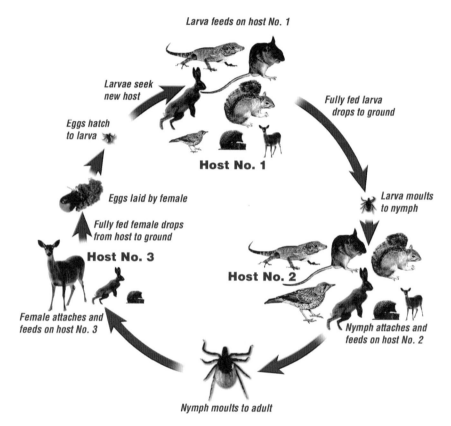

FIGURE 1-1 The life cycle of a three-host tick, such as *Ixodes* and *Dermacentor* sp., illustrating the common host for each stage. In this example, beginning prior to the first host, the eggs hatch to larvae and then feed on the first host. After the larval feeding is complete, the larvae drop from the host and molt to the nymph stage. At this stage, the nymph attaches and feeds again. It then drops off of the second host and molts to an adult. The adult tick attaches to a third host for a final meal. Following the final meal, the tick drops off and eggs laid by a female tick restart the process.

SOURCE: Reprinted with permission of Dr. Jeremy Gray.

as each of these life stages requires a blood meal from a vertebrate host. Ticks are highly adaptive to environmental change. In warmer climates, the life cycle duration may be less than a year. In colder climates, ticks can go months or years without feeding when the hosts are not available; the life cycle can encompass 3 years or longer. Numerous vertebrate species, such as rodents, deer, and rabbits, participate in zoonotic cycles that maintain infectious organisms in nature. Typically, a tick becomes infected with a virus, bacterium, or protozoan by feeding on an animal (reservoir host) that has the infection in its blood or by transovarial transmission of infected ova from an infected adult female tick. Ticks, in turn, transmit pathogens to reservoir animals in their salivary secretions while feeding.

This unusual lifestyle requires extraordinary evolutionary adaptation of the pathogen to the hosts, both vertebrate animals and ticks. Each of the tick-borne infections is initiated by the inoculation of the pathogen in saliva secreted by the feeding tick. Acquiring a blood meal occurs in a short feeding period only by soft ticks. Hard ticks feed for a period of days. Thus, ticks have evolved salivary components with pharmacologic activities of anticoagulation to maintain blood flow in the feeding site and modulation of inflammation and immunity to prevent deleterious host responses to the tick. The pathogen is transmitted via the tick saliva secreted during feeding (Kaufman and Nuttall, 1996), which has pharmacologically active substances (e.g., antihemostatic, vasodilatory, anti-inflammatory, and immunosuppressive) to aid in effective transmission. Infectious inocula can benefit from the local effects of the saliva, and through this transmission severe or fatal illness can result.

The local tick bite site lesion is useful for diagnosis of Lyme disease (erythema migrans) and *R. parkeri* infection (eschar). A multiple circular rash (Lyme disease); inflammation of the head and neck (tularemia); maculopapular, sometimes petechial, rash (Rocky Mountain spotted fever); and maculopapular, sometimes vesicular, rash (*R. parkeri* infection) occur frequently. Cutaneous lesions are observed less often in other tick-borne diseases in the United States.

Ticks have been recognized as a source of infections for humans for more than 100 years. In the United States, more than a dozen infectious diseases are transmitted by ticks (Table 1-1). The most common tick-borne diseases in the United States include Lyme disease, babesiosis, anaplasmosis, ehrlichiosis, relapsing fever, tularemia, Rocky Mountain spotted fever, and other rickettsioses. The geographic distributions of TBDs vary depending on the prevalence of the pathogen and vectors and the ecological system in which they are embedded. Additionally, tick-borne infectious diseases vary tremendously in their severity of illness. Severity of illness corresponds to visceral involvement (e.g., interstitial pneumonia and encephalitis) in Rocky Mountain spotted fever and human monocytotropic (or monocytic)

**TABLE 1-1** Tick-Borne Infections in the United States[a]

| Disease | Agent | Vector(s) | Intracellular/ Extracellular[b] | Chronic/ Prolonged/ Acute | Life-threatening |
|---|---|---|---|---|---|
| Lyme borreliosis | Borrelia burgdorferi | Ixodes scapularis, Ix. pacificus | E | Acute >> Chronic | No |
| Babesiosis | Babesia microti | Ix. scapularis | I | Prolonged | Seldom |
| Rocky Mountain spotted fever | Rickettsia rickettsii | Dermacentor variabilis, D. andersoni, Rhipicephalus sanguineus | I | Acute | Yes |
| Maculatum disease | R. parkeri | Amblyomma maculatum, A. americanum | I | Acute | No |
| Human monocytotropic ehrlichiosis | Ehrlichia chaffeensis | A. americanum, D. variabilis, Ix. pacificus | I | Acute | Yes |
| Ewingii ehrlichiosis | E. ewingii | A. americanum, D. variabilis | I | Acute | No |
| Human granulocytotropic anaplasmosis | Anaplasma phagocytophilum | Ix. scapularis, Ix. pacificus | I | Acute | Yes |
| Tick-borne relapsing fever | Borrelia turicatae, B. hermsi | Ornithodoros turicatae, O. hermsi | E | Prolonged | Yes |
| Tularemia | Francisella tularensis | D. andersoni, D. variabilis, A. americanum | I/E | Acute | Yes |
| Powassan/Deer tick virus encephalitis | Powassan and deer tick viruses | Ix. scapularis, D. andersoni | I | Acute | No |
| Colorado tick fever | Colorado tick fever virus | D. andersoni | I | Acute | Rare |
| Southern tick-associated rash illness (STARI) | unknown | A. americanum | unknown | unknown | No |

[a] Worldwide, there are approximately 865 species of ticks (Keirans and Durden, 2005), of which four species, *I. scapularis, I. pacificus, I. ricinus,* and *I. persulcatus,* are the primary vectors for Lyme disease, babesiosis, and human anaplasmosis. Other tick-borne illnesses that may occur in the United States include *Rickettsia* sp. 364D strain carried by *D. occidentalis* on the Pacific coast, *E. muris*-like organisms in the upper midwestern states, *Babesia duncani,* and *B. divergens*-like infections. The most frequently imported travel-associated tick-borne illness is African tick bite fever caused by *R. africae. Rickettsia massiliae,* a potential human pathogen, has been identified in *Rh. sanguineus* ticks in the United States, but not yet in humans. *Coxiella burnetii,* the agent of Q fever, occurs in ticks, but transmission in the United States is associated with inhalation of aerosols from animal parturition.
[b] E=extracellular; I=intracellular.

ehrlichiosis. These illnesses, human granulocytotropic anaplasmosis, and tularemia can also manifest clinically as sepsis. Rocky Mountain spotted fever, however, is among the most virulent infectious diseases known, and human monocytotropic ehrlichiosis, human granulocytotropic (or granulocytic) anaplasmosis, tick-borne-relapsing fever, and tularemia are life-threatening diseases. Currently no documented cases of mortality are associated with *Rickettsia parkeri*, *Ehrlichia ewingii*, and southern tick-associated rash illness (STARI), and only very rare cases are associated with *Borrelia burgdorferi* (Kugeler et al., 2011). More than half of the tick-borne diseases in the United States are emerging infectious diseases—many of which have been recognized only in the past two decades. Given the growing list of tick-borne diseases, one would predict that there are others involving zoonotic cycles yet to be discovered.

Many TBDs such as ehrlichioses, anaplasmosis, Lyme disease, and Rocky Mountain spotted fever are on the rise as animal reservoirs and tick vectors have increased in number and range and humans have inhabited areas where reservoir and tick populations are prevalent (Ismail et al., 2010). From a public health standpoint, this disease trend is of growing concern. Also of growing concern is our incomplete knowledge and understanding of the complex interactions of ticks, hosts, pathogens, and habitats and the potential impact of climate change. Improvements in our knowledge of this group of emerging and re-emerging diseases and their dynamics will be needed to reduce the risk of infection and the burden of these diseases.

## THE GENESIS OF THE WORKSHOP

The U.S. Senate and House included in the Appropriation Bill in September 2009 the following:

> The Committee encourages the [NIH] Director, in collaboration with the Director of NIAID, to sponsor a scientific conference on Lyme and other tick-borne diseases. The Committee believes that the conference should represent the broad spectrum of scientific views on Lyme disease and should provide a forum for public participation and input from individuals with Lyme disease. (U.S. Congress, House, 2009)

In March 2010, the National Institutes of Health (NIH) and the National Institute of Allergy and Infectious Diseases (NIAID) contracted with the Institute of Medicine to form a committee to plan the workshop and summarize the viewpoints in a workshop report. NIAID charged the committee to hold a workshop that discussed the state of the science, but that did not include a discussion of treatment guidelines. The committee was to provide opportunity for public input into the activity.

## THE COMMITTEE APPROACH

The Committee on Lyme Disease and Other Tick-Borne Diseases: The State of the Science met on April 29, 2010, in a planning session that was open to the public. Federal agencies conducting research in the field were invited to make brief presentations to the committee. These presentations were followed by a public comment period during which interested members of the research, advocacy, and patient communities were invited to make brief remarks. Individuals also were encouraged to submit comments to the project's e-mail address.

Following the initial meeting, the committee decided that it needed to provide additional opportunities for input from patients and groups not represented by the individuals who attended the planning meeting. The committee held four listening sessions on June 2, 15, 18, and 25, 2010, to hear from residents of the Southeastern United States (Georgia, North Carolina, South Carolina), the Southwest and West (Arizona and California), the Midwest (Iowa, Michigan, Minnesota, and Wisconsin), and members of the Native American population, respectively. The publicized target populations served as guidelines for those registering for the listening sessions, and the committee did not exclude anyone who wished to register but did not fit into one of the groups. A multiplicity of viewpoints with diverse ideas for workshop topics and speakers were expressed in the listening sessions, e-mail submissions, and planning meeting. Appendix C summarizes the public input into the agenda of the workshop.

The committee recognized the limitation of a 2-day workshop, which meant that not all proposed topics or speakers could be accommodated. The development of the agenda was driven primarily by topics that would cover the state of the science in tick-borne diseases: surveillance, burden of disease, diagnosis, diagnostics, at-risk populations, environmental and host interactions, pathogenesis, and prevention, as well as the human face of the disease. Per NIAID's charge to the committee, discussion of treatment guidelines was excluded from the workshop. With any complex scientific discipline it is difficult to limit discussion on a disease without some references to treatment. The committee further excluded the topics of physicians' discipline by state medical boards and insurance reimbursements from the workshop. Although these topics are of concern for many patients and clinicians, they fell outside the scope of the state of the science.

In addition to the speaker presentations, the committee commissioned 10 papers to gather further information on the state of the science of tick-borne diseases. The papers address a number of areas, including diagnostics, emerging infections, tick-transmitted microbes, vaccines, environmental contribution to tick-borne diseases, atypical Lyme disease, global burden of disease, case definitions, and a patient perspective. The patient perspective paper addresses the human aspect of tick-borne diseases. All of the commissioned papers are included in Appendix A. The Committee also requested information from federal agencies that conduct research or have programs associated with tick-borne diseases in their current research programs on tick-borne diseases. The information is summarized in Appendix B. Finally, the committee recognized that even with a generous allotment of time for discussion, a number of comments would not be able to be expressed during the workshop. The additional comments sent to the committee by e-mail are summarized in Appendix E.

Upon reviewing the presentations and comments during the workshop and in the pre-workshop listening sessions, the committee acknowledged that the language and terminology used to describe various facets and manifestations of Lyme disease and coinfecting conditions are inconsistently applied. Rather than offering its own interpretation of terms and definitions used by the various presenters, the committee has transcribed the terms as they were used by the workshop participants. This does not imply that the committee believes that terms such as "post-Lyme disease," "post-treatment Lyme disease," "persistent Lyme disease," and "chronic Lyme disease" are or are not interchangeable, differ in meaning or value, or have differing scientific validity. Similar confusion exists regarding terminology related to recurrent and relapsing Lyme disease with or without reinfection. As highlighted by many presenters, a standard lexicon that is consistently applied and understood would improve and advance research efforts regarding Lyme disease and other TBDs and likely improve patient care.

This workshop summary report is a reflection of what occurred during the workshop held on October 11–12, 2010. As part of the charge, the committee invited individuals with diverse viewpoints to present and participate at the workshop. The committee recognizes that not all viewpoints to fully discuss the nuances of the state of the science were represented at the meeting, nor with the number of topic areas could a point–counterpoint discussion occur. This workshop was designed to not reach concensus but to discuss a range of ideas. The committee did not weigh the scientific evidence on any topic, but it did ask the presenters to supply the references for their remarks. Where the references were available, they were included. Furthermore, the summary report should not be interpreted as a consensus of the Institute of Medicine, the committee, or its sponsors. The views presented, including the key knowledge gaps and research opportunities, are those of the individual speakers.

The reader will note that the workshop report is organized into eight additional chapters, which summarize the committee's preliminary introductions to the respective chapter and the corresponding presentations. The presentations from speakers and sessions may be presented in a different order than that reflected in the agenda. Chapter 2 provides a broad overview of tick-borne diseases from a systems perspective. Chapter 3 provides the societal and patient perspective of Lyme disease. Chapter 4 reflects the ecology, tick biology, and host interactions discussions. Chapter 5 provides a broad overview of the surveillance, spectrum, and burden of tick-borne diseases. It further includes a discussion of at-risk populations. Chapter 6 reviews the latest research on pathogenesis of four tick-borne diseases: Lyme disease, anaplasmosis, ehrlichioses, and rickettsial diseases. Chapter 7 reviews the state of the science on diagnostic tools for tick-borne diseases and the challenges for physicians in the treatment of these diseases. Chapter 8 provides a short overview of the prevention, including vaccines and non-pharmaceutical measures. Chapter 9 summarizes the viewpoints from participants on the research gaps, opportunities, and priorities for the field of tick-borne diseases.

# 2

# An Overview of Tick-Borne Diseases

A SYSTEMS APPROACH TO UNDERSTANDING TICK-BORNE
DISEASES: PEOPLE, ANIMALS, AND ECOSYSTEMS

*Richard S. Ostfeld, Ph.D., Cary Institute of Ecosystem Studies*

Throughout the 20th and 21st centuries, the number of infectious diseases in humans has been increasing as approximately 335 human infectious diseases have emerged since 1940 (Jones et al., 2008; Figure 2-1). Approximately 60 percent of those diseases are zoonotic, of which 72 percent are transmitted from wildlife and the remainder are transmitted from domestic animals. Furthermore, approximately 30 percent of emerging infectious diseases are vector-borne, which include tick-borne diseases (TBDs). Currently, there is incomplete and inadequate knowledge about key factors pertaining to persistence of reservoir, transmission, and host responses. More research is needed to better understand these diseases and to improve strategies to protect human health.

Lyme disease, one of the tick-borne diseases in the United States, emerged in the later half of the 20th century. It was first described in United States in the mid-1970s, although cases were reported in Europe in the late 1800s and early 1900s. The annual incidence of reported cases of Lyme disease has grown significantly from its initial recognition through 2008. By 1982, the Centers for Disease Control and Prevention designated Lyme disease as a notifiable disease, but even with this designation, an unknown number of cases remain unreported. Lyme disease is also found in Europe, where it is one of the fastest growing zoonotic diseases.

No. of EID events  • 1    ● 2–3    ● 4–5    ● 6–7    ● 8–11

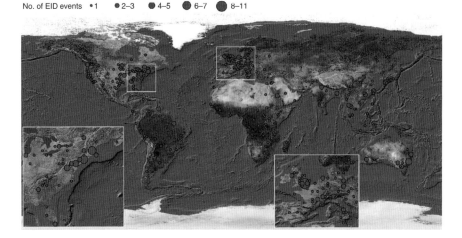

FIGURE 2-1 Global richness map of emerging infectious diseases from 1940 through 2004 showing clustering in the northeastern United States, western Europe, Japan, and southeastern Australia.
SOURCE: Reprinted by permission from Macmillian Publishers LTD: Nature, Jones et al., copyright 2008.

Reducing the burden of Lyme disease and other TBDs requires two main strategies: treatment of currently infected patients and prevention of transmission. Prevention is the ultimate goal to reduce the number of infections and clinical manifestations of TBD. Critical to any prevention measure is a fundamental understanding of the tick, its hosts, the pathogen, and the dynamic interplay of these components. Armed with that understanding, we can target the life stages, habitats, and other features of the organisms that confer a high risk of Lyme disease and other TBDs. Because effective vaccines are not currently available to humans, prevention strategies can be grouped into two approaches. The first focuses on human behavior such as the use of repellants and protective clothing, avoidance of risky activities and habitats, and so forth. The second is environmental and includes interventions that target ticks, their hosts, and the pathogens they transmit.

In most of northeastern United States, the black-legged tick, or *Ixodes scapularis*, is the primary vector for the transmission of *Borrelia burgdorferi*, the spirochete bacterium that causes Lyme disease. The *Ixodes* tick is a three-host tick, and its life cycle includes three post-egg stages: larva, nymph, and adult. At each stage, the tick takes a single blood meal from a vertebrate host. The tick then drops off the host and molts into the next stage: larvae into nymph, nymph into adult (see Figure 2-2). After a single

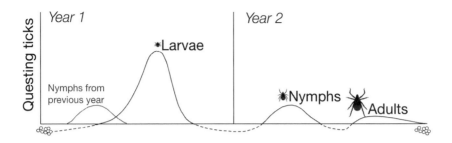

FIGURE 2-2 In its 2-year life cycle, the black-legged tick develops from egg to adult, taking a single blood meal at each stage in its development.
SOURCE: Unpublished, reprint courtesy of Dr. Jesse Brunner.

blood meal during which the males and females copulate, the adults also drop off, the females lay eggs, and both adults die to complete the life cycle.

Larval ticks hatch uninfected with Lyme disease spirochetes because of the lack of transovarial transmission of the pathogen from ticks through their eggs. However, the larval ticks will feed on virtually any warm-blooded vertebrate they encounter while questing on the forest floor. If they happen to feed on a host infected with Lyme disease spirochetes, the larvae may become infected. In that case, they will molt into an infected nymph capable of transmitting the infection to its next host, including humans.

Lyme disease and other TBDs are most likely to be transmitted to humans during the nymphal stage. The primary reasons are the frequent high prevalence of infection among nymphal ticks, the very small size of the nymphs, and the fact that nymphs reach their peak activity in late spring and early summer when human outdoor activity also peaks. The size of the nymphal population peak and the prevalence of infected nymphs are critical in determining the risk of human exposure to Lyme disease and other TBDs.

After Lyme disease was discovered in the 1970s, conventional wisdom held that only a few hosts determine how many infected nymphs would appear in a given year, with white-tailed deer being the predominant one. Even today, many research articles suggest that white-tailed deer are the definitive host of the black-legged tick. This theory is true for some environments.[1] For example, in a recent study on Monhegan Island, Maine, Rand and colleagues (2004) hunted to reduce a deer herd from approximately

---

[1] The committee notes evidence also supports the theory of deer being the definitive host. A mainland study in the same area as Monhegan documented a strong relationship of adult tick numbers and deer density (Rand et al., 2003), and studies by others (Wilson et al., 1988; Daniels et al., 1993) revealed similar tick reduction in the presence of alternative hosts for adult ticks.

100 to zero in a few years. By the end of the study, larval and nymphal tick populations had also declined to near zero. However, this is likely because humans and their pets were the only host species available on the island for adult black-legged ticks after the removal of the deer.

Other studies that have controlled deer populations and monitored tick populations have found a different outcome when other host species for the black-legged tick were present. For example, Stafford et al. (2003) significantly reduced a deer herd at two sites in southern Connecticut. At one site, the nymphal tick population declined steadily, and the researchers found a significant correlation in the size of the deer and nymphal tick populations. However, they found no significant correlation between deer and nymphal tick populations at the other site. Similarly, Deblinger et al. (1993) reduced the deer population on the northern coast of Massachusetts by 40 percent per year. Initially, the nymphal tick population declined significantly. However, by the end of the study the nymphal tick population had recovered and returned to the population level at the beginning of the study. Other studies have found no correlation between deer density and nymphal tick density in New York (Ostfeld et al., 2006) or between deer density and Lyme disease incidence in New Jersey (Jordan et al., 2007).

There are three primary reasons why the association between deer populations and black-legged ticks is often weak or variable. First, the black-legged tick is a host generalist in all three of its host-seeking life stages. Larvae and nymphs are known to feed on 41 species of mammals, 57 species of birds, and 14 species of lizards, while adults are known to feed on at least 27 species of mammals and 1 species of lizard. Second, when the population of a host species drops, ticks can aggregate on the remaining hosts. In the study reported by Deblinger et al. (1993) the number of ticks per deer rose as the researchers reduced the deer population. The same phenomenon may occur with other (non-deer) hosts for adult ticks as well, but has yet to be studied. Third, there is no correlation between the abundance of larval ticks in one year and the abundance of nymphal ticks (Ostfeld et al., 2006). A disconnect is apparent between the factors affecting larval tick populations and those affecting nymph populations—and therefore the risk of Lyme disease. So even if deer abundance determines subsequent larval abundance, this might not be relevant to Lyme disease risk.

An important note is that all three life stages feed on a number of different hosts. Rather than making assumptions about which hosts are fed upon by black-legged ticks, scientists need to determine empirically the role that the different host species play in producing the nymph population. The size of the larval cohort does not predict the size of the nymphal cohort—the cohort that is responsible for transmission of the pathogen. The critical issues are how many of the larvae are able to find a host that will support successful feeding and how many hosts will infect the larval tick so that it becomes an infected nymph. Understanding the interactions between the various host species and the larval tick is critical.

A particular host species might encounter ticks at a typical rate based on its body size, the way it uses space, or some other factor that scientists do not yet understand. However, some ticks that encounter a host will be unable to feed because they will be groomed off and killed in the process—host permissiveness. The combination of encounter rates and permissiveness determines the number of larvae on a host—known as body burden—during the larval period. Furthermore, each host species may provide a different quality or quantity of blood to feeding larval ticks, affecting their rate of molting success and over-the-winter survival. Different host species also have different reservoir competence levels: that is, different probabilities that they will infect feeding larvae with a tick-borne pathogen.

Ostfeld and colleagues (Keesing et al., 2009) captured six types of birds and mammals—representing a range of taxonomic groups and body sizes—in August, when larval black-legged ticks were feeding. The animals were held in the laboratory for about 4 days, until all naturally acquired ticks had dropped off; the researchers then placed 100 larval ticks on each host and followed their fate. There was significant variation in permissiveness among the host species. Approximately 50 percent of larval ticks that attempted a blood meal on white-footed mice succeeded, and dropped off in a replete state. Only 3.5 percent of larval ticks attempting a blood meal on an opossum succeeded, however, with the rest killed while trying to feed. Similarly, there was a significant variation in larval tick burden among species. When species were captured from the wild and the number of attached ticks determined, it was found that the average mouse hosts about 25 larval ticks, the average gray squirrel about 150 larval ticks, and the average opossum about 250 larval ticks. From these data, the encounter rate of larval ticks with hosts and the proportion of ticks that do not feed successfully as a result of low permissiveness can be estimated. The white-footed mouse grooms off and kills an average of 50 larval ticks per week, while gray squirrels groom off and kill approximately 843 larval ticks and opossums 5,686 larval ticks.

These species also vary in reservoir competence, with infected white-footed mice infecting approximately 90 percent of larval ticks that feed on them, and the other species, such as the white-tailed deer, raccoons, and opossums, infecting very few larval ticks (see Figure 2-3). Although white-footed mice, and secondarily eastern chipmunks, are ideal hosts for both feeding and infecting larval ticks with tick-borne pathogens, opossums, gray squirrels, and probably other hosts are not, which reduces the risk of human exposure to Lyme disease from these hosts. Thus, the composition of the host community for black-legged ticks in nature may determine risk for human Lyme disease.

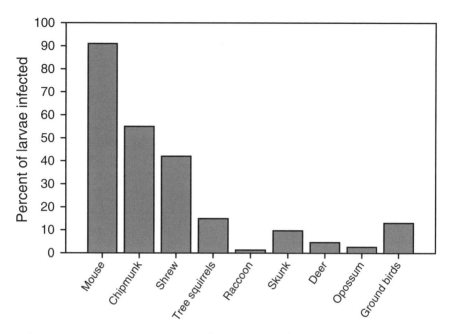

**FIGURE 2-3** Reservoir competence of common *Ixodes* ticks in potential hosts in which high rates of larval infection reflect a greater risk of pathogen transmission during subsequent feeding cycles.
SOURCE: Updated from LoGiudice et al., 2003.

Vertebrate host populations are reduced when land is developed and habitats become fragmented. Primarily the large body animal species, which require large amounts of space to live, and the predatory species disappear. Small, omnivorous species, such as the white-footed mouse, tend to dominate small forest fragments. Based on the host competence data and host permissiveness studies, one likely outcome is an elevated risk of Lyme disease transmission in small forest fragments but not in larger forest fragments. In suburban Duchess County in southeastern New York, there was a significant negative correlation between the size of a forest fragment and the prevalence of Lyme disease infection in the nymphal tick population (Allan et al., 2003). In forest fragments smaller than about two or three hectares, the risk of human exposure to *B. burgdorferi* rose by a factor of three or four. Public health officials could use this information to develop avoidance and intervention mechanisms by identifying landscapes that are likely to be the riskiest for transmission to humans.

Scientists do not yet know whether these findings apply to other tick-borne diseases such as human babesiosis, which emerged in 1966, and granulocytic anaplasmosis, which emerged in 1994. Hampering the research is the lack of a complete list of the natural reservoirs for the pathogens that cause those tick-borne diseases. However, initial work is beginning to test the role of various mammalian and avian hosts in infecting feeding larval ticks with the pathogens of these two emerging TBDs.

### Knowledge Gaps and Research Opportunities

Ostfeld identified a number of key questions that remain for future study:

- *Which factors other than the size of forest fragments predict the abundance of ticks and the prevalence of Lyme disease?* Some studies show that certain types of edges between forest and non-forest habitats influence the risk of Lyme disease transmission. Other studies show that the types of matrixes surrounding forest patches are important. The degree of isolation of these fragments can also influence the vertebrate host community. Understanding these factors and their impact will require much more research.
- *Do Lyme disease, anaplasmosis, and babesiosis share common risk factors?* If different hosts play different roles in infecting ticks with the pathogens that cause these diseases, that would suggest that the environmental determinants of risk of Lyme disease versus other tick-borne diseases are decoupled.
- *Which animal hosts of* Ixodes scapularis *ticks are of critical importance in determining the tick population density?*
- *Which local and landscape features affect human use of forests and other habitats, and hence their contact with ticks?* Although the density of infected nymphs in small forest fragments might be high, this finding may not be tremendously important for Lyme disease if people prefer to use more extensive forests for recreation. The decoupling of entomological risk and human behavior will mean that different educational and environmental interventions are needed to reduce risk.

### DISCUSSION

During the discussion, the participants and Ostfeld focused on the roles of various hosts, ticks, and habitats in the transmission of *B. burgdorferi* to humans and how this knowledge can be used to predict the occurrence of new areas for tick populations and to develop public health strategies aimed at reducing transmission of the disease.

## The Role of Migratory Birds in Tick Distribution

Several studies (Klich et al., 1996; Smith et al., 1996) have shown the nymphal tick burdens on migratory birds in the northeastern and midwestern United States and in Canada, where researchers have hypothesized that migratory birds are responsible for moving significant numbers of ticks long distances into areas where populations might not otherwise occur or for increasing the number of ticks in an already populated area. Ostfeld noted that this is another emerging frontier for research. Some evidence suggests that the ticks that are moved around by migratory birds tend to have low infection prevalence because, with a few exceptions, migratory birds are not highly competent reservoirs. However, the research is not complete and the data is limited.

## Reservoir–Competent Hosts

The need for ongoing research to identify why some host species have low or zero reservoir competence was suggested by some participants who cited the fact that lizards are not competent hosts. Ostfeld noted that the reason for low reservoir competence can vary by species. In the case of lizards, circulating proteins prevent infection. In other cases, such as opossums or gray squirrels, it is unknown whether low reservoir competence is a function of that complement system, which is innate or of induced immunity, including antibody production.

## Environmental Factors Affecting Tick Populations

One participant questioned the relationship between the population size of larval ticks and the opportunities for feeding on hosts. Ostfeld noted that researchers have found that acorn abundance is a reliable predictor of infected nymphal ticks 2 years later. In studies in New York, increased acorn production both attracts white-tailed deer and boosts populations of white-footed mice, with a subsequent increase in the abundance of larval ticks (Ostfeld et al., 1996; Jones et al., 1998).

## Transovarial Transmission

Studies in the late 1980s assessed questing larval ticks for prevalence of infection with spirochetes. The rate of infected larval ticks was approximately 1 percent, but the techniques used were not highly specific to *B. burgdorferi* (Piesman et al., 1986). One participant questioned whether the larvae's role in transmitting disease to humans has been underrecognized.

Ostfeld noted that other spirochetes are known to have a more efficient transovarial transmission, and the 1 percent rate noted in these studies may be these other spirochetes. The evidence of the lack of transovarial transmission comes from experimental studies that were done with adult ticks feeding on hosts known to be infected with *B. burgdorferi* spirochetes. The larval ticks that hatched from the eggs of infected ticks were not infected.

### Land-Use and Public Health Strategy

The relationship of tick and host habitat to the transmission of disease to humans was an area of considerable interest in which participants and Ostfeld discussed land-use strategies and the potential influence on public health. One participant asked whether there is an inherent geographic or landscape scale limit on the spread of Lyme disease. Ostfeld noted that it is possible to sample various areas to estimate tick abundance and to use Landsat imagery to examine the correlates. With these estimates, scientists can make models of how the ticks will spread. The problem is that the risk maps are created on a dynamic system, which results in underestimating the suite of potentially favorable conditions under which ticks can occur. As a result, ticks may inhabit areas that the risk maps do not indicate as favorable.

The research presented suggests an opportunity for engaging with regional planners in terms of forest fragmentation, observed one participant. Ostfeld concurred that engaging various county- and city-level government agencies is an area for future collaboration. The challenge lies in translating ecological observations into actual policy at the local, regional, and county levels, and more discussion is needed to determine how to integrate these observations into zoning and planning.

Other participants focused on specific strategies such as placing signage in high-risk areas or using pesticides. Ostfeld agreed that both of these strategies had promise. For example, the Tick Task Force in Duchess County has placed signs at trail heads and in public parks. The signs not only point out that the danger of exposure to pathogen-bearing ticks is high but also offer advice on how to reduce risk through personal protection measures. Targeted pesticide usage is an area of further discussion, Ostfeld noted. This strategy would benefit public health by targeting application in areas where both the incidence of infected ticks and human use are high—such as school fields—while reducing the collateral damage from overuse of pesticides.

# 3

# The Social Construction and Human Face of Tick-Borne Disease

## THE SOCIAL CONSTRUCTION OF LYME DISEASE

*Robert A. Aronowitz, M.D., University of Pennsylvania*

The apparent consensus about a treatable disease caused by a spirochete found in New England in the mid-1970s turned out to be anything but a simple story. The American definition and diagnosis of Lyme disease has generated considerable controversy. Disease definitions are often negotiated balances between two ways of understanding illness: as a specific disease or as an individual idiosyncrasy. Although biological processes place limits on how diseases can be defined, what counts as a (new) disease often depends on values, interests, and contingent historical events. As the history of Lyme disease suggests, the definition of a disease often results in winners and losers, and controversy among the stakeholders is apt to follow.[1]

To place the discovery of Lyme disease in the United States in context, it is helpful to review earlier events in Europe. As early as 1910, European clinicians described a rash they called erythema chronicum migrans following a tick bite. In the 1930s, the disease was connected to meningitis, and people had strong suspicions that it was bacterial in origin, pointing to *Rickettsia* in particular. There was even speculation that spirochetes might be involved, although the evidence seemed weak. After World War II, European clinicians used penicillin to fight the illness, and it generally was

---

[1] The committee notes that other accounts of the history of Lyme disease exist, such as the book, *Borrelia: Molecular Biology, Host Interaction and Pathogenesis* Samuels and Radolf (2010), and the original research articles such as Steere et al., 1980b.

thought to work. At the same time, different groups, primarily dermatologists and syphilologists, linked different syndromes, such as acrodermatitis chronica atrophicans and Bannwarth's syndrome, that are now considered part of the Lyme disease complex. These Europeans were already viewing the illness that Americans would later call Lyme disease as a systemic disease.

The first U.S. case report of erythema migrans appeared in Wisconsin in the 1970s. In 1976, physicians at the naval base in Groton, Connecticut, reported the first cluster of erythema migrans cases in the *Journal of the American Medical Association* (Mast and Burrows, 1976). Although this report received little attention, a Danish doctor participating in dermatology grand rounds at Yale connected the cases to erythema chronicum migrans in Europe. A prospective study was mounted in 1976 that identified erythema migrans in new cases.

During this same period, Yale rheumatologists had begun investigating undiagnosed illnesses among children and adults in and around Lyme, Connecticut, focusing especially on an apparent clustering of joint and other problems in children. These clinicians suspected some kind of juvenile rheumatoid arthritis, but that illness was not known to cluster geographically. About 25 percent of the patients had a history of a rash, but that sign did not appear prominently in these early case descriptions. By 1976 the Yale researchers had postulated a new condition, which they first called "Lyme disease arthritis" (Medical News, 1976; Steere et al., 1977), now known as Lyme disease.

The Yale rheumatologists considered Lyme disease to be a new rheumatological condition because it was unlike any previously described condition, and swollen joints were one of the most prominent signs. In addition, referral patterns reinforced the rheumatological identity of the disease. Later the fact that Lyme disease represented a new synthesis of previously separate diseases provided another rationale for declaring it a new illness, reinforced by the accompanying professional rewards and media and medical interest. Some observers noted that changing ecological conditions in and around the Northeast may also be associated with the occurrence of Lyme disease.

Framing Lyme disease as new disease rather than an American variant of an existing one had consequences. Early investigations focused on viruses as the prime etiological suspect. Thereforth, many cases were not treated with antibiotics, as was common in Europe.[2] Newness brought fear, uncertainty, and controversy over the proper definition, diagnosis, and treatment of Lyme disease, as did various biological and sociological factors. The

---

[2] The committee notes that some reports from the 1980s demonstrate the effectiveness of antibiotic therapy (Steere et al., 1980b).

timing of the disease's emergence coincided with the evolution of the AIDS epidemic. There was geographical risk of contracting the disease, as well as an apparent tendency for it to disproportionately affect certain populations, such as residents, especially children, of suburban areas. Diagnosis came primarily from clinical criteria, due to the imprecision of laboratory tests. Finally, because of the emergence of this new disease and the associated clinical manifestations, patients were concerned and frightened.

Disputes about the definition and diagnosis of Lyme disease helped spawn the debate about chronic Lyme disease that continues today. The controversy also spurred dispute about the benefits and risks of a vaccine against the disease that was developed during the 1990s and early 2000s. This dispute partly concerned the vaccine's benefits and risks; however, the core issue remained the legitimacy of chronic Lyme disease as a sequela of infection with *Borrelia*. In particular, some people contested the diagnostic criteria employed during clinical trials for the vaccine, seeing them as much too narrow and reminiscent of the orthodox view of Lyme disease as an acute, treatable, and self-limited disease rather than a disease that could become chronic.

The decision by vaccine developers to opt for a narrow-case definition seemed perfectly sensible from one perspective: Such a definition increased the power of clinical trials to detect a positive effect from the vaccine. However, vaccine promoters failed to understand and anticipate what was at stake in the controversy over Lyme disease. To patient advocates, evidence of the efficacy of the vaccine simply reinforced the fallacy inherent in narrowly defining the disease. This dispute played out when investigators of two clinical trials, who published the results in the *New England Journal of Medicine*, found very little, if any, asymptomatic seroconversion among people vaccinated during the trials (Steere et al., 1997; Sigal et al., 1998). To promoters of the vaccine, this was evidence of its efficacy over and above the 75–85 percent reduction in clinical cases of Lyme disease seen during the trials. The fact that asymptomatic seroconverters were not subject to clinician and patient bias during referral and diagnosis underscored this finding.

However, critics who thought the trial was designed to reinforce the orthodox view of Lyme disease argued that no asymptomatic seroconversion occurred because the vaccine induced everyone who was asymptomatic to become symptomatic. No data could reconcile these two points of view: They were simply incommensurate. Indeed, regulatory hearings on the vaccine suggested that its promoters and critics inhabited different universes.

Immediately after winning regulatory approval for the vaccine, the manufacturers launched an extensive advertising campaign built largely on provoking fear of the disease and raising awareness of the vaccine among consumers. In so doing, the manufacturers again misjudged what was at stake in the Lyme disease controversy: not solely or perhaps even primarily fear of the disease, but rather fear among those favoring a broader definition of Lyme disease that the vaccine could cause a chronic Lyme disease-like syndrome and evidence of vaccine efficacy could be understood to delegitimize chronic Lyme disease. In addition, Lyme disease does not reflect the typical characteristics of a disease against which to vaccinate. Many vaccines are developed for diseases that are communicable and potentially severe and are designed to reduce or prevent the spread of the disease through herd immunity. Because Lyme disease is not contagious, the vaccine would not generate herd immunity; it would prevent infection only in vaccinated individuals. Furthermore, the perception by a few that Lyme disease was an acute, self-limiting condition tended to reduce the impetus to vaccinate widely. In different ways, both those who adhere to an orthodox view of Lyme disease and those who advocate for inclusion of the experience of chronic, persistent symptoms within the diagnostic umbrella had reservations about widespread use of the vaccine.

Interestingly, people on both sides of the debate seemed to share the assumption that suffering is legitimate only if linked to a "real" disease. The controversy arises partially over who determines whether the suffering among patients with chronic, persistent symptoms is legitimate, and perhaps more generally a societal concern over the reach of medical authority.

In conclusion, Aronowitz noted that the history and sociology of Lyme disease suggest several lessons:

- Recognizing a new disease has no hard-and-fast rules: what counts often depends on historical events and participants' interests and values.
- Participants in such controversies need to tone down efforts to amplify fear of a disease, while avoiding overly optimistic pronouncements about it—a difficult balance to achieve.
- Clinicians and researchers need to accept the diversity of diagnostic names and possible natural histories of a disease and to decouple disease naming and diagnosis from treatment decisions.

## THE HUMAN FACE OF TICK-BORNE DISEASE INFECTIONS

*Pamela Weintraub*

Pamela Weintraub is the features editor at *Discover* magazine and author of the book *Cure Unknown: Inside the Lyme Epidemic.* Her presentation is not intended to reflect the views of all patients, but rather to draw on her personal experiences with Lyme disease, and her interviews with both Lyme disease patients and researchers to provide a commentary and a basis for discussion of how research takes place in a context of human experience. What follows is a first-person narrative.

Lyme disease entered my life in 1993, when my husband, Mark, our two sons, and I moved to Westchester County, New York. Our lovely property abutted a spruce forest, and we reveled in our new contact with nature, which included squirrels, raccoons, mice, and other animals and birds.

From that point on we all became increasingly sick. First there were headaches, joint pains, and an inexplicable weariness. With time the symptoms intensified and multiplied. My knees became so painful that I had to sit down to descend stairs on my bottom one step at a time. I developed dysphasia (impaired speech and verbal comprehension). I had so much trouble swallowing that I choked on my food. I developed peripheral neuropathy: My arms and legs buzzed gently at first, and then increasingly painfully, until it felt like electricity was running through me. The headaches became relentless. My eyes were painfully sensitive to light. I spent hours each day in a darkened room in bed.

Meanwhile Mark, an avid tennis player, began stumbling and bumping into walls. An award-winning journalist, he began struggling with memory and groping for words. He was forced to leave his job after realizing that he had spent hours trying to read a single simple paragraph.

Our youngest son, David, began to sleep so much that he could not do his homework or see his friends, and eventually could not get to class. In the end he was sleeping 15 hours a day. Hardest hit was Jason, our oldest, who suffered profound fatigue and shooting pain starting at age 9, late in the summer of 1993. The doctors called these normal "growing pains," so my son tried to keep going.

Then in 1998 he developed a huge erythema migrans rash over his torso. I called the doctor's office and was told not to bring him in. Because the rash wasn't in the shape of a bull's eye, it wasn't Lyme disease, they said. After that rash, Jason became increasingly ill and never seemed to get well. By 2000, at age 16, he was functionally disabled. He couldn't think, walk, or tolerate sound and light. On medical leave from high school, he spent his days in the tub, drifting in a mental fog while hot water and steam eased his pain. A raft of specialists at New York City's top teaching hospitals suggested diagnoses from migraine aura to parvovirus. Each diagnosis elicited a treatment, but none of them worked.

"What about Lyme disease?" I asked from time to time. "There are too many symptoms here and he is way too sick for Lyme disease," responded the pediatrician, who told us he felt it was all psychological. Thankfully, the psychiatrist who we ultimately consulted, who literally wrote the book on child and adolescent psychiatry, disagreed. At his insistence the pediatrician drew 14 vials of blood testing for hormonal imbalance, mineral deficiency, anemia, and a host of infections, including one tick-borne disease: Lyme disease. A week later the pediatrician called to tell us that a Western immunoblot had come back positive for Lyme disease, with 8 of 10 bands highly lit.

Finally, the head of infectious disease at Northern Westchester Hospital weighed in with his opinion. Jason probably had been misdiagnosed for years, he said. I will never forget the way he phrased his grudging diagnosis: "I will give it to you," he said, as if we had earned some coveted prize that others whose confusing array of multisystem ailments could be explained in some other way, would never get.

Unaware of the political turmoil surrounding this tick-borne disease, I didn't yet understand how rare it was for a doctor like him to diagnose late-stage Lyme disease in New York State. However, when Jason didn't get well after 8 weeks of intravenous Rocephin, the doctor consigned him back to psychiatry.

The situation would have stretched anyone's credulity. Our formerly straight-A, basketball-playing son, after contracting Lyme disease, being misdiagnosed for years, and finally receiving antibiotic therapy for 2 months, had now developed a bizarre, unrelated psychiatric disorder whose symptoms were coincidentally exactly the same as those of Lyme disease. Perhaps it is possible to believe that kind of explanation when served up by experts talking about other people's children, but it is the rare parent who would accept that decree for her own child, especially when her psychiatrist had never seen this form of psychiatric disease in his life.

Mark and I, by now both quite ill ourselves, faced a choice. Accept this unlikely story and give up on our son's future, or find one of the Lyme disease doctors said to treat more aggressively, in opposition to the mainstream views we had followed for years to the current tragic state of affairs.

In the summer of 2000 we bundled our boy into the car and headed up to New Haven, Connecticut, and the practice of the embattled pediatrician Charles Ray Jones. Jones examined and tested Jason and told us he was so sick because he had contracted not only Lyme disease but two common coinfections: babesiosis and anaplasmosis. Epidemiologically it seemed like a reasonable call, given the many vacations we had taken on Martha's Vineyard and Cape Cod, where babesiosis was ripe. Jones treated Jason with standard doses of doxycycline for anaplasmosis and Lyme disease, and Mepron and Zithromax for babesiosis.

Two weeks later, after years of free fall, our son got out of the bathtub and began throwing a basketball around the family room. Two years later he was playing varsity basketball for his high school, and today he holds a B.A. from Brown University and is a graduate student at Boston University earning his M.F.A. in film.

Although my book *Cure Unknown* is partly a memoir, it really focuses on what I found after I had dealt with my family's health problems sufficiently for me to sit back and peer through the eyes of the skeptical, investigative science journalist I had been for decades before Lyme disease swept us away. From 2000 to 2008, I interviewed Lyme disease patients, Lyme disease doctors, and dozens of academic scientists, including most of those at the forefront of research, and many of those speaking at this forum. I met large numbers of patients with classic incontrovertible presentations of Lyme disease who, like Jason, would probably have been cured with early treatment, but who were instead diagnosed late—often very late—in the game.

Patients routinely reported going to their primary care doctors with the tick in hand and being told to throw it away and return only if symptoms emerged. Many patients told me of doctors who insisted that a Lyme disease rash had to look like a literal bull's eye. Patients reported going to doctors with a tick bite, early flu-like symptoms, and sometimes even the erythema migrans rash, and being told to wait for a positive test before they could be treated. A significant percentage who had tested positive had been told they could still not be treated for Lyme disease until they developed gross, objective signs of disease, such as swollen knees or inflamed nerves—in other words, until they had advanced to the late stage of disease, when treatment was more likely to fail.

Other patients with known exposure and signs and symptoms of Lyme disease failed to test positive on their Western blots, according to criteria of the Centers for Disease Control and Prevention. Take me. I had a positive enzyme-linked immunosorbent assay (ELISA) test, and four positive bands on a Western blot, plus evidence of two additional *Borrelia burgdorferi* proteins—six bands in all. Yet I still had to step outside the bounds of the medical mainstream to find a practitioner who recognized this band pattern as Lyme disease.

Patients in the South with a trademark rash and other objective signs of disease would similarly be told there was no Lyme disease in their state and be turned away. Such patients in aggregate constitute what I think of as the chronic Lyme disease population. Instead of getting early treatment, these Lyme disease patients had been diagnosed months or years too late. They were eventually treated for late-stage Lyme disease in accordance with the guidelines of the Infectious Diseases Society of America, and they had failed that treatment.

Completing this community of patients are the coinfected: those with babesiosis, anaplasmosis, ehrlichiosis, or some other tick-borne infection. Surveys around the country report that ticks can transmit these well-known human diseases, yet primary care physicians almost never consider or test for them, even if they seriously consider Lyme disease. I think they need to determine the suite of possible diseases Lyme disease patients may be carrying because, like Jason, those patients can be very sick and resistant to treatment specifically because their illness isn't just Lyme disease.

Mark Klempner of Boston University found that a cohort of chronic Lyme disease patients was as impaired as patients with congestive heart failure or osteoarthritis, and more impaired than those with Type 2 diabetes or a recent myocardial infarction. Brian Fallon of Columbia reported pain equivalent to post-surgical pain, and fatigue as severe as in multiple sclerosis.

Patients can suffer stabbing, boring, shooting pains in their arms and legs, or impaired vision and hearing from damaged nerves. They can suffer heart damage. Even more devastating are the cognitive and memory deficits. After testing hundreds of patients, Leo Shea, a neuropsychologist at New York University, found specific deficits in concentration, short-term memory, and processing speed.

Fallon has traced these impairments to blood flow and metabolism deficits in the brain. Some scientists have called the impact of these impairments mild, but that does not remotely capture the agony of falling behind in school or feeling perpetually foggy and confused. Many patients report getting lost while driving around their own neighborhood, and some patients told me they could no longer remember enough to perform the specific details of their jobs.

For me the fatigue was the worst symptom. During the years I had Lyme disease, I collapsed in a heap every afternoon while my children were in school, my exhaustion overwhelming and profound. Studies minimize these "subjective" symptoms as almost irrelevant. However, a lack of external evidence does not mean that such internal devastation cannot be reliably measured and shouldn't be given weight as perhaps the most important outcome of all.

For parents, unresolved pediatric Lyme and tick-borne diseases are a nightmare, as they bear the heartache of watching their children suffer, along with helplessness and despair when the medical community all too quickly dismisses their complaints. After a child has been allowed to slip through the cracks of early diagnosis and treatment, the stage is set for isolation and alienation as she drops clubs, sports teams, friendships, and often even school.

In the wake of a child's decline, schools often push psychiatric interpretations, forcing inappropriate labels and help. When a child doesn't respond to wrong-headed strategies, the schools may accuse parents of poor skills or even Munchausen by proxy—a diagnosis that has fallen into disrepute among top psychologists and psychiatrists but that still manages to rear its head as an accusation where mothers and Lyme disease are concerned.

What a chasm I found between the patients I interviewed and some of the physicians at Northeast teaching hospitals. One well-known academic told me that virtually all Lyme disease patients are diagnosed early these days, and that treatment response is guaranteed for the rare patient who slips through the cracks to late-stage disease. If the patient doesn't respond, he or she never had Lyme disease, the doctor said.

When during grand rounds or training sessions such doctors suggest that patients are malingerers, too wimpy to handle stress, middle-aged suburban women with somatoform disorder, or hypochondriacs in search of the disease du jour, they have poisoned the chance of timely diagnosis by predisposing primary care physicians to seek psychiatric explanations first. With early treatment off the table, such patients wander from family doctor to clinic to teaching hospital, from one specialist to the next, and then off the grid.

My family found our way to doctors who diagnosed infections clinically and treated empirically while providing symptomatic relief for chronic disease. These were the best of the Lyme disease doctors. They treated our babesiosis and addressed our Lyme disease relapses, and over the course of years brought us back to health. We found them compassionate and responsible. However, being the patient of such a doctor is stressful. He or she may be under investigation, and will rarely take insurance for fear of being profiled as an outlier and further stigmatized. That makes the patient's financial stress extreme.

Other patients default to outright quackery: dangerous chemicals, lethal levels of heat applied to internal tissues, risky doses of salt. Some patients spend life savings on trips to India for a black-box therapy said to be based on stem cells. A diaspora of the desperate and broke, many of these patients have come to the end of the line.

Being sick is hard enough, but being so sick for so long and also being a suspect, having your physical pain, your integrity, and your very sanity called into question as you travel the medical landscape begging for help: That is a crushing course of events. No one suggests that the cancer patient is fictitious, or that the heart patient is a sociopath. But in the case of Lyme disease and other tick-borne diseases, the brutality of such rejection on top of real physical illness has traumatized the patient community. No wonder patients are in such turmoil.

The three largest patient advocacy organizations have boycotted this forum because they say it is biased against them. To quote their press release, they remain skeptical that it will lead to a true understanding of patients' needs. The history of the patient experience has robbed them of faith that anyone in government will understand their pain or truly address their plight.

Nearly 35 years ago, Polly Murray reported the strange set of symptoms in her town of Lyme to the Connecticut Department of Health. Murray noted the loneliness of her journey back in 1976, but decades later new patients travel the same lonely path, as if Murray and many others had never paved the way. Too many of us still spend years seeking help for what was in the beginning incontrovertible, classic, and curable Lyme disease, only to reap the whirlwind of late diagnosis and failed treatment even in the most endemic areas of the United States.

In interviews with hundreds of these patients, I found that relapsing-remitting illness was the overriding experience. Antibiotics were over-whelmingly the strategy these patients preferred for fighting back. However, which drug might work for which patient was highly variable, suggesting an extremely complex scenario.

I had relapsing–remitting disease. I was infected for some 7 years before diagnosis. I would get better after antibiotic treatment but then relapse like clockwork after 2 to 3 months. I went through such draining cycles for 4 years before a recovery was sustained. Can we really dismiss this common experience as coincidence or a psychiatric disease?

I have heard it said that all Lyme disease patients want are more anti-biotics, but that isn't true. Patients just want to get well, and will embrace any therapy that cures them. No reasonable person would argue that the answer sought by science should be endless antibiotic treatment, even if infection remains chronic at a low level, as evidence suggests. To help these patients, medicine must acknowledge their pain, and science must deal with the complexity.

Anyone who follows bioscience knows that pioneer Leroy Hood is building the medicine of the future that any patient group this varied needs: data-driven "P4 medicine," for predictive, preventive, personalized, and participatory. As Benjamin Luft of State University of New York–Stony Brook has suggested, only a systems-biology approach can target the full spectrum of strains, infections, and immune cascades for every patient with tick-borne disease. Academic scientists are embroiled in a dumbed-down fight with patients about the chronicity of infection even as a revolution in bioscience has reframed the questions we need to ask.

To paraphrase Tolstoy: Every early-stage Lyme disease patient is pretty much the same, while each chronic patient takes a singular journey of one. This discomforting fact has undermined the patient narrative. But with the advent of proteomics, genomics, epigenomics, and other 21st-century tools—with greater powers of vision—the story told by bioscience and the story told by patients can finally converge.

## DISCUSSION

The challenge of diagnosis of reported symptoms have been frustrating for patients and clinicians. Primary areas of discussion during the work-shop included the polarization that has developed between some patients, particularly those experiencing chronic symptoms, and clinicians; the need to improve communication and understanding between clinicians and patients; and patients' desire to focus greater discussion and research efforts on the care needs of those experiencing chronic symptoms.

Acknowledgment of patient experiences also may help keep barriers from forming between patients and clinicians or social institutions, such as schools, or break down existing ones. In response to a question about how best to support a teenager with debilitating symptoms, Weintraub observed that it helps teens to receive validation that they feel sick, as well as having the flexibility to make accommodations based on how they feel (e.g., deferring a test for a day if the student does not feel well).

In response to a participant's comment about the apparent stigma attached to Lyme disease within the medical community, Ms. Weintraub noted that stigma and a bias against Lyme disease do exist and can result in delays in diagnosis and treatment, as reflected in her son being undiagnosed for years. In addition to the stigma, the vitriol of the fight gives many physicians pause. To avoid the angry atmosphere, they may wish to stay out of the fray, especially where long-untreated or late-diagnosed and complicated presentations of illness are concerned. However, she also noted that the multiple manifestations of the disease in many cases can contribute to the confusion surrounding it, likewise resulting in delays in diagnosis and initiation of treatment. As one family physician observed, patients with chronic symptoms tend to present as 1 sick person with 10 different diseases, whereas a patient with early or uncomplicated late-stage Lyme disease tends to present as an otherwise healthy person with 1 disease. Another participant noted the absence of an integrated model of care, resulting in the need for patients to obtain care from many different specialists. The result in any case can be mutual frustration on the part of patients and their clinicians at the failure to resolve or alleviate the symptoms experienced by the patients, as well as the difficulties patients experience in obtaining care. This frustration, perhaps combined with poor communication, in turn may lead to anger and polarization.

Weintraub observed that all this polarization is very destructive and perhaps a primary reason why little progress has been made in advancing the treatment of patients with chronic symptoms. With others, she pressed the need to move past the sound bites issued by the two extremes to appreciate and focus on the complexity and nuance of the work to be done. Many people with great expertise in the academic community are doing that and working to move the science of diagnosis and treatment forward, she noted. Two participants observed the need for substantial funding for research to help address some of the current knowledge gaps and to promote early diagnosis, as well as prevention and vaccine development.

Several participants, while noting the hope for future patients observed by Jacobs and others, emphasized the desire that focus also remain on or return to the quality of life of those individuals currently experiencing symptoms. One participant highlighted the current gap in communications, noting that how information is provided on the Internet can vary, with implications for how those to whom it is disseminated (e.g., schools, insurance companies) will respond to the disease. The same participant called for a centralized source of information on the latest research to facilitate patient/family efforts to obtain such information. Another participant called for better communication between patients and their physicians, noting the damaging effect of this disconnection between two groups who have worked together on other illnesses. By working together in creative ways, physicians and patients may help to advance the science and understanding of the disease processes and chronic manifestations to permit earlier diagnosis and better treatment outcomes.

Participants also expressed concern about the underuse of the current population of patients and families as a rich data source in terms of bioinformatics, and perhaps a biorepository, to advance research into tick-borne diseases and the efficacy of various treatments. Weintraub responded that retrospective assessment of patients would be informative, but that it is important to move forward as well. She noted the availability of new tools to advance the diagnosis of infection and understanding of the pathophysiology of the diseases. It is important to look at what clinicians treating Lyme disease are doing, but to do so in the context of the new technologies. The goal is to move toward a definitive diagnostic tool and targeted treatment. Weintraub counseled that if the diseases can be diagnosed definitively in their earliest stage and treated effectively, then the occurrence of chronic, persistent symptoms will be eliminated or greatly reduced.

# 4

# Emerging Infections, Tick Biology, and Host-Vector Interactions

Today ticks inhabit almost every continent, with the number of species worldwide topping 850. Ticks have proven resilient and persistent in the environment, and the fossil records suggest that they originated 65–146 million years ago (see Olsen and Patz; Paddock and Telford, Appendix A).

The recognized number of important diseases transmitted by ticks has been growing over the past 30 years (see Paddock and Telford, Appendix A). The emergence and increased incidence of several major tick-borne diseases (TBDs) has been attributed to specific human activities and behaviors that disrupt ecosytems (see Paddock and Telford, Appendix A). Increases in human population and demographic shifts have brought dramatic changes in the distribution and composition of natural habitats, as people modify the land to create living spaces for agriculture or for recreation (see Munderloh and Kurtii, Appendix A). These changes mean that people and animals interact at many more interfaces, creating new opportunities for the transmission of zoonotic diseases, including TBDs. For example, habitat fragmentation can alter the movement of hosts that carry TBDs, the dynamics of disease transmission, and biodiversity (see Appendix A). Global environmental changes and other abiotic and biotic factors also help shape the ecology of TBDs and their emergence and reemergence.

Fortunately, new molecular tools and analytical techniques such as gene sequencing and analysis have enabled scientists to gain insights into tick biology and have resulted in a better understanding of TBDs. New technologies have also revealed a diverse microbial community associated with ticks that include viruses, bacteria, protozoans, and fungi. These microbes may act as symbionts (interacting closely, often to the benefit of the tick), pathogens, and transient commensals (colonizing the tick without marked detrimental effects), or as pathogens (see Clay and Fuqua, Appendix A).

In this chapter, five scientists examined the natural history of ticks and their wildlife and domestic hosts; outlined the contributions of animal health experts to understanding human TBD; explored genetic diversity among pathogens, vectors, and hosts; and showed how scientists investigate the microbial community found within the ticks to better understand the human risk for tick-borne diseases.

## EMERGING AND REEMERGING TICK-BORNE INFECTIONS: GENETIC MANIPULATION OF INTRACELLULAR TICK-BORNE PATHOGENS

*Ulrike G. Munderloh, D.V.M., Ph.D.*
*Department of Entomology, University of Minnesota*

Ticks are efficient vectors of multiple pathogens due to their potential interactions with several different vertebrate hosts during their life cycle. As a result, they have the opportunity to acquire a large array of different types of organisms that are present in the blood of these hosts. The microbial community in ticks includes viruses, bacteria, protozoa, and fungi, and serve as symbionts, commensals, and pathogens. In fact, the organisms that comprise the tick microbiome vastly outnumber recognized human pathogens. This microbial community can influence the acquisition, transmission, and virulence of human pathogens. Furthermore, as the tick feeds for extended periods, it interacts with its vertebrate host and has the ability to suppress the host's immune system by dampening down the immune response and binding up antibodies that the host might have made in an attempt to rid itself of the blood-sucking parasite. These attributes ensure that a pathogen can be acquired from or transmitted to a bite site that is suppressed and immunologically inactive.

*Anaplasma phagocytophilum* shares a vector, the black-legged tick, with Lyme disease spirochetes, a vector that is expanding its range, which helps to explain the increasing incidence of human granulocytic anaplasmosis. The white blood cells, specifically the neutrophils, are infected in reservoir mammalian hosts in the peripheral blood, and in lungs, heart, spleen, and gut. Animals also serve as models to account for the multiple signs of disease that infected people may present. There is a need to understand how these pathogens can survive and flourish in a broad range of mammalian hosts and a number of organs within the host, as well as in vector ticks. This can be done with new techniques to analyze how microbes use their genomes during passage in mammals and ticks. Live imaging can further reveal in real time how arthropod-associated pathogens and symbionts interact with their hosts, and point to ways to disrupt these interactions through genetic manipulation and mutagenesis. Molecular analysis is revealing the remarkable diversity of, and possible genetic exchange taking place within, this microbial community, which illuminates its capacity to adapt rapidly to new environments.

One hypothesis is that differential microbial gene expression may play a role in the pathogen's adaptability to the markedly different environments in the mammalian host and tick vector. Gene expression was studied in cell lines that focused on the life cycle of *A. phagocytophilum* and represented the tick, the human endothelium, and the human granulocyte. Gene expression varied depending on the host cell line. For example, the outer membrane protein 1A is expressed quite well in mammalian cell lines, but not in the tick cell line. The outer membrane efflux protein, and the major surface protein 4, are seemingly expressed in tick cells, but not at all in mammalian cells. The heat shock protein is primarily expressed in mammalian cells, but less so in tick cells, perhaps reflecting the lower incubation temperature in the tick. However, a "housekeeping" gene required by the organism seems to be equally expressed in all cell lines, independent of their origin.

Mutational analysis is another technique to probe the biology of the pathogens and symbionts. Approximately 40 percent of the genome of *A. phagocytophilum* has no known function, and gene knockouts can reveal the function of those genes. Further explorations can be accomplished by overexpressing genes to obtain sufficient samples for biochemical and immunological characterization, and by studying promoters and gene regulation *in vivo*. Genetic analysis reveals that human pathogens are closely related to the symbionts of ticks, yet the symbionts do not infect humans or animals.

We have found that a single-plasmid construct encoding the Himar 1 transposase and a transposon could be used to mutagenize *A. phagocytophilum* when introduced into the bacteria by electroporation. The transposon is inserted randomly into the genome of the recipient bacteria by a "cut-and-paste" mechanism. This approach produces mutants that are then screened for their ability to replicate in tick cells, an endothelial cell line, or HL-60 cells (a human promelocytic cell line that can be differentiated into granulocytes). In experiments using two separate mutants of *A. phagocytophilum* with identified genomic insertion sites, we characterized the effect of gene disruption on the phenotype of the pathogen. One mutant that has an insert in the o-methyltransferase gene does not infect tick cells or even bind to them, but it does grow well in HL-60 cells. A second mutant has an insert into a large gene expressed only in the mammalian cells. This organism is able to grow in tick cells but no longer infects HL-60 cells, although it can infect laboratory hamsters.

Spotted-fever group rickettsiae cause reemerging TBDs. The incidence of Rocky Mountain spotted fever caused by *Rickettsia rickettsii* has significantly increased since 2000 and has geographically shifted from the Rocky Mountain states to the South Central and southeastern United States. Pathogens in the spotted fever group occur in a wide range of ticks, including *Dermacentor andersoni* and *D. variabilis* (the Rocky Mountain wood tick and American dog tick, respectively), *Rhipicephalus sanguineus* (the brown dog tick), and *Amblyomma maculatum* (the Gulf Coast tick), whereas *Ixodes scapularis* carries a rickettsial symbiont that does not cause infection in animals and humans. We have successfully created a family of Himar 1 constructs that carry selectable and fluorescent markers to probe this group of pathogens. This has demonstrated that rickettsia, which were thought to only penetrate a tick's midgut, and then somehow move into other organs through the hemolymph, actually travel from the midgut through tracheal air tubes throughout the tick's body (Baldridge et al., 2007).

Recently, it was found that *Rickettsia felis*, which is transmitted by fleas, carries plasmids (Ogata et al., 2005). Since this initial finding, plasmids have been found in most *rickettsia*, including *R. monacensis, R. peacockii, R. massiliae, R. amblyommii, R. hoogstraalii,* and *R. helvetica.* Plasmids have thus far not been found in highly pathogenic species such as *R. rickettsii* and *Rickettsia prowazekii*, and the reasons for this true absence or lack of detection are unclear. Because plasmid-encoded genes are conserved across many species, the working hypothesis is that plasmids play an important role in the biology of *rickettsia.* Many genes on rickettsial plasmids are related to genes in other rickettsial species. However, there are genes on rickettsial plasmids that do not occur in other *rickettsia* but are found in unrelated bacteria. These findings suggest that rickettsial plasmids participate in horizontal gene transfer in these species. The genome of *R. peacockii,* which is the closest relative to virulent *R. rickettsia,* has a plasmid that encodes a cluster of genes related to the glycosylation island of *Pseudomonas aeruginosa* that are likely involved in phospholipid biosynthesis. The chromosome of *R. peacockii* encodes a gene important in phospholipid biosynthesis that has been mutated, and it is possible that the plasmid-encoded genes compensate for that mutation. Plasmids of different rickettsial species carry other genes that are only distantly related. For example, the parA proteins of *R. peacockii* and *R. felis* are most closely related to those of *E. coli* and *Pseudomonas*, whereas the small heat shock proteins Hsp-1 and -2 are tightly aligned with the rickettsial phylogenetic lineage.

The discovery of diverse plasmids in different *Rickettsia* species suggested their potential use as transformation vectors, a method that could greatly facilitate genetic analysis and accelerate understanding of pathogeneis. We developed a series of shuttle vectors starting with a recombinant version of pRAM18, one of the plasmids from *R. amblyommii,* bearing fluorescent and selectable markers. The regions of the plasmid encoding the *parA* and *DnaA* genes, which are important in plasmid maintenance and replication, along with a selectable and fluorescent traceable marker, were subcloned into pGEM. Subsequently, screening of a pRAM18 library yielded evidence of another *R. amblyommii* plasmid, pRAM32, and the section containing the *parA* and *DnaA* genes was subcloned into pUC, another commercially available plasmid. This produced a family of constructs: the original recombinant, large-size pRAM18, its smaller derivatives, and the smaller pRAM32 construct. With all four of these constructs, transformants were obtained by electroporation of *R. monacensis*, *R. montanensis*, and *R. bellii.* The recombinant rickettsial pRAM18 plasmids were maintained as plasmids in rickettsial populations, as were the much smaller pGEM- and pUC-based constructs.

In conclusion, Munderloh noted that the Himar 1 transposase system is useful for random mutagenesis and gene knockouts in obligate intracellular bacteria, but it has proven not to be very efficient. Despite this shortcoming, Himar 1 transposon mutagenesis has enabled the study of gene function in organisms that traditionally have been difficult to manipulate genetically. In combination with plasmids used in complementation assays, existing constructs will enable investigators to make headway toward a functional genomic analysis of these bacteria. In this way, drugs targeting specific genes could be developed, or vaccine strains with attenuated virulence might be created that would generate a protective immune response without causing illness. The tools generated for rickettsial organisms could be useful for other pathogenic bacteria.

## NATURAL HISTORY OF TICKS: EVOLUTION, ADAPTATION, AND BIOLOGY

*Tom G. Schwan, Ph.D., M.S., Laboratory of Zoonotic Pathogens, National Institute of Allergy and Infectious Diseases*

Ticks belong to the Phylum *Arthropoda* and the Class *Arachnida*. They are not insects. Although they have an exoskeleton and jointed appendages, they have eight legs, do not fly, and do not have a head, a thorax, or an abdomen. Ticks also differ vastly from most insects in that they are important vectors for many pathogens. Among those insects that feed on blood, such as mosquitoes, black flies, sand flies, tsetse flies, and fleas, only the adults—and often only females—feed on blood. That means that only adults can acquire an infectious blood meal from infected animals that serve as reservoirs for pathogens, such as rodents. In contrast, ticks are obligated blood feeders at all stages of their life-cycle, which makes them adept at transmitting pathogens at various stages.

There are three families of ticks: *Ixodidae, Argasidae,* and *Nutalliellidae. Ixodidae* has 12 genera, while *Argasidae* has 4. *Nutalliellidae* consists of a single species. The ixodids are hard ticks and evolve through three stages: larva, nymphal, and adult. Argasids are soft ticks that also undergo multiple stages: larval, multiple nymphal stages, and mature adult. In contrast to hard ticks in which the adults feed only once, soft tick adults can feed multiple times. Not much is known about the evolution of ticks, as fossil ticks found in amber dating back 94 million years look like ticks of today (Klompen and Grimaldi, 2001).

*Ixodid* ticks have a life cycle of 1 to 3 years and are typically less able to fast and survive without a blood meal. In contrast, *Argasidae* have an expanded life cycle that may take many years to complete. These ticks are able to fast for long periods of time between blood meals. *Ornithodoros parkeri* females, *O. tholozani* nymphs, and *O. moubata* nymphs can live 10 to 11 years between meals (Schwan, unpublished) and may even outlive their vertebrate hosts by many years.

Ticks can be three-, two-, or one-host arthropods. For three-host ticks, larvae feed on a host, fall off, and molt into a nymph. The nymph then attaches to another host, feeds, and falls off, and finally the adult attaches to a third host and feeds. This group includes the hard tick *I. scapularis,* the vector for Lyme disease *Borrelia.* In the case of two-host ticks, some larvae and nymphs feed on a single host and then attach to a second host to reach adulthood. No North American ticks are two-host ticks. One-host ticks attach to a host as larvae, and then feed and mature to the adult stage on the same host. *Rhipicephalus (Boophilus) microplus* and relatives, which are cattle ticks, are classic one-host ticks. Deer, elk, and goats can have high numbers of *Dermacentor albipictus,* also a one-host tick, and hunters in North America often encounter these ticks.

There are approximately 870 species of ticks. Within this group, some ticks are widely distributed and feed on many different types of hosts, while other ticks are very host specific. *I. scapularis,* for example, is found throughout the eastern United States and feeds on 50 to 70 different hosts, while *Argas monolakensis,* an argasid, is found only on islands in Mono Lake, California, in high density and feeds only on the California gull. All ixodid ticks feed for long periods of time, while most argasids are fast feeders, although the larvae of some feed for many days. The latter is the case with *A. monolakensis,* which can exsanguinate gulls during the feeding.

In 1893, it was demonstrated that blood-feeding arthropods could be biological vectors of a pathogenic organism (Smith and Kilborne, 1893). Ticks are effective vectors and, sometimes, effective reservoirs. In some species, adult females can transmit the pathogens to their offspring as a result of transovarial transmission. Infected ticks can also pass an organism from one development stage to subsequent stages in its life cycle, which is termed transstadial transmission. Because ticks feed on blood at every stage, live a long time, and can transmit pathogens to their offspring or next life cycle, they are capable of sustaining pathogens for long periods of time and they are exquisitely adapted to serve as reservoirs for pathogens and as effective transmitters. Moreover, all TBDs in North America are zoonoses—transmitted from animals to humans. However, the O. *moubata* tick can directly transmit B. *duttonii*, the pathogen that causes relapsing fever in East Africa, from person to person. In North America, O. *hermsi* ticks are nocturnal and fast feeding, and usually feed on people sleeping in tick-infested cabins.

Relapsing fever occurs in Africa, but it also occurs in the western United States, where it is underdiagnosed and underreported. The disease causes significant mortality in some regions of Africa, especially among pregnant women. Relapsing fever is usually not fatal in North America, but the risk of mortality increases for fetuses during pregnancy.

### Knowledge Gaps and Research Opportunities

Schwan noted that the research needed in the future falls into two key areas:

- The number and training of medical acarologists and tick biologists are declining, and scientists who do investigate TBDs often focus only on Lyme disease–related questions. Support for the training of tick biologists with wide-ranging interests and broad research portfolios are essential to ensure continued progress on the full spectrum of TBDs.
- Field research on TBDs is particularly important: Analysis of ticks in the lab, using technologies such as polymerase chain reaction (PCR), is not enough.

### WILDLIFE AND DOMESTIC HOSTS: THEIR IMPORTANT ROLES IN MAINTAINING AND AMPLIFYING PATHOGENS AND THEIR CHANGING DYNAMICS

*Howard Ginsberg, Ph.D., U.S. Geological Survey
and the University of Rhode Island*

Ticks and their hosts can be influenced by environmental factors, and complex interactions influence the transmission of TBDs. This can be illustrated by Lyme disease in eastern North America, which is dependent primarily on one vector and one pathogen, B. burgdorferi. Several factors influence the transmission of tick-borne illnesses in North America, including

- *Tick density*, which affects the probability that both humans and reservoir hosts for B. burgdorferi—such as small rodents and birds— will be exposed to the bacteria.
- *Host factors*, including the diversity of hosts and their competence as reservoirs for pathogens.
- *Spatial patterns*, primarily the geographic distribution of I. scapularis ticks, the vectors for B. burgdorferi. That distribution can vary in the field meter by meter because of various microspatial factors.
- *Temporal patterns*, primarily the length of the season during which ticks and their hosts are active.

Tick density influences the probability of exposures of both human and reservoir hosts of the pathogen. The probability that a host will be exposed to a pathogen that causes a tick-borne disease, given the density of ticks, can be expressed as $P_e = 1-(1-k_v)^n$ whereas $P_e$ is the probability of being bitten by at least one infected vector, $k_v$ is the proportion of vectors infected with the pathogen, and n is the number of vector bites (Ginsberg, 1993). When the results are plotted for different rates of infection, it is an asymptotic curve, such that a 25 percent infection rate, which is common for nymphal ticks in endemic areas, means that by 5 to 10 tick bites, the probability of exposure is near one. On Fire Island, a barrier island that runs parallel to the south shore of Long Island, New York, most mice are bitten by 30 to 200 ticks per season. If a mouse is bitten by 100 ticks in an average season and a successful intervention decreases the number of bites to 20, there will still not be an effect on whether the mouse is going to be exposed to the pathogen. Therefore, trying to manage Lyme disease by developing strategies in the natural environment is difficult. Human risk, however, is lower because most individuals are bitten by only a few ticks in a given year. If the number of tick bites is lowered, then the probability of being exposed to the pathogen is lowered. Thus, managing the environment to minimize human–tick encounters is an easier approach than trying to manage the natural cycle.

A number of factors control the density of ticks. For example, the number of primary hosts in a region, such as deer, seems to determine the mean number around which the number of ticks fluctuates. However, broad fluctuations of the tick population occur from year to year. Tick populations in Westchester County north of New York City, Prudence Island in Narragansett Bay, and Fire Island off Long Island have similar yearly fluctuations, which suggests that whatever controls these fluctuations is occurring on a regional scale (Ginsberg et al., 1998). However, weather alone apparently does not explain Lyme disease incidence as correlations with weather factors have variable results (McCabe and Bunnell, 2004; Ostfeld et al., 2006). The relationship between ticks and weather is complex and requires examination of conditions in the leaf litter where the ticks reside rather than simply measuring weather from an airport station. Furthermore, the amount of time that a tick spends below a certain humidity level affects both its survival and activity (Rodgers et al., 2007).

How the ticks interact with hosts can influence the number of ticks that acquire a pathogen from infected host animals, including the proportion of hosts that are infected, the reservoir competence of various species of hosts, and the distribution of larval and nymphal ticks on those hosts. Hosts, especially mammals and birds, vary significantly in their reservoir competence. Some domestic animals, such as dogs, are competent reservoirs for Lyme disease. However, domestic animals probably do not play a large role in the transmission cycle of Lyme disease because they spend much less time in the woods than do wild animals. There are exceptions: for example, on Monhegan Island, Maine, Norway rats are an invasive species that are competent reservoirs and run wild (Smith et al., 1993). Furthermore, the reservoir competence of hosts can vary significantly between laboratory and field studies (Table 4-1). In the laboratory, investigators study reservoir competence by putting infected ticks on animal hosts, or by injecting the animals with *B. burgdorferi*. A week or two later, the investigators put uninfected tick larvae on the now-infected animals and determine what percentage of the larvae acquire the bacteria. In field studies, by contrast, investigators put uninfected larvae on wild animals and determine how many acquire the infection. The results can vary between the laboratory and the field for reasons that are not well understood. For example, when robins were infected in the lab, they proved to be highly competent reservoirs for *B. burgdorferi*, with 82–92 percent of tick larvae acquiring the pathogen. By contrast, when uninfected tick larvae were placed on robins from the field, only 16 percent of the larvae acquired the bacteria (Richter et al., 2000; Ginsberg et al., 2005).

The reservoir competence of *B. burgdorferi* can also vary by geographic area depending on the diversity of the available hosts. Some of these host species are competent reservoirs and others are not. On Fire Island, uninfected *I. scapularis* larvae feed on a variety of host species—some good reservoirs and some not—with small rodents being the primary competent reservoirs. However, the community of hosts is not very diverse, so a high percentage of tick nymphs become infected. In a more ecologically diverse community, the variety of hosts for *B. burgdorferi* dilutes the impact of rodents as hosts (LoGiudice et al., 2003). That, in turn, affects the probability that people will acquire Lyme disease, although the effect is complex.

**TABLE 4-1** Reservoir Competence of Selected Vertebrate Species for *Borrelia burgdorferi* (Using Xenodiagnostic *Ixodes Scapularis* Larvae)

| Common Name | Lab/Field | Reservoir Competence (%) | Source |
|---|---|---|---|
| White-footed mouse | L | ~75 | Donahue et al. (1987) |
| | F | 89 | Mather et al. (1989a) |
| | F | 56 | Ginsberg et al. (unpub.) |
| Meadow vole | L | ~70 | Markowski et al. (1998) |
| | F | 62 | Markowski et al. (1998) |
| Chipmunk | F | 20 | Mather et al. (1989b) |
| White-tailed deer | F | 1 | Telford et al. (1988) |
| American robin | L | 92 | Richter et al. (2000) |
| | L | 82 | Ginsberg et al. (2005) |
| | F | 16 | Ginsberg et al. (2005) |
| Northern cardinal | F | 9 | Ginsberg et al. (2005) |
| Gray catbird | F | 0 | Mather et al. (1989a) |
| | F | 4 | Ginsberg et al. (2005) |
| Eastern fence lizard | L | ~7 | Tsao et al. (2008) |
| Five-lined skink | L | >20 | Levin et al. (1996) |
| Dog (beagle) | L | 78 | Mather and Ginesberg (1994) |
| Norway rat | F | 72 | Smith et al. (1993) |

SOURCE: Ginsberg, unpublished.

For example, dilution works in the Northeast because small rodents, the primary host for *B. burgdorferi*, are very good reservoirs. In the South, lizards, the primary hosts for *Ixodes scapularis*, are not good reservoirs, so expanding the diversity of hosts in that region could actually increase the incidence of Lyme disease.

Vector diversity can also affect the likelihood of human disease. On Fire Island in the early 1980s, the American dog tick and the black-legged tick were the most common kinds of ticks. In the later 1980s and 1990s, the lone star tick, *A. americanum*, became more abundant, and the pathogens *E. chaffeensis*, *E. ewingii*, and *R. amblyommii* began to present risk for human disease (Mixson et al., 2006).

Spatial patterns include the geographic distribution of competent hosts and vectors. For *I. scapularis*, its distribution is common in the northern and much of the southern United States, but the cases of Lyme disease that are reported to the Centers for Disease Control and Prevention (CDC) are predominantly from the northern states. Thus, tick density alone does not determine these rates. One factor that might be important is the host competency. As noted above, mammals residing in the North are highly competent reservoirs for *B. burgdorferi*, while in the South the abundant lizards are not good reservoirs. A second spatial factor can be the genetic distribution of ticks. For example, one genetic lineage of *I. scapularis* ticks occurs in both the northern and the southern United States, but numerous other lineages occur in the South but not the North (Beati, unpublished). Whether genetic lineages differ in host preference and vector competence is unknown.

Temporal patterns are also likely to be affected by geographic trends. In the Northeast, for example, adult *I. scapularis* lay eggs, and uninfected larvae hatch in midsummer and feed on infected hosts. Infected nymphs then emerge the following spring and take a blood meal, emerging as adults in the fall. That means the nymphs and larvae present in any given year represent different populations. Nymphs infect hosts with *B. burgdorferi* bacteria, which the larvae acquire feeding on these same hosts slightly later in the season; the transmission cycle is very efficient. If the seasonal cycles of larvae and nymphs overlapped even more, transmission could be less efficient. If nymphs emerged significantly earlier in the season and larvae considerably later, animal hosts could lose their infectivity during the interim period. Understanding the temporal relationship between these stages is therefore critical to understanding why Lyme disease is common in some areas and not in others. For example, understanding how a longer growing season affects the active season of various stages of the tick could inform how changing climate might affect human disease.

In a multilaboratory investigation of geographical patterns, standardized samples of host communities and the distribution of ticks on the hosts in four regions around the country are being collected to determine which genetic groups are present, and whether they correlate with ecological factors. Hypothesis testing and ecological modeling may help to determine why Lyme disease results in some areas with many infected ticks, while others have few. The results may shed light on how the distribution of Lyme disease might change in the future.

As discussed previously in the report, there are changing dynamics that will affect human disease. For example, tick distribution is expanding up the Hudson Valley in New York, into northern New Jersey, down into the Southeast, and into Illinois, and modeling suggests that the tick will expand further into Canada. Expanding tick distribution alone does not necessarily mean more human disease, but it is an important contributor. Another factor may be expanding host distribution. For example, if lizards expand north, the incidence of Lyme disease may decrease. Similarly, introduced species may influence disease transmission if they are competent hosts. Finally, changing active seasons of the ticks as a result of longer growing seasons may affect the transmission dynamics.

## Knowledge Gaps and Research Opportunities

The key areas for future work Ginsberg noted include the following:

- The effect of physical factors on the distribution and abundance of ticks.
- The effect of changing climate on the distribution of vertebrate hosts of tick-borne pathogens.
- The factors that influence the infectivity of those hosts in the field versus in the laboratory.
- The influence of the length of the active season on tick phenologies, or life cycle events.
- Geographic patterns in the genetic structure of tick populations.
- Efficient targeting and integration of techniques for managing human exposure to ticks. For example, land-use planners and landscape architects could design communities and developments to reduce human exposure to ticks, even if they are relatively abundant. Such an approach would require a relatively modest investment.

## DISCUSSION

King questioned the panel about what role pheromones may play in tick-borne disease. Munderloh noted that different species of ticks produce different types of pheromones for aggregation and for stimulation of mating. In addition, the composition of saliva is vastly different between *I. scapularis* and *D. variabilis*. Aggregation hormones play a major role in some ticks, such as *D. variabilis*, but play a lesser role in *I. scapularis*. It would be difficult because of the divergence of ticks to make generalizations. Ginsberg noted that there is active research on the use of pheromones to enhance tick management methods by attracting ticks to the pesticides, but nothing is commercially available.

Schutze questioned if freezing weather for longer than 3 days could affect the number ticks and thus the number of tick-borne illnesses that season. Ginsberg noted that laboratory studies suggest that the temperature has to be significantly below freezing before it has an effect. However, this may not be true in the field as ticks have adapted to finding places in the soil and under the surface that provide a measure of protection. Munderloh further noted that deep snow cover is protective because just underneath the snow cover some areas are barely below freezing.

Emerging infectious diseases seem to have a trajectory over time, where the incident rates increase and then plateau. Drawing from this observation, one participant questioned through pathogen, tick, or host dynamics what the limit will be on Lyme disease in the Northeast. Ginsberg noted that making any predictions will be difficult because Lyme disease is still spreading into new areas, and the increased reporting reflects this fact. The participant further questioned whether there is any long-time series of infection rates in hosts and ticks at multiple locations. Ginsberg noted that infection rates vary significantly. On Fire Island, the infection rate can fluctuate from 4.5 percent to more than 30 percent from year to year. Although these are preliminary observations, he noted that the fluctuations may be related to reservoir host populations.

Walker asked if there is any effect of the prevalence of the pathogen in the ticks relative to the virulence of the pathogen. For example, this may be the case with *D. variabilis* that carry *R. rickettsii* and *A. cajennense* in South America that carry *R. rickettsii* in areas where the diseases are prevalent, but the tick numbers are relatively low. Schwan noted this question has not been well studied. Relapsing fever spirochetes may be detrimental to the tick if the ticks ingest a significant number of spirochetes, but this is anecdotal information. Higher environmental temperature increased the mortality of *D. andersoni* ticks when infected with *R. rickettsii* (Niebylski and Peacock, 1999).

Another participant questioned whether a host adapts over time to become an incompetent reservoir as its immune response adapts. For example, in a newly endemic area, the same species might be a good reservoir because it has not developed that type of immune response. Ginsberg noted that this might occur in nature and there may also be differences during the life cycle of the hosts, such that juveniles have a different reservoir competence than do adults. The participant further questioned if one of the reasons for the lack of overlap of the distribution of reported cases of Lyme disease and the distribution of the black-legged tick is the result of underreporting. Ginsberg noted that this could be one explanation but that the use of flagging techniques to collect ticks have found results that are comparable to CDC results about human cases.

## COMPARATIVE MEDICAL IMPORTANCE OF A ONE-HEALTH APPROACH TO EMERGING TICK-BORNE DISEASES

*Edward B. Breitschwerdt, D.V.M., College of Veterinary Medicine, North Carolina State University*

A "One Health" approach recognizes the need for veterinarians, human health professionals, and environmental scientists to work together given the dynamic interface among people, animals, and the environment. This approach is increasingly important for zoonotic diseases, such as TBDs, which rely on animals as reservoirs. Numerous exchanges of knowledge, such as using animals as sentinels for human diseases, reveal the importance of a One Health framework for understanding TBDs. Use of this approach is likely to achieve advances in health care for the 21st century "by accelerating biomedical research discoveries, enhancing public health efficacy, expeditiously expanding the scientific knowledge base, and improving

medical education and clinical care" (http://www.onehealthinitiative
.com/mission.php).

Animals, especially dogs, because of their close proximity to humans
and the fact that they often present with similar signs of tick-borne disease,
are often sentinels for human TBDs (Elchos and Goddard, 2003). For
example, the symptoms of dogs infected either naturally or in the laboratory with *R. rickettsii* are nearly identical to those of humans with Rocky
Mountain spotted fever. In the context of one medicine, veterinary medicine
and human medicine can both provide key insights into TBDs. In a 2003
case study, a farm family's dog died, despite treatment with antibiotics, after
a delayed diagnosis of ehrlichiosis. Two weeks later the farm's 46-year-
old owner developed fever, headache, vomiting, and back pain. Because
recognizing tick-borne illness in people is difficult, her family physician diagnosed muscle sprains and acute cystitis. The woman received two drugs,
including a sulfonamides, which are contraindicated for the treatment of
rickettsial diseases. She died 3 days later as a result of vasculitis. The CDC
determined that she had had Rocky Mountain spotted fever. A week later
the family's second dog developed febrile illness and was quickly placed
on doxycycline. A diagnosis of Rocky Mountain spotted fever was made
based on seroconversion to *R. rickettsia*, as confirmed by the CDC (Elchos
and Goddard, 2003).

In a second case study, an outbreak of Rocky Mountain spotted fever in
the Bronx, New York City, in 1987 occurred most likely after a female tick
was carried in by a dog that had traveled to an endemic area (Salgo et al.,
1988). The tick, carrying *R. rickettsii*, presumably transmitted the pathogen
transovarially to the next generation of baby ticks, which led to the outbreak of human disease. Today, as a result of improved acaricide products
that are safer and more effective and tick-borne disease educational efforts
by veterinarians, an urban outbreak is much less likely.

Surveillance and diagnostic advances in veterinary medicine continue to
inform human tick-borne disease management and vice versa. Veterinarians
routinely use a rapid, on-site surveillance test to determine whether dogs
have been exposed to *Ehrlichia* sp., *Borrelia burgdorferi* (Lyme disease),
or *A. phagocytophilum;* results from that testing have helped shed light on
where human diseases caused by these pathogens can occur. Surveillance for
*E. canis*, *E. chaffeensis*, and *E. ewingii* antibodies in dogs helped uncover
that there is a high prevalence of brown dog ticks infected with and transmitting transmit *E. canis* in Arizona (Figure 4-1). The surveillance found a
cluster of *Ehrlichia* in dogs in Minnesota and Wisconsin, which made sense
after the CDC recently found an *Ehrlichia muris*–like infection in immunocompromised people in that region. Moreover, highly sensitive molecular
tests for tick-borne organisms have helped to define the importance of coinfection and have clarified the pathogenesis and pathophysiology of TBDs.

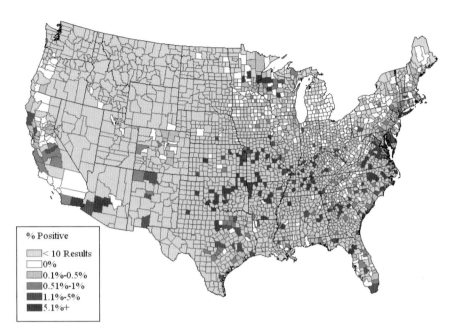

**FIGURE 4-1** National prevalence data of *Ehrlichia* antibodies in dogs.
SOURCE: Reprinted from Veterinary Parasitology, 139, Bowman et al., Successful or currently ongoing parasite eradication programs, 138-148, Copyright 2009, with permission from Elsevier.

PCR analysis of peripheral blood samples has been useful in the diagnosis of *Ehrlichia* in dogs and humans. A recent report of *E. chaffeensis* in lemurs was confirmed by PCR (Williams et al., 2002).

Similar insights from naturally occurring infection in animals have enhanced understanding of human diseases due to other tick-borne pathogens. For example, *A. phagocytophilum* can cause illness in cats, dogs, horses, and humans in the same geographic area, with thrombocytopenia (low platelet count) the most consistent abnormality revealed by laboratory tests across species. Coinfection with *B. burgdorferi* is common because the same tick transmits both organisms. There is some experimental evidence of chronic infection of *A. phagocytophilum* in dogs (Scorpio et al., 2010), and this finding suggests the need to look at human illness caused by this pathogen. Notably, the discovery of human anaplasmosis occurred decades after veterinarians at the University of California identified the causative agent, then described as *Ehrlichia. equi* in the mid-1960s. Experimentally,

*E. equi* was transmitted to cats, dogs, and nonhuman primates to test how pathogenic the organism would prove to be across species lines. From these results a species of *Ehrlichia* was subsequently linked to human granulocytic ehrlichiosis (Bakken et al., 1994). This human pathogen was sequenced and found to be closely related phylogenetically to the *E. equi* reported decades earlier (Chen et al., 1994). Subsequent phylogenic studies resulted in reclassification of *E. equi* to the genus *Anaplasma* taxonomic unification of this agent with that of human disease, and speciation of *A. phagocytophilum* (Dumler et al., 2001).

Underscoring the need for a One Health approach, shortly after the discovery of human granulocytic anaplasmosis, researchers found by using DNA sequencing that dogs and horses with neutrophilic morula in Sweden were infected with a genetically identical segment of approximately 1,400 base pairs of the 16S rRNA gene to the *Ehrlichia* pathogen reported by Chen (Johansson et al., 1995). These results underscore the need for a One Health approach. As a result of sharing information across disciplines, across species, and across continents, granulocytic anaplasmosis was subsequently confirmed in cats and dogs in the northeastern United States and human anaplasmosis was reported in Sweden, Germany, Austria, and many other European and Asian countries.

Another opportunity for which veterinary research can provide insight into human disease is by using dogs as a naturally occurring model of disease. For example, in a recent study, whole blood and serum were collected from 731 dogs from a single veterinary hospital in Baxter, Minnesota. Clinical disease and a positive PCR test for *A. phagocytophilum* were more likely to occur in dogs previously infected with *B. burgdorferi*. The *A. phagocytophilum* and *B. burgdorferi* seroprevalence in dogs in this region was very high (55 percent, or 405 of 731 dogs tested) (Beall et al., 2008). For both of these pathogens, a dog was as likely to be healthy after having been exposed to and infected with these organisms than to present for disease manifestations. However, if these dogs had antibodies to both *A. phagocytophilum* and *B. burgdorferi*, then statistically the animals were clinically ill. Moreover, diagnostic documentation of *A. phagocytophilum* DNA in the blood was associated with illness. There is a high correlation between canine exposure to ticks that transmit *A. phagocytophilum* and *B. burgdorferi* and the likelihood that a person will be infected by ticks in the same environment. As veterinarians routinely screen for antibodies to these organisms, they can educate the client about the risk of TBDs in their pets and family members.

*Bartonella* is an alpha-proteobacterium and is phylogenetically related to other tick-borne pathogens in the genera *Anaplasma*, *Ehrlichia*, and *Rickettsia*. This may be the most important genus of bacteria infecting both people and animals that scientists can study in the next decade. These organisms can be intraerythrocytic in humans, rodents, and cats alike. Unfortunately, unlike tick-borne organisms that have a tropism for only neutrophils (*A. phagocytophilum* or *Ehrlichia ewingii*) or macrophages (*E. canis* or *E. chaffeensis*, or primarily *Bartonella*), bacteria seem to invade erythrocytes, endothelial cells, and microglial cells as well as CD34 progenitor cells in the bone marrow. Currently, only circumstantial evidence supports tick transmission of *Bartonella*. Similarly, *Bartonella* underscores the need for One Health research because lice, fleas, sand flies, and possibly ticks can transmit pathogens in this genus of bacteria (Angelakis et al., 2010; Dietrich et al., 2010). In addition, people can become infected through animal bites, scratches, needle inoculation, and potentially through in utero transmission (Breitschwerdt et al., 2010; Oliveira et al., 2010). Gray squirrels, ground squirrels, and groundhogs can also serve as reservoirs for *Bartonella*—most likely different species of the bacterium. Meanwhile the spectrum of chronic human disease linked to this genus is expanding (Breitschwerdt et al., 2008, 2010a; Sykes et al., 2010).

Dogs and humans with bartonellosis share similar clinical manifestations, including culture-negative endocarditis (endocarditis without etiology), peliosis hepatis, bacillary angiomatosis, myocarditis, arthritis, encephalitis, immune-mediated thrombocytopenia, and immune-mediated hemolytic anemia (Chomel et al., 2009; Breitschwerdt et al., 2010a). Peliosis hepatis and bacillary angiomatosis occur in HIV-infected individuals and in dogs that are immunosuppressed due to cancer chemotherapy or immunosuppressive drug therapy (Yager et al., 2010). Furthermore, 32 percent of people with extensive contact with arthropods and animals are infected with sheep *Bartonella*, squirrel *Bartonella*, dog *Bartonella*, or cat *Bartonella*. Individuals who are not engaged in such contact show no reported infection using PCR analysis (Maggii et al., 2010).

Together Breitschwerdt noted that these findings for TBDs emphasize that collaboration among practitioners of veterinary and human medicine, along with overlapping surveillance systems, would be highly beneficial to both people and animals. Furthermore, there is a critical need to understand the role of vector-borne organisms as a cause of chronic disease in animals and humans. Finally, public education is important in preventing illness and death from acute infectious TBDs, such as anaplasmosis, ehrlichiosis, and Rocky Mountain spotted fever.

## VARIATION OF *BORRELIA* SUBSPECIES: IMPLICATIONS FOR HUMAN DISEASE

*James H. Oliver, Jr., Ph.D., Institute of Arthropodology and Parasitology, Georgia Southern University*

Today, *B. burgdorferi* sensu lato complex includes 18 named and 1 not named yet spirochete species. Several of these subspecies are known human pathogens. In Europe, *B. afzelii* and *B. garinii* are among the most important genospecies causing human illness. In the United States, *B. burgdorferi* sensu stricto is considered to be the only causative agent of Lyme borreliosis until recently, when *B. bissettii*–like spirochetes were detected in people. Most of what is known about *B. burgdorferi* has been reported in the northeastern and midwestern states. For the southeastern United States, fewer studies have been conducted. To begin to investigate the differences in the southeastern United States, a number of working hypotheses of borreliosis have been proposed:

- There is greater genetic diversity among *B. burgdorferi* s.l. in the southeastern United States.
- Infectivity and pathogenicity of southern *Borrelia* vary more than northeastern strains.
- Several "populations" of vector *I. scapularis* are distributed in the eastern and central United States. Tick behavior, life cycles, and *Borrelia* incidence vary among the populations and are determined by climate, local vegetation, suitable reservoirs or hosts, and the genetic profile of the *Borrelia* strains.
- The largely non-human-biting *I. minor* and *I. affinis* are often infected with *B. burgdorferi* s.l. and serve as enzootic vectors of *Borrelia*.
- Adult *I. scapularis* bite humans in the southeastern United States, but nymphs rarely do.
- There is a wider diversity of vertebrate hosts of ticks in the southeastern United States, particularly reptiles, which probably serves to dilute incidence of *B. burgdorferi* in *I. scapularis*.
- Birds are a major vehicle for long-distance transport of ticks and *Borrelia*.
- Recent evidence suggests that one of the key determinants of spirochete–host association is the host complement system.

The 18 recognized genospecies of the *B. burgdorferi* sensu lato complex are listed in Table 4-2. Some have debated whether *B. burgdorferi* occurs in the southern states. Evidence in birds and animals of several subspecies

**TABLE 4-2** Seventeen Recognized Genospecies of *Borrelia burgdorferi* Sensu Lato Complex

| Genospecies | Distribution | Author | Reference |
|---|---|---|---|
| *B. afzelii* | Europe | Canica et al. (1993) | Scand J Infect Dis. 25:441-8 |
| *B. Americana* | U.S. | Rudenko et al. (2009) | J Clin Microbiol. 47:3875-3880 |
| *B. andersonii* | U.S. | Marconi et al. (1995) | J Clin Microbiol. 33:2427-34 |
| *B. bavariensis* | Europe | Margos et al. (2009) | Appl Environ Microbiol. 75:5410-6 |
| *B. bissettii* | Europe, U.S. | Postic et al. (1998) | J Clin Microbiol. 36:3497-504 |
| *B. burgdorferi ss* | Europe, U.S. | Baranton et al. (1992) | Int J Syst Bacteriol. 42:378-83 |
| *B. californiensis* | U.S. | Postic et al. (2007) | Int J Med. Microbiol. 297:263-271 |
| *B. carolinensis* | U.S. | Rudenko et al. (2009) | J Clin Microbiol. 47:134-141 |
| *B. garinii* | Europe, Asia | Baranton et al. (1992) | Int J Syst Bacteriol. 42:378-83 |
| *B. lusitaniae* | Europe | Le Fleche et al. (1997) | Int J Syst Bacteriol. 47:921-5 |
| *B. japonica* | Japan | Kawabata et al. (1993) | Microbiol Immunol 37:843-8 |
| *B. sinica* | China | Masuzawa et al. (2001) | Int J Syst Evol Microbiol. 51:1817-24 |
| *B. spielmanii* | Europe | Richter et al. (2006) | Int J Syst Evol Microbiol. 56:873-81 |
| *B. tanukii* | Japan | Fukunaga et al. (1996) | Microbiol Immunol 40:877-81 |
| *B. turdi* | Japan | Fukunaga et al. (1996) | Microbiol Immunol 40:877-81 |
| *B. valaisiana* | Europe, Asia | Wang et al. (1997) | Int J Syst Bacteriol. 47:926-32 |
| *B. Yangtze* | China | Chen-Yi Chu et al. (2008) | J Clin Microbiol. 46:3130-3133 |

NOTE: *B. bavariensis–B. garinii* related; *B. yangtze–B. valaisiana* related.
SOURCE: Oliver, unpublished.

has found *Borrelia* in that area, including Georgia, Florida, South Carolina, and Missouri. These subspecies include *B. americana*, *B. carolinensis*, and *B. bissettii*. Furthermore, isolated genes from European *Borrelia* genotypes have been found in samples from birds and animals (Oliver, unpublished). In analyzing 112 subcultures from more than 300 isolates in those four states, 52 strains of *B. burgdorferi* have been found. Of those 52 strains, 15 had identity to the B31-type strain found in the northeast, while 37 had identity to other *B. burgdorferi* sensu stricto strains, including those from California and Europe (Oliver, unpublished). These data were based on two genomic loci, the 5S-23S intergenic spacer and the 16S rDNA.

An analysis of six genomic loci from *B. burgdorferi* strains in nymphal *I. minor* ticks found on a single Carolina wren in South Carolina underscores the great diversity of those strains. In nymphal ticks on a Carolina wren, two different genetic groups of *B. americana* were described. By pooling data from numerous *I. minor* larvae on the same bird, two other new subspecies of *Borrelia* were isolated (Oliver, unpublished). The fact

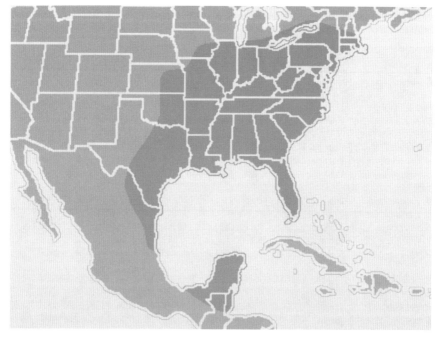

FIGURE 4-2 Birds are efficient transmitters of *Borrelia* strains over great geographic distances. For example, the range of Carolina wrens alone encompasses nearly half the United States.
SOURCE: Image courtesy of Ken Thomas, www.kenthomas.us.

that birds are efficient transmitters of *Borrelia* strains over great geographic distances promises to make these strains more widespread. The range of Carolina wrens alone encompasses nearly half the United States (Figure 4-2).

Among ticks that serve as vectors for *B. burgdorferi*, and among their animal hosts, there is significant genetic diversity. For example, we isolated 53 *Borrelia* strains in *I. scapularis*, 43 in *I. dentatus*, 27 strains in *I. affinis*, and 27 in *I. minor*. In addition, Borrelia strains were cultured from three primary rodents that serve as reservoirs of *Borrelia* in the south: *Peromyscus gossypinus*, the cotton mouse, had 70 strains; *Sigmodon hispidus*, the cotton rat had 26 strains; and *Neotoma floridana*, the eastern wood rat, had 35 strains (Oliver, unpublished).

There is also significant genetic diversity among *Borrelia* subspecies found to infect these bird and animal hosts. For example, in examining *Borrelia* isolates from five animals in South Carolina and Georgia—including a cotton rat, two cotton mice, a wood rat, and a downy woodpecker—the researchers found both American and European strains, including sensu stricto, *B. carolinensis,* and *B. garinii.* In examining *Borrelia* isolates in 16 birds from St. Catherine's Island, a small island south of Savannah, some birds carried only one genospecies while others carried three (Oliver, unpublished).

All these findings contradict recent dogma that *Borrelia* does not occur in the southern United States. In fact, *Borrelia* strains are spreading throughout the region. The question remains whether these strains cause human disease.

In summary, Oliver noted that more than 300 *B. burgdorferi* sensu lato have been isolated from Georgia, Florida, South Carolina, and Missouri. The largest numbers of isolates are *B. burgdorferi,* followed by *B. bissettii* from Georgia, South Carolina, and Florida, and then *B. andersonii* from Missouri, with *B. carolinensis* and *B. americana* recently described from Georgia and South Carolina. Most of the isolates have one genospecies, but 25 cultures contain more than one genospecies. Isolates from three sites in Georgia and two in South Carolina have genes from at least two European genospecies, *B. garinii* and *B. afzelii. I. scapularis, I. affinis,* and *I. minor* are the most common vectors of *B. burgdorferi* sensu lato in Georgia, Florida, and South Carolina.

Based on these findings and other research, Oliver noted a number of hypotheses for future research:

- The infectivity and pathogenicity of *Borrelia* strains vary more in the southern states than in the northeastern states.
- The behavior and life cycle of ticks and the incidence of Borrelia vary among tick populations, based on climate, seasonality, local vegetation, suitable reservoir hosts, and the genetic profile of the *Borrelia* strains.
- *I. minor* and *I. affinis* are often infected with *B. burgdorferi.* Although those ticks rarely bite humans, they serve as enzootic vectors of *Borrelia.* That is, they keep *Borrelia* populations high in the environment. *I. dentatus,* also a common vector of *B. andersonii,* bites humans infrequently.
- Unlike in the Northeast, *I. scapularis* nymphs rarely bite humans in the southern United States. However, contrary to belief, adult *I. scapularis* do bite humans in the South.
- The southeastern United States has a wider diversity of vertebrate hosts, particularly reptiles, than does the northeastern United States, which may dilute the risk of human exposure.
- The diversity of *Borrelia* associated with rodents is much lower than that associated with birds.

- Genetically diverse strains of *Borrelia* often occur within the same individual tick or vertebrate host. Other investigators have shown that *Borrelia* has the recombination system needed for horizontal genetic exchange.

## DISCUSSION

One participant questioned the accuracy of the tick distribution maps because many counties do not have an entomologist. Oliver noted that the distribution maps are incomplete because the collection of specimens is voluntary and relies on volunteers to send in samples. Another participant asked what a person should do given that the information on tick distribution is incomplete. Oliver noted that tick identification needs to be done. He said that most ticks do not transmit *Borrelia* and even if it is a species that does, the infected rate is low. Another participant noted that the lone star ticks *A. americanum*, do not carry *B. burgdorferi*, but may carry *B. lonestari*, which can cause Southern Tick-Associated Rash Illness (STARI). Oliver noted that STARI is not a well-understood area in the tick-borne disease field. He has found spirochetes on darkfield illumination, but has not been successful in culturing these.

Another participant noted that Columbia, Maryland, has one of the highest incidences of Lyme disease in the state. He asked the panel what communities can do to intervene in the tick life cycle, such as installing deer-feeding stations. Ginsberg noted that in highly endemic areas there is generally a need to provide an integrated approach that is tailored to the specific ecological conditions in the area. Four-poster feeding stations have been studied over a broad range of environments and have average effectiveness in controlling nymphal ticks; however, they will not do a complete job of prevention. There is a need to integrate different management methods, including education and environmental controls.

## CONCLUDING THOUGHTS ON EMERGING INFECTIONS, TICK BIOLOGY, AND HOST–VECTOR INTERACTIONS

*Lonnie King, D.V.M., M.S., M.A., College of Veterinary Medicine, Ohio State University*

Because many TBDs are zoonotic, animal and human health experts urgently need to collaborate and to develop an integrated surveillance system that includes domestic animals, wildlife, ticks, and people. Wider and more effective surveillance could allow animals to serve as sentinels and surrogates for human risk and exposure to TBDs. Indeed, without robust diagnostics and surveillance systems, TBDs are likely to remain underreported, and the true incidence and burden of these infections underappreciated.

In fact, surveillance conducted in Florida, Georgia, Missouri, and South Carolina suggests that the current map of the distribution of *B. burgdorferi* may be incomplete. Studies of the distribution, host, and diversity of isolates of *B. burgdorferi* in the Southeast also suggests the possibility that human risk in this region may be underrecognized and that the epidemiology is certainly poorly understood. The impact of regional differences in tick populations, hosts, habitats, and pathogens on human disease—and of genetically distinct subpopulations of those pathogens—deserve further study.

Although scientists know that ticks are coinfected with multiple microbes and pathogens, further research is needed to understand the roles and activities of these microbes and their interrelationships. Possible genetic exchange within this microbial community also needs further investigation, given that it could lead to new diseases.

Finally, comprehensive cross-disciplinary approaches to studying TBDs, and to improving prevention and treatment, are essential.

# 5

# Surveillance, Spectrum, and Burden of Tick-Borne Disease, and At-Risk Populations

An understanding of the science of Lyme disease and other tick-borne diseases (TBDs) begins with the surveillance, spectrum, and burden of disease.

In addition to case definitions used for surveillance purposes, even terminology used to describe a condition can have an impact on the perceptions and recognized burden of a disease. As an example, what some refer to as "post-Lyme syndrome" others call "chronic Lyme disease." The lack of consistency, understanding, and application of accepted definitions and terms are major obstacles to a better understanding of this disease and its long-term outcomes.

The availability, use, and interpretation of diagnostic tests also influence the validity and accuracy of surveillance findings. This can substantially impact the reported patterns and burden of disease. Diagnostic methods now used for most tick-borne illness are antibody based and have not improved much throughout the past two decades.

Ticks can often transmit more than one pathogen. For example, *Ixodes* ticks can simultaneously or sequentially infect their hosts with *Borrelia burgdorferi*, *Anaplasma phagocytophilum*, and *Babesia microti*. How often this occurs—and what it means for the presentation and severity of tick-borne diseases—is not well understood. As a result of changes in climate, the geographic distribution of tick vectors may also change the currently recognized demographic patterns, seasonality, and, ultimately, the incidence of tick-borne diseases.

In this chapter, five researchers explored the current state of knowledge of the incidence, patterns, and severity of key tick-borne diseases in the

United States and their impact on patients. These researchers also explain what efforts to track these diseases among people, and the movement of the pathogens in the environment, reveal about how infection moves from animals to people, especially among vulnerable populations.

## LANDSCAPE OF LYME DISEASE: CURRENT KNOWLEDGE, GAPS, AND RESEARCH NEEDS

*Gary P. Wormser, M.D., New York Medical College*

Lyme disease is the most commonly reported vector-borne infection in the United States. *B. burgdorferi* is the only recognized pathogen to cause Lyme disease in the United States, and can be differentiated into 16 to 45 subtypes that may vary in infectivity and/or in pathogenicity (Wormser et al., 2008a; Crowder et al., 2010). In Europe, *B. burgdorferi* also causes Lyme disease, but other species of *Borrelia,* such as *Borrelia afzelii* and *Borrelia garinii,* also are responsible for Lyme disease. Because different species are responsible for infection in the two locations, the clinical syndromes associated with Lyme disease also differ between the United States and Europe.

The reported incidence rate of Lyme disease has increased steadily from 10,000 cases in 1992 to approximately 30,000 cases in 2009 (CDC website) (Figure 5-1). Twelve states in the Northeast, Mid-Atlantic, and North Central regions of the United States account for nearly 95 percent of these reported cases. New Hampshire (a 37-fold increase) and Maine (a 19-fold increase) have seen the largest proportionate increases in the number of cases during the past 10 years. New York has the largest absolute number of reported cases of Lyme disease, but is only fifth in the incidence of Lyme disease—the number of cases per 100,000 residents. Connecticut has the highest reported incidence.

In the United States, *B. burgdorferi* are transmitted exclusively by *Ixodes* ticks, which may transmit pathogens that cause other infections as well, including babesiosis, human granulocytic anaplasmosis, and flavivirus Powassan-like encephalitis. Of the diseases transmitted by *I. scapularis,* flavivirus Powassan-like encephalitis virus is the least well characterized. One recent study suggested that 2–5 percent of adult *Ixodes scapularis* ticks collected from two sites in Westchester County, New York, in 2008 contained Powassan virus (Tokarz et al., 2010). Approximately 4 percent of those ticks also contained *B. miyamotoi,* a relapsing fever-like *Borrelia.* Whether *Borrelia miyamotoi* causes human infection is unknown, and the clinical manifestations, if it does, are likewise unknown. Both Powassan virus and *B. miyamotoi* deserve of additional research efforts.

A number of animals act as reservoirs for *Borrelia* species, including mice, other small mammals, and some birds. Although deer serve as hosts

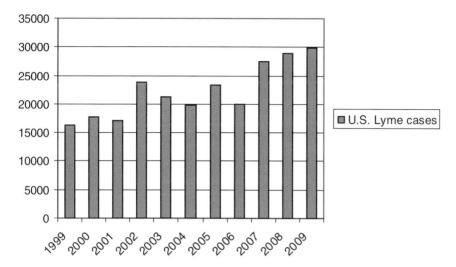

FIGURE 5-1 The reported incidence rate of Lyme disease has steadily increased in the United States since its emergence in the early 1980s.
SOURCE: Gary Wormser, unpublished.

for *Ixodes* ticks, they are not competent reservoirs for *B. burdorferi*. A number of prevention strategies have been demonstrated to decrease the incidence of Lyme disease. Reducing the number of ticks through the use of acaricides on land, mice, or deer is one approach for preventing Lyme disease. Modifying landscapes and building fences to keep deer away from inhabited areas can also reduce human exposure to ticks. Some investigators have reported that simply clearing leaf litter can reduce the number of ticks by approximately 90 percent (Schulze et al., 1995). Personal protective measures have been shown to reduce exposure to ticks. These measures include covering up as much as possible when outdoors, using insect repellents on exposed skin (Vasquez et al., 2008), bathing within 2 hours of tick exposure, and performing daily tick checks (Connally et al., 2009).

Absent from this arsenal of personal protective measures is a human Lyme disease vaccine. A first generation Lyme disease vaccine was introduced in 1998 by GlaxoSmithKline and was approximately 80 percent effective against Lyme disease. The reasons for the withdrawal of the vaccine from the market in 2002 are multifactorial and would be difficult to enumerate in this section. Subsequently, little work has been done to develop a new human vaccine. There is interest in developing a Lyme disease vaccine for mice, because they are the host reservoir for this infection. In laboratory experiments, *Borrelia* infection rates can be substantially reduced by feeding antibacterial compounds to mice (Dolan et al., 2008). Limiting the pathogen burden in the host reservoir, either through vaccination or anti-bacterial treatment, would likely reduce the proportion of ticks that become infected and therefore are capable of transmitting Lyme disease to humans. However, the long-term feasibility of such an approach is unknown.

Lyme disease has several stages. *Early localized Lyme disease* manifests as a single skin lesion known as erythema migrans (EM). *Early disseminated Lyme disease* consists of multiple erythema migrans skin lesions in addition to possible cardiac and neurological manifestations, such as seventh cranial nerve palsy and meningitis. *Late Lyme disease* is most often associated with arthritis in large joints, less commonly with neurological and cardiac manifestations, and in Europe, acrodermatitis, a chronic skin condition.

From 1992 to 2006, 248,074 cases of patients with Lyme disease were reported to the U.S. Centers for Disease Control and Prevention (CDC). Of these patients, 69 percent had EM, 32 percent had arthritis, and 12 percent had neurological manifestations (Bacon et al., 2008). In contrast, during a vaccine trial that monitored 267 patients before and after they became ill, approximately 73 percent had erythema migrans, approximately 1.5 percent had arthritis, and 18 percent had developed a nonspecific viral-like syndrome (Steere et al., 1998). Other studies have suggested that 10 percent of patients believed to be infected with *B. burgdorferi* present with a viral-like syndrome, but the clinical manifestations and patterns of disease progression have not been well characterized (Aucott et al., 2009). Furthermore, approximately 7 percent of individuals in the vaccine trial study developed an asymptomatic infection based on documented seroconversion. At this time, the natural history for asymptomatic infection, and whether it is the same as that for untreated erythema migrans, is unknown. This area needs further study.

In 2008, the CDC/Council of State and Territorial Epidemiologists (CSTE) surveillance case definition for Lyme disease was made more encompassing to allow the documentation and tabulation of other manifestations reportedly associated with Lyme disease. The definition of a *confirmed case* remained the same: either erythema migrans, or late manifestations of the disease with laboratory evidence of infection. However, a definition for a *probable case* was added of physician-diagnosed Lyme disease with laboratory evidence of infection using a two-tier test. That is, any disease a physician designates as Lyme disease is a probable case if supported by laboratory test results. In 2009, clinicians reported 8,500 probable cases of infection, for a confirmed-to-probable ratio of 3.5 to 1.

CDC and CSTE also added two definitions for a *suspected case*: (1) EM with no known exposure to ticks and no laboratory evidence of infection, and (2) laboratory evidence of infection in the absence of clinical information. These changes were a constructive attempt to build the knowledge base regarding the spectrum of illness among persons that the community considers to have Lyme disease.

Current serological testing for Lyme disease presents a number of challenges. First, serology testing using Western blots during early Lyme disease and in patients with erythema migrans is not sensitive. Second, the over-reading of weak bands on a Western blot by many commercial laboratories results in a high percentage of false-positive reports, although no studies have been done to document the percentage. Third, residents of some high-risk regions may demonstrate background seropositivity, leading them to test positive for Lyme disease on IgG Western blots even though they are completely well or have confirmed illness due to other etiologies. In one study, more than 50 percent of individuals who tested positive for Lyme disease on Western blot had no history of having had Lyme disease (Hilton et al., 1999). Finally, there are some patients who, after successful treatment and resolution of early Lyme disease symptoms, maintain persistent antibodies to *B. burgdorferi*.

Serologic findings lag the presence of erythema migrans. In a study of 252 patients in the United States with erythema migrans, serologic testing, including whole cell sonicate enzyme-linked immunosorbent assay (ELISA), two-tier testing, and the second generation serologic assay, C6 showed low sensitivity during the first 7 days of infection when erythema migrans is present. By 20–30 days after the onset of illness, the frequency of a positive C6 serologic test rises to approximately 100 percent of all patients (Wormser et al., 2008b). Although the dissociation of symptoms and laboratory results may appear insignificant, erythema migrans can resemble southern tick-associated rash illness (STARI), which appears after the bite of a lone-star tick (*Amblyomma americanum*). In fact, cases of STARI have been reported in Maryland and New Jersey, where *B. burgdorferi* infection is also common. The ability to differentiate STARI from *B. burgdorferi* infection clinically and in the laboratory would be helpful. Currently, the etiology, disease burden and patterns, and clinical manifestations (other than a rash) of STARI are unknown.

*Borrelia burgdorferi* spirochetes are thought to move from the site of a tick bite to other parts of the skin and organs through hematogenous dissemination. Blood cultures of approximately 40 percent of untreated patients in one study, tested up to 1 month after erythema migrans first appeared, yielded *B. burgdorferi* regardless of the size or duration of the rash (Wormser et al., 2005).

Approximately 73 percent of Lyme disease patients have symptoms in addition to a skin lesion when they first seek treatment, including arthralgias (joint pain), myalgias (muscle pain), fatigue, malaise, neck pain, and headache. Approximately 25 percent of patients continue to report milder symptoms even after treatment, although their skin lesions have long since resolved. The median frequency of reported symptoms at 6 months is approximately 11.5 percent in eight U.S. randomized treatment trials (Cerar et al., 2010).

Three long-term outcome studies of patients with Lyme disease found that among healthy controls, who did not have Lyme disease, 15–43 percent reported fatigue, 16–20 percent reported headaches, up to 27 percent reported joint pain, and 19 percent reported muscle aches. These findings call into question whether the percentages of Lyme disease patients who continue to have symptoms more than 6 months after treatment exceed the percentages of the general population reporting the same symptoms. Furthermore, if the percentages among those reported to have Lyme disease are above the background rates, the causes of the long-term symptoms among Lyme disease patients remain unknown. A number of factors are associated with long-term symptoms, including how severely ill patients are when they first seek care (Nowakowski et al., 2003), the presence of neurologic manifestations (Eikeland et al., 2011), prior or current psychiatric conditions (Solomon et al., 1998), and greater sensitivity to symptoms (i.e., patients who are more aware of their symptoms will report them over a longer length of time). There are limited data suggesting that coinfection with untreated babesiosis and autoimmune events, such as the production of antineural antibodies, are correlated with long-term symptoms.

Some of the controversies surrounding Lyme disease reflect the fact that the disease means different things to different people. To some, Lyme disease is insidious and ubiquitous: Such patients commonly present with nonspecific symptoms, are diagnosed based on clinical judgment because diagnostic tests are insensitive, and require antibiotic treatment for months to years. To others, Lyme disease occurs focally, depends on exposure to infected ticks, and usually is linked to objective clinical manifestations. Positive laboratory tests are needed to support a diagnosis for symptoms other than EM, and the disease typically responds to antibiotic treatment.

## Knowledge Gaps and Research Opportunities

There are a number of research opportunities to begin to answer questions regarding outstanding issues associated with Lyme disease:

- Create a network of investigators and clinical trials for Lyme disease and other TBDs, and promote opportunities for collaborative research.
- Create a repository for specimens of serum and cerebrospinal fluid from patients with tick-borne diseases.
- Formalize definitions of tick-borne diseases and instruments for evaluating and following patients in different clinical groups.

- Conduct broad-based studies of chronic Lyme disease, fibromyalgia, chronic fatigue syndrome, and other medically unexplained syndromes, free of any preconceived ideas on cause, perhaps led by the Institute of General Medical Sciences.

## LYME DISEASE: APPROACHES TO UNDERSTANDING A MULTIDIMENSIONAL DISEASE

*Benjamin J. Luft, M.D., State University of New York–Stony Brook*

Lyme disease is an emerging and diverging disease. Increasingly, clinicians are starting to recognize that it is a disease that may affect many organ systems in subtle ways and have a biological, social, and societal impact for the patient. The acknowledgment that Lyme disease may be a complex and chronic illness requires a comprehensive, multidisciplinary and patient-centered perspective. Patients are not interested in whether their illness is caused by *Borrelia burgdorferi* or another genotype of *Borrelia*. They want to be well again.

Clinicians and researchers need to understand that the disease and its impact may intimately affect the severity and progression of symptoms. Because of the complexity of this disease, there is a need to develop better biological and clinical instruments to evaluate and measure the effectiveness of outcomes of treating its various manifestations. Furthermore, there is a need to develop a universally accepted phenotype of the disease. More than a quarter century after the discovery of Lyme disease, infectious disease specialists, neurologists, and psychiatrists still hold different conceptions of the disease. This may be due in part because they are focused on a particular organ system (i.e., their specialty), or they may be seeing the patient at a different phase of the illness. The natural history varies greatly from person to person, leading to an absence of consensus about what is "active" disease and what is disease impact.

The management of chronic illness, with its waxing and waning symptoms, poses a challenge to our traditional office-based, single-specialty approach to management. Furthermore, few centers are equipped to address the full gamut of medical, psychological, and social aspects of Lyme disease in a coordinated fashion. Because of the complexities and unknowns, third-party payers are not responsive to the needs of Lyme disease patients. As a result, reimbursement for disease management is denied because the symptoms are not accepted as the "disease," and the patient is presented with a significant bill and marginalized from standard medical care.

The complexity of Lyme disease is unraveling. Currently, 37 species of *Borrelia* have been identified throughout the world, 12 of which are believed to cause Lyme disease. Some have been cultivated in the lab, while others have been detected only by using polymerase chain reaction (PCR). In general, *B. burgdorferi* is the sensu stricto species that results in Lyme disease in the United States, while *B. afzelii, B. garinii,* and *B. burgdorferi* cause Lyme disease in Eurasia. The species diversity of *Borrelia* has important research implications, such as the appropriate number of the patients needed for studies, the geographic locations of study sites, and the appropriate power for meaningful statistical analysis.

The structure of OspA and OspC, the major outer surface proteins of *Borrelia burgdorferi,* and epitopes—the part of *B. burgdorferi* antigens recognized by the immune system—have been mapped. These data have allowed for further characterization of the pathogen at different stages along the life cycle of the tick and disease transmission. In an early study (Wang et al., 1999; Qiu et al., 2002), OspC variation was used to determine the variants of *B. burgdorferi.* Most ticks were host to between one and nine variants of *B. burgdorferi.* In a subsequent study (Seinost et al., 1999) that looked at patients and their skin isolates, ticks transmitted only a subset of *B. burgdorferi* variants, and even fewer of these variants actually made their way into the blood of patients. That means that only a relatively small number of *B. burgdorferi* strains actually cause invasive disease. The structure of OspC did not differ significantly among strains except that the electrostatic force at the head of the protein appears to be much stronger in invasive strains (Kumaran et al., 2001). The VMP protein in *Borrelia hermsii* strains that become invasive, and can cause relapsing fever, has a similar characteristic. These findings deserve further study.

At least 46 genotypes of *B. burgdorferi* have been identified and more than 34 percent of ticks carry at least 2 of the genotypes, while 5 percent have more than 3 (Qiu et al., 2002, 2008; Crowder et al., 2010). Some genotypes persist longer in mice and affect the severity of disease in humans. However, it is not known whether there is synergy or antagonism among a patient's immune responses to different genotypes. Using a combination of broad-range PCR and mass spectrometry, *Borrelia* genotypes were identified in New York, Connecticut, Indiana, and California (Coulter et al., 2005). The genotypes varied among the four states. For example, 31 genotypes were found to occur in New York and 19 in Connecticut (see Figure 5-2). Although the two states are neighbors, they shared only 15 of the genotypes, with the remainder being found in only one of the states. Such variation suggests that people can contract different types of Lyme disease depending on where they live, and they may respond differently to antibiotic treatment.

Although there is no current research that indicates antibiotic resistance varies from strain to strain, multicentered therapeutic trials will be required to assess the efficacy of treatment over a broad array of patients exposed to various genotypes and their variants, as well as other concomitant

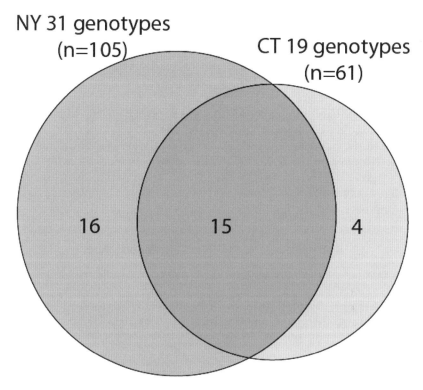

**FIGURE 5-2** *Borrelia burgdorferi* genotype variation between regions. New York has 31 genotypes, but only 16 of them are unique to that state. Connecticut has 19 genotypes, with 4 unique to that state.
SOURCE: Coulter et al., 2005.

pathogens. These studies will need to be double blinded, placebo controlled, and amply powered to make a definitive assessment of efficacy. Furthermore, diagnostic tests for Lyme disease will need to consider genotypic variants of *B. burgdorferi*, as well as whether concomitant infection with other pathogens can lead to false-positive or false-negative results.

Recently, multilocus genetic sequencing was used to produce a family tree of *Borrelia* to determine whether *B. burgdorferi* could continually acquire new genetic information from other species and strains. After sequencing 17 *B. burgdorferi* genotypes, the organism's core genome (i.e., the genes that occur in all strains of the organism) and its pangenome (i.e., the full complement of genes) could be characterized. From these results, it appears that the genome is open to a large gene repertoire, can adapt to evade host immunity and vaccination, and had the ability to develop antibiotic resistance. In addition, there is the opportunity for lateral gene transfer between genotypes, which will determine the effectiveness of any treatment.

Understanding the genome of *B. burgdorferi* is a potential avenue to refine diagnostic tools. In one experiment, researchers identified *B. burgdorferi* genes that were positively selected (varied from strain to strain) as a result of immune pressure. From this information, an array that included more than 500 recombinant proteins was developed. Sera from patients tested using the two-tiered testing protocol found that approximately 54 percent of the patients sera yielded results that were diagnostic for Lyme disease (Coulter et al., 2005). When the protein microarray was used to test the patients' sera, all patients tested positive for antibodies to *Borrelia*. These results suggest that seronegative Lyme disease, whether early or late, does not exist, and the findings simply reflect inadequate diagnostic tests.

### Knowledge Gaps and Research Opportunities

A number of areas are important for future research, including

- Developing accurate methods for identifying *B. burgdorferi* phenotypes;
- Using appropriate animal models, such as the C3H persistent infection mouse model, to assess new approaches to diagnosis and treatment;
- Developing better biological and clinical instruments to evaluate and measure the effectiveness of outcomes of treating its various manifestations;
- Establishing standard operating procedures for developing criteria for acute and chronic Lyme disease; and
- Gathering information and biological samples from patients at various stages of their disease, and using technology to evaluate those samples.

### DISCUSSION SESSION

One clinician participant noted that chronic fatigue syndrome is a clinical condition of prolonged and severe fatigue of at least 6 months' duration for which other causes have been excluded. He stated that in his clinical experience there is a relationship between chronic fatigue syndrome and Lyme disease in which some patients who meet the case definition for chronic fatigue syndrome may have seronegative Lyme disease. This was identified as a research gap.

Another clinician participant noted that in his practice there is a spectrum of acute and chronic Lyme disease, and, although work on acute disease is important, there needs to be a further emphasis on the research needs of chronic illness. For example, the National Institutes of Health (NIH) trials showed 22 standardized measures of fatigue, pain, mental health, and physical health with patients with chronic illness that was not being adequately studied. The Zhang et al. study suggests that individuals with chronic manifestations of Lyme disease have costs of approximately $16,000 a year. He concluded by noting the need for a multidimensional program to help individuals with chronic manifestations. This discussion was expanded by other participants who suggested that research on this issue has not made substantial progress and a mechanism is needed to allow for innovative approaches to investigating the various stages of Lyme disease.

Another discussion focused on whether a protein assay could be produced to detect *B. burgdorferi* in all stages of disease for the general market. Luft commented that the technology could be developed to identify seroreactive proteins and detect disease in all stages. He also noted that, in addition to the development of such technology, a disease phenotype needs to be developed that would unify the research as technology moves forward.

## THE INCREASING HEALTH BURDEN OF HUMAN BABESIOSIS: CLINICAL MANIFESTATIONS, COINFECTION, AND RESEARCH NEEDS

*Peter J. Krause, M.D., Department of Epidemiology and School of Public Health, Yale School of Medicine*

Babesiosis is an infection caused by intraerythrocytic protozoa of the genus *Babesia*. Transmission is primarily through the tick, *Ixodes scapularis*, but also may occur via blood transfusion, and rarely from mother to child perinatally. The health burden of the disease is significant and increasing in the United States (Vannier et al., 2008).

Babesiosis diagnosis is made on the basis of epidemiological, clinical, and laboratory information (Vannier et al., 2008). A person must live or have recently traveled to an endemic area or have recently received a blood transfusion. Babesiosis-compatible symptoms include fever, chills, sweats, headache, and fatigue. Most patients become ill approximately 1 to 2 weeks after a tick bite, although symptoms may appear up to 9 weeks after *Babesia* transmission through blood transfusions (Ruebush et al., 1981; Gubernot et al., 2009; Leiby, 2011). Symptoms usually last 1 to 2 weeks but can persist much longer in immunocompromised individuals (Krause et al., 2008). Laboratory confirmation of the diagnosis usually is made by microscopic identification of the organism on a thin blood smear supplemented with amplification of *Babesia* DNA using PCR and detection of antibody with immunofluorescence assay (IFA) or Western blot assays (Figure 5-3) (Krause et al., 2002; Vannier et al., 2008).

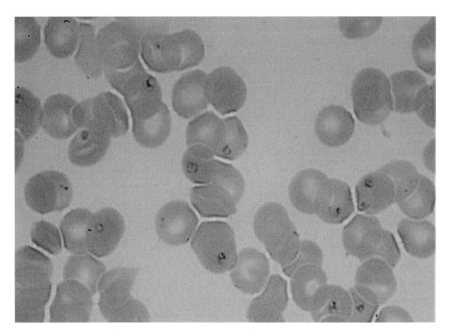

FIGURE 5-3 Ring forms of *Babesia microti* in human blood smear (× 1,000).
SOURCE: Courtesy of Peter Krause.


More than 100 *Babesia* species have been documented in a wide variety of wild and domestic animals; however, only a few of these species are known to infect humans (Vannier et al., 2008). *Babesia microti* is the most important of these because it causes endemic disease in the northeastern and northern Midwest United States (Vannier et al., 2008). Several cases of WA-1 (*Babesia duncani*) and CA-1 have been reported in Washington state and California (Persing et al., 1995; Conrad et al., 2006). *Babesia divergens*–like human illness has been reported in Kentucky, Missouri, and Washington state (Herwaldt et al., 1996; Beattie et al., 2002; Vannier et al., 2008). Both *B. microti* and *B. duncani* have been transmitted through transfusions of whole blood, packed red blood cells, and platelets (Ruebush et al., 1981; Gubernot et al., 2009).

In Europe, babesiosis follows a more sporadic pattern, with fewer cases being reported than in the United States, although a higher proportion of these cases are severe (Zintl et al., 2003; Vannier et al., 2008). Nearly all have occurred in people who are asplenic, raising the possibility that milder cases in immunocompetent people are not being identified. The primary agent is *B. divergens*, a cattle *Babesia*, but *B. microti* and *Babesia venatorum* (EU-1) also have been described (Herwaldt et al., 2003; Zintl et al., 2003; Hildebrandt et al., 2007). In Asia, *B. microti*–like organisms have been reported to cause human infection in Japan, Korea (KO-1), and Taiwan (TW-1) (Shih et al., 1997; Wei et al., 2001; Kim et al., 2007).

The National Academy of Sciences cited babesiosis, ehrlichiosis, and Lyme disease as emerging threats to human health in the United States in a 1992 report (Lederberg et al., 1992). From 1991 to 2009, Connecticut experienced a marked increase in the number of cases of babesiosis (Connecticut State Department of Health) (Figure 5-4). Although similar trends have been reported in Massachusetts, New Jersey, New York, and Rhode Island, the actual numbers of infections are underestimated (Krause et al., 2003; Vannier et al., 2008). This increase is likely due to the expansion of the *Babesia* endemic range, increased recognition of babesiosis by clinicians and the public, and more widely available diagnostic testing. In a 10-year prospective study (1991–2000) of residents of Block Island, Rhode Island, case finding and serosurvey were conducted to determine the number of people with symptomatic and asymptomatic *B. microti* and *Borrelia burgdorferi* infection. About 50 *B. microti* and 75 *B. burgdorferi* infections per year were diagnosed for a ratio of 1 to 1.5 (Krause et al., 2003), reflecting the proportion of local ticks infected by these pathogens. Similar rates of hospital admissions for babesiosis were recorded for Block Island and southeastern Connecticut. These results suggest that in some areas endemic for both pathogens, the incidence of Lyme disease and that of babesiosis

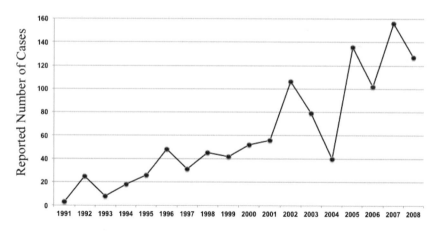

FIGURE 5-4 The reported incidence of babesiosis in Connecticut has increased from 1991 until 2008.
SOURCE: Peter Krause, unpublished.

are comparable. In recognition of the growing importance of babesiosis, the CDC and CSTE designated babesiosis as a national notifiable disease beginning in January 2011.

The health burden of disease includes both the number and severity of cases. Babesiosis is characterized by a wide range of disease severity, from asymptomatic to fatal. Approximately 25 percent of adults and 50 percent of children are asymptomatic when infected with B. microti (Krause et al., 2003). Typical clinical symptoms include chills, sweats, headache, fatigue, myalgia, arthralgia, anorexia, nausea, and cough (Krause et al., 2002, 2008; Vannier et al., 2008). Fulminant illness and death occur in 3–5 percent of otherwise healthy people and up to 25 percent of those who are immunocompromised or suffering from certain premorbid conditions (see discussion later in the chapter) (Hatcher et al., 2001; Vannier et al., 2008; Gubernot et al., 2009; Leiby et al., 2011). Healthy individuals with mild to moderate babesiosis can clear the infection without treatment, although antibiotic therapy can shorten the duration of illness (Krause et al., 1998).

Babesiosis is currently the most commonly reported transfusion-associated pathogen in the United States (FDA, 2008). More than 70 cases have been reported since the first report in 1979, with associated mortality of 10–28 percent (Gubernot et al., 2009; Leiby et al., 2011). Severity of transfusion-transmitted disease is presumably greater than tick-transmitted disease because blood recipients are more likely to be immunocompromised than those who acquire infection through tick transmission. Estimates of risk of transfusion transmission vary widely depending on geographic location, from approximately 1 case per million units of blood administered to as high as 1 in 604 units (Gerber et al., 1994; Tonnetti et al., 2009).

Human coinfection with B. microti and B. burgdorferi can occur because both pathogens share a common tick vector and mouse reservoir. Several studies suggest B. microti may increase B. burgdorferi disease severity, but B. burgdorferi appears to have little effect on the severity of B. microti infection. In a prospective study of 240 patients with Lyme disease, 26 (11 percent) were coinfected with B. microti (Krause et al., 1996). Patients experiencing both Lyme disease and babesiosis had significantly more symptoms than those with Lyme disease alone, and the duration of illness was longer. Borrelia burgdorferi DNA was detected in the blood of a higher percentage of coinfected individuals than in the blood of people infected with B. burgdorferi alone, suggesting that coinfected patients may be more likely to experience disseminated complications of Lyme disease, such as arthritis and neurologic problems, than those with Lyme disease alone. This study only assessed acute disease and did not include long-term follow-up of these patients, however. Although similar results are noted with other coinfections, including Lyme disease and human granulocytic anaplasmosis (HGA) (Belongia et al., 1999; Krause et al., 2002; Steere et al., 2003), further studies are needed regarding long-term complications of coinfection.

In conclusion, the health burden of babesiosis may be approaching that of Lyme disease. The incidence and geographic dispersion of Lyme disease are greater than those of babesiosis, but the differences are smaller than generally recognized and appear to be decreasing. Babesiosis is the most commonly reported transfused pathogen in the United States. At certain endemic sites, the incidence of Lyme disease and babesiosis are similar. Babesiosis causes more life-threatening disease than Lyme disease does, and coinfection may increase the severity of Lyme disease.

## Knowledge Gaps and Research Opportunities

A number of questions offer research opportunities pertaining to babesiosis:

### Epidemiology

- Where is babesiosis enzootic and endemic now and in the future?
- What is the incidence of babesiosis at the state, national, and international levels?
- How fast is the incidence of babesiosis increasing?
- What is the frequency of transfusion-transmitted babesiosis?
- How often and where do pathogens other than *B. microti* cause babesiosis?

### Pathogenesis

- What is the pathogenesis of babesial illness?
- Are there *B. microti* substrains with varying pathogenic potential?
- What are the primary immune factors responsible for clearing babesiosis?
- What are the mechanisms that worsen the severity of babesiosis with aging?

### Clinical Manifestations

- What are the long-term complications of babesiosis?
- How does coinfection with babesiosis and other co-transmitted pathogens influence transmission in the reservoir host and disease in humans?

### Diagnosis

- Can scientists develop better biomarkers for babesiosis, including antibody, nucleic acid amplification test technologies, and culture?

*Treatment/Prevention*

- How can transfusion-transmitted babesiosis be prevented?
- What new antiparasitic therapies are available for babesiosis?
- Is the use of partial-exchange transfusion to treat severe cases of babesiosis equivalent to full-exchange transfusion?

## EHRLICHIA AND ANAPLASMA: SURVEILLANCE, COINFECTION, AND RESEARCH NEEDS

*J. Stephen Dumler, M.D., Johns Hopkins School of Medicine*

*Ehrlichia* and *Anaplasma* are pathogens within the Anaplasmataceae family; they are obligate intracellular bacteria similar to *Rickettsia*. At least three species of *Ehrlichia* and *Anaplasma* are known to cause human disease. *Ehrlichia chaffeensis* causes human monocytic chrlichiosis (HME) by infecting monocytes in peripheral blood and macrophages in tissues. *Anaplasma phagocytophilum* causes HGA by infecting neutrophils. *Ehrlichia ewingii*, the cause of ewingii ehrlichiosis, resembles *Ehrlichia chaffeensis* genetically and serologically, but resembles *Anaplasma* phenotypically because it also lives inside neutrophils. HGA occurs predominantly in northern states where the black-legged tick, *Ixodes scapularis*, serves as the vector for both *Anaplasma phagocytophilum* and *Borrelia burgdorferi*. HME occurs predominantly across the South Central and Southeast United States, mirroring the range of the lone-star tick, *Amblyomma americanum*, the vector for the pathogen that causes the disease.

All these pathogens cause an undifferentiated febrile illness with typical laboratory findings. The incidence of ehrlichiosis is less than that of Lyme disease; however, the disease still carries a substantial burden. Cases of all forms of ehrlichiosis have been increasing since HME was first identified in the mid-1980s (Figure 5-5). Since 2000, there has been a significant spike in the number of reported ehrlichiosis cases, although, as with other tick-borne diseases, they are underreported.

HME and HGA often present with severe headache, myalgias, and a variety of other constitutional symptoms, such as nausea and vomiting. Rashes occur relatively infrequently, differentiating these illnesses from Rocky Mountain spotted fever and Lyme disease. Many patients—especially those with HME—also have some degree of central nervous system involvement. Approximately 20 percent of patients with HME have meningoencephalitis. Some immunocompromised patients, such as those with HIV, develop overwhelming infection.

Common laboratory findings include leukopenia (low white blood cell count) and/or thrombocytopenia (low platelet count). Furthermore, there is

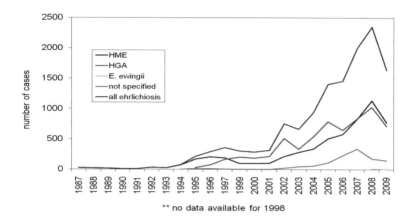

FIGURE 5-5 The incidence of reported ehrlichiosis and anaplasmosis in the United States has increased since 1986 when HME was first identified.
SOURCE: Steve Dumler, unpublished.

often evidence of mild hepatic (liver) injury, based on elevated serum levels of the hepatic enzymes ALT and AST.

Nearly half (48 percent) of the patients reported with HME from 2000 to 2007 were admitted to a hospital, while approximately 36 percent of patients with HGA were hospitalized during that period (CDC, unpublished data). The case fatality rate was approximately 2 percent for HME, and 0.5 percent for HGA. Life-threatening complications reported among these patients include acute respiratory distress syndrome, disseminated intravascular coagulation, meningitis, meningoencephalitis, and renal failure.

One way to analyze how often people are infected is to look at cross-sectional seroprevalence studies. The seroprevalence for HME in Tennessee ranges from 3.3 percent to 12.5 percent, depending on the diagnostic test used to detect the pathogen, while it is substantially lower in Arkansas at 1.3 percent. For HGA, the seroprevalence ranges from 0.6 to 0.9 percent in Connecticut to 14.9 percent in northwest Wisconsin. These results suggest a significant number of individuals are becoming infected in these locations. In contrast, the number of infections based on disease surveillance data is significantly lower. For HME, they range from 300 cases per 100,000 persons in Tennessee to 400 cases per 100,000 persons in Missouri (Standaert et al., 1995; Olano et al., 2003). For HGA, they range from 50 cases per 100,000 persons in Connecticut to 60 cases per 100,000 persons in northwest Wisconsin (Bakken et al., 1998). Based on these figures, the ratio of symptomatic disease to infection ratio is 3–30:100 for HME and .4–6:100 for HGA. Even if the seroprevalence data reflect old and new infections, the difference between the two findings suggests either that many infected individuals are asymptomatic or subclinical, or that the diagnostic tests used to classify them are problematic.

Globally, *Anaplasma* seroprevalence is high: 8.9 percent in Asia, 7.2 percent in Europe, and 4.5 percent in North America, although these studies were conducted in endemic or high-risk regions (Dumler, 2005). The seroprevalence among individuals with confirmed Lyme disease who are also seropositive for *Anaplasma* is much higher than in cross-sectional studies. That raises two questions: Are these patients being appropriately diagnosed, and/or are there problems with serologic testing?

There are a number of common pathologic features among patients with HME and HGA. There is activation of the mononuclear phagocyte system, with macrophage infiltrates in tissues and hemophagocytosis; individuals with HME often have granulomas in the bone marrow. Pancytopenia—reflecting low leukocyte counts and low platelet counts—is likely due to consumption, sequestration, or destruction of these elements in the periphery, because bone marrow production tends to be normal in these patients. Pancytopenia can predispose patients to hemorrhage or opportunistic infections, both of which occur in HME and HGA. Some HME patients have significant hepatitis and with histopathologic appearance of apoptotic hepatocytes, a feature observed with cytokine-mediated diseases. Less frequent complications, such as acute respiratory distress syndrome, stem from interstitial pneumonitis and diffuse alveolar damage—probably from systemic proinflammatory response. Such inflammatory responses also appear with meningoencephalitis in patients with severe HME and among those who experience a toxic-shock–like syndrome with either disease.

It is not clear to what degree disease severity can be attributed to the host or the pathogen. HGA patients have a mean white blood cell count of $3.7 \times 10^3$ per microliter, yet the average proportion of infected leukocytes in less than 1 percent. In contrast, the mean leukocyte count among healthy adults is $7.8 \times 10^3$ per microliter (Dumler, 2005). Thus, HGA patients lose many more white blood cells than can be accounted for by infection alone. On the other hand, the severity of HGA and HME is linked to the amount of time that elapses between the onset of illness and treatment, and the infections respond rapidly to antimicrobial therapy, suggesting that the microbe is responsible for at least some components of the disease.

Based on animal models, a consensus is beginning to emerge that these diseases are immunopathologic. In a mouse model using *Ehrlichia muris* or *Ixodes ovatus ehrlichia*, natural killer T cells mediate *Ehrlichia*-induced toxic-shock–like syndrome, likely via interactions with antigen-presented cells (Mattner et al., 2005). In a second mouse model study, natural killer cells promote immunopathology and defective anti-Ehrlichial immunity, possibly by decreasing the protective immune response (Ismail et al., 2007). Similarly, mice infected with *Anaplasma phagocytophilum* develop lesions as a result of immunopathological mechanisms from natural killer and natural killer T cells rather than bacteria-mediated injury (Martin et al., 2001).

The hypothesis that HGA may be an immunopathologic disease as a result of macrophage activation and hemophagocytic syndromes was tested in a cohort of 42 well-corroborated HGA patients. High levels of triglycerides, significantly elevated levels of ferritin, and a variety of cytokines classically seen with hemophagocytic syndromes and macrophage-activation syndromes were found. Furthermore, severity was directly related to the levels of triglycerides, ferritin, and interleukin-12 in these patients, as well as to the the ratio of IL-10 to interferon gamma as a reflection of the interplay between the TH1 and TH2 axis.

The immunologic tests used to diagnose HME and HGA are problematic. They rely on specific antigens to detect antibodies to the pathogens, and the presence of disease is considered confirmed if there is seroconversion or a fourfold rise in antibody titer. However, patients typically do not have detectable antibodies at the time they are diagnosed, so clinicians must decide to treat before the diagnosis has been confirmed. In fact, according to the CDC, only 11 percent of reported HME cases and only 8 percent of reported HGA cases were based on either seroconversion or a fourfold rise in antibody titers. Instead, 73 percent of reported HME cases and 53 percent of reported HGA cases relied on a single serum antibody test result as the laboratory basis for the diagnosis.

Information on the sensitivity and specificity of serologic tests is limited. For HME, the Immunoglobulin G (IgG) or IFA has greater than 80 percent sensitivity, but information on the test's specificity is lacking. For HGA, the sensitivity of IgG IFA is 82–100 percent, but that of immunoglobulin M (IgM) IFA is just 27–37 percent, which makes it less reliable as a diagnostic test. The specificity of these assays in detecting HGA can be as low as 82 percent, although this improves if patients infected with *Ehrlichia chaffeensis* are omitted because of serologic cross-reactivity.

### Knowledge Gaps and Research Opportunities

A number of questions require additional research, including

- *What is the natural history of HGA?* Do patients with HGA have persistent health problems after recovering from acute infection? A retrospective study in Wisconsin looked at individuals during the 12 months after they had been diagnosed with HGA. HGA patients had significantly more fever, shaking chills, sweats, and fatigue, as well as

higher levels of bodily pain and lower levels of relative health than
did individuals in a control group.

- Clinical study groups are needed to obtain a critical mass of patients,
  standardize approaches, and develop sample repositories.
- *Why does the severity of HGA vary so widely?* Is the severity of
  disease determined by host or pathogen? What are the microbial
  determinants and human genetic predispositions? What is the true
  pathogenesis and immunopathogenesis of HGA and pathogen-
  defined injury to tissues and organs?
- *How accurately are HGA cases identified?* Are existing acute-phase
  diagnostics sufficient? Does the poor predictive value of serology
  hamper effective diagnosis? How often does coinfection with other
  tick-transmitted pathogens occur? What are the short- and long-term
  consequences of proven coinfection?

## RICKETTSIA DISEASES: SPECTRUM OF DISEASE, SPATIAL CLUSTERING, AT-RISK POPULATIONS, AND RESEARCH NEEDS

*Captain Jennifer H. McQuiston, D.V.M., M.S.,*
*U.S. Centers for Disease Control and Prevention*

Worldwide, numerous *Rickettsia* species are human pathogens that
can be transmitted to humans by ticks, other arthropods, and fleas. In the
United States, *Rickettsia rickettsii,* which causes Rocky Mountain spotted
fever, is the primary agent for human rickettsial disease. Increasingly, other
*Rickettsia* pathogens are being reported, including *Rickettsia parkeri* and
*Rickettsia phillipi;* the latter causes 364D rickettsiosis. *Rickettsia massiliae*
is also found in the United States, but there is no current evidence for
transmission to humans. Travelers may bring infections caused by other
Rickettsia species into the country as well, particularly *Rickettsia africae*
and *Rickettsia conorii.*

In the United States, several ticks serve as vectors of spotted fever group
*Rickettsia*: the American dog tick, *Dermacentor variabilis,* in most of the
eastern half of the United States; the Rocky Mountain wood tick, *Dermacentor andersoni;* in the west, is the vector for *R. rickettsii.* The brown dog
tick, *Rhipicephalus sanguineus,* where it is increasingly appearing as a vector of *R. rickettsii.* The Gulf Coast tick, *Amblyomma maculatum,* transmits
*R. parkeri* in the Southeast. Finally, the Pacific Coast tick, *Dermacentor
occidentalis,* which lives primarily in the Pacific Northwest, is associated
with 364D rickettsiosis.

*Rickettsia* pathogens cause a spectrum of illnesses. Rocky Mountain
spotted fever is the most documented *Rickettsia* infection in the United
States and was first recognized in the late 1800s. It infects endothelial cells,

which line blood vessels, causing damage to the vasculature. Patients with Rocky Mountain spotted fever typically present with fever and headache, and approximately 90 percent of them also have a rash.

Rickettsial infections generally respond to treatment with tetracycline-based antibiotics, such as doxycycline, if administered in a timely manner. However, if untreated, the disease progresses, affecting most organ systems and causing death in up to 10 percent of cases. Furthermore, patients who recover may experience long-term health effects, including impaired hearing from neurologic damage; cognitive deficits; and gangrene of fingers and toes caused by damage to blood vessels.

Rocky Mountain spotted fever is the most potentially fatal known rickettsial illness. Prior to the advent of antibiotic therapy, the fatality rate ranged from 20 to 90 percent in published case series. The fatality rate in more recent studies ranges from 3 to 20 percent (Conlon et al., 1996; Buckingham et al., 2007; Martinez-Medina et al., 2007). In national surveillance summaries, fatality rates decreased from about 4 percent (Dalton et al., 1995) in the 1980s to 0.5 percent during 2000 to 2007 (Openshaw, 2010). This decrease may in part be due to changes in the national surveillance system and the differences in how physicians are diagnosing Rocky Mountain spotted fever. Among confirmed cases, the mortality rate from 2000–2007 remained at 3 percent. Reducing these deaths is important because it is a wholly preventable infectious disease, and prompt antibiotic treatment will further reduce fatalities.

Other spotted fever rickettsial diseases generally result in less severe illness. *Rickettsia parkeri* and 364D *Rickettsia* cause an eschar-associated illness, fever, and a rash. These patients, however, may not come to a public health official's attention unless an individual grows concerned or a physician pursues additional testing, for example, to rule out cutaneous anthrax or black widow spider bites.

Testing for *Rickettsia* relies on detection of antibodies. As *Rickettsia* infect the endothelial cells lining blood vessels and do not circulate in the blood, PCR using whole blood is not often useful to detect the pathogen except during severe, fulminant infections. During the early stages of illness, PCR can detect *Rickettsia* in skin biopsy tissue taken from a rash site, but most physicians are reluctant to take such a biopsy. IFA is the predominant diagnostic test used by healthcare providers and relies on *R. rickettsii* antigens, but cross-reacts with antibodies to other *Rickettsia* species. Single serum samples cannot be used to confirm infection because an antibody is long lived, and single positive tests may reflect past infection. Furthermore, a single serologic test may appear negative in the first week of infection, before an antibody has had time to rise to a detectable level. Infection is best confirmed using two serologic tests spaced a few weeks apart, and documenting a rise in antibody titers associated with acute infection.

Serologic tests also have less specificity than PCR, meaning that a positive serologic test indicates only that the patient is infected with a spotted fever *Rickettsia*, but does not identify which one. In 2010, the CTSE changed the name of the reporting category to spotted fever rickettsioses to more accurately describe the data being collected relative to this lack of ability of the serologic test to determine the specific *Rickettsia*.

The CTSE, in collaboration with the CDC and public health officials from state heath departments, determines which diseases to include in the national notifiable disease list and the criteria for inclusion of individual cases. Cases reported to the CDC represent only the tip of the iceberg because cases can be missed at the physician, local, or state level. What these reports have shown, however, is that the reported incidence of spotted fever rickettsiosis has increased steadily (Figure 5-6), although some of the increase may reflect a change in case definition in 2004 to include cases diagnosed by serologic tests such as enzyme immunoassays for IgM antibodies in addition to IFA. However, there are other possible explanations, including environmental changes, increasing exposure to ticks, or a rising number of ticks. The parameters of the surveillance system do not allow a determination of the contribution of each factor to the reported increase in incidence.

Although people living anywhere in the continental United States are at risk for Rocky Mountain spotted fever, there is spatial clustering of cases in the South Central and Southeast regions. Five states—Arkansas, Missouri, North Carolina, Oklahoma, and Tennessee—account for more than 64 percent of reported cases (Openshaw, 2010). These cases can be analyzed

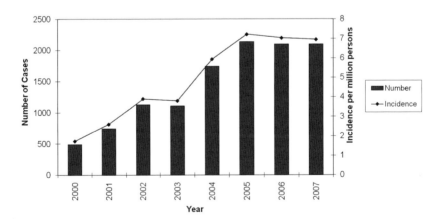

**FIGURE 5-6** The number of cases and the incidence rate of spotted fever rickettsiosis has increased since 2000.
SOURCE: Jennifer McQuiston, unpublished.

further to determine whether there is a geographic difference in the severity of the disease. West Tennessee reports the highest proportion of patients who are hospitalized with complications or die from Rocky Mountain spotted fever. North Carolina, by contrast, sees less hospitalization and lower case fatality rates than the national average. Current information is insufficient to determine the cause of the geographic differences. For example, the differences could result from a different strain of *Rickettsia* or from differences in diagnosing or reporting. This represents a current research gap.

Risk factors for Rocky Mountain spotted fever include poverty and age. Although many individuals associate tick-borne diseases with higher socioeconomic status, because persons in this group engage more frequently in outdoor leisure activities, states with the highest incidence of Rocky Mountain spotted fever fall below the median socioeconomic status for the United States. This may reflect a lack of education about these diseases and prevention strategies, inability to treat their dogs for ticks, and lack of access to health care. The influence of poverty on incidence rates remains a major research gap.

Although the incidence of Rocky Mountain spotted fever increases with age, it is worth noting that the case fatality rates are highest among children ages 9 or younger. One reason for the higher number of fatalities may be the reluctance of physicians to prescribe doxycycline, a tetracycline-based antibiotic that greatly reduces mortality rates, to children. In a survey of healthcare providers in Tennessee, more than half reported that they would prescribe a non-tetracycline antibiotic for suspected Rocky Mountain spotted fever in a child under age 8. This may be due to the idea that tetracycline-based antibiotics stain developing teeth. Current research suggests that doxycycline does not stain teeth, and even if it does, the parents and the patients might well decide that the risk is outweighed by the decreased risk of death.

American Indian populations are also at higher risk of contracting Rocky Mountain spotted fever, with approximately 16 cases per million people versus a national average of 7 cases per million. The rate among American Indians is also about four times that of other racial groups, and American Indians die from their infections at four times the rate of other racial groups. The reasons for these high rates are unclear. Two theories are that cultural differences could put American Indians at higher risk of exposure to ticks, or underlying health disparities could predispose them to severe disease.

In 2002, an outbreak of Rocky Mountain spotted fever began in eastern Arizona—a region where the disease had never before occurred. Although ticks are not often associated with desert climates, this outbreak was linked to the brown dog tick, which can survive in hotter, drier climates. The outbreak was associated with tribal lands with large numbers of stray dogs, which supported large numbers of ticks. Since 2002, there have been 95 human cases of Rocky Mountain spotted fever (and climbing) and 9 deaths among about 30,000 people. Compared to the national case rate, this translates to 527 cases per million on the reservation versus the national rate of 7 per million. The epidemiology of Rocky Mountain spotted fever also differs markedly in this region. The median patient age is only 8 years old, and more than half the fatalities have occurred among children younger than age 4. That makes Rocky Mountain spotted fever a significant contributor to childhood mortality on affected reservations.

The brown dog tick is of continued interest to public health officials because it has also been associated with urban outbreaks of tick-borne diseases. For example, in 2009, more than 1,000 suspected cases of Rocky Mountain spotted fever occurred in urban Mexicali, Mexico. As in Arizona, this outbreak was associated with the brown dog tick, high numbers of stray dogs, and intense transmission in home and peridomestic environments. It is of interest to know whether the brown dog tick might be contributing to Rocky Mountain spotted fever in other parts of the country as well, but just not recognized as the vector in these cases.

## Knowledge Gaps and Research Opportunities

Areas for future study are described below:

### Diagnostics

- Develop diagnostic assays, both serologic and molecular, that can identify patients during acute illness and differentiate the causative *Rickettsia* species.
- Better assess the sensitivity and specificity of new commercial serologic assays, including the IgM enzyme immunoassay.
- Improve surveillance and research on human infections caused by tick-borne *Rickettsia* species other than *R. rickettsii*.

### Emergence

- Explore the role of the brown dog tick in the ecology of Rocky Mountain spotted fever.
- Understand the ecological cycle of *R. rickettsii* in the brown dog tick, including the role of dogs as a possible reservoir.
- Improve surveillance of infections caused by other species of spotted fever *Rickettsia*.
- Given that ticks are acutely sensitive to moisture, precipitation, and temperature, investigate the role of climate change in the emergence of spotted fever rickettsiosis.

*Special Populations*

- Investigate preventable factors that contribute to higher mortality from Rocky Mountain spotted fever among children and American Indian populations, and in certain geographic areas.
- Clarify links between *Rickettsia* infection and low socioeconomic status.
- Investigate differences in pathogenicity among *Rickettsia* strains in different geographic areas.
- Develop new antibiotics and prevention strategies specifically for rickettsial infections, particularly for pregnant women and high-risk populations for whom antibiotics are contraindicated.

## DISCUSSION SESSION

In the discussion session following the presentations of Krause, Dumler, and McQuiston, participants focused primarily on three areas: surveillance, chronic disease, and ongoing research into other potential pathogens.

The differences in severity of Rickettsia spotted fever diseases are an understudied area. One participant noted that the distribution map of Rocky Mountain spotted fever bears a remarkable resemblance to the distribution of *Amblyomma americanum*, the Lone Star tick, and asked whether there is any new information about the relationship of the Lone Star and *R. amblyommii* to human disease. Dr. McQuiston noted that there is increased interest in the *Rickettsia* species that are found in Lone Star ticks. No cases of *R. amblyommii* infection have been confirmed in humans, but some serologic data suggest it could play a role in mild human illness. CDC and other investigators are currently interested in whether the milder form of *Rickettsia* spotted fever in North Carolina could be related to *R. amblyommii* infections.

A number of participants commented on the problems with diagnostics, clinician education, and surveillance. One participant noted that many physicians with whom she interacts know very little about TBDs and therefore are not ordering appropriate diagnostic tests. This lack of knowledge, according to the participant, results in the underreporting of surveillance data. Krause concurred and noted that one of the greatest challenges for diagnosis is awareness of these diseases. In regions where babesiosis has been present for many years, physicians are more familiar with the symptoms and usually order the appropriate diagnostic testing, but even here, *Babesia* testing may not be ordered in a timely fashion because of the nonspecific nature of the symptoms. Physicians practicing in areas where the pathogen recently has been introduced are unlikely to have the same knowledge of babesiosis and may not order the appropriate testing.

Another participant noted the lack of confidence among the public about the serological tests for diagnosing tick-borne infections. Dumler noted that in Rickettsial and Babesia there are a few laboratories that are working on serodiagnostics to clarify the confusing issues, such as cross-reactions between *E. chaffeensis* and *A. phagocytophilum*. Dumler stressed that in the future there will be good methods that could be validated using well-corroborated patient serum samples.

Weber furthered the discussion on surveillance by commenting that research at the 11 largest hospitals in North Carolina indicates that in some instances only 15 percent of reportable diseases are actually reported to state agencies and the CDC. In light of this, he suggested that, in addition to other methods targeted toward underreporting, active surveillance methods are considered to strengthen and improve knowledge of incidence of tick-borne diseases.

Another participant shifted the discussion from surveillance to research on disease mechanisms by noting that there is considerable research on acute infection, but less on chronic infection, such as that reported for babesiosis. Krause agreed with the need for more research on long-term effects of babesiosis, but he indicated that these studies are more difficult to do. A number of unanswered questions also remain about acute infections. Dr. Krause noted the need for more information on pathogenesis of acute infections, such as exploring the role of cytokine expression in immunopathogenesis (Krause et al., 2007).

Another participant was interested in whether *Babesia* could be transmitted through organ transplantation and whether a person who had been cured of *Babesia* should be an organ donor. Although the panel was unable to cite a report that demonstrated this type of transmission, Krause commented that the possibility of transmission through organ donation is likely and worthy of further research.

Another clinician participant questioned the length of persistent PCR positivity in *Babesia* infection and its relationship to Lyme disease. Krause noted that the presence of amplifiable babesial DNA may persist for longer than 2 years, but such persistence was not necessarily indicative of active parasitemia (Krause et al., 1998). The question that still needs to be answered is whether amplifiable *Babesia* DNA from blood correlates directly with active infection.

## PANEL DISCUSSION SESSION

The panel focused on three main themes: surveillance, coinfection, and reinfection and relapse. Although the topics varied, overall the panel indicated that research lagged far behind the needs of the community, and that further research was at the core of addressing these deficiencies.

Surveillance systems, such as the National Notifiable Disease List, are passive in nature. One participant asked whether there is a need to enhance the surveillance for tick-borne diseases by supplementing the current efforts with an active surveillance program. McQuiston suggested an enhanced surveillance model that would focus on specific geographic regions and use data obtained from active surveillance to extrapolate and more accurately quantify the national disease burden. Such surveillance methods, although promising, are not without barriers. Such barriers included inadequate physician education and knowledge of disease presentation and the availability of funding to adequately implement such programs. The panel recognized that an adequate active surveillance model would require physicians to be able to identify and diagnose illness. For this system to be effective, physicians, patients, and, potentially, patient advocacy organizations would need to be able to identify classical and less common manifestations of the respective diseases. This ability was seen as especially important in cases of Lyme disease where the classic presenting signs and symptom of erythema migrans may be absent in up to 20 percent of infected individuals. Inadequate funding was mentioned as a barrier to research, particularly for research on *Rickettsia*, *Ehrlichia*, *Babesia*, and *Anaplasma* infections, which generally receive less funding than Lyme disease research does. For example, an active surveillance program in Tennessee has an estimated cost of $120,000 for four counties for a year.

The panel also discussed the usefulness of actively surveying the disease vectors and their hosts. McQuiston indicated that, in terms of *Rickettsia*, the level of antibody in semi-domesticated dogs could indicate areas that pose a higher risk for human disease and that these data currently are being used to encourage surveillance in these areas. For example, it was noted that in eastern Arizona, when there is a seroprevalence of approximately 5 percent among the canine population, there may not be a significant rate of transmission to humans. Cases of human infection begin to present when host seroprevalence rates rise above this baseline (in the affected region of Arizona, human cases were noted with a canine seroprevalence background of more than 70 percent (McQuiston, 2011). Krause mentioned a survey designed to test ticks for *Anaplasma*, *Babesia*, and *Borrelia* and to create national prevalence maps that highlight areas with a high concentration of infected ticks. He stated that these types of studies would be very helpful in understanding where *Babesia* and *Anaplasma* infections were occurring. He also noted that testing of the ticks will result in public health officials having a better understanding of the geographic distribution of pathogens and how the disease is changing over time as it is not a one-to-one correlation between ticks and pathogens.

The use of surveillance data to identify potential at-risk populations was briefly discussed. There do not appear to be significant racial differences among infected persons, except for Native Americans who appear to be at greater risk for *Erlichia chaffeensis* and Rocky Mountain spotted fever. In addition, McQuiston commented that some data show race-related factors and disease severity, such as more severe Rocky Mountain spotted fever disease in African-Americans with a glucode-6-phosphate dehydrogenase (G6PD) deficiency and more severe babesiosis in some children with sickle-cell disease. Because data on disease in minorities is lacking, however, correlating these associations on a national scale is difficult.

Because many ticks are coinfected with more than one pathogen, human coinfection is of growing concern. Luft noted the need to broadly examine the issue, pointing out that some data suggest that pathogens may act synergistically to worsen health outcomes. Wormser said that his laboratory is interested in coinfection, but there is difficulty determining which patients are coinfected, have sequential infection, or simply have an abnormal laboratory test. He noted there is a need for research to improve diagnostic assays to distinguish different pathogens and the immunologic responses they invoke. The issue of coinfection within the tick and tick biology is an area for further research, noted Luft. Currently, it is difficult to discern which pathogen has infected an individual. He noted that the technology available today should help researchers study these coinfections systematically. A participant noted that there are interactions among microbes within ticks, including the pathogenic and nonpathogenic microbes. In ticks infected with related *Rickettsia* pathogens, nonpathogenic *Rickettsia* agents may inherit more pathogenic properties.

The influence of multiple pathogens within the host vector has been understudied. Krause noted that in experiments in the *Peromyscus leucopus* mouse, the effect of coinfection can vary according to the timing with which these organisms are introduced (e.g., simultaneous infection by a single coinfected tick or sequential infection from a second tick bite). He further noted that at least *Babesia* and *Borrelia* may affect each other in the natural reservoir host, which has implications in terms of the transmissions of these diseases. Some evidence shows that *Borrelia* may enhance the transmission or the infection intensity of *Babesia* in the reservoir mouse. Understanding the various interactions of multiple pathogens, both in the vector and in the pathogen reservoir hosts, could provide insight into the natural history of the disease, disease epidemiology, and disease transmission.

Finally, the panel discussed its opinions on reinfection and relapsing disease. In terms of Lyme disease, the panelists held divergent views on whether the disease was capable of relapsing or whether persistent symptoms following treatment indicated subsequent reinfection following a cure. Wormser noted that between 1 to 4 percent of patients become reinfected with the *B. burgdorferi*. In a study of 17 patients from whom the pathogens were cultured and genotyped, it was found that none of the new pathogens were the same genotype as those that caused the prior infection. Luft agreed that reinfection does occur, but given the nature of Lyme disease, it was likely the disease was a relapsing process characterized by periods of active and inert disease. Krause noted that in his study on the Block Island cohort, he did not find evidence of relapsing disease (Krause et al., 2006). Approximately 10 percent of the population reported a repeat episode, and several lines of evidence indicated that it was due to reinfection as opposed to relapse. First, the subsequent reported infection episodes occurred during the tick transmission season and not during the winter when tick transmission is greatly reduced. Second, people with repeated infections had a high degree of exposure to ticks. Third, the location of repeated erythema migrans rash lesions were at different body sites than the initial infection. Fourth, repeated episodes did not occur within a year of the initial episode and usually were separated from the first by several years. For most relapsing illnesses, subsequent episodes occur in the first month or two after the initial illness. Finally, one component of the study was an annual serosurvey. Most of the patients had clearance of their initial antibody test, and one would not expect this if there was a persistence of infection. Furthermore, when patients presented with a second infection, their responses were amnestic immunologic responses with a high IgG concentration and an absence of an IgM response.

With the exception of babesiosis in immunocompromised individuals (Krause et al., 2008), little evidence supports the idea of relapse in tickborne diseases. Dumler noted that there is not clear evidence of persistent infection of *Ehrlichia* and *Anaplasma* in humans. Most infection in humans with either *Ehrlichia* or *Anaplasma* are either self-limited or are cured with appropriate treatment. Relapses of either agent appear to be a very rare occurrence, and most subsequent presentations of disease are the result of new infections. McQuiston commented that there is also a lack of data in terms of *Rickettsia* infection, but most Rocky Mountain spotted fever infections are acute infections that either are self-limited, and fatal, or resolve with antibiotic treatment. She indicated that although rare, most permanent or long-term consequences are the result of damage sustained by the body during the course of the acute infection. However, it was mentioned that difficulty in isolating the pathogen does not indicate an absence of persistent infection. There is a *Rickettsia* species, *Rickettsia prowazekii*, that causes epidemic typhus and has been shown to persist in the body for very long periods of time and to reappear decades later in a form of disease called Brill-Zinsser disease. This type of event has not been observed with *Rickettsia rickettsii* infections, however.

In closing, some members of the panel noted the need for a consensus on the terminology and case definitions used to report and discuss tickborne diseases. Some members of the panel indicated that many surveillance efforts were hindered not only because many physicians did not understand the clinical manifestations of disease but also because there was a lack of commonality in defining these diseases.

## GENETIC AND ACQUIRED DETERMINANTS OF HOST SUSCEPTIBILITY AND VULNERABLE POPULATIONS

*David Jay Weber, M.D., M.P.H., University of North Carolina School of Medicine and School of Pubic Health*

Tick-borne diseases result from the interaction of tick biology (host[s], climate, and species), tick exposure (e.g., residence, occupation, and recreation activities), and human biology (e.g., age, gender, and treatment). Acquiring a tick-borne disease is the result of a two-pronged process of exposure and infection. Each of these processes plays a role in acquisition of disease and determination of risk.

The risk of exposure is dependent on two variables: proximity to the tick environment and barriers to tick interaction. Proximity to the tick environment is a measure of the distance to and amount of time in the tick environment. Living in a rural area puts one at greater risk than does living in an urban area; however, this risk is not equal across all areas. Wooded areas, for example, carry greater risk of exposure to ehrlichiosis than pastures because they have a higher prevalence of host animals (Standaert et al., 1995). The geographic region in which persons reside is crucially important because the presence of tick-borne diseases is highly geographically dependent. In the United States, Lyme disease, babesiosis, and Rocky Mountain spotted fever (RMSF) all have important geographic predilections.

In terms of occupation, people who work outdoors are at higher risk for tick exposure than are office workers, although different outdoor occupations vary in their risk for tick-borne diseases. For example, general outdoor laborers were shown to be at a greater risk for Lyme disease (Schwartz et al., 1994), farmers for tick-borne encephalitis (Cisak et al., 1999), and forestry workers for Lyme disease, tick-borne encephalitis, and anaplasmosis (Cisak et al., 1999, 2005; Adamek et al., 2006). Recreational activities may also increase one's risk of exposure because many outdoor activities place participants within the tick environment. For example, an increased risk of Lyme disease has been demonstrated for gardeners and orienteers (Fahrer et al., 1991, 1998) whose activities take place in open, outdoor areas. In some cases, one's ability level as well as one's recreational preference may influence the level of risk associated with a particular activity. For example, Standaert and colleagues (1995) found that poor golfers are at an increased risk of ehrlichiosis due to the greater amount of time spent in the higher, thicker grass of the rough compared with those who play primarily from the manicured grass of the fairway and green. Finally, interspecies relationships also can influence one's exposure to disease. Pet owners may be at increased risk of Lyme disease (Schwartz et al., 1994) and RMSF (Demma et al., 2006) because of ticks that have fallen from domesticated animals or household pets.

The relative effectiveness of barriers to tick interaction varies with proximity to the tick environment. In low-proximity areas, these barriers are less important because the overall exposure risk is low. For example, among those in wooded rural areas (high proximity), those with unfenced backyards are at greater risk than those whose property is at least partially enclosed (Connally et al., 2009). Moreover, evidence has shown that practicing personal, protective measures, such as wearing long sleeves and pants, taping pants or tucking them into boots, and the use of insect repellents or insecticides such as permethrin-treated clothing can reduce risk of tick exposure by up to 93 percent (Vaughn and Meshnick, 2011).

Although exposure to a tick is a necessary part of the development of tick-borne disease, it is not sufficient to produce disease as an individual needs to be infected by the pathogenic agent. Like exposure, many factors can affect one's risk of becoming infected with a pathogen and developing severe or fatal disease. Many risk factors are associated with behavioral and biological indicators of the exposed individual or of the tick environment. Behavioral factors associated with increased risk of infection include failure to perform regular tick checks after interacting in the tick environment (Smith et al., 2001; Connally et al., 2009) and lack of use of tick insect repellents (Standeart et al., 1995; Smith et al., 2001). Biological risk factors that have been identified for RMSF include being Caucasian (Dalton et al., 1995) or of Native American descent (Holman et al., 2009), being male (Dalton et al., 1995), and being between the ages of 5 and 9 years old (Dalton et al., 1995). Age has also been indicated as a risk factor for Lyme disease particularly for individuals ages 10 to 19 (Smith et al., 2001). In addition to behavioral and biological indicators, the nature of some infections may play a role in the risk of infection. For instance, because *Babesia* species primarily infect red blood cells, there has been evidence indicating a higher risk of infection among blood transfusion recipients than the general population (White et al., 1998; Cable and Leiby, 2003).

Beyond the risk for infection, some factors have been associated with the likelihood of severe disease and hospitalization. For RMSF, risk factors for severe disease and hospitalization include being American Indian (McQuiston et al., 2000); the geographic location in which the infection occurs, particularly in North Carolina and Oklahoma (Adjemian et al., 2009); and the use of chloramphenicol instead of tetracycline-based antibiotics (Dalton et al., 1995). In addition, in terms of *Babesia* species, splenectomy (Sun et al., 1983; White et al., 1998) and immunosuppression from HIV or cancer (Vannier et al., 2008) have been shown to increase one's risk of severe disease. Research indicates that genetics also may predispose individuals to severe disease. Genetic predispositions include the presence of a toll-like receptor (TLR)-9 in Crimean-Congo fever (Engin et al., 2010a), homozygosity for CCR5 delta 32 in tick-borne encephalitis (Kindberg et al., 2008), and HLA-DR4 and DR2 in Lyme disease (Steere et al., 1990; Kalish et al., 1993).

Research further indicates that some tick-borne diseases carry additional risk factors for fatal disease. In the case of RMSF, anything that delays treatment by as little as 4–5 days, including the absence of rash or headache and the presence of fever, results in a higher risk of fatal disease. In addition to the fact that many doctors are not trained to recognize early-stage disease, off-season presentation and no history of tick attachment contribute to delayed diagnosis and treatment and may further increase the risk of fatalities (Hattwick et al., 1978; Dalton et al., 1995; Kirkland et al., 1995; Holman et al., 2001). Age also seems to be a factor in determining the risk of fatal infection. Individuals younger than age 5 and older than 40 appear to be at increased risk of dying from RMSF than are healthy individuals between 6 and 39 years old (Dalton et al., 1995; Holman et al., 2001; Chapman et al., 2006b). In addition, a high risk of fatal disease has been associated with increased serum creatinine on presentation and the presence of neurological involvement (Conlon et al., 1996) as well as with being African American with a G6PD deficiency (Walker et al., 1983). This is not to say that all genetic predispositions are indicative of severe or fatal disease. For example, TLR-2 heterozygous for SNP Arg753Gln may provide increased protection against late-stage *Borrelia burgdoferi* infection (Schroder et al., 2005).

Despite the advantages of knowing the aforementioned high-risk associations, it is important to recognize that these data are not without limitations. Determining risk factors for tick-borne disease requires sufficiently sophisticated tests to detect disease accurately, and the development and conduct of surveillance studies capable of multivariate analysis to delineate independent risk factors that may be thrown together or overshadowed in case-control studies. Furthermore, despite disparate indications, it is difficult to isolate risk factors for exposure from risk factors for infection, and for this reason, many case-control studies measure exposure rate based on the number of infections reported rather than recording the total number of actual tick exposures or tick bites, an outcome measure that may not always be appropriate. In spite of these limitations, there are sufficient scientific data to develop policies that would lead to risk reduction and to design safe and cost-effective intervention studies to reduce exposure and disease. Furthermore, these data can be used to develop educational programs for healthcare providers regarding recognition and proper treatment of TBDs. In conclusion, additional research is needed, especially on genetic factors to further define risk factors for infection and severe or fatal TBDs.

## AT-RISK POPULATIONS FOR BABESIA

*Peter J. Krause, M.D., Department of Epidemiology and
School of Public Health, Yale School of Medicine*

As discussed earlier in the chapter, babesiosis is associated with a number of clinical syndromes, including asymptomatic infection; viral-like illness (fever, chills, sweats, headache, fatigue); persistent, relapsing illness; and fulminant illness and death. Adults over age 50 are at risk for more severe disease manifestations (Ruebush et al., 1981; Vannier et al, 2008). As the U.S. population ages, babesiosis will have an increasingly important impact on the health of this segment of the population. Immunological problems associated with aging or comorbid diseases, such as lung, renal, or liver disease, contribute to the difference. Patients with AIDS, malignancies, or splenectomy are at increased risk for persistent, relapsing illness (Gubernot et al., 2009). Complications of babesiosis that are seen more frequently in immunocompromised people consist of acute respiratory distress syndrome, disseminated intravascular coagulation, congestive heart failure, coma, and renal failure (Leiby et al., 2011).

The specific mechanisms that lead to increased severity of babesiosis continue to be the subject of investigation. A DBA/2 mouse model has been developed to investigate age-related severity of babesiosis (5). Edouard Vannier and I are carrying out a study to elucidate genetic factors that may account for severe babesiosis in people over age 50.

We previously carried out a retrospective case-control study of human *Babesia microti* infection among 14 highly immunocompromised patients who experienced persistent, relapsing babesiosis and 49 control subjects who experienced a typical course of babesiosis infection that resolved after 1 to 2 weeks (Gubernot et al., 2009). The subjects were enrolled between 1991 and 2005 and resided in Connecticut, Massachusetts, New York, Rhode Island, and Wisconsin. Eleven of the 14 patients with severe relapsing disease had malignancies, including 8 with B-cell lymphoma, while 10 were asplenic. Patients with B-cell lymphoma were given Rituximab, a monoclonal antibody directed against the protein CD20 on B cells. For the patients with relapsing illness, the percentage of infected red blood cells ranged from 2 to 75 percent, compared with 0.5 to 10 percent for the control group. The group with relapsing illness required 2–10 courses of anti-*Babesia* antibiotic to clear infection while the control group required only a single course of antibiotic. The median length of therapy was 13 weeks for the relapsing illness group (range 4–102 weeks) and 1 week (range 0.5–1.5 weeks) for the control group. About a quarter of the relapsing illness group died compared to none in the control group. Resolution in the immunocompromised patients required several courses of anti-*Babesia* therapy, but once a therapy was found to be effective, duration was a critical factor for success. All the patients who cleared infection were given a minimum of 6 weeks of therapy, including therapy that continued for at least 2 weeks beyond the first noted absence of parasites on thin blood smear. These results indicate that people who suffer from broad-based immunosuppression are at risk of persisting, relapsing *Babesia microti* infection and require prolonged antibabesial therapy. They also suggest that B cells and anti-*Babesia microti* antibodies are important in clearing *Babesia* infection, although differences in the relative contribution of T cells and B cells in clearing infection requires further study.

One of the first well-recognized risk factors for severe babesiosis was asplenia (Krause et al., 2002). The spleen removes red blood cells that are infected or senescent, and macrophages and other immune factors present in the spleen may help to eliminate intraerythrocytic pathogens. Interestingly, asplenia does not always result in severe *Babesia* illness. This suggests that *Babesia* strains with different virulence also may contribute to disease severity. An editorial in the *New England Journal of Medicine* suggested that individuals who lack a spleen should avoid owning property or visiting an area that is highly endemic for *Babesia microti* because such activities could potentially be life threatening (Persing et al., 1995). Clinicians treating patients who lack a spleen, have a malignancy, are HIV infected, or are immunocompromised for other reasons should provide information and counseling regarding the potential for life-threatening babesiosis in regions that are highly endemic.

### Knowledge Gaps and Research Opportunities

There are several critical questions that offer research opportunities pertaining to the effect of babesiosis on populations at risk for severe and fatal outcome:

1. What are the causes of life-threatening babesiosis in people who are over 50 but otherwise healthy, and how can they best be treated and the problem prevented?
2. What are the causes of life-threatening babesiosis in people with asplenia, HIV, malignancy, and pre-morbid conditions, and how can they best be treated and the problem prevented?
3. Why do people who acquire babesiosis through blood transfusion experience more severe babesiosis, and how can they best be treated and the problem prevented?

### DISCUSSION

During the discussion of the At-Risk Populations Panel, panelists and participants presented a number of points that addressed an array of topics, including public health communication, research potential and barriers, transmission in at-risk communities, and disease severity.

King posed the question of how to develop public health messages to educate the public on tick-borne diseases and disease prevention strategies. Weber noted that targeted messages need to be directed to high-risk populations, but public health messages may not be very useful. Targeting the outdoor workforce population might be particularly effective because the workforce model could permit the development and enforcement of preventive policy measures. Public health messages are apt to be less effective because it is difficult to compel behavioral changes, such as wearing long sleeves even on hot days or routinely checking for ticks. Instead, Weber suggested the need to continue to develop permethrin-impregnated clothing and other technological advances to limit exposure.

One participant questioned whether it is possible for *Babesia* to be transmitted through national blood donation programs. Krause observed that, although the chance of acquiring babesiosis from a blood transfusion likely is very low, *Babesia microti* is the most common infectious agent transmitted through the blood supply in the United States (FDA, 2008). This has attracted the attention of the CDC and the NIH as a potentially significant public health problem. Screening for potential active *B. microti* infection in blood donors currently relies on self-reporting by the blood donor regarding a history of prior infection and results in lifetime prohibition from donation for those who report having had babesiosis.

In addition, the Food and Drug Administration has approved a screening program at the Rhode Island Blood Center that uses laboratory-based *B. microti* screening, including antibody analysis and PCR, to test donor blood for use in newborn infants and persons with sickle-cell disease (Gubernot et al., 2009; Young and Krause, 2009). The purpose of this study is to observe whether the screening will affect the infection rate in these populations. Although confident this type of screening will be effective in reducing the incidence of transfusion-transmitted babesiosis, Krause indicated that further assessment is necessary to develop a laboratory-based screening protocol that will optimally balance the need to minimize the risk of *B. microti* transmission with the need to minimize discarding blood or blood products that may not be actively infected. Any screening system developed will need to address the issue of screening in endemic and non-endemic areas. A variety of screening approaches may be necessary to meet the needs of different populations with varying levels of risk. Use of pathogen reduction technologies to destroy *Babesia* within donated blood units is another potential option for reducing transfusion transmitted babesiosis (Gubernot et al., 2009).

Another participant questioned the potential of the *Babesia* pathogen to infect cells other than erythrocytes. Although human *Babesia* currently is believed to infect only red blood cells, further research may include investigation of the possibility of alternative sites of infection during various stages in the pathogen life cycle. Neurologic manifestations of *Babesia*, such as coma, have not been shown to be the result of *Babesia* infection of neuronal tissue and may occur because of electrolyte imbalance or other side effects of the overall infection.

The disease severity of *Babesia duncani* and its implication for treatment was another topic of discussion. In response to a participant's question, Krause indicated that *B. duncani* infections that have been reported have been more severe than *B. microti* infections (Persing et al., 1995). He added that although it is generally true that initially the most critical manifestations of a disease receive the most attention, there is evidence in a hamster model that *B. duncani* is a significantly more severe disease than *B. microti* is (Wozniak et al., 1996). Krause advocated aggressive treatment for patients diagnosed with *B. duncani*, including the possibility of exchange transfusion to replace infected red blood cells and remove toxic by-products of infection.

Finally, one participant asked whether there may be some utility in investigating antibiotic alternatives to cure *Babesia*. Krause indicated that there is limited evidence that the anti-malarial drug Artemisinin may be useful in clearing a babesial infection, but that more research is needed to determine the effectiveness of this and other alternative therapies, including new drugs and herbal remedies (Krause et al., 2008).

### Concluding Thoughts on Surveillance, Spectrum, and Burden of Tick-Borne Disease, and At-Risk Populations

*Gordon Schutze, M.D., Baylor College of Medicine*

Creating a repository for specimens of blood and cerebrospinal fluid from patients with tick-borne diseases can improve the accuracy of diagnostic tests and disease diagnosis. Such a repository needs to include demographic information on patients and information on their diagnosis, treatment, and outcome. A well-funded network of researchers investigating tick-borne diseases could maintain such a repository, which also would enable them to advance knowledge of these diseases.

Clinicians clearly need new methods for diagnosing tick-borne diseases, given the genetic diversity among different strains of a pathogen (e.g., *Borrelia burgdoferi*) and the realization that new species may be responsible for a larger burden of disease than previously recognized (e.g., *Rickettsia parkeri* in spotted fever rickettsiosis). Clinicians also need better tests to accurately differentiate between patients with acute tick-borne illness and those previously infected with tick-borne disease.

# 6

# Pathogenesis

The pathogenesis of a disease describes the mechanisms by which it develops, progresses, and either persists or is resolved. Understanding pathogenesis of an infectious disease at the cellular and molecular levels is critical for discovering, developing, and implementing methods to prevent infection, and to improve patient outcomes after treatment.

By determining which microbial molecules establish infection by binding to and entering human cells or tissues, for example, scientists can develop vaccines against tick-borne diseases (TBDs)—as they already have for influenza. The pathogenesis of tick-borne diseases can also reveal why some individuals are more prone to severe disease, or fail to resolve infection.

Scientists rely on several methods to study the pathogenesis of TBDs. These include *in vitro* studies, based on cultured cells; animal studies, based on tracking animals with a disease; and patient studies, based on clinical trials and specimens from biopsies and autopsies. While no one approach can represent the full spectrum and complexity of human disease, the ability to "reduce" or "control" the number of variables by using *in vitro* and animal models allows more rapid and less equivocal determination of key variables in disease progression—knowledge required to improve prevention, diagnosis, and treatment of TBD in patients.

Animal models have been especially useful in shedding light on the key features of tick-borne infectious diseases. These models include naturally occurring infectious disease, such as neuroborreliosis in horses and Rocky Mountain spotted fever in dogs, and infections introduced into animals such as mice. Mice are particularly helpful in revealing the pathogenesis of infectious disease because scientists can study mice that differ only in a single gene, and because they can use imaging to track the progression of infection and cellular trafficking in real time.

In this chapter, six scientists presented the state of the science regarding the pathogenesis of tick-borne infections—specifically those caused by pathogens in the *Anaplasma, Borrelia, Ehrlichia,* and *Rickettsia* genera.

## PATHOGENESIS OF *BORRELIA BURGDORFERI* INFECTION AND DISEASE

*Janis J. Weis, Ph.D., Department of Pathology, University of Utah School of Medicine*

In humans, the bite of the infected tick is required for introduction of the pathogen through healthy skin. This extracellular pathogen starts in the dermal tissue where it begins to adapt to life in the mammalian host by changing the expression of its surface glycoproteins. At the same time, the bacterium stimulates responses of inflammatory cells and their secreted mediators that cause acute-phase lesions such as the classical erythema migrans (EM) lesion. The bacterium also activates proteases and other induced host cell molecules to allow for dissemination through the blood and into other tissues, including secondary skin lesions, joints, the heart, and nervous tissue (Coleman et al., 1997; Gebbia et al., 2004; Rosa et al., 2005).

Differences in the severity and spectrum of disease among patients infected with *Borrelia burgdorferi* is one of the hallmarks of Lyme disease (Steere and Glickstein, 2004). The reasons for this variation include both genetic differences among strains of the bacterium and differences in the host responses. On the bacterial side, genetically distinct strains, identified by ribosomal spacer types and outer surface protein C (OspC) heterogeneity, have been associated with invasive versus localized cutaneous disease (Wang et al., 2002; Wormser et al., 2008a). Furthermore, *B. burgdorferi* is characterized by a large and complex plasmid content, some of which are essential for infection and others which can vary among strains (Rosa et al., 2005). Similarly, the host response has significant differences in the host response. Among human patients, approximately 60 percent of infected patients who do not receive early treatment develop clinical arthritis (Steere et al., 1987). This difference between those patients who do and those who do not develop arthritis reflects, at least in part, genetic differences in host response. These effects can be studied using inbred strains of mice with defined genetic differences and with clearly reproducible difference in the severity of carditis and arthritis following *B. burgdorferi* infection (Barthold et al., 1990).

The use of gene knockout mice has begun to unravel the genetic contribution to the spectrum of the disease. Severely combined immunodeficient C3H/HeJ mice (SCID)—which lack B and T lymphocytes—develop severe arthritis and carditis independent of the number of *B. burgdorferi* used to experimentally infect the mice. In contrast, C57BL/6 mice with the same SCID mutation develop only mild arthritis and carditis, again independent of the infectious dose (Barthold et al., 1992). These results suggest that although B cells and T cells are important in clearing *B. burgdorferi*, the adaptive immune response (mediated by B and T lymphocytes) itself does not drive severe disease. Furthermore, C57BL/6 mice with mild disease and severely affected C3H mice have equal numbers of bacteria in their ankle tissues, evidence that arthritis severity does not correlate with the bacterial load (Ma et al., 1998; Morrison et al., 1999).

Understanding how *B. burgdorferi* traffic to and colonize various tissues is important in shedding light on the reasons for differences in the organ-specific manifestations and severity of disease. *B. burgdorferi* expresses outer surface proteins that selectively interact with endothelial cells, platelets, chondrocytes, and extracellular matrix via specific interactions with integrins, glycosaminoglycans, fibronectin, and collagen (Coleman et al., 1997; Gebbia et al., 2004; Coburn et al., 2005). These interactions are important in homing to and colonization of tissues, including the skin, joint, and heart. Bacterial ligands, such as DBPA/B, p66, BBk32, and OspC, promoting heart and joint invasion have been identified by genetic and immunological techniques (Coburn et al., 2005). These receptor-ligand interactions also contribute to inflammatory responses in resident cells (Behera et al., 2005, 2006a).

The host response to *B. burgdorferi* plays a key role in disease pathogenesis. *B. burgdorferi* does not produce toxins or proteases that are directly responsible for tissue damage upon colonization. In contrast, the bacterium produces multiple molecules that activate host responses and can lead to localized and generalized inflammatory pathogenic responses. Most of these host responses normally function to contain or clear infections and are components of the innate defense and/or inflammatory response (Liu et al., 2004; Benhnia et al., 2005; Behera et al., 2006a; Oosting et al., 2010). Although their purpose is to clear infection, if continually activated, they lead to lesion development and disease.

Numerous signaling pathways have been identified that are responsible for Lyme disease arthritis (see Table 6-1). The $Pam_3Cys$-lipid-modified proteins of *B. burgdorferi*, which are abundantly expressed by the bacteria, are the best characterized. These lipoproteins interact with the host, specifically through toll-like receptor (TLR)-2 and TLR-1 heterodimers, and activate signaling through the adaptor molecule MyD88. This signaling pathway results in activation of numerous proinflammatory cytokines, chemokines, and matrix metalloproteinases (Hirschfeld et al., 1999; Alexopoulou et al., 2002). In addition, the bacterial flagellin and peptidoglycan also activate host TLRs, again connecting to the MyD88 pathway (Bolz et al., 2004;

**TABLE 6-1** Numerous Signaling Pathways Have Been Implicated in Pathogenesis

| B. burgdorferi Ligand | Host Receptor | Signaling Pathway | Type of Response |
|---|---|---|---|
| Pam₃Cys- outer surface lipoproteins (Osps) | TLR2/TLR1 | MyD88 & NF-kB dependent, MAP Kinases | Pro-inflammatory cytokines, MMPs chemokines, anti-inflammatory (1, 2, 18) |
| Flagellin | TLR5 | MyD88 | Cytokines, etc. (33) |
| Peptidoglycan | TLR2, NOD2 | MyD88 | Cytokines, etc. (29) |
| RNA | TLR7 & 2nd unidentified PRR | MyD88 dependent and IRF 3 dependent | Type I IFN ($\alpha/\beta$)(26, 30) |
| Secreted molecules | Unknown | IRF3 | Type I IFN ($\alpha/\beta$)(26) |
| BBB07 | $\alpha3\beta1$ integrin | Endosome | Cytokines, MMP(5) |
| Diacyglycolipid- BbGL-IIc | CD1d | iNKT-TCR | IL-2, IFN$\gamma$(19, 20) |

Liu et al., 2004; Behera et al., 2006a; Shin et al., 2008). The result of this MyD88 stimulation is production of pro-inflammatory products such as cytokines, chemokines, and matrix metalloproteinases.

Using knockout mice that lack individual components of the pathways, the contribution of specific pathways to control of infection and resolution of disease can be studied. The TLR/MyD88 pathway is important for host defense and for controlling the bacteria numbers in tissues. However, knockout mice that lack either TLR2 or MyD88 still develop arthritis (Wooten et al., 2002; Bolz et al., 2004; Liu et al., 2004; Behera et al., 2006a). These results suggest that although this pathway is important for host defense and control of the bacterial numbers, it is not essential for arthritis development. Consequently, global gene expression profile analysis was used to find pathways specific to arthritis development (rather than host defense) in C3H and C57BL/6 mice. These experiments focused on early time points in pathogenesis, 1 week after infection prior to the arrival of inflammatory cells in joint tissue. As noted previously, C3H mice had severe ankle swelling beginning at week 1, while C57BL/6 mice had minimal swelling. In C3H mice, there is an early and transient induction of genes associated with an interferon signature profile at one week that decreases by week 2. Furthermore, immunodeficient (lacking interleukin-10 or IL-10) C57BL/6 mice showed a delayed increase in the same interferon panel that remained elevated through the infection (Crandall et al., 2006).

One hypothesis was that type I interferons (IFNs), which are normally associated with host response to viral infections, are important for the development of arthritis following B. burgdorferi infection. To test that hypothesis, the C3H mice were treated with an antibody that blocked the receptor for type I IFNs. Arthritis was reduced by 50 percent in these C3H mice given a single injection of interferon-blocking antibody before infection (Miller et al., 2008). A second study with mutant CH3 mice deficient in interferon receptors confirmed the involvement of type I IFNs. These studies provide functional evidence for the involvement of type I IFNs in the development of arthritis. This result was unexpected as most bacteria known to induce host type I interferon are intracellular, whereas *B. burgdorferi* are extracellular. Notably, this type I interferon pathway can be induced by at least three distinct ligands from *B. burgdorferi*, some of which function independently from the MyD88 adaptor molecule pathway (Petzke et al., 2009; Miller et al., 2010).

Importantly, the host responses and inflammatory pathways have organ-specific differences. In contrast to arthritis, which is characterized by infiltration of neutrophils, carditis is characterized by influx of macrophages and T lymphocytes at the base of the heart where *B. burgdorferi* infiltrates connective tissue (Barthold et al., 1990; Ruderman et al., 1995; Bockenstedt et al., 2001). Also unlike arthritis, the numbers of infectious bacteria in the heart are correlated with the severity of inflammation (Morrison et al., 1999). Furthermore, T lymphocytes help resolve Lyme disease carditis by production of interferon gamma and other cytokines, which in turn activate the macrophages to clear *B. burgdorferi* from the heart, and therefore suppress the carditis (McKisic et al., 2000; Olson et al., 2009). Disruption of this interferon gamma pathway in C57BL/6 mice results in more severe carditis.

### Knowledge Gaps and Research Opportunities

Weis noted three key questions for future study:

- What is responsible for the variability in individuals' response to infection by *Borrelia burgdorferi*?
- Why do some symptoms persist in some patients?
- What is responsible for the pathogenesis of neuroborreliosis in patients?

### DURATION OF SPIROCHETE INFECTION FOLLOWING ANTIBIOTIC TREATMENT IN ANIMALS

*Linda K. Bockenstedt, M.D., Yale University School of Medicine*

Bacterial infections have a number of outcome determinants, including pathogen factors, host genes, host co-morbid conditions, host immunity, and the effects of antibiotics. A current debate is how effective antibiotics are *in vivo* against *B. burgdorferi*. Antibiotic treatment failures occur occasionally in all animal models of Lyme borreliosis and in humans. Evidence for treatment failure comes from persistence of *B. burgdorferi* DNA after treatment for Lyme disease arthritis and, in animal models, the ability to culture spirochetes from tissues. Several studies have found that *B. burgdorferi* DNA can be detected in tissues for extended periods of time after antibiotic treatment of laboratory animals even though cultures of tissues may be negative (Straubinger et al., 1997; Bockenstedt et al., 2002; Hodzic et al., 2008). This raises the question of how to interpret the significance of *B. burgdorferi* DNA in tissues.

In our published study (Bockenstedt et al., 2002), we used xenodiagnosis with ticks to determine whether bacterial DNA detected in mouse tissues after antibiotic treatment indicated the presence of spirochetes that could replicate and cause infection. In this approach, uninfected laboratory-reared ticks were allowed to feed on mice that had previously been infected with *B. burgdorferi* and treated with antibiotics (doxycycline or ceftriaxone). Immunofluorescent staining was then used to determine whether the ticks had acquired *B. burgdorferi* spirochetes. The results were equivocal in that spirochete forms were detected microscopically in the tick midguts, but, on further study, these spirochetes appeared to be attenuated because genes on specific plasmids required for *B. burgdorferi* infectivity could not be detected by polymerase chain reaction (PCR) (Bockenstedt et al., 2002).

Similarly, spirochetes could not be cultured from tissues of mice that had been treated with antibiotics. No other method was used to assess viability and infectivity of the spirochetes visualized in ticks. However, larval ticks that had fed on antibiotic-treated mice could not transmit *B. burgdorferi* infection to uninfected mice. In a subsequent study (Hodzic et al., 2008), ticks used for xenodiagnosis of ceftriaxone-treated mice were able to transmit *B. burgdorferi* DNA to uninfected immunodeficient SCID mice, which lack T and B cells, and are highly susceptible to *B. burgdorferi* infection. In addition, *B. burgdorferi* DNA could be detected in some SCID mice that had received tissue transplants of skin from antibiotic-treated mice. Although viable spirochetes could not be cultured from the ticks, the antibiotic-treated donor mice, or the recipient mice, rare spirochete forms were visualized microscopically in specific connective tissues of some donor mice (Hodzic et al., 2008). These findings raised two questions. First, does the persistent DNA indicate continued infection, or is it simply residual debris? Second, are the rare residual spirochete forms viable and infectious?

To begin to address these questions, we used two-photon (multiphoton) confocal microscopy to directly visualize the location and motility of spirochetes in living, anesthetized mice in real time. C57BL/6 MyD88-deficient mice were infected with *B. burgdorferi* strain 297, a strain previously isolated from a Lyme disease patient but subsequently genetically modified to express a green fluorescent protein. The C57BL/6 mice are relatively disease resistant, but deficiency in MyD88 results in higher bacterial load so that infected mice have 100- to 1,000-fold more spirochetes in the skin and other organs, thus enhancing the ability to image the spirochetes. After 21 days of infection to allow dissemination of spirochetes throughout the tissues, mice were treated with either ceftriaxone or doxycycline. Multiphoton microscopy was then used to image spirochetes in ear skin and tendons, two easily accessible sites where spirochetes often reside. After imaging, mouse tissues were tested by culture to detect viable organisms, PCR to detect residual spirochete DNA, and direct fluorescent antibody (DFA) staining to detect residual spirochete antigen.

In the experiments using ceftriaxone, mice were treated twice daily with ceftriaxone for 5 days or sham treated. We began analyzing mice during the antibiotic treatment period and up to 9 days after completion. Spirochetes could not be cultured from tissues of mice treated with antibiotics at any time point. Multiphoton microscopy revealed a large number of spirochetes moving in the ear skin of sham-treated mice, but after just two doses of ceftriaxone (1 day of treatment), only a few spirochetes remained in antibiotic-treated mice. Fewer spirochetes were seen in the tendons of sham-treated mice, and only two stationary spirochetes were found in the tendon of one mouse treated with two doses of ceftriaxone (Bockenstedt et al., 2011). The spirochetes in the tendons of sham-treated mice were less motile than those in the skin. With the exception of mice analyzed after one day of antibiotic treatment, no spirochetes could be visualized in ear skin or tendons of antibiotic-treated mice at any time. At the end of the experiment, however, DFA revealed green fluorescent material adjacent to the ear cartilage in all of the antibiotic-treated mice.

In the doxycycline experiments, mice were given a one-month course of antibiotics supplied in drinking water to maintain serum levels above the minimal concentration necessary to inhibit *B. burgdorferi* growth *in vitro*. This method of antibiotic administration sustains therapeutic serum drug levels analogous to levels achieved in humans treated with oral doxycycline. Mice were analyzed between 2 and 10 weeks after the last dose of antibiotics. Similar to the ceftriaxone-treated mice, spirochetes could not be cultured from mice treated with doxycycline. Ticks used for xenodiagnosis also tested negative by culture after feeding on antibiotic-treated mice. In sham-treated (control) mice, multiphoton microscopy revealed motile spirochetes in the skin, as well as large, amorphous collections of fluorescent debris near ear cartilage, a finding not seen in uninfected mice. Similar nonmotile fluorescent material adjacent to the ear cartilage was also visualized in the treated mice (Bockenstedt et al., 2011), and these mice tested positive for *B. burgdorferi* DNA by PCR in both skin and joints.

To determine whether the amorphous fluorescent material contained viable and infectious spirochetes, ear tissue was transplanted into MyD88-deficient mice, which may provide a "permissive" environment for attenuated organisms. When analyzed up to 5 months after the transplant, sera from mice transplanted with tissues from antibiotic-treated mice only showed reactivity to single bands on immunoblots. Sera from mice transplanted with tissue from sham-treated mice, in contrast, showed a banding pattern typically found in mice and humans infected with *B. burgdorferi.* Neither viable spirochetes nor spirochete DNA were observed in mice that had received tissue transplants from treated mice. In contrast, mice that received ear transplants from sham-treated mice did have spirochete DNA and were culture positive (Bockenstedt et al., 2011). In a separate experiment, infected immunocompetent C57BL/6 mice given a month-long course of oral doxycycline were evaluated similarly for persistent infection by skin transplantation into MyD88-deficient mice. Only one of the five mice that received ear transplants from an antibiotic-treated donor mouse developed a serologic response to *B. burgdorferi* as indicated by a single immunoblot band. Mice that received transplants from sham-treated donor mice, in contrast, developed evidence of infection, as revealed by tissue culture, PCR, and serologic conversion (Bockenstedt, unpublished observations).

Bockenstedt noted that a number of conclusions can be drawn from this work:

- *Antibiotics are effective in eliminating B. burgdorferi infection in immunocompetent C57BL/6 mice and even immunodeficient C57BL/6 MyD88-deficient mice.* Because C57BL/6 mice are relatively disease resistant, similar studies are in progress in immunocompetent and MyD88-deficient C3H mice, a mouse strain background that is more susceptible to *B. burgdorferi*-induced infection and disease.
- *Spirochete debris may persist for some time after B. burgdorferi-infected MyD88-deficient mice are treated with antibiotics.* More extensive analyses need to be performed to determine whether such debris occurs in different tissues throughout the host and whether this debris could serve as a nidus for stimulating inflammation.
- *Tissue transplants containing the debris may elicit an antibody response in the new host, but if the donor mice were treated with antibiotics, the tissue transplants induce responses to only one or two B. burgdorferi proteins.* Only mice that receive transplants from sham-treated mice become infected, as shown by tissue culture, PCR, and seroconversion. Transplants from mice treated with antibiotics do not introduce infection into recipient mice.

## DISCUSSION

The discussion session focused on the pathogenesis of Lyme disease and how these studies inform us about human disease. A participant questioned if the spirochetes were able to change their morphology and "hibernate" under periods of stress. Bockenstedt noted that there are changes in the morphology of spirochetes when they are exposed to different stressful conditions in culture. For example, if the spirochetes are nutrient deprived, they can actually stop making peptidoglycan and fold up on themselves. However, the same phenomenon has not been observed *in vivo*.

Schutze questioned whether the observed residual pieces of organisms could stimulate an inflammatory cascade. Bockenstedt noted that this material does contain DNA, which might stimulate an inflammatory cascade through TLRs. The fluorescent material in the tissue specimens has not been isolated for testing, and there may be other components in the sample that would trigger inflammation. However, the current research has not been able to answer these questions.

Another participant inquired about the genetic differences between the C57BL/6 and the C3Hmice and what these differences meant for TBDs. Dr. Weis noted that some genes transcend the genetic differences among the mice strains, for example, MyD88, TLR-2, and interleukin 10. Mutations in those genes on either the C57BL/6 or the C3H background would result in a compromise either in host defense, resulting in elevated levels of bacteria in tissues, or in the case of IL-10, an increase in inflammation (Brown et al., 1999, 2008; Wooten et al., 2002). The MyD88-deficient knockout mice are particularly interesting because the bacterial number in tissues is significantly elevated compared to bacteria loads in wild-type mice (Bolz et al., 2004). She further noted that there is no indication of a change in the bacteria, but rather that they persist longer because the host cannot clear the bacteria.

Research is currently being done to understand the difference in arthritis severity between C57BL/6 and C3H mice through the use of genetic intercross populations. Weis noted that she has identified at least 12 different loci that are different between these two mice strains (Ma et al., 2009). One area of research will be to look for genes that regulate type I interferon because there is a difference in the induction of type I interferon in infected joints between the two mouse lines.

## ANTIGENIC VARIATION AS A MECHANISM FOR PERSISTENT BORRELIA INFECTION

*Steven J. Norris, Ph.D., Department of
Pathology & Laboratory Medicine,
University of Texas Medical School at Houston*

Pathogens can vary in their ability to be invasive and toxic to an organism (see Figure 6-1). For example, *Clostridium botulinum* is very toxigenic and produces a powerful neurotoxin, but is not invasive. In contrast, *C. perfringens*, which causes gas gangrene, is both highly invasive and

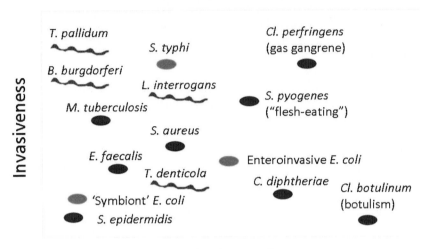

**FIGURE 6-1** The relationship between invasiveness and toxigenesis. SOURCE: Norris et al., 2010.

highly toxigenic. A group of pathogens, including *Treponema pallidum* and *Mycobacterium tuberculosis* that produce no known toxins, are highly invasive organisms that can persist for the lifetime of the host.

Lyme disease *Borrelia* is a highly motile organism. In animal models, *B. burgdorferi* disseminates early during infection into numerous tissues, including skin, joints, heart, bladder, and spleen, and persists in the tissues for up to 2 years. The persistence of infection in humans is not well understood, but likely can last months to years; however, the *Borrelia* produces no known toxins or enzymes that cause tissue damage. Thus, Lyme disease *Borrelia* falls into the group of highly invasive, non-toxigenic pathogens.

To cause persistent infection, *B. burgdorferi* must have multiple ways of evading a host's immune response (see Norris et al., 2010). One common mechanism is protective niches through sequestration of the pathogen in dense tissue, such as tendons. A second cellular process is through down-regulation of antigen expression. During infection of the mammalian host, *B. burgdorferi* down-regulates the expression of the surface protein antigen OspA. This protein is important during the tick part of the *B. burgdorferi* life cycle, but the organism usually does not express OspA at high levels during mammalian infection. A third mechanism is the inhibition of a host's innate immune response. For example, *B. burgdorferi* inhibits the complement cascade by complement regulator-acquiring surface proteins. A fourth mechanism is antigenic variation, which causes a change in a surface structure that usually occurs at a higher rate than expected from mutation. Antigenic variation and, specifically, the *vls* gene system will be the focus of this presentation.

A 28-kilobase linear plasmid of *B. burgdorferi* B31 called lp28-1 contains a variable membrane protein-like sequence locus, which resembles a similar system in the relapsing fever spirochete, a prototypical antigenically variant pathogen. The plasmid contains both an expression site called *vlsE* and a set of silent cassettes upstream from *vlsE*. Alignment between the expression site and the silent cassettes reveals regions of sequence identity or relative invariant sequence and other regions of variation. Approximately 92 percent of the genetic sequences of the silent cassettes are identical to those of the central part of the expression site. In contrast, the areas of variation are important in determining the structure of the antigen expressed by the *vls* system.

The initial hypothesis was that each of the silent cassettes could exchange into the expression site, and therefore result in approximately 15 variants of the antigen. Subsequently, however, segmental recombination via a gene conversion mechanism was discovered in which the silent cassettes donate genetic sequences of different lengths and locations into the expression site. This recombination event appears to occur only within the mammalian host and has not been detected in standard liquid culture or in ticks. The recombination process continues as long as mammals are infected and can theoretically produce as many as $10^{32}$ different sequences of amino acids. Most variations in sequences consist of only one or two amino acids. In fact, so much variation occurs that it is rare to find the same *vlsE* sequence twice in a given tissue 28 days after infection (Zhang et al., 1997; Zhang and Norris, 1998; Coutte et al., 2009). The VlsE protein is anchored to the outer membrane of the organism, with the variable regions being accessible on the surface of the protein. Thus, the sequence differences in those regions provide a mechanism so that the organism can effectively evade the immune response through continuously changing the amino acid sequence of the exposed region.

The invariant regions also elicit a host immune response during infection, one of which is now used to diagnose Lyme disease (see Chapter 8). The IR6 region of the protein, also called C6, induces a particularly high antibody response in humans and other animals. This region is not the only reactive invariant region, but the one that is best characterized. Overall, it is not understood how this protein can permit evasion of the immune system while also inducing a high antibody response.

In a landmark study, the portion of the *B. burgdorferi* plasmid lp28-1 that carries the *vls* locus was deleted (Bankhead and Chaconas, 2007). These modified organisms could not infect immunocompetent mice, which quickly eliminated them within 3 weeks. These results indicate that this locus is required in enabling *B. burgdorferi* to evade a mammal's adaptive immune response.

Little is known about the mechanism of *vlsE* recombination. Although it involves gene conversion, it does not require RecA—a protein commonly involved in recombination. The *vlsE* gene conversion is greatly reduced in *Borrelia* strains lacking the Holliday junction resolvase, which is encoded by proteins RuvA and RuvB (Dresser et al., 2009; Lin et al., 2009). As noted above, *vlsE* recombination occurs during animal infection but has not been detected during standard test-tube cultures of *B. burgdorferi*. Recent work has made progress in understanding what occurs during *vlsE* recombination using tissue explants from skin, heart, liver, spleen, and bladder. Explants were cultured on Gelfoam and then inoculated with *B. burgdorferi* to mimic what happens in mammalian tissue. After 16 days, the tissue retained normal appearance, although with loss of some lymphocytes. There was multiplication of *B. burgdorferi*, which was dependent on the type of tissue and the culture medium. Because *vlsE* recombination is a rare event, occurring in about 1 of $10^6$ cells per generation, a PCR technique was used that distinguished between the parental and recombinant sequences in the region of the central cassette sequence where most of the replacements would change the sequence. In three of the four explant samples, the specific PCR amplicon indicative of recombination was detected. The first explant showed a recombination with cassette 7, while the second and third explants showed a recombination in cassette 2 and cassette 1, respectively. While still preliminary, this method may provide a model to study antigenic variation *in vitro*.

The *vls* antigenic variation system appears to be present in all Lyme disease *Borrelia* but exhibits a high degree of sequence diversity. In comparing 13 strains of *B. burgdorferi*, these *vls* sequences vary more than any other homologs in Lyme disease *Borrelia* (unpublished data). The identity and similarity in *vlsE* sequences is as low as 54 and 69 percent, respectively. That contrasts with the 69 and 79 percent values for OspC—touted as one of the most heterogeneous proteins. These results indicate that the *vls* system is under a high degree of evolutionary pressure and selection. Differences between the *vls* loci in different strains are therefore substantial and may be responsible for differences in the infectivity and virulence of the strains. There are 22 silent cassettes in *B. burgdorferi* strain 64B as opposed to the 15 in the initially characterized strain, B31. These 22 silent cassettes have three frameshifts. Strain 29805 has 17 silent cassettes, with a single long open reading frame. Finally, Far04 of *Borrelia garinii* contains 18 silent cassettes. However, most of the frameshifts in this strain occur between silent cassettes rather than interrupting them. This meta-analysis called into question many theories about how the *vls* system works because invariant regions are not as conserved between different species and strains as expected. One possible next step will be to replace the *vls* system in one strain with the *vls* system of other strains to observe the effect on pathogenesis.

This work provides several conclusions. First, the *vls* system of antigenic variation is an important mechanism allowing Lyme disease *Borrelia* to evade a host's immune system—and allowing infection to persist. Second, while the *vlsE* gene conversion process is not well understood, it is known to involve the RuvAB Holliday junction resolvase. Third, the tissue explant model may allow investigators to identify the factors required to regulate and carry out *vlsE* recombination. Finally, the *vls* system shows greater sequence diversity among different *Borrelia* strains than any other genetic component, including OspC.

### Knowledge Gaps and Research Opportunities

Norris noted the following key questions for future study:

- What are the *cis*- and *trans*-acting factors—that is, DNA segments and proteins—that regulate and carry out *vlsE* recombination?
- Can investigators use tissue explant models to study the mechanisms of immune evasion and other aspects of the pathogenesis of Lyme disease?
- Do differences in the *vls* antigenic variation systems in *Borrelia* correlate with distinct manifestations of the disease, such as arthritis and neurologic effects?
- How can a *Borrelia* protein that induces strong antibody responses— now used to diagnose Lyme disease—help the organism evade a host's immune system?
- What other mechanisms of immune evasion are involved in persistent infection by Lyme disease *Borrelia*?

### COLLAGEN SEQUESTRATION AS A MECHANISM FOR PERSISTENCE OF *BORRELIA BURGDORFERI*

*Stephen W. Barthold, D.V.M., Ph.D., University of California, Davis*

The persistence of *B. burgdorferi* in mammals is integral to the bacteria's natural cycle of infection. Unlike relapsing fever *Borrelia*, which requires antigenic variation to maintain high levels of spirochetes in the blood (spirochetemia) for transmission by rapidly feeding soft ticks, *B. burgdorferi* needs to survive for long periods of time in its reservoir mammalian hosts for transmission by slower feeding hard ticks. This is an inefficient mechanism of transmission, which requires that the *Borrelia* spirochetes disseminate widely in its reservoir host in order to maximally populate and persist in the skin, which is the host–vector interface. Persisting spirochetes become intercalated within collagen fibers of the skin and other tissues, which appears to be a unique mechanism of host immune evasion. After persisting in collagen-rich tissues, especially skin, *B. burgdorferi* can emerge and replicate as a host's antibodies to the bacteria's key antigens wane. In humans and animals, such periodic emergence of persisting spirochetes allows inflammation to recur periodically. Despite the fact that persistence is a key characteristic of *B. burgdorferi*, the mechanisms underlying that attribute are not well understood.

Humans are not competent reservoirs hosts because their infections are localized and multifocal, rather than disseminated and uniform, as occurs in small rodents. Erythema migrans occurs relatively early in infection after an infected tick has fed, transmitted the bacterium, and dropped off. The rash results from a person's adaptive immune response: infiltration of lymphocytes, plasma cells, and other types of cells. The EM is a transitional point in the infection. With the evolution of the host immune response, the erythema migrans will spontaneously resolve, but spirochetes persist in the same tissue, without eliciting inflammation. Thus, one of the earliest clinical signs of Lyme disease, erythema migrans, signals the onset of the immune phase of persistent infection, when spirochetes are sequestered in collagen with minimal or no inflammation.

Various laboratories have found adhesions on *B. burgdorferi* that are specific to ligands in the host's extracellular matrix (Cabello, 2007). For example, an undefined *Borrelia* protein was found to adhere *in vitro* to type I collagen lattices stripped of glycosaminoglycans (Zambrano et al., 2004). The adherence allowed the bacterium to invade the collagen lattices, where it underwent a burst of replication. Studies in the mouse model suggest similar activity *in vivo* (Barthold et al., 2006). For example, SCID mice are being used to study the infection process by accentuating events in the absence of adaptive immunity and then interrupting these events with the transfer of immune components back into the mouse through passive immunization or adoptive transfer.

Based on mouse model studies, there are two phases of infection (Barthold et al., 2010). The first is the pre-immune phase, when *B. burgdorferi* spirochetes disseminate in blood (spirochetemia) and the extracellular matrix. In this phase, spirochetes populate extracellular matrix of loose connective tissue throughout a host's body, particularly skin, vessel walls, nerves, muscle, and myocardium (the heart's muscular wall). Arthritis and carditis occur during this phase. In the second phase (adaptive immune phase), spirochetemia ceases and there is a generalized reduction of spirochete populations in the host's tissues. Disease, including the inflammation characteristic of arthritis and carditis, also resolves with the evolution of the immune response. This occurs in immunocompetent mice, mice deficient in T cells, and SCID mice reconstituted by adoptive transfer of naïve lymphocytes. Inflammation can also be resolved with passive transfer of immune serum from persistently infected immunocompetent C3H mice into SCID mice (Barthold et al., 2006). Using the antibodies from immune sera to screen an expression library, a number of antigens have been identified that may be important in disease resolution, including decorin-binding protein (Dbp) A, and arthritis-related protein (Arp), found on linear plasmid 28-1, upstream from the *vlsE* locus of *B. burgdorferi* strain B31, and elsewhere in other strains. After hyperimmunizing mice with non-lipidated recombinant DbpA and Arp proteins, and transferring the resulting hyperimmune serum into SCID mice, there is resolution of both carditis and arthritis (Barthold et al., 2006). Transfer of immune serum from infected C3H mice into SCID mice mimics what happens in immunocompetent animals: a global 10- to 100-fold reduction in spirochetes occurs. Transferring immune serum into immunocompromised MyD88 mice can produce an even greater reduction in spirochetes. However, as occurs during the evolution of the host immune response in immunocompetent mice, complete elimination of spirochetes is ineffective and spirochetes persist within collagen fibers of skin, tendons, and vascular adventitia.

In the initial pre-immune phase of infection, spirochetes are ubiquitous and present in loose connective tissue all over the body, around the vessels and nerves, in the dermis, in the myocardium, and in the muscle. As the adaptive immune response begins, most of these spirochetes will be cleared; however, as the immune response evolves, translocation of spirochetes occurs. Spirochetes move from sites of inflammation, where they are eliminated by host immune factors, into a "safe zone" of the more collagenous type I milieu of adjacent tendons, ligaments, and vessel walls. This translocation coincides with formation of multifocal colonies of spirochetes, similar to that seen *in vitro* within collagen lattices. This phenomenon of spirochete proliferation is not specific to mice, but appears to occur in other mammals, such as during neuroborreliosis in horses. In these examples, spirochetes appear to be responding to the adaptive inflammatory environment that they encounter during the first stage of infection.

To understand the role of DbpA/B and Arp proteins in the translocation process, SCID mice were infected with B31 spirochetes from which either the Dbp A and B locus or the Arp locus had been knocked out. Similar to the normal infection, spirochetes were observed in the adventitia, the myocardium, and the media of the vessels. However, when the infected SCID mice were treated with immune serum from normal persistently infected mice, the antibodies cleared the DbpA/B-spirochetes from all three sites and the animals became PCR- and culture-negative. In contrast, in SCID mice infected with Arp-spirochetes and treated with immune serum from normal infected mice, large numbers of Arp-spirochetes remained in all three sites, each mouse was still spirochetemic, and carditis worsened. These findings reveal very specific interactions between spirochetes and different types of tissue.

In the immune phase of persistent infection, when spirochetes are sequestered within collagen and inflammation is absent, spirochetes seem to be no longer motile and are not replicating. Initial analysis of their RNA transcription profiles also reveals transcriptional changes—such as down-regulation of flagellin, for example. This apparently dormant persistent state within dermal collagen allows spirochetes to wait for a tick vector to initiate feeding. This dormancy is maintained by the host immune response. For example, passively transferred immune serum administered to SCID mice will induce this state of persistence without inflammation, but if the antibody is allowed to decay, spirochetes become active again, disseminate, and reinduce inflammation. In persistently infected immunocompetent mice, biologically active antibodies (those that induce disease regression and spirochete reductions in tissues) peak at 60 days and then progressively decline. Thus, the host immune response wanes, despite the presence of persisting spirochetes. This suggests that persisting spirochetes, by virtue of their collagen-sequestered dormant state, are not apparent to immune surveillance. Despite these findings, scientists are far from a complete understanding of the process by which *B. burgdorferi* spirochetes persist and evade immune clearance.

### Knowledge Gaps and Research Opportunities

Barthold noted that a number of key questions need future study:

- Does collagen have a specific *B. burgdorferi* ligand?
- What is the role of innate immunity in the sequestration and persistence of *B. burgdorferi*?
- What is the role of adaptive immunity in the sequestration and persistence of *B. burgdorferi*?
- What replicative and metabolic activity do sequestered *B. burgdorferi* undergo?
- What is the antibiotic tolerance of sequestered *B. burgdorferi*?

### DISCUSSION

Following the presentation, a number of participants questioned the panelists about the studies of persistence in animal models. The range of the type of questions asked is summarized for the reader.

One participant noted that it is stated frequently that *Borrelia burgdorferi* is an extracellular bacterium, but wanted the speakers to discuss the studies that show that *Borrelia* is found intracellularly under certain conditions. Barthold said he consistently observes extracellular forms of spirochetes, fully elongated and in association with collagen, but any intracellular organism are observed in a macrophage, where they are believed to be killed. Norris agreed, but noted that in rare instances *Treponema pallidum*, also a spirochete, can become an intracellular bacterium.

Another participant questioned how neurologic symptoms occur if the bacterium is just in collagen, even if it is associated with neural tissue. Barthold noted that mice do not get central nervous system disease, possibly because they don't have much connective tissue in their brain. However, central nervous system disease is seen in larger mammalian species that have more collagen in their meninges and perivascular spaces. Under those circumstances, Barthold has observed spirochetes in the collagenous areas and along the perivascular spaces into the brain. Because there is a dearth of good analysis of human neuroborreliosis cases, it is not known if the spirochetes are located in other areas. He noted that a tissue bank or biorepository would be very valuable to allow for these types of analysis.

Another participant noted that the studies by Bockenstedt had affirmed that 28 days of doxycycline was effective in treating the newly infected immunocompetent mice, but that the transplant debris only tested positive in one out of five mice, or 20 percent. The individual questioned if studies were planned that looked at animals where treatment was delayed. Bockenstedt noted that she is planning to do such studies in which infection is first established and allowed to progress to a persistent stage before administering antibiotics. These experiments will be done in C3H immunocompetent and C3H MyD88-deficient mice. She further commented on where spirochetes can be seen by multiphoton imaging in wild-type mice and MyD88-deficient mice that have been infected for 6 months. She noted that while spirochetes may be more difficult to find in immunocompetent mice at 6 months of infection in comparison to earlier periods, they are always found in extracellular collagen-rich matrixes, not inside cells.

Gerber noted a need to understand the phenotypic expressions of disease in humans and to identify the physiological, metabolic, and genetic determinants that affect disease expression. She questioned if the research involving C3H and C57BL/6 mice had incorporated both males and females and what metabolic differences (e.g., fat metabolism, obesity, propensity to develop tumors) had been identified. Weis noted that both male and female mice are used and there is not a gender difference in the arthritis severity. For many experiments, female mice are used for simplicity, but the results are consistent with male mice. To begin to understand the metabolic differences, Weis suggested the use of Genome Wide Association Studies in humans infected with *Borrelia burgdorferi* and displaying different symptoms.

These studies have provided clues to genes involved in hypertension, diabetes, and other conditions regulated by a complexity of traits.

## PATHOGENESIS OF *EHRLICHIA* AND *ANAPLASMA* INFECTION AND DISEASE

*Nahed Ismail, Ph.D., M.Sc., Department of Pathology, Meharry Medical College*

*Ehrlichia* and *Anaplasma* are small obligate, intracellular gram-negative bacteria with a characteristic dimorphic appearance and cell wall ultrastructure. They reside in cytoplasmic endosomes generally within hemopoietic cells that have evolved in close association with ticks and reservoir hosts. There are several species of *Ehrlichia* and *Anaplasma*, with *E. chaffeensis* being the causative agent of human monocytic ehrlichiosis (HME) and *A. phagocytophilum* being the causative agent for human granulocytic anaplasmosis (HGA). In the mammalian hosts, including infected humans, the primary target cells of *E. chaffeensis* and *A. phagocytophilum* are, respectively, monocytes and neutrophils.

*E. chaffeensis* is a small bacterium with a 1.2–1.5 mb genome. Unlike classical gram-negative bacteria, this pathogen lacks both peptidoglycan and lipopolysaccharide (LPS), but it uses cholesterol acquired from the host to maintain membrane integrity. A similar mechanism is used by *Anaplasma*. The *E. chaffeensis* P28 outer membrane protein family stimulates specific antibody responses in humans. P28 is also immunoprotective: Antibodies against it protect mice from fatal infection. However, the presence of a large family of P28 proteins may also enable the bacteria to evade the host's immune system and adapt to different hosts such as ticks and mammals. Several secreted *Ehrlichia* proteins have tandem repeats associated with interaction between the pathogen and the host. Furthermore, several proteins with eukaryote-like ankyrin domains, which influence transcription and translation of genes in the host, have been described. The mechanism for delivering secreted proteins into the host cell cytosol is not completely understood but in part uses the type IV secretion system (TFSS).

*Ehrlichia* and *Anaplasma* have developed mechanisms for evading a host's immune response. For example, *Ehrlichia* down-regulates cytokines essential for stimulating a protective Th1 phenotype of acquired immune response and subsequent elimination of the bacteria. These cytokines include IL-12, IL-15, IL-18, and MHC class II. *Ehrlichia* and *Anaplasma* also down-regulate the TLR2 and TLR4 receptors that the innate immune system uses to recognize and respond to *Ehrlichia*. Furthermore, *Ehrlichia* and *Anaplasma* also down-regulate several bactericidal mechanisms of monocytes and neutrophils, including degradation of p22$^{phox}$, inhibition of superoxide generation, and inhibition of phagolysosomal fusion. To survive and replicate inside cells, the bacteria induce apoptotic inhibitors or decrease expression of apoptotic inducers.

As discussed in the previous chapter, HME can manifest as either a mild, self-limited disease or a severe fulminate disease with a toxic shock–like syndrome. Patients with severe HME usually have multiorgan dysfunction that progresses to multiorgan failure. Although their symptoms may be nonspecific, patients with severe HME also present with marked leukopenia, lymphopenia, marked thrombocytopenia, and elevated liver enzymes. There is a disconnection between the number of bacteria in the blood of HME patients and the severity of the disease. This suggests that the pathogenesis of the disease and the outcome of infection have a significant immune-mediated component. The first task is therefore to characterize the molecular and cellular immune mechanisms that contribute to *Ehrlichia*-induced toxic shock. The long-term goal is to develop both a vaccine and an immune-based therapy.

A well-established fact is that protective immunity against several intracellular bacteria is mediated by Th1 cells that promote cell mediated immune responses (O'Garra and Murphy, 2009). Stimulation of T cells occurs when bacteria is phagocytosed by the host antigen-presenting cells (APCs), processed into small peptides and presented to naïve CD4+T cells and CD8+ T cells in the context of MHC class II and I, respectively. Following activation, T cells differentiate into either Type-1 or Type-2 cells depending on costimulatory signals cytokine environment. Intracellular bacteria stimulate IL-12 production by APCs to induce Th1-type cells that produce large amounts of IFN-γ. IFN-γ produced by Th1 cells activate macrophages to kill the bacteria, activate the bactericidal mechanisms of neutrophils, and enhance or stimulate an antibody response, mainly IgG2a antibodies. The latter allows opsonization (i.e., engulfing and digesting) of extracellular bacteria, and the killing of intracellular bacteria.

Immunocompetent mice have been used to understand how host defenses interact with the bacteria and contribute to resolution or progression of disease. Although *E. chaffeensis* does not accurately recapitulate human infection and disease, the related *Ixodes ovatus Ehrlichia* (IOE), which is highly virulent, and *Ehrlichia muris*, which is mildly virulent, do recapitulate key features and have been used in a series of elucidating studies. The disease is dose dependent. For example, mice receiving a large dose of IOE intradermally died on day 10 post-infection, while mice receiving a low dose of IOE survived (Stevenson et al., 2006). Specifically, the mice that died developed focal necrosis, apoptosis, and toxic shock–like syndrome. However, as in humans, despite severe tissue injury, these mice did not have evidence of overwhelming infection.

The immune mechanisms responsible for fatal disease were examined.

CD4 T cell proliferation and the frequency of CD4 Th1 cells were decreased, which, as noted, are very important in clearing *Ehrlichia* and intracellular bacteria from the host. The mice that died also had a concomitant increase in proinflammatory and anti-inflammatory cytokines TNF-alpha and IL-10—both implicated in tissue injury (Ismail et al., 2004, 2006). Furthermore, there was a marked expansion of CD8 T cells producing TNF-alpha in the mice that died. Mice that lacked CD8+T cells survived a lethal low-dose infection with IOE compared to similarly infected wild-type mice (Ismail et al., 2007). Survival of IOE-infected CD8+T cell deficient mice was associated with enhanced bacterial elimination, increased numbers of CD4+Th1 cells, decreased TNF-alpha production, and decreased tissue injury. These data suggest that CD8 T cells play a pathogenic role during severe and fatal monocytic ehrlichiosis by mediating apoptosis of CD4 T cells, decreasing Th1-type responses, and immunopathology.

Although fatal ehrlichiosis is associated with an increase in pathogenic CD8+T cells, which possibly mediate leukopenia and low CD4+T cell count, the mechanism by which *Ehrlichia* induced this pathogenic response is not yet known. It is well known that early interactions occur between the host's antigen-presenting cells and innate lymphocytes, such as when natural killer (NK) and natural killer T (NKT) cells influence the subsequent acquired immune response against intracellular pathogens. Unlike conventional CD4+ and CD8+T cells, NKT cells recognize endogenous host self-ligands as well as foreign microbial ligands (e.g., glycolipids, lipoprotein, or even cholesterol) presented by antigen-presenting cells through a receptor called the CD1d molecule, which is a non-polymorphic MHC class I-like molecule. For gram-negative bacteria that have LPS such as *Salmonella*, NKT cells are stimulated via signals mediated by endogenous self-ligands presented in the context of CD1d and signals generated by toll-like receptors (TLRs are pattern recognition receptors). In contrast, alpha protobacteriae, including *Ehrlichia* that lack LPS, appear to have a specific bacterial ligand that directly stimulates NKT cells (Mattner et al., 2005). NKT cells are essential for eliminating the bacteria, thus NKT-deficient mice succumb to an overwhelming bacterial infection (Stevenson et al., 2006). Moreover, NKT cells prevent chronic joint inflammation after infection with *Borrelia*. A recent study has shown that Lyme disease patients seem to have a low number of NKT cells and low migration of those cells to joints, which was postulated to be an etiologic factor that contributes to arthritis in Lyme disease patients. One recommendation from this study was to propose enhancing the stimulation of NKT cells, and their migration to peripheral tissues, so they would suppress joint inflammation (Tupin et al., 2008).

One question that remained was whether NK cells are functionally similar to NKT cells, or whether they have different roles during infection. In fatal ehrlichiosis, NK cells expand in the liver by day 7 post-infection and produce most of the cytokines produced during fatal ehrlichiosis, including TNF-α, IFN-γ, and IL-10 (Stevenson et al., 2010). Furthermore, these NK cells are also highly cytotoxic. The next step was to show a causal association between NK cells and development of immunopathology and fatal disease. After depleting NK cells from mice, there was a significant decrease of the systemic cytokine production, mainly IL-10 and TNF-alpha, and a decreased number of apoptotic cells and necrotic foci, suggesting that NK cells directly or indirectly mediate tissue injury during fatal ehrlichiosis. Even more surprising, the absence of NK cells enhanced the elimination of bacteria (Stevenson et al., 2010). That suggested, conversely, that NK cells inhibit effective elimination of bacteria. Together, those findings suggest that interaction of virulent *Ehrlichia* with antigen-presenting cells following high-dose lethal infections results in strong stimulation of cytotoxic NK cells. These data suggest that NK cells are possibly the main inducers of the harmful/pathogenic immune responses seen in ehrlichiosis, including generation of pathogenic CD8+T cells and development of CD4+Th1 hyporesponsiveness. The mechanism by which NK cells promote pathogenic responses following ehrlichial infection is not completely known, however, it is possible that this occurs via stimulation of IL-10 production, as well as via pro-inflammatory cytokines. Human patients with fatal HME had increased Th2 immunosuppressive cytokines, mainly IL-10, as compared to those with mild disease (Ismail et al., unpub. data). Patients with fatal outcomes also had a higher level of NK and monocyte chemokines, IP-10 and MCP-1, and decreased T cell chemokines, including RANTES. In addition, these patients had increased pro-inflammatory cytokines, including IL-1 alpha, IL-6, and TNF-alpha, and increased neutrophil chemokines, including IL-8 and granulocytic colony-stimulating factor.

In conclusion, cytokine dysregulation and expansion of pathogenic NK and CD8 T cells are the main immunopathological mechanisms in ehrlichiosis that mediate tissue injury and organ dysfunction. On the other hand, hyporesponsiveness of CD4+ T cells, decreased number of CD4+T cells, and a late-stage apoptosis (programmed cellular death) of CD4+T cells also contribute to severity of disease, possibly by failure to control continuous microbial stimulation of NK and CD8+T cells. These findings are consistent with Dumler's findings in a murine model of HGA, in which pathogenic innate responses consisting of uncontrolled macrophage activation, NK, and NKT play a role in the immunopathology caused by *Anaplasma phagocytophilum* infection in mice.

## Knowledge Gaps and Research Opportunities

Ismail noted the following areas are critical ones for future study:

*Understanding the Bacteria*

- The regulatory mechanisms that control the developmental cycle of *E. chaffeensis*;
- Proteomic analysis of the biphasic forms of *E. chaffeensis*, to identify the determinants of invasiveness and virulence;
- The mechanistic details of how the T4SS and other secretion mechanisms secrete *Ehrlichia* and *Anaplasma* effectors, and their subcellular sites of action; and
- Identification of effector candidates—including ankyrin-motif bearing proteins and cognate partners secreted via T4SS or other secretion apparatus. This will provide a molecular basis for understanding pathogen subversion of host defense, and disease.

*Understanding the Host*

- Immune defense mechanisms and regulation at the peripheral sites of tick-borne *Ehrlichia* infection, such as the skin, liver, and lung;
- The relative contribution of specialized Langerhans cells, hepatocytes, Kupffer cells, and endothelial cells to immune surveillance, immunity, and pathology;
- Local factors influencing dendritic cell, NK, and T cell recruitment and differentiation;
- The mechanisms controlling the cross-presentation of endosome/phagosome-derived *Ehrlichia* antigens to CD8+T cells; and
- The role of regulatory T cells in controlling immune responses to *Ehrlichia*.

*Potential Therapeutics*

- Molecular and cellular profiles of mild and fatal infections in patients with HME;
- Collection of human samples, such as blood, cerebral spinal fluid, and tissues;
- Development of screening tests, including biomarkers, to identify individuals at early stages of infection, and those at risk for progressive disease;
- Studies of the efficacy of highly promising interventions in animal models of disease; and

- Characterization of host defenses and immune responses in models of tick-transmitted *Ehrlichia* and *Anaplasma* infections that mimic mild and severe HME and HGA.

## PATHOGENESIS OF RICKETTSIAL INFECTIONS

*Gustavo Valbuena, M.D., University of Texas*

*Rickettsia* are small, obligate intracellular bacteria in the Class *α-Proteobacteria*. Ticks serve as both vectors and primary reservoirs of spotted fever group *Rickettsia* as they can transmit the *Rickettsia* between stages and transovarially to the next tick generation. In general, small mammals act as amplifying hosts and human infections are accidental. The main target tissue in mammalian hosts, including humans, is the endothelium, which lines the interior of the vascular system.

Taxonomically, *Rickettsia* can be subdivided into four groups: typhus, spotted fever, transitional, and ancestral. In North America, the spotted fever group and the typhus group are of most concern. *Rickettsia rickettsii* cause the most severe rickettsiosis in North America, Rocky Mountain spotted fever. However, the newly discovered *R. parkerii* also produces an important disease syndrome, although apparently less severe than that produced by *R. rickettsia*.

Ticks can survive for long periods while harboring *Rickettsia*, although the organisms may decrease the fitness of the tick. When a tick attaches to a host, the *Rickettsia* are "reactivated"—a poorly understood process that requires 12 to 18 hours and results in the *Rickettsia* acquiring an infectious phenotype. Because hard ticks take several days to feed on a vertebrate host, they produce substances that inhibit the host's immune and coagulation systems, possibly allowing infection to become established.

*Rickettsia* enter endothelial cells rapidly through a process of receptor-induced endocytosis: enzymes produced by the bacteria rapidly lyse the endocytic vacuole and move into the cytoplasm, where they replicate (Weiss, 1973). Several mechanisms are likely involved in damaging the endothelium. The first is cell death, necrosis (Silverman, 1984), in which the replicating *Rickettsia* lyse the cell. Second, there is evidence of increased oxidative stress as cells respond to the intracellular infection (Rydkina et al., 2004). Third, although cells could also die through apoptosis, there is evidence that rickettsia can inhibit apoptosis to favor its own survival (Bechelli et al., 2009). In addition, during the infection, *Rickettsia* induce increased production of nitric oxide and several lipid mediators derived from the cyclooxygenase system, particularly COX-2 (Rydkina et al., 2010).

Once infection is established, endothelial cells acquire an activated phenotype that can trigger coagulation and activate the host's inflammatory response. The endothelial cells can express cytokines and other immuno-modulatory substances, and adhesion molecules, which recruit leukocytes to the infection sites (Valbuena and Walker, 2009). The inflammatory response is mediated, in part, through NF-kappa B, an important transcription factor that regulates many immune response genes (Sahni et al., 1998). Other mechanisms in the host's inflammatory response include synthesis of inflammatory cytokines, including IL-1 and IL-8. When endothelial cells interact with immune cells, especially if the latter are producing interferon gamma and TNF-alpha, as in the case of NK cells or CD8 T cells, the endothelial cells become activated and kill *Rickettsia*. A goal is the harness the mechanisms that allow the endothelium to kill the pathogen for use in treating disease.

There are a number of reasons why Rocky Mountain spotted fever often becomes severe and results in a high case fatality rate. Endothelial cells normally form a barrier in the vasculature and balance the movement of fluid between the intravascular and extravascular spaces. The disruption of this barrier due to rickettsial infection of the endothelium affects these functions and results in leakage of fluid. When this occurs in organs such as the brain or lungs, the disease can rapidly progress. Rocky Mountain spotted fever may also be severe because it is a systemic infection involving cells that regulate the coagulation and immune systems. Furthermore, clinicians often confuse Rocky Mountain spotted fever with viral illnesses—for example, influenza in North America and dengue fever in Latin America. This confusion can have severe consequences because early suspicion of spotted fever can result in effective treatment with the antibiotic doxycycline. However, once patients develop the full spectrum of disease, physicians may refer them to higher level hospitals, which may treat the patients with newer broad-spectrum antibiotics—to which *R. rickettsia* are frequently constitutively resistant. Another barrier to combating Rocky Mountain spotted fever is that current diagnostic tests rely on antibodies, which are produced after the infection has already disseminated.

## Knowledge Gaps and Research Opportunities

Valbuena noted that the number of key areas for future study include:

- Determination of the mechanism by which *Rickettsia* are reactivated in the tick to an infectious state. (The fact that the bacteria must be reactivated allows for public health intervention. For example, because ticks must remain attached to a host for at least 6 to 8 hours to transmit *R. rickettsii*, people at risk for exposure could prevent infection by checking their bodies daily for ticks.)

- Further definition of the cells that are initially infected and the underlying early pathology. *Rickettsia* could be transmitted directly into vessels and cause rapid systemic infection or, alternatively, the bacteria could move into lymphatic vessels, and from there into local lymph nodes, triggering an early response of the immune system.
- Understanding of the preference of *Rickettsia rickettsii* to infect endothelial cells *in vivo*, given that they can infect numerous cell types *in vitro*.
- Better understanding of the roles of autophagy and of the activated innate intracellular mechanisms is needed.
- Identification of the metabolic pathways used by *Rickettsia* during growth and replication in the cytosol.
- Identification of genes and proteins differentially expressed and required for growth in mammalian hosts versus tick vectors.
- Identification of the *R. rickettsii* antigens that stimulate a protective immune response. This will be essential for development of a vaccine against Rocky Mountain spotted fever.
- Development of better animal models including those that better recapitulate the natural mode of transmission via tick bite and include human tissue and immune systems.
- Study of *Rickettsia* from a systemic approach that considers the response of the vector to the host, the response of the host to the vector, the response of the vector and host to the bacteria, and the response of the bacteria to the vector and host.

Three overall priorities for addressing rickettsial diseases were highlighted:

- *Diagnostics*. People now die of these diseases because clinicians have no effective way to diagnose them at the early stages of disease when antibiotic treatment is most effective.
- *More studies of the disease pathogenesis*. These would allow scientists to develop treatments for severe disease, such as when complications arise because of delayed treatment.
- *Vaccine development*. This would allow prevention of infection and disease in endemic areas and for individuals at high risk of exposure.

## DISCUSSION

One participant asked how much is known about the intracellular tick-borne pathogens in the tick and the triggers for reactivation. Valbuena noted that in the *Rickettsia*, research has observed that all tissues in the ticks are infected. Thus when the ticks bite, their salivary glands are already infected.

Those rickettsiae in the salivary glands undergo a mechanism of reactivation by a process that is still poorly understood. He further noted that in nature *Rickettsia* can be transmitted through stages of the tick life cycle, as well as to the next generation by transovarial passage. In general, ticks do not require an amplifying host, unlike *Ehrlichia*, to maintain the infection in nature. Ismail noted that studies in animal models of HME and patients infected with *E. chaffeensis* have identified infection-induced production of chemokines, which are attractants for monocytes and other host target cells such as neutrophils. The influx of these cells into the skin would provide a niche for further replication of ehrlichiae within the mammalian host. However, it is not yet clear whether a similar process occurs in infected ticks.

Another participant asked if there may be a potential therapeutic approach by targeting the mechanism where the infected host has to get the pathogen back to the tick. Ismail noted that in the knowledge gaps there is a need to study different parameters of the immune responses at multiple time points in humans, reservoir host (e.g., white-tailed deer), and vector host. This would include examining the different stages of infection to see how the bacteria progress from initial infection until the tick again acquires the bacterium.

Gerber asked if Valbuena had done dose responses and then looked at the CD4 or CD8 T cell response in mice. Valbuena noted that these experiments were done in Walker's laboratory. In the mouse model, when *R. conorii,* which is similar *to R. rickettsii*, is injected at a relatively low dose into the mouse, the animals become ill but do survive and establish a solid immunity. If these mice are subsequently challenged with extremely high doses, they will not succumb to the disease. In contrast, a very high dose will result in death of a naïve animal. These results may imply that a dysregulation in the immune response occurs when the dose is too high but also indicate that protective immunity, as a basis for a vaccine, is feasible. Ismail stated that for *Ehrlichia* infection, they noted that the dose can control the magnitude of immune responses and determine the outcome of infection. For example, a strong correlation between the dose of *Ehrlichia* and decreased CD4+T cell count and apoptotic death of activated CD4 T cells and NKT cells had been established in murine models of fatal monocytotropic ehrlichiosis. In fact, when mice were treated with doxycycline, the number of NKT cells could be restored.

## CONCLUDING THOUGHTS ON PATHOGENESIS

*Guy Palmer, D.V.M., Ph.D., College of Veterinary Medicine,*
*Washington State University*

The overriding lesson from these scientists is the yin and yang of the immune response to tick-borne pathogens in the *Anaplasma, Borrelia,*

*Ehrlichia*, and *Rickettsia* genera. On the one hand, the immune response controls the number of pathogens and helps people and other animals avoid massive systemic infection. On the other hand, the immune effectors themselves—especially those of the innate immune system—cause inflammation and tissue damage. These lessons apply to both early and persistent phases of infection, corresponding to acute and chronic disease.

Scientists have clearly identified the innate immune system, and specific immune effectors, as mediating inflammation in Lyme disease. In fact, the mechanisms underlying inflammation and damage can be organ specific. That is, the mechanism producing arthritis differs from that leading to carditis.

Studies based on genetically defined lines of mice have clear relevance to pathogenesis in humans, as individual patients may suffer severe symptoms in some organs and not in others. Comments from patient advocates throughout the discussion—and indeed throughout the workshop—underscored this variation in symptoms. Presenting scientists and discussants alike emphasized the need for better markers of the progression in severity and chronicity of tissue damage. This is a notable translational gap between basic research on the science of Lyme disease and help for patients.

The persistence of *B. burgdorferi* infection is complex and involves both antigenic variation and sequestration. That is, the bacteria's ability to generate novel variants that display new antigens on their surface allows them to escape the host's adaptive immune system. How these variants may alter the response of cells and tissues and inflammatory immune responses remain unanswered questions. Other knowledge gaps include how the bacteria's repertoire of surface proteins varies among strains, and how those variants affect disease.

The evidence that infectious spirochetes sequester in sites protected from antibodies also raises important questions. Are these spirochetes truly quiescent in replicating and in stimulating inflammation? How similar are these spirochetes to "persister" cells described in bacterial infections? Do these sequestered bacteria reemerge during actual infection—as suggested by passive serum transfer experiments? Experimental approaches can likely help close these knowledge gaps, but applying the findings to human infection will again prove challenging.

Unlike passive techniques such as PCR, scientists can use imaging to detect viable organisms. Imaging has therefore provided new answers to vexing questions regarding whether or not infection persists even after antibiotic therapy. These questions concern the migration of bacteria to and from transmission sites, and the responses of cells to viable as well as nonviable bacteria. Indeed, the detection of "remnant" material at infection sites raises questions about whether an antigenic stimulus persists even after viable, replicating bacteria are killed. The use of imaging technology may also allow scientists to examine host pathogen interactions concerning the progression of Lyme disease in deeper tissues such as the joints and heart.

Infection with rickettsial pathogens, including those in the *Anaplasma, Ehrlichia, Orientia,* and *Rickettsia* genera, can progress so rapidly that patients require immediate hospitalization and intensive care—along with antimicrobial therapy—to prevent death. The acuteness and severity of these infections highlight the need for better educating medical professionals in regions where the organisms are endemic. Investigators also need to better define these endemic regions and determine the risk that infectious bacteria and their animal hosts as they shift their range and distribution, and the likelihood that new pathogens will emerge.

Finally, we need more accurate tools for clinical and laboratory diagnosis of these diseases. The reasons underlying differences in the severity and rapidity of progression in patients is a major scientific gap—both on the pathogen side (diversity of species and strains) and the host side (genetic background and immune status).

With only a few exceptions, the pathogenesis of the broad group of rickettsial diseases is understudied—typical of many neglected diseases of significant but underappreciated significance for public health. Workshop presenters and discussants emphasized all these challenges.

However, two experimental models reveal the progress that scientists can achieve. Experiments using the *Ixodes ovatus Ehrlichia* are some of the best so far and underscore the dominant theme of the session: that the immune system is responsible for controlling infection but also producing the severe toxic shock–like syndrome when that control gets out of hand. A better understanding of immune mechanisms and effectors is critical to improving therapy once infection has progressed to severe acute disease.

Research on *Rickettsia* in the spotted fever group has similarly begun to elucidate the pathogenesis of severe disease. Progress in developing animal models illustrates the possibilities. Still, the knowledge gaps regarding the pathogenesis of the rickettsial pathogens are numerous and wide, and the need for experiments that lay the groundwork for translating that knowledge to human disease is strong.

In fact, such translational studies are essential for the full spectrum of tick-borne pathogens. To avoid a "translational canyon" between experimental studies and human treatment and prevention, scientists should consider studying *B. burgdorferi* in naturally occurring models, such as neuroborreliosis in horses and *Rickettsia rickettsii* and *Ehrlichia canis* in dogs. The use of "humanized" organs such as human skin in mouse models—as noted by Valbuena—can accelerate scientists' understanding of pathogenesis, and speed the application of that understanding to treating patients and preventing infection.

# 7

# Diagnostics and Diagnosis

Diagnostics and diagnosis, which are at the heart of the controversy surrounding tick-borne diseases (TBDs), have different connotations. Diagnostics provide a cluster of objective measures directed toward identifying the cause of a disease. After scientists discover the causative agent of an emerging infectious disease, such as *Borrelia burgdorferi* or *Ehrlichia chaffeensis*, they develop, evaluate, and refine diagnostic tests over time. Diagnosis, by contrast, rests on a patient's history and symptoms and observed physical and laboratory findings. Ultimately, accurate diagnosis requires knowledge of the epidemiology, clinical manifestations, and diagnostic tests of a disease.

Lyme disease presents a significant challenge to this standard approach. The presentation of symptoms may not align directly with the diagnostic laboratory test results. Necessary and sufficient conditions for the diagnosis may not be met, and yet the constellation of findings might lead one to make a diagnosis. At the time of acute presentation to a health professional, serologies may not be definitive. Conversely, serology may be positive, but symptoms may not match the serological picture. This suggests opportunities to develop laboratory measures that are reliable, valid, and sensitive to change and that may help to define the phases/stages of Lyme disease, such as acute, post-acute, chronic, and recurrent.

In this chapter, three researchers explored the limitations of existing tests for Lyme borreliosis and other tick-borne diseases and suggested promising new approaches to diagnostics that can improve the diagnosis of those diseases, and four clinicians discussed the challenges and needs for improving diagnosis in the medical office.

# DIAGNOSTICS FOR LYME DISEASE:
## KNOWLEDGE GAPS AND NEEDS

*Maria Aguero-Rosenfeld, M.D., New York Medical College
and Bellevue Hospital Center*

Microbiologists share some of the concerns that patients have about the current diagnostic tests for Lyme borreliosis and other tick-borne diseases. The laboratory diagnostic challenges stem from the organism's complex antigenic composition and its variation in expression depending on the environment where the organism is located. *Borrelia burgdorferi* has both linear and circular plasmids along with chromosomal DNA, and, in contrast to many other bacteria, a large portion of its genes are in plasmid DNA. The plasmid genes encode outer membrane components allowing the pathogen the flexibility of switching on and off antigens depending on the environment. This mechanism allows the pathogen to survive during the inactive tick stage (wintering) and to replicate during blood feeding on a suitable host.

Unlike other spirochetes, *B. burgdorferi* can be cultured *in vitro*. However, researchers are just beginning to understand the difference between immune responses to antigens expressed *in vivo* and antibodies detected using antigens from *B. burgdorferi* cultured *in vitro*. The *Borrelia* pathogen expresses some antigens as it first comes in contact with the host mammal leading to the early antibody response. Then, as more antigens are presented, the mammalian host develops the corresponding immune response in a sequential fashion. The intensity and type of antibodies developed depend on the duration of disease prior to antimicrobial treatment, the host immune system, and, perhaps, pathogenetic properties of the microorganism. Researchers have found that there are antigens expressed *in vivo* and others expressed *in vitro*. Therefore, the assays that are used to identify antibodies need to include those antigens expressed *in vivo*.

Two methods are available for directly detecting the presence of the pathogen in humans: culturing and polymerase chain reaction (PCR). Both of these have had mixed results in detecting *B. burgdorferi* (Table 7-1). Culturing spirochetes from a patient's blood or synovial fluid has been difficult because the concentration of spirochetes is low. The key to this approach would be to optimize the culture methods that could allow scientists to detect these spirochetes efficiently. Microbiologists attain the best results from culture when using skin from a patient's erythema migrans rash.

Modifications to the medium used to culture a patient's blood have had mixed results. The sensitivity of the test depends on the volume of cultured blood and evidence of early disease dissemination, when the organism is most likely to be present in the bloodstream. However, only 40 percent

**TABLE 7-1** Sensitivity of Direct Methods of Detection of *Borrelia burgdorferi*

| Disease Stage | Sample | Culture (%) | PCR (%) |
|---|---|---|---|
| Early disease— Erythema migrans | Skin | >50 (up to 86) | 69 (up to 88) |
| | Blood | >40 | 21 |
| Early disseminated— Neuroborreliosis | CSF | No data (US) | 38-67 |
| Late disease— Arthritis | Synovium | Anecdotal | 78 (up to 96 of untreated patients using 4 primer sets) |

SOURCES: Wang et al., 2002; Aguero-Rosenfeld et al., 2005; Mygland et al., 2010.

of patients in the early stages of infection test positive for *B. burgdorferi* in their blood. European scientists can sometimes detect *B. burgdorferi* spirochetes in patients' cerebrospinal fluid (CSF). The differences between being able to detect *Borrelia* in the blood or CSF may be a function of the *Borrelia* genotype. For example, the European *Borrelia garinii* is more neuroinvasive, which means that it is more often present in the cerebrospinal fluid, where it can be detected in culture.

The second technique for directly detecting *Borrelia* in patients is PCR, which amplifies specific sequences of spirochete DNA in samples of skin, synovial fluid, or blood. The efficiency of PCR depends on primers, number of sets used, sample type, and quality of the sample. In general, this detection method is more successful for *B. burgdorferi* when several different genetic sequences are amplified on DNA extracted from the skin of patients with erythema migrans and synovial fluid from the joints of patients with untreated Lyme disease arthritis. Obviously, PCR will have a higher yield on those samples with more spirochetes. Only a few U.S. scientists have used PCR to examine for spirochete DNA in cerebrospinal fluid where evidence of borreliae was seen in up to 60 percent of patients with early neuroborreliosis in one study. PCR is more sensitive in detecting infection in patients with untreated arthritis, as spirochete's DNA is present in 78–96 percent of these patients. However, the high yield of PCR in CSF of patients with early neuroborreliosis and in synovial samples of patients with untreated arthritis was obtained when several PCR primer sets were used. Direct testing works well if applied to the best samples at the right time. Drawbacks are the unavailability of PCR in most clinical settings and the need to biopsy the skin or to perform a joint tap, which many primary care physicians do not do.

Because of the drawbacks of those two methods for directly detecting *B. burgdorferi*, most clinicians continue to rely on detecting antibodies to the pathogen when testing patients for Lyme disease. The first generation of assays in the 1980s did not use antigens that were effective in detecting antibodies in patients' sera. These tests often failed to confirm that patients were infected with *B. burgdorferi* or gave positive results in patients who did not have Lyme disease.

In the mid-1990s, two-tier testing became the standard serological approach, and improvements were made on the antigen composition used in first- and second-tier tests, which produced better results. However, the two-tier approach is ineffective in detecting antibodies to *B. burgdorferi* during the acute phase of infection. Only 29 percent of patients later found to be infected with the pathogen have antibodies detected during the initial period. The sensitivity of the two-tier approach rises markedly during later stages of infection (Table 7-2).

The first step in the two-tier approach, the enzyme-linked immunosorbent assay (ELISA) test, has high sensitivity, but low specificity. That is, patients infected with *B. burgdorferi* are very likely to yield positive results on that test. However, ELISA also produces false positives, suggesting that some people are infected with the pathogen when they actually are not. For this reason, microbiologists apply the second step to confirm the results for those patients who test positive on the ELISA test. The Western immunoblot, by contrast, has high specificity: Most of the people who test positive for antibodies to *B. burgdorferi* are infected. The criteria for a positive result on this test are fairly stringent: Two of 3 specified bands on an IgM immunoblot or 5 of 10 specified bands on an IgG immunoblot must be detected for the specimens to be diagnostic. The IgM immunoblot should be used only within the first 4 weeks of illness, while the IgG immunoblot can be used at any stage in Lyme disease. If patients test positive on the ELISA but negative on the Western blot, they are considered not to have specific antibodies against *B. burgdorferi*.

One of the most immunodominant antigens in early disease is outer surface protein C (OspC). Antibodies to this antigen are among the first to appear after infection occurs. Another key result is evidence of antibodies to VlsE, which shows reactivity as early as 8 days after patients become ill. The addition of VlsE to both first- and second-tier tests has improved their performance. An increment in immunoreactive bands is observed in

**TABLE 7-2** Performance of Two-Tier Testing

| Early Disease Erythema Migrans | Early Dissem. (neurological) | Late Disease (arthritis, neurological) | Reference |
|---|---|---|---|
| Acute 29–54%<br>Conv. 65–88% | Acute 87%<br>Conv. 82% | 97–100% | Bacon et al., 2003 |
| Acute 31%<br>Conv. 64% | 63% | 100% | Branda et al., 2010 |
| 27.1–63.8% | Acute 80%<br>Conv. 75% | 94.7–100% | Wormser (in preparation) |

the IgG immunoblots of sera of patients with neuroborreliosis and Lyme disease arthritis.

One scientific gap is the testing of cerebrospinal fluid for antibodies. Europeans measure intrathecal production of antibodies by measuring antibodies in CSF and comparing these results against the concentration of antibodies in the serum to produce a ratio. U.S. scientists have not had a sufficiently large population in which to evaluate the efficacy of this approach because fewer cases of neuroborreliosis are documented in the United States as compared to Europe and CSF sampling is not routinely done in patients with Lyme disease. The absence of this type of testing is a gap in diagnostics for neuroborreliosis caused by *B. burgdorferi* in the United States.

Besides the lack of sensitivity in detecting early *Borrelia* infection, the two-tier test cannot distinguish between active Lyme disease and past infection or reinfection. Promising new tests to address this problem are on the horizon. European researchers have advanced the use of recombinant antigens. Furthermore, a combination of immunodominant antigens in a bead format could be used instead of whole-cell lysates. For example, scientists at the Centers for Disease Control and Prevention evaluated the use of VlsE and pepC-10 (a synthetic peptide derived from OspC) in a kinetic ELISA. More recently C6, a synthetic peptide based on a component of VlsE, has been approved as a source of antigen in first-tier enzyme immunoassay (EIA). Three studies (Bacon et al., 2003; Steere et al., 2008; Wormser et al., unpub.) compared the C6 testing protocol with the standard two-tier method. The C6 testing protocol has performed comparably in accurately detecting the presence of antibodies to *B. burgdorferi* in sera of patients with acute EM, but it was slightly less effective in the case of neurological Lyme disease. Overall, the specificity of C6 testing protocol is lower than that of the two-tier testing protocol. False positives remain a significant concern as U.S. laboratories now perform more than 2 million tests for Lyme disease annually, with at least 1 percent of these tests generating false positives. Thus, current test protocols produce approximately 20,000 false positives each year, a problem that may increase with wider adoption of the C6 testing protocol.

In conclusion, education is crucial to the diagnostics for both the clinician and the community. The positive predictive value of a test relies on the test being applied to the appropriate patient. Furthermore, physicians need to be educated on the availability of the tests and their limitations. Clinicians sometimes order tests on patients with a low probability of infection, making the results difficult to interpret. In the diagnostic laboratory, education and training are also important for laboratorians as individual interpretation of the test often results in over-reading of the Western blots, in particular IgM immunoblots.

## Knowledge Gaps and Research Opportunities

Aguero-Rosenfeld identified a number of key areas for future work:

- Development of programs to educate practitioners on the appropriate use of laboratory tests for Lyme disease.
- Improvement of direct methods for detecting *B. burgdorferi* in samples from patients. For example, scientists could improve and automate culture techniques and use PCR to target several gene sequences.
- Development of immunoassays containing a combination of recombinant or peptide antigens of importance, such as VlsE and OspC, in a bead format or other comparable method that would allow measuring the quantity of antibodies to individual antigens.
- Development and evaluation of assays on cerebrospinal fluid that can support a diagnosis of neuroborreliosis.
- Development of an algorithm that enables laboratory tests for *B. burgdorferi* infection to determine the stage of disease or duration of infection.
- Establishment of a repository of well-characterized samples from Lyme borreliosis patients for use in evaluating new assays.
- Recombinant antigens and peptides such as C6, including variations in gene sequences, require further evaluation for sensitivity and specificity.

## IMPROVED DIAGNOSTICS AND NOVEL APPROACHES TO TICK-BORNE DISEASES

*Juan P. Olano, M.D., University of Texas Medical Branch*

Diagnosis of infectious diseases is based on the same techniques for nearly all infectious agents: antibody detection, antigen capture, and culture and detection of nucleic acids with or without amplification. Antibody detection (serological techniques) is the most common diagnostic method used in infectious diseases, but as reiterated throughout the workshop, a serologic diagnosis is frequently rendered too late to be of clinical value for therapeutic decisions because the immune response requires time to develop so that pathogen-specific circulating antibodies can be reliably detected. More recently, great progress has been made following the development of PCR and other nucleic acid amplification techniques for detection of pathogens in blood and other tissues. Most types of diagnostic tests used to diagnose Lyme disease are also used to diagnose other tick-borne infections, including rickettsial diseases, ehrlichioses, and anaplasmosis. *Rickettsia* disease differs pathologically from those of *Ehrlichia* and *Anaplasma* in that it infects the microvascular endothelium, and therefore levels of circulating rickettsiae are usually low, posing a challenge for diagnosing rickettsioses during the acute phase of the disease. The indirect immunofluorescence assay (IFA) is considered the gold standard for diagnosis of rickettsial infections due to its high sensitivity and specificity when paired serum samples obtained 2–3 weeks apart are tested. However, its sensitivity is very low when single serum samples obtained in the acute phase are used. As with the diagnostic tests for *Borrelia burgdorferi*, the presence of IgM antibodies can be detected 5 to 7 days after the onset of symptoms, but the specificity of these tests is low. They produce false positives as other bacterial, viral, and parasitic infections can cross-react with the antigens. Similarly, IgG antibodies have rising titers after 7–10 days, but there is cross-reactivity within the spotted fever and typhus group rickettsiae. Diagnostic titers continue to rise, and, by day 30, approximately 100 percent of the patients have detectable circulating antibodies. As a result of the delayed diagnosis, appropriate treatment may be delayed, and case-fatality ratios are higher in the absence of specific antibiotic therapy.

There are a number of other diagnostic tests for rickettsial diseases. Western blots allow for early detection of IgM antibodies to lipopolysaccharide antigens, but they still have low specificity, and cross-reactions occur between the spotted fever and typhus group rickettsiae. Detection of diagnostic IgG bands parallels the IFA detection rates. Cross-adsorption studies can be used to distinguish between the various species, but the tests are cumbersome and expensive. Dot blot enzyme immunoassay has similar sensitivity as IFA but also allows for the use of multiple antigens.

The rash associated with rickettsial disease is caused by infection of the endothelial cells lining the microvessels in the skin. When the rash is present in the acute phase of the disease, detection of rickettsiae by immunohistochemistry of skin biopsies has a sensitivity of ~60–80 percent.

Nucleic acid amplification techniques (mostly DNA), including PCR and real-time PCR, are used in selected research laboratories around the world for detection of circulating rickettsiae (inside macrophages or circulating endothelial cells that have detached from their microvascular niche). These tests are not commercially available, and their sensitivity and specificity have not been evaluated systematically. The agents of human monocytic ehrlichiosis (HME), *Ehrlichia ewingii* ehrlichiosis (EEE), and human granulocytic anaplasmosis (HGA) infect mononuclear phagocytes, including circulating monocytes (HME) and neutrophils (EEE and HGA). Therefore, detection of these pathogens in blood is theoretically more sensitive compared to rickettsioses. However, the diagnosis of these diseases presents similar difficulties as described for rickettsiae. Direct observation of the pathogens in peripheral blood smears is usually insensitive (more so for HME than HGA) due to the lower abundance of circulating target cells for HME. Diagnosis relies primarily on IFA, and its sensitivity and specificity is similar to the rickettsioses. Other serological tests include Western immunoblotting using native or recombinant antigens. Antibodies against tandem repeat protein (TRP) 120 and TRP 42 provide diagnostic bands to differentiate *Ehrlichia chaffeensis* from other *Ehrlichia* spp., while the 42, 44, and 49 kDa proteins help in distinguishing HGA from other ehrlichiae.

Similar to *Rickettsia*, there are a number of other diagnostic approaches for ehrlichioses and anaplasmosis. Immunohistology is available, but not widely applied outside the research setting. Conventional and real-time PCR assays have been developed and evaluated in small series of cases. Sensitivity varies widely, from 50 to approximately 100 percent, depending on several factors including primers used, time of testing during the course of the disease, use of pre-test antibiotics, etc. Specificity for PCR is very high provided there is no amplification contamination. All amplification techniques are available at selected research laboratories and are not commercially available. Currently, several new technologies provide platforms for improving the performance of conventional serological assays and are based on antigen capture using pathogen-specific antibodies in microfluidic settings followed by different detection techniques, including electrochemiluminescence and microretroreflectors.

Electrochemiluminescence is a highly sensitive technique that uses ruthenylated antibodies that in the presence of tripropylamine and an electrical current release photons. For rickettsial pathogens, its analytical sensitivity *in vitro* and *in vivo* using animal models is ~1,250 to 1,500 organisms/mL. Microretroreflector detection is based on reflection of light off a gold-coated surface. As rickettsiae are captured by antibody-coated magnetic beads or nanogold particles, their deposition on a reflective surface dims the amount of light bouncing off that surface. This variations are detected using conventional optics. Other antigen-capturing systems being evaluated with microfluidic systems include the use of microporous substances to increase the capturing surface area.

Improved serological assays using protein microarrays is another promising technology. In short, all open reading frames of the *R. rickettsii* genome have been cloned, expressed, and blotted onto microarray spots. The serological response is then analyzed and response patterns are delineated. This technique could improve both sensitivity and specificity for diagnosis of rickettsioses, ehrlichioses, and anaplasmosis. Promising preliminary results have been observed with rabbit and dog sera and a few human samples available for testing.

In conclusion, Olano noted that despite advances in antigen-capturing systems, detection technologies, automation, and nucleic acid amplification techniques, commercially available tests for the diagnosis of human rickettsioses, anaplasmosis, and ehrlichioses by nucleic acid amplification have not been developed. Aside from IFA, all these tests are available only at selected research laboratories around the United States and the world. Thus, the gap between the laboratory bench and the patient bedside in diagnosing tick-borne diseases remains wide. As better detection platforms are refined and become increasingly available, microfluidic technology, automation, nanotechnology, and point-of-care testing will result in accurate, fast, and inexpensive diagnosis of these diseases.

## POTENTIAL BIOMARKER APPLICATIONS FOR LYME DISEASE: ALIGNING MULTIPLE SYMPTOMS WITH BIOLOGICAL MEASURES

*Afton L. Hassett, Psy.D., University of Michigan Medical School*

Biomarkers are cellular, biochemical, and molecular characteristics by which normal and abnormal processes can be recognized or monitored. Their identification has numerous clinical applications, such as improving diagnostic accuracy; assessing disease activity, prognosis, and efficacy of treatment; and tailoring treatment to the individual. However, studies that fail to properly characterize the patients studied (i.e., phenotyping) hamper progress. For example, a recent review of research on biomarkers for autoimmune diseases found that some investigators had failed to control for patients' age or gender, while others had not controlled for medication use, other medical and psychological comorbidities, or the stage of disease (Tektonidou and Ward, 2010). These factors, and several others, must be accounted for as each can influence biological measures.

Currently, there are no credible biomarkers for post-Lyme disease despite ongoing efforts in this area. For example, in a series of studies, researchers using the CD57 marker for natural killer cells found that patients with post-Lyme disease had fewer natural killer cells, suggesting that the marker could be used to assess treatment outcomes (Stricker and Winger, 2001, 2003; Stricker et al., 2002). However, a more recent study using a combination of CD56 and CD16 surface markers in conjunction with CD3 markers showed that natural killer cell counts did not differ between post-Lyme disease patients and healthy controls or patients who had recovered from Lyme disease after treatment (Marques et al., 2009).

In another study, heightened anti-neural antibody reactivity was found in 49.4 percent of post-Lyme disease patients compared with control groups who had recovered from Lyme disease (18.5 percent) or were healthy (15 percent) (Chandra et al., 2010). The heightened reactivity was not greater compared to patients with systemic lupus erythematosus (73.3 percent). A similar reactivity was observed in an earlier study evaluating ongoing neurologic Lyme disease (Sigal and Williams, 1997). This antibody reactivity supports the hypothesis that a sustained immune response may contribute to persistent neurologic dysfunction in Lyme disease patients, even after the pathogens are eliminated (Sigal and Williams, 1997). Other ongoing and/or promising research includes

- Immune system abnormalities (e.g., persistent activation, cytokine-induced sickness behavior);
- Proteomics—proteins produced specific to post-Lyme disease;
- Neuroendocrine dysfunction;
- Neuroimaging (microglial activation, neural network differences); and
- Genetic predisposition.

Charting a scientific inquiry into the nature of post-Lyme disease may rely on understanding the symptoms of the condition, which include arthralgias, musculoskeletal pain, radicular pain, paresthesia, fatigue, neurocognitive impairment, and mood disturbances. These symptoms are the very same symptoms observed in conditions such as fibromyalgia and chronic fatigue syndrome, which are currently thought to result from disturbances in the central nervous system processing of sensory information. These conditions are frequently referred to as "central sensitivity" syndromes. Thus, to understand the persistent symptoms of post-treatment Lyme disease, there is a need to understand the commonalities between these symptoms and those associated with central sensitivity syndromes. Moreover, aspects of the underlying pathophysiology of central sensitivity syndromes will likely inform biomarker research.

We begin with the most prominent symptom—pain. Findings from the past decade of neuroscience research suggest there are at least three types of pain. The first, peripheral pain, includes acute injury, osteoarthritis, rheumatoid arthritis, and cancer pain, and is "nociceptive," meaning that a stimulus in the periphery (e.g., inflammation, mechanical malfunction, or tissue damage) is causing the pain. This type of pain responds to interventional procedures, non-steroidal anti-inflammatory drugs, and opioids. Second, neuropathic pain stems from damage to or dysfunction of peripheral nerves and can include diabetic neuropathic pain and postherpetic neuralgia. Neuropathic pain responds to both peripheral and central interventions. Third, "central," or non-nociceptive, pain results from disturbances in central nervous system processing and leads to diffuse hyperalgesia (increased response to painful stimuli) and allodynia (painful response to normal stimuli). Examples of central pain conditions include fibromyalgia, interstitial cystitis, and irritable bowel syndrome. Individuals can have a combination of these types of pain. For example, about 15 percent of patients with rheumatoid arthritis also have fibromyalgia: that is, they have both inflammatory pain and central pain. Even patients with well-controlled rheumatoid arthritis, as evidenced by a lack of inflammation, may continue to have persistent pain. In these cases, it appears that augmentation of central nervous system pain processing accounts for the persistent experience of pain.

Another common symptom in central sensitivity syndromes is fatigue, which is thought to have a peripheral or central origin. It has been proposed that peripheral fatigue is predominantly due to physical exhaustion and may be attributed to organ-system dysfunction (Silverman et al., 2010). This type of fatigue occurs commonly in patients with rheumatoid arthritis, cardio-respiratory diseases, and myasthenia gravis. By contrast, central fatigue is more cognitive in nature and is attributed to central nervous system dysfunction. Classic examples of central fatigue include chronic fatigue syndrome, fibromyalgia, and irritable bowel syndrome, although central fatigue can also accompany rheumatoid arthritis, lupus, and cancer. Importantly, the difficulty with memory and concentration reported by a myriad of patients with various systemic diseases may be a function of central fatigue.

As with many other medical conditions, a stress-diathesis model for the etiology of central sensitivity syndromes is widely accepted. Such a model purports that genetic and environmental factors likely contribute to central sensitivity syndromes in equal measure. A series of case-controlled studies suggest that in predisposed individuals these syndromes can be triggered by peripheral pain conditions (e.g., rheumatoid arthritis and lupus [Clauw and Katz, 1995], physical trauma [Buskila et al., 1997; McBeth, 2005; Miranda et al., 2010], or catastrophic events, such as war [Clauw et al., 2003]) and infections. Pertinent to Lyme disease, infections in general have been shown to trigger central sensitivity syndromes in approximately 10 percent of patients. More specifically, 5 to 30 percent of patients with enteric infections later manifest irritable bowel syndrome (Bayless and Harris, 1990; Saito et al., 2002; Thabane and Marshall, 2009). Similarly, urinary tract infections appear to later lead to interstitial cystitis and painful bladder syndrome (Warren et al., 2008). In the Dubbo population-based prospective cohort study of patients infected with three very different viruses—Epstein-Barr virus, Ross River virus, and *Coxiella burnetii*, the bacterium that causes Q fever—approximately 9 percent of infected patients continued to present with a chronic fatigue–like syndrome even after the agent was cleared (Nickie et al., 2006). More recently, there was a case report of a central sensitivity syndrome triggered by H1N1 influenza (Vallings, 2010).

Similarly, various TBDs appear to trigger some central sensitivity syndromes. For example, approximately 39 percent of patients with human anaplasmosis developed chronic fatigue syndrome despite no serological evidence of persistent infection (Ramsey et al., 2002). In two prospective studies of patients with Lyme disease, 13 percent of patients eventually met the diagnostic criteria for fibromyalgia (Hassett et al., 2009), and 32 percent of patients eventually developed a fibromyalgia-like central sensitivity syndrome (not all met the criteria for fibromyalgia) (Hassett et al., 2010). Findings from studies conducted in Europe vary broadly, with anywhere from 2 to 48 percent of Lyme disease patients reporting symptoms after treatment consistent with central sensitivity syndromes (Cerar et al., 2010; Ljostaf and Mygland, 2010). The discrepancies in the European studies are likely due to differences in how the symptoms were measured. Biomarker research in central sensitivity syndromes could be highly pertinent to patients with persistent symptoms after treatment for Lyme disease. A recent study showed a decrease in natural killer cell cytotoxicity, and three different measures of CD26—an antigen located on cellular surfaces associated with immune regulation—accurately discriminated chronic fatigue syndrome patients from controls (Fletcher et al., 2010). Immune system biomarker research in irritable bowel syndrome has had mixed results, but there is some support for a dysfunctional mucosal immune response in these patients (Barbara and Stanghellini, 2009). For fibromyalgia, immune system research has suggested that IL-1β, IL-6, IL-8, and TNF-α contribute to central pain (Abbadie et al., 2003; Wang et al., 2008). The challenge, as noted earlier, is that many of the studies failed to control for variables such as obesity, autonomic nervous system dysfunction, and depression that are commonly observed in these populations and that have prominent effects on cytokine expression.

Studies involving twins have helped to reveal potential genetic biomarkers for central sensitivity syndromes. For example, one Swedish study (Kato et al., 2008) relied on a twin registry to investigate four somatic disorders (chronic widespread pain, chronic fatigue, irritable bowel syndrome, and recurrent headache) and two psychiatric disorders (major depressive disorder and generalized anxiety disorder). Multivariate twin analyses found a common genetic pathway for all six illnesses, but there were two distinct latent traits. One latent trait loaded heavily on the psychiatric disorders, while the other loaded on the somatic illnesses and not the psychiatric disorders. The somatic disorders were also affected by specific gene influences that were unique to each disorder. In family studies, first degree biological relatives of people with fibromyalgia had an eightfold higher risk of having fibromyalgia than did people without the familial link. There was also familial aggregation with mood disorders, but this was less pronounced (odds ratio of 2) (Arnold et al., 2004). Many of the genes thought to be involved in pain processing are also associated with mood disorders. This could help explain why pain and depression commonly co-occur. Psychiatric comorbidity is also common in patients with post-Lyme disease syndrome.

For example, in a study using gold-standard assessment interviews, 45 percent of patients with post-Lyme disease syndrome were found to meet the criteria for major depressive disorder (Hassett et al., 2009). Moreover, that percentage was higher than that found in patients with fibromyalgia and those with medically unexplained symptoms. Causality could not be determined in that study because of its cross-sectional design, thus it is not clear if the depression predisposed patients to post-Lyme disease syndrome, or if post-Lyme disease patients are depressed because they have a difficult illness that has disrupted their lives.

In a prospective study of newly diagnosed Lyme disease patients, baseline depression, anxiety, and other medical and psychological factors were measured and the patients were followed over time. After antibiotic treatment, approximately 32 percent of the patients developed chronic symptoms ascribed to Lyme disease. Chronic symptoms were predicted by the severity of the Lyme disease symptoms at baseline (Hassett et al., 2010). Furthermore, positive affect was perhaps the best predictor of who would develop chronic symptoms, such that patients with high levels of positive affect when first diagnosed were less likely to have persistent symptoms. Level of positive affect at baseline was unrelated to the severity of their symptoms at baseline. That finding reinforces numerous studies (Horan and Dellinger, 1974; Adames et al., 1986; Bruel et al., 1993; Zautra et al., 2005; Connelly et al., 2007) linking positive affect to positive outcomes from surgeries and lower sensitivity to pain. The results from this prospective study suggest that the high rates of depression among patients with post-Lyme disease are more likely to be due to living with a chronic condition than to a predisposing factor for symptom chronicity. However, patients with chronic symptoms after treatment for Lyme disease may have an underlying genetic or immunologic vulnerability that predisposes to both chronic pain and other symptoms including depression and anxiety.

In research looking for fibromyalgia biomarkers, numerous investigators have explored stress-response system functioning. Dysregulation of the hypothalamic–pituitary–adrenal (HPA) axis is frequently observed in central sensitivity syndromes. The nature of the reported abnormalities varies, but hyporesponsiveness of the HPA axis is found in 20 to 25 percent of the patients (Heim et al., 1998; Dedert et al., 2004; Van Den Eede et al., 2007; Wingenfeld et al., 2008). Further, in repeated-measure studies, a flat awakening cortisol level (McBeth et al., 2005; McLean et al., 2005; Weissbecker et al., 2006) and flat diurnal variation (Crofford et al., 2004; Dedert et al., 2004; Weissbecker et al., 2006) were observed in people with central sensitivity syndromes. In healthy individuals, cortisol peaks about 45 minutes after awakening as daily activities are initiated and then declines throughout the day. However, people with post-traumatic stress disorder and central sensitivity syndromes tend to have a low flat cortisol level, as if the HPA axis has lost its resiliency.

Although this pattern suggests an interesting biomarker for these patients, numerous cortisol studies have not accounted for depression, anxiety, childhood sexual or physical abuse, religiosity, positive affect, or other factors that can have a large effect on patients' cortisol levels. For example, a Swedish study (Tjernberg et al., 2010) found a higher cortisol response on an adrenocorticotropic hormone stimulation test among post-Lyme disease patients. The investigators, however, did not assess subjects for depression, even though it has been associated with such a response, so the significance of the finding is unclear. These results underscore the need to control for these potential confounding factors with thorough patient phenotyping.

In addition to the HPA axis, the autonomic nervous system is an important part of the stress-response system. For individuals with fibromyalgia and other central sensitivity syndromes, another common pattern has emerged. Patients with central sensitivity syndromes tend to have high baseline sympathetic arousal, decreased parasympathetic activity, and an attenuated response to stressors (Adeyemi et al., 1999; Cain et al., 2007; Gockel et al., 2008).

In evaluating these findings on stress response among people with central sensitivity syndromes, it is important to note that even when studies reveal mean differences between patients and controls, there is substantial overlap between the two groups. The fact that cortisol levels are correlated with momentary pain in fibromyalgia patients also suggests that the pain may be causing the autonomic nervous system dysfunction, rather than vice versa. Finally, people with baseline hypo- or hyperactivity of these stress response systems may be more likely to develop central sensitivity syndromes after exposure to stressors, including even routine events such as cessation of exercise or restrictions on sleep.

Recent studies of potential neural biomarkers for central sensitivity syndromes have shown that a number of factors influence an individual's sensitivity to pain. Neurotransmitters such as Substance P, nerve growth factor, and glutamate and other excitatory amino acids facilitate pain, while neural transmitters like norepinephrine, serotonin, dopamine, opioids, GABA (gamma-aminobutyric acid), adenosine, and cannabanoids inhibit pain. High levels of facilitatory neural transmitters and low levels of inhibitatory transmitters are linked to hyperalgesia, or higher sensitivity to pain. For fibromyalgia patients, there are elevations of neurotransmitters that facilitate pain and low levels of those that inhibit pain. Only the opioid levels appear to be appropriate in these patients, which may explain why opioids are not effective for relieving fibromyalgia pain.

Finally, neuroimaging has contributed significantly to our understanding of pain in fibromyalgia. In a 2002 study using functional magnetic resonance imaging (MRI), fibromyalgia patients showed activation of 12 cortical areas following pressure applied to the thumb bed. Controls need approximately twice the level of pressure applied to elicit the same pain response as demonstrated by a similar activation pattern as seen in the fibromyalgia group (Gracely et al., 2002). Finally, proton magnetic resonance spectroscopy imaging studies suggest that patients with fibromyalgia tend to have increased levels of glutamate in the insula and that these levels are associated with sensitivity to pain.

In summary, research suggests that

- Although depression is common among people with post-Lyme disease, it does not explain the symptoms nor predict which patients with active *Borrelia burgdorferi* infection will later develop post-Lyme disease. These individuals could have a genetic vulnerability to central sensitivity syndromes, which might offer a productive approach to better identify those at risk.
- Good biomarkers for post-Lyme disease are not yet available. However, conceptualizing the disease as having roots in central nervous system dysfunction could help chart the way toward identifying such biomarkers.
- Promising areas to explore for biomarkers for post-Lyme disease include immune abnormalities, proteomics, genetics, neurotransmitter levels, stress-response system functioning, and neuroimaging.

### Knowledge Gaps and Research Opportunities

Hassett noted that a state-of-the-art biorepository is essential to finding biomarkers for post-Lyme disease. To meet this research goal, the following features need to be considered:

- A repository should include a wide range of samples, including serum, plasma, cerebrospinal fluid, organ tissue, heart rate variability, imaging studies, and genetic information.
- The patients whose samples would be included in the biorepository must be carefully phenotyped. That detailed information should be collected and made available in regard to clinical characteristics of their Lyme disease, other medical comorbidities, psychiatric comorbidities, psychological factors, symptom profile and severity, and functional status.
- The biorepository would have high-quality maintenance and provide open access to all researchers.
- A conference or workshop convened specifically to hear all viewpoints regarding the attributes of such a biorepository would help make it a reality.

## DISCUSSION

One participant noted that recent studies (Gomes-Solecki et al., 2007; Sillanpaa et al., 2007) suggest that the C6 testing paradigm is not as sensitive as it needs to be and was highly dependent on the particular *Borrelia* strain used during development. The participant questioned whether the test would have a higher sensitivity if it used the same *B. burgdorferi* strains that are in the patient's geographic region. Aguero-Rosenfeld noted that the C6 assay that is commercially available in the United States as a Food and Drug Administration (FDA) approved test uses *B. burgdorferi* American genotype. While other researchers have looked into incorporating different sequences, the U.S. commercial test uses *B. burgdorferi* sensu stricto. What was not discussed in detail in the three studies (Bacon et al., 2003; Steere et al., 2008; Wormser et al., unpublished) described earlier is that two of the studies used in-house developed C6 assays. More recent, unpublished results suggest that the sensitivity of C6 is better than reported by Bacon et al. Aguero-Rosenfeld further noted the need for including other components, such as OspC and VlsE, to potentially improve these assays.

Another clinician noted that for research purposes, specificity of the testing is the goal, but many clinicians are more interested in sensitivity. They do not want to overtreat, but as noted during the workshop, complications can result when patients are not properly diagnosed. Aguero-Rosenfeld noted that the diagnostic test needs to combine the right antigen with less cross-reactivity. That would result in a test that has high sensitivity and high specificity. She further noted that the testing available today does not have the specificity needed and it can be difficult to find a balance between sensitivity and specificity.

Another participant questioned why IgM is only useful for diagnosis in early disease. Aguero-Rosenfeld noted that in very well-characterized Lyme disease patients, IgM positivity remained up to a year or more after a patient was well. She noted that IgM antibody-validated diagnostic criteria were restricted to acute Lyme disease in the first month of illness. Furthermore, IgM immunoblot reading and interpretation is prone to yield false-positive results when weak reactivities are scored and reported.

## PANEL: CHALLENGES FOR CLINICIANS IN DIAGNOSIS AND MANAGEMENT OF CHRONIC ILLNESS MANIFESTATIONS: KNOWLEDGE GAPS

*Sam T. Donta, M.D., Professor of Medicine (ret.),*
*Infectious Diseases, Falmouth Hospital, MA*

The clinical challenges involving Lyme disease are multifaceted, and research is needed to support the challenges in clinical diagnosis, diagnostic tools, and treatment. As most individuals will agree, the diagnosis of acute Lyme disease is relatively straightforward. The challenges arise in the diagnosis of "chronic Lyme disease" or "post-Lyme disease." The criteria for chronic disease include fatigue, musculoskeletal symptoms, and neurocognitive impairments involving memory, concentration, and mood. Minor criteria include an array of nonspecific symptoms such as headaches, eye and/or ear symptoms, jaw/tooth pain, Bell's palsy, disequilibrium, dyspnea, and others.

One difficulty that clinicians face is the absence of objective, measurable evidence for these symptoms. Unless a patient has an observable sign such as Bell's palsy, a swollen joint, or a rash (EM), the clinician cannot easily attribute the patient's symptoms to Lyme disease. A second difficulty arises in distinguishing the array of symptoms from those associated with other multisymptom illnesses such as chronic fatigue syndrome (CFS), fibromyalgia, or Gulf War syndrome. Clinicians are hard-pressed to say whether a patient's complex of symptoms is caused by Lyme disease or some other etiology. For example, MRI findings in patients considered to have chronic Lyme disease can show signals that are confused or overlap with multiple sclerosis. Single-photon emission computerized tomography scans also can be positive. At the same time, patients press clinicians to provide an explanation, a diagnosis, for their symptoms.

Research is needed to define what is happening in terms of the pathogenesis of Lyme disease. It is important to understand "what about the organism is doing what," as well as to understand how the host is responding. Greater focus needs to be placed on the former.

The bacteria are very difficult or impossible to find in the patient, even during the acute phase of the disease. Improvement in direct detection techniques may permit documentation of the bacteria in the future, but until that occurs, it is difficult to say definitively that a patient has Lyme disease or, conversely, that a patient no longer has Lyme disease following antibiotic therapy.

Another fertile area of research surrounds the mechanisms involved in Lyme disease (i.e., the ways in which the bacteria trigger the associated symptoms). One possibility is direct toxicity, in which a toxin produced by the bacteria perturbs the local nerve involved or the central nervous system, as is the case with tetanus and botulism. A toxin or other antigen might trigger the production of antibodies and an autoimmune reaction in the patient, although no evidence indicates this is the case in Lyme disease. Tetanus toxin, botulinum toxin, and other toxins bind to gangliosides in the nervous system, causing direct interference with nerve transmission, thus providing a precedent for other toxins to act in an analogous fashion. The fact that certain antibiotics can eliminate the symptoms patients experience supports the hypothesis that the continuing presence of the organism is responsible for the symptoms.

A third difficulty in diagnosing chronic Lyme disease is the lack of criteria for ELISA and Western blot results in those patients. The criteria that exist were developed for "late Lyme disease" and may not apply to patients farther removed from the initial infection. Our study of patients with chronic Lyme disease illustrates the difficulty in the diagnostic criteria as one third of the patients show neither a positive ELISA nor a positive Western blot. The number of positive Western blots increases when IgM is included. In addition, the IgM immunoblot tends to disappear following successful treatment with tetracycline (Donta, 1997), although not for all patients.

Considering the presence of IgM antibodies to be indicative of early disease, but to be considered a false positive in later disease, is illogical; perhaps IgM does persist as a sign of continuing, unresolved infection. A patient with IgM reactivity to the 23 kDa OspC protein and symptoms indicative of chronic Lyme disease definitely has been exposed to *Borrelia*, because there is no other identified cause of any cross reactivity. The number of bands should not be what provides the laboratory support for the clinical diagnosis, but rather it is the specificity of the reaction that is important. The numbers were established for surveillance criteria, which are much more restrictive, and then translated into clinical criteria. Regardless, the current laboratory antibody-based tests are adjunctive to the clinical picture.

Neurologists routinely persist in the assertion that the cerebrospinal fluid of patients with neuro-Lyme disease will be positive for the bacteria. This misconception needs to change. The amount of IgG synthesis in the spinal fluid of those patients rarely is more than that found in the serum. All of these tests are fraught with difficulties.

In summary, symptom-based treatments are important, but they do not address the underlying pathology. A patient's response to antibiotic treatment can be important as a diagnostic tool. More research involving clinical trials is needed for diagnostic tools, including direct antigen detection, and for vaccine development, as well as additional clinical antibiotic trials.

*Brian A. Fallon, M.D., M.P.H., Columbia University Medical Center
and the New York State Psychiatric Institute*

Helping patients with chronic persistent symptoms requires understanding who the patient is, the chief complaint, the history of this person's disease, and the history of treatment. Clinicians' ability to help such patients depends on their experience with other similar patients and on what is known from the literature about the particular patient population. Before reviewing what is known about this patient group from the literature, it is important to emphasize that researchers and clinicians often have very different goals. Researchers aim to answer a specific question in a very tightly controlled setting, while clinicians aim to relieve suffering for an individual person and to help that person return to an active life. The clinical setting is filled with numerous confounding variables, and diagnostic and treatment decisions are often based on different levels of probability rather than on certainty. Treatment decisions also often reflect a cost–benefit analysis.

Turning to the literature pertaining to patients with chronic persistent symptoms, Fallon noted a number of areas need additional research. A European study compared patients with neurologic Lyme disease to those with erythema migrans, 3 years later, and found that 50 percent of those with neuroborreliosis experienced persistent symptoms versus 16 percent of the EM patients (Vrethem et al., 2002). These results suggest that rather than focusing solely on early EM, follow-up studies on chronic symptoms, should focus on the subpopulation of patients who present with neurologic or other disseminated symptoms.

Children are an at-risk population—another subpopulation that needs further research. A 2003 study found that 43 children with a history of cranial nerve palsy experienced more neck pain, behavioral changes, arthralgias, nerve sensations, and memory problems compared to age-matched controls (Vazquez et al., 2003). The study found no difference in functional impairments between the two groups, which raises the question of whether there is a difference between the effects on children and adults.

Finally, a study of Lyme disease encephalopathy at Columbia showed that most of the cognitive impairments the patients experienced were mild to moderate, primarily affecting verbal memory, working memory, and verbal fluency. Interestingly, the patients experienced only mild psychopathology; while some depression and anxiety were reported, these were not prominent (Fallon et al., 2008). Many patients (72 percent of Lyme disease patients versus 22 percent of controls), however, demonstrated sensory loss on their neurologic exams. On the rheumatologic exam, many patients had multiple-joint involvement compared to very few joints involved in the control group. Few of the Lyme disease patients exhibited multiple trigger points, suggesting that fibromyalgia was not a significant problem, at least if it is defined based on trigger points.

Future studies of patients with chronic symptoms should focus on the most prominent problems they report, which are pain, fatigue, and physical disability. When examining the patient's treatment history, 70 percent of the patients screened for participation in the Lyme disease encephalopathy study had had at least 2 months of prior intravenous antibiotic therapy, and many of them had had significant oral treatment (Fallon et al., 2008). These facts suggest that many people continue to experience persistent symptoms despite having received a significant amount of antibiotic therapy.

Despite a large number of patients screened with persistent symptoms, few of them met the strict criteria for inclusion in the Columbia study. Only 1 percent had objective cognitive impairments, a positive IgG Western blot, prior intravenous therapy, and documentation of prior Lyme disease. We learned that a requirement of IgG Western blot positivity at time of enrollment for studies of patients with chronic symptoms following Lyme disease will exclude a large number of patients with good clinical histories, thus hampering enrollment and narrowing the generalizability of the findings.

Ten percent of patients in the Lyme disease encephalopathy sample had a history of co-infections. There was no difference in the incidence of human granulocytic anaplasmosis between the Lyme disease patients and the controls, but *Babesia* IgG was positive in 27 percent of the Lyme disease patients versus none of the controls. There was a high rate of *Bartonella* IgG positivity in the Lyme disease patients, but also in the controls, suggesting that exposure to Bartonella is common in the population.

Cerebrospinal fluid findings across four studies of patients with persistent symptoms following Lyme borreliosis showed elevated protein in 25.8 percent, 7.3 percent, and 12.1 percent of the patients, respectively (Klemper et al., 2001; Krupp et al., 2003; Fallon et al., 2008).

Brain imaging studies at the National Institutes of Health (NIH) reported that 55 percent of the patients with post-treatment Lyme disease exhibited hyperintensities on MRI (Morgen et al., 2001). Another study comparing the Lyme disease encephalopathy patients with controls well-matched for age, sex, and education showed no difference in the white matter hyperintensity density (DelaPaz et al., 2005). The study did find that the patients who had had Lyme disease were more likely to have blood flow deficits in their brains, as well as metabolic differences on positron emission tomography imaging, compared with the well-matched controls (Fallon et al., 2009). Prior work found the blood flow deficits to be reversible with intravenous ceftriaxone therapy (Logigian et al., 1997).

With respect to pathophysiology, *Borrelia* act directly and can invade neural cells *in vitro* (Livengood and Gilmore, 2006); there are also indirect actions, such as the induction of local cytotoxins or inflammatory mediators (reviewed in Fallon et al., 2010). European studies show that pro-inflammatory cytokines are increased, and chemokines, excitotoxin, and quinolinic acid are increased in patients with neuroborreliosis (Weller et al., 1991; Halperin and Heyes, 1992; Widhe et al., 2004; Rupprecht et al., 2005).

A rich field of research is psychoneuroimmunology, in which studies have suggested that individuals with risk factors for inflammatory disorders and for psychiatric disorders are more likely than those without them to experience chronic peripheral inflammation and chronic activation of the brain cytokine pathways following infections, leading to subjective health complaints similar to those in Lyme disease and a number of other disorders (Dantzer et al., 2008). Anti-neural antibody reactivity is increased in patients with persistent symptoms following treatment for Lyme disease (Alaedini and Fallon, 2010; Chandra et al., 2010). Approximately 50 percent of patients enrolled in two independent studies (Klemper et al., 2001; Fallon et al., 2008) of patients with chronic, persistent symptoms had elevated levels of anti-neural antibodies, indicating there is an abnormally activated immunological process at work in some of these patients with chronic symptoms.

A summary of the possible explanations for chronic, persistent symptoms in patients following treatment for Lyme disease includes: persistent infection in some patients; reinfection from a later tick bite; reactivation of a latent, dormant infection; widely distributed effects from a small amount of physiologically active but attenuated spirochetes; or post-infectious phenomena, such as spirochete-triggered immune abnormalities, neurotransmitter/receptor changes, or damage from prior infection. The symptoms also could be related to an unrecognized concurrent process, such as another TBD, another non-tick-borne infection, or another disease (e.g., depression or hypothyroidism).

There is a danger that persistent symptoms following treatment for Lyme disease will be labeled as somatoform. In part this may be due to clinicians' assumptions that 2 to 4 weeks of antibiotic therapy is always curative and that any symptoms after minimal antibiotic treatment are due to other causes. It may also reflect a clinician's failure to recognize that any infection may have a course of post-infectious symptoms that can continue for a year or more. In addition, some clinicians may experience hostility or frustration toward patients with chronic illnesses or may misinterpret the patient's presentation with anxiety and multi-systemic, nonobjective symptoms as indicative of a psychiatric etiology.

*Richard F. Jacobs, M.D., University of Arkansas for Medical Sciences and Arkansas Children's Hospital Research Institute*

One of the challenges that clinicians face in the diagnosis and management of tick-borne diseases (TBDs) in children is a poor understanding of the true incidence and geographic distribution of the diseases. The more information is known about the different variations of these organisms, the greater the realization will be that what has been taught about geographic distribution is not true. Another challenge is the similarity in the multisystem presentation among the TBDs. In addition, diagnostics are limited in acute illness, and the rates of chronic illness and morbidity are unknown. There is information about neuroborreliosis in adults, but aside from a few studies in children, there are no data on any of the TBDs that are sufficiently reliable to tell parents what the potential chronic neurologic or other sequelae may be.

Children are different; they are not little adults. They are still developing, and they have a very different central nervous system from adults, as well as a developing immune system. For this reason, it is important to recognize and study children as a distinct population. Furthermore, it is also important to keep in mind that the duration of any long-term effects of disease in this population will last 50 to 70 years.

Jacobs noted there is a need to provide enhanced educational information to clinicians—not only pediatricians, but also family physicians, advanced practice nurses, and physicians' assistants—about the clinical manifestations of and other information regarding tick-borne illnesses. Conventional wisdom about spotted fever rickettsiosis (Rocky Mountain spotted fever) indicates that young children have a lower mortality rate, but a much higher infection rate, than do older adults (Dalton et al., 1995), although this generalization is not completely accurate. In addition, the fatality rate increases dramatically among cases in which treatment was not started until after the fifth day following the onset of symptoms (Dalton et al., 1995). Therefore, it is important to make treatment decisions presumptively and empirically based upon a patient's clinical presentation.

Experience with *Ehrlichia chaffeensis* led to the recognition of a set of symptoms associated with ehrlichial infection. Fever and rash are common, but a host of other signs and symptoms occur as well: myalgia, headache, vomiting, diarrhea, and puffy eyes (Schutze and Jacobs, 1997). The physical presentation of ehrlichiosis has a large differential diagnosis, including a significant overlap with Rocky Mountain spotted fever (Buckingham et al., 2007), but the clinical laboratory triad of thrombocytopenia, leukopenia with lymphopenia, and elevated hepatic enzymes suggests human monocytic ehrlichiosis and warrants doxycycline therapy at admission (Schutze and Jacobs, 1997), given the importance of prompt treatment in reducing mortality.

Compounding the challenges of diagnosis and prompt treatment, different pediatric diseases within the differential for tick-borne illnesses, such as Kawasaki syndrome and meningococcemia, require very different therapies, but on a similarly urgent time line. The clinical challenge is that the diagnostics and clinicians' understanding about the ecosystem and the organism do not allow them to separate these clinically.

Consider a child with a rash on her arms, legs, face, hands, and feet, along with fever, headache, and pleocytosis in her CSF. Rocky Mountain spotted fever and ehrlichiosis certainly are on the list of differential diagnoses. But the child had disseminated meningococcemia, which carries a 20 to 40 percent mortality rate had it not been treated with a third-generation cephalosporin on admission. This example highlights both the difficulty and the urgency of separating these diseases clinically.

The clinical challenge is compounded by the short incubation period of the TBDs. Antibody testing is not useful in the acute management of Rocky Mountain spotted fever or human monocytic ehrlichiosis. Both infections, as well as others, respond to treatment with doxycycline, however, so physicians are taught to administer doxycycline.

In terms of knowledge gaps, more data and understanding are needed on the genetics, predisposing factors, and epidemiology associated with tick-borne illnesses. In addition, more information is needed about the organisms, acute and persistent infections, diagnostics, spectrum of disease, and chronic manifestations and outcomes. In addition to the dearth of information in these areas for adults, there is virtually no knowledge of most of these infectious diseases as they relate to the unique attributes of children.

Lessons have been learned about the different impacts of acute disease from babies exposed to herpes simplex virus, different disease manifestations from children with tuberculosis, age-related immune responses to vaccinations, unknown central nervous system effects (autism-spectrum disorders), age-related exposures and adaptive immunity (Kawasaki's disease), and central nervous system growth and development (use of folic acid to prevent neural tube defects). But much of the biology remains a mystery.

Jacobs noted the United States needs a study group to explore tick-associated and tick-borne infections in children. Two models currently exist. The NIH/National Institutes of Allergy and Infectious Diseases Collaborative Anti-Viral Study Group has operated for 30 years. Thirty-two sites now study rare diseases. The study of TBDs can follow the same model. The National Children's Study, now NIH funded, involves randomly selected, geographically dispersed counties in the United States. that will follow pregnant women and their babies until the children are 20 years old. The study provides an opportunity to collect information in a repository, including biological samples and detailed historical information, and is charged to look at priority exposures and examples. Infectious agents are already listed as one of the study areas. The National Children's Study provides a wonderful opportunity to use a currently NIH-funded, 20-year-long prospective study to focus some attention on TBD.

*Matthew H. Liang, M.D., M.P.H., Harvard Medical School
and Harvard School of Public Health*

In unselected, non-specialty (primary care) practices, atypical manifestations of common illnesses are much more common than typical manifestations of uncommon illnesses. Primary care physicians build their practices on their patients' trust in and access to them, both of which are necessary for fine-tuning a diagnosis or refining a treatment. The usual strategy is to identify treatable illnesses, make a working presumptive diagnosis, treat, and assess the outcome. If the treatment is not working, the physician may get more information, refine the diagnosis, and/or change the treatment. The process can be threatened, or lulled into complacency, by the primary care physician's familiarity with the patient and the underlying probability that the illness is benign rather than serious. These factors sometimes make it difficult to keep an open mind about a patient with a persistent problem.

The presentation of Lyme disease in clinical practice is variable. Thirty-nine percent of patients ultimately considered to have Lyme disease do not meet the Centers for Disease Control and Prevention (CDC) criteria, and approximately 40 percent had negative Lyme disease serology and an acute viral-like illness without objective findings. Nearly one-third of the patients had a rash that did not meet the criteria for EM, and only 19 percent of those with EM exhibited the stereotypical bull's-eye appearance (Aucott et al., 2009).

Given the variability, it is helpful when patients can provide the actual tick or a good description of a fed tick, as well as a time line to indicate how long the tick had been on them. A tick has to feed for 48 to 72 hours to transfer *Borrelia* to the host. The finding of a tick that is not well fed decreases the probability that it infected the patient. Clinicians also look for EM or forme-frustes, although EM can look like almost anything and is often mistaken for spider bites.

Generally clinicians would treat empirically because of the importance of early treatment and the assumption that there is little to lose because treatment can always be stopped. This presupposes the treatment has minimal negative effects. As mentioned previously, doxycycline is a common default treatment for suspected tick-borne illness; however, there are some downsides, including dental staining.

A prime area for intervention is educating people about prevention. Successful education requires understanding and reversing the thought barriers that prevent people from receiving and acting upon the message. There is, as already noted, a 48- to 72-hour time window within which to find a tick before it can infect the host, and a nightly shower provides ample opportunity to interrupt the life cycle. In theory, improved education will increase prevention and decrease the occurrence of Lyme disease.

A 5-year study randomized 29,000 people traveling by ferry to Nantucket (Daltroy and Phillips, 2007). The study group was exposed to an entertainment-based information session about Lyme disease and steps to prevent it. Participants also received a card with a Braille dot on it the size of a tick and a plastic shower card similar to those used for breast self-exam, tweezers, and a map of the island where ticks were prevalent. The study showed a reduction in Lyme disease in the group who received the message, both among year-round residents and among visitors, who constitute a high-risk population.

A population-based retrospective cohort study of 38 patients in a particular location in Ipswich, Massachusetts, who had been treated for Lyme disease showed 13 patients with ongoing symptoms of arthritis or recurrent arthralgias, neurocognitive impairment, neuropathy, or myelopathy (Shadick et al., 1994). The individuals with these sequelae tended to have higher IgG antibody levels to the spirochete and also to have received treatment later following infection. One of the 13, a 76-year-old woman, had been worked up by Lyme disease experts, had received two courses of ceftriaxone, and was negative for objective central nervous system findings. She died and at post mortem a Dieterle silver stain demonstrated two spirochetes, one in the cortex and another external to a leptomingeal brain vessel (Shadick et al., 1994).

Another study of approximately 6,000 year-round residents of Nantucket showed patients who had been diagnosed with Lyme disease and continued to be symptomatic following treatment, but the study presented few objective findings. This reinforces the challenges that clinicians face in the diagnosis and treatment of patients with chronic persistent symptoms following Lyme borreliosis.

In treating such patients, it is important to ensure that a thorough history and physical exam are conducted and that they have received sufficiently long courses of the appropriate doses and types of antibiotics. Beyond that, at a certain point the diagnosis matters less than treating the symptoms in an effort to maintain and improve function. In addition, it sometimes is necessary to assist patients in revising their expectations as well.

## DISCUSSION

Much of the discussion focused on the challenges associated with the diagnosis of TBDs, both in patients with acute illness and in those experiencing persistent symptoms following an initial diagnosis of and treatment for Lyme disease. A second focus of discussion centered on the occurrence of Lyme borreliosis and other TBDs in children.

One participant questioned the reliability of screening tests, such as white blood cell count and standard neurological exam, to evaluate patients with chronic symptoms. Liang felt that these tests are not particularly useful and noted that there is tremendous variation among practitioners in terms of their approach to patients with persistent symptoms.

With regard to diagnosing TBDs in children, Jacobs noted that practitioners have come to rely on a clinical presentation of multisystem disease, in which the clinician must determine which systems are involved and create a differential diagnosis that is treatable. He reiterated the approach discussed by Krause, in which clinicians learn to look at particular presentations on screening tests (e.g., anemia, with thrombocytopenia) in acute infection to help make a diagnosis. The presence of multisystem disease and a specific picture of laboratory results together can generate a presumptive diagnosis and the initiation of treatment. Jacobs stressed, however, the need to develop better diagnostic testing that would permit more definitive diagnosis of TBDs.

Another participant questioned the practice of those clinicians who use the absence of direct markers of an infecting organism following treatment as evidence of the treatment's success given the absence of, or the current inability to identify and test for, markers for the presence of infecting organisms prior to treatment as well.

With respect to cognitive dysfunction, one participant asked about the ability of brain SPECT scanning to distinguish hypoperfusion brain damage and cognitive dysfunction caused by TBDs from that caused by long-term excessive use of medication. Fallon agreed that certain medications can confuse the interpretation of SPECT scans. Cocaine use, although not a medication, can cause heterogenous hypoperfusion consistent with vasculitis, which appears similar to that seen in Lyme disease patients who have had SPECT scans. He also stated that despite the power of such imaging tools for research purposes, the use of SPECT scanning as a clinical tool is of questionable reliability because rarely are systematic methods used to evaluate the scans against healthy populations, making variation in readings across clinicians likely and interpretations of clinical significance difficult.

A question was posed about the implications of multiple phenotypes or strains of *Borrelia* and other organisms for the development of new, improved diagnostics. It has to do with moving forward into the new diagnostics. Fallon reiterated that 17 different isolates of *Borrelia* in the United States have been sequenced and their antigens are now known. He mentioned the possibility of using that information to study a wide sample of patients and perhaps trying to correlate some of their clinical profiles, clinical histories, and/or treatment outcomes with these actual antigenic profiles. Doing so would require a very large study of many patients followed up with good bioinformatics over a long period of time, but the ability is there to do it.

With respect to the experience and impact of Lyme disease and chronic persistent symptoms in children, Jacobs emphasized how difficult it is to have to tell concerned parents that there is simply no solid information about the long-term effects and impact of the disease on the child.

A participant observed that it seems as if the numbers of children experiencing symptoms and being diagnosed with illnesses such as fibromyalgia or chronic fatigue syndrome have risen since the last generation and asked whether schools could be surveyed to obtain information on the school-age population and the kind of symptoms and difficulties they are experiencing. Jacobs discussed the current National Children's Study as an example of a study looking at the complex interactions among the environment, infectious agents, and genetics. He expressed the need to tap into the new area of bioinformatics, which can provide detailed information on participants, and combine that information with access to environmental samples from the National Children's Survey, as well as human samples in a biorepository. Such a data repository would provide a very rich source of information to probe once there are better diagnostics, better biomarkers, or a better understanding of which imaging system or type of testing to do.

A question was raised regarding concerns about privacy and confidentiality, among citizens and schools, as well as publicized knowledge of being located in a tick-endemic area. Jacobs acknowledged the possibility of such concerns, but that generally when members of a community are or become vested in a project, the schools and other community organizations follow. Another participant indicated that the interest level in participating in such a trial would be high in that community.

Related to questions about the long-term impact of Lyme disease and other TBDs on children as they develop and mature, a request for greater consideration of gender differences and issues specific to women in these diseases was made by one participant. She specifically mentioned the impact of hormonal fluctuations (e.g., during adolescence and puberty, pregnancy, and menopause) on symptoms. Questions were also raised about congenital transmission of the diseases as well as their impact on fertility. Donta noted that there are changes in the severity of symptoms experienced by women not only with Lyme disease but also with various chronic conditions, such as chronic fatigue syndrome, as hormone levels fluctuate. In addition there is a gender difference in Lyme disease, perhaps related to the presence of estrogen and progesterone receptors in glial and neural cells. Jacobs reiterated the need for a large-scale, long-term study, such as the National Children's Study, involving bioinformatics, although he acknowledged that the results would not be available in time to help inform the parents of children currently experiencing symptoms. Nevertheless, such a study would provide hope that the present large knowledge gaps will be filled in the future.

## CONCLUDING THOUGHTS ON
## DIAGNOSIS AND DIAGNOSTICS

*Lynn Gerber, M.D., Center for the Study of Chronic Illness
and Disability, George Mason University
David H. Walker, M.D., Department of Pathology,
University of Texas Medical Branch at Galveston*

Many participants in this session noted that diagnosis of tick-borne diseases remains problematic. This could be ameliorated using a three-pronged approach: (1) education of clinicians about which diagnostic tests to use, when to use them during the course of the disease, and how to interpret these results; (2) developing and applying new technology for serological assays to close the gap between bench and bedside using microfluidic technology, automation, and nanotechnology to achieve accurate, fast, and inexpensive diagnostic tests; and (3) consensus building to establish criteria for clinical phases of disease in children and adults, possibly describing necessary and sufficient criteria for arriving at common nomenclature, such as in systemic lupus erythematosus, chronic fatigue syndrome, and fibromyalgia, among others.

Clinicians need better education regarding the limitations of existing tests, and how to interpret the results. Some 10–20 percent of healthy people in some regions may already carry antibodies to a particular organism, such as *Rickettsia rickettsii* or *Ehrlichia chaffeensis*. The antibodies might stem from exposure to a related organism that caused a subclinical infection. In that situation, a clinician who does not realize that a patient with acute febrile illness has had antibodies for a long period might wrongly diagnose rickettsiosis or ehrlichiosis on the basis of a single acute serologic test. In fact, clinicians often fail to do a follow-up serologic test to determine whether the concentration of antibodies to a tick-borne disease in a patient is rising.

Clinicians need to understand that testing patients with a low likelihood of a tick-borne disease strongly undermines the test's positive predictive value. When clinicians do test such patients, a substantial proportion will be false positives. Lengthy menus of tests also present a barrier to effective diagnosis of tick-borne illness by clinicians who are not familiar with the advantages and disadvantages of many laboratory assays.

Some clinicians also use serologic assays for IgM antibodies that have not been validated through well-documented series of cases. The soaring incidence of reported spotted fever rickettsial infections—few of which have been confirmed by methods specific to *R. rickettsii*—is one result.

Some presenters in this session emphasized that patients with tick-borne diseases do not develop antibodies to an infectious organism until some time after the onset of illness, because of the nature of the immune response. That means existing tests that may be highly reliable later in the disease are insensitive early on. It also means that diagnosing a tick-borne infection requires knowledge of a patient's geographic and seasonal exposure to ticks as well as the clinical manifestations of tick-borne diseases.

Despite these diagnostic shortcomings, tick-borne diseases such as human ehrlichioses and anaplasmosis likely have undiagnosed incidence equal to that of Lyme borreliosis. And they and Rocky Mountain spotted fever carry the threat of a fatal outcome, which Lyme disease does not.

New methods that can determine which species of *Rickettsia* or *Babesia* a person has encountered are particularly important. Some participants noted that investigators also need to develop tests that can shed light on the etiology of southern tick associated rash illness (STARI), whose erythema migrans resembles that of Lyme disease but is not caused by *B. burgdorferi*.

Creating biorepositories and a network of clinical studies, such as those now supported by the National Institute of Child Health and Human Development, would greatly enhance the opportunity to improve diagnostics by providing wider access to stored specimens as well as clinical information. Sera from documented cases of tick-borne diseases—during both acute and convalescent phases—would enable scientists to validate new serologic tests. Such repositiories would aid in enabling investigators correlate symptoms and biological findings and help develop evaluative and treatment outcome criteria. It might help determine whether children, for example, have a different course of illness, given that their central nervous and immune systems are still developing.

Samples of whole blood and cerebrospinal fluid, tissue biopsies, and other specimens would allow scientists to validate the use of PCR for amplifying nucleic acids and to identify and validate novel methods of detecting tick-borne pathogens. The recently sequenced genomes of different strains of *B. burgdorferi* also promise to allow scientists to develop new diagnostics and ultimately, preventive measures. The community affected by Lyme borreliosis and other tick-borne diseases seeks guidance on prognosis and treatment, and that has not yet been achieved.

Throughout the workshop, during podium presentations and comments and questions from the floor, participants employed descriptive terminology pertaining to Lyme disease in different ways. This presented several challenges to discussants in that it was not always clear that the topic under discussion was addressing acute, chronic, recurrent phases of illness or other co-infections. Better descriptors would provide a uniform vocabulary for clinicians, researchers, and patients. They would also provide a basis for building and validating a comprehensive, sensitive battery of tools for evaluating both objective and patient-reported outcomes for tick-borne diseases. Improved descriptors should include both signs and symptoms: that is, information that is both objective and self-reported, and that includes physical findings, serological measures, and psychological measures, among others.

Further exploration of the stress response to tick-borne pathogens could help expand our understanding of the pathogenesis and natural history of Lyme disease. One approach is to investigate the role of the hypothalamic–pituitary–adrenal axis and the cortisol response in people with chronic Lyme disease symptoms that resemble those of other chronic fatigue or pain syndromes. Another would be to determine whether there is a genetic vulnerability to central sensitivity syndromes, which might offer a productive approach to better identify those at risk. Good biomarkers for post-Lyme disease are not yet available. However, conceptualizing the disease as having roots in central nervous system dysfunction could help chart the way.

# 8

# Prevention

The societal burden of tick-borne diseases (TBDs) is substantial. In the United States alone, every year this group of diseases produces tens of thousands of illnesses, many of which are severe and result in hospitalization, long-term sequelae, including disabilities or deaths. Research efforts have been focused on ameliorating the symptoms and consequences of disease through treatment. However, the development, deployment, and evaluation of strategies to prevent the occurrence of TBDs should also be a major area of scientific inquiry. This is one aspect of the debate about tick-borne diseases where there is no controversy. Prevention of disease is far preferable to treating the short- and long-term consequences once they occur.

The incidence rate of all of the diseases discussed in this workshop has been on the increase. They have also been expanding in geographic range, and new human tick-borne pathogens continue to be recognized. These trends result in an ever-larger number of persons requiring treatment, placing a greater financial impact on the healthcare system and individual patients, and, ultimately, a greater burden on society. The escalating burden of TBDs is a clear demonstration that the available prevention measures have been ineffective. Whether this is because they simply do not work or because they have been underused is far less clear. But a wider array of simple and effective prevention modalities would be very beneficial and would, it is hoped, change the current trajectory of TBD incidence.

Prevention measures can be divided into two categories: Pharmacologic preventive measures such as antibiotic prophylaxis or vaccines, and non-pharmacologic interventions such as behavior change or tick-targeted strategies (e.g., tick checks or tick reduction). In this workshop, information was presented for both categories, but there was not enough time to cover the entire range of available or potential approaches. Two presentations addressed current and future opportunities for vaccine development. One presentation addressed the role and effectiveness of behavior change and another addressed vector-control strategies.

## CURRENT VACCINES FOR TICK-BORNE DISEASES AND VACCINE DEVELOPMENT

*Jere W. McBride, Ph.D., M.S., Center for Biodefense and Emerging Infectious Diseases, University of Texas Medical Branch at Galveston*

Currently, no tick-borne disease vaccines for humans are licensed in the United States. The U.S. Food and Drug Administration licensed a vaccine for Lyme disease in 1998 and it was withdrawn from the market in 2002. While the vaccine—based on outer surface protein A (OspA) emulsified in aluminum hydroxide adjuvant—prevented transmission of *Borrelia burgdorferi* from ticks to humans by killing spirochetes in ticks, three doses were needed to provide 80 percent protection against infection. A number of problems contributed to the withdrawal of the vaccine. The antibody titers did not persist for long time periods, which required individuals to receive multiple boosters to maintain protective immunity. Furthermore, a number of autoimmune-related side effects, including arthritis and neuropathology, were reported to possibly be associated with the vaccine (Schuijt et al., 2011). A short stretch of amino acids in OspA with the potential for molecular mimicry with human LFA-1 (lymphocyte function associated antigen) was identified as a possible cause for the autoimmune-related responses, but this finding remains controversial (Steere et al., 2001; Ball et al., 2009). In Europe, current efforts are focused on developing vaccines with a modified OspA that does not contain the sequence linked to autoimmune responses. Other vaccines for *Borrelia* are in varying stages of development as either single- or multiple-antigen vaccines that include OspB, OspC, or DNA-binding protein HU-alpha.

Experimental veterinary vaccines for bovine anaplasmosis and infection and treatment strategies for heartwater—an ehrlichiosis of ruminants—demonstrate that vaccines for human rickettsial diseases are feasible. To develop such vaccines, however, some basic research on these emerging infectious diseases needs to be done, including:

- Defining immunoprotective pathogen proteins;
- Understanding and defining pathogen antigenic variation;
- Understanding variations in pathogenicity;
- Understanding protective immune mechanisms;

- Developing appropriate animal models;
- Understanding host influence on pathogen phenotype and transmission;
- Defining pathogen and host gene expression during infection to identify vaccine candidates;
- Understanding molecular host-pathogen interactions that can be blocked by the host immune response; and
- Identification and development of vector vaccine components.

A number of studies have elucidated a host's protective immune mechanisms against *Ehrlichia* and *Anaplasma*. For example, humoral and cellular immune mechanisms have been shown to be important in controlling acute bacteremia in *Ehrlichia* (Winslow et al., 2000; Feng and Walker, 2004); passive transfer of antibodies against the pathogen's outer membrane proteins can protect a host (Winslow et al., 2000); and interferon gamma (IFN-γ) is important in activating a host's monocytes and clearing infection (Feng and Walker, 2004). Furthermore, in mice, lymphocytes (CD4 and CD8) protect against fatal infection (Feng and Walker, 2004), and the major histocompatibility complex (MHC) class II is important for pathogen clearance (Ganta et al., 2002). For *Anaplasma*, while protective adaptive immune responses include cellular and humoral immune mechanisms, the innate immune mechanisms appear to be dispensable for control of the infection (von Lowenich et al., 2004). Elimination of *A. phagocytophilum* is mediated by antibodies and IFN-γ (Sun et al., 1997; Akkoyunlu and Fikrig, 2000; Wang et al., 2004). High-antibody titers are associated with immunity, although antigenic variation provides an immune evasion mechanism for the pathogen (Barbet et al., 2003; Granquist et al., 2010).

For *Ehrlichia*, some proteins are promising for vaccine development. Initial efforts have focused on immunoreactive proteins, surface-exposed proteins, and effector proteins that either play a role in arthropod infection and transmission, induce both cell-mediated and humoral immunity, or are recognized by the acute-stage immune response. Initial experiments to molecularly characterize potential effector proteins have shown they contain tandem repeats (TRPs). Thus far, 12 TRPs have been identified as being encoded by the *Ehrlichia chaffeensis* genome. Of these 12, 8 are predicted to be secreted. Two of those TRPs—TRP120 and TRP47—have mucin-like properties: that is, they have high serine/threonine content, and are strongly acidic. These tandem repeat proteins are of high interest because TRPs in other microorganisms have been associated with immune resistance, antigenic diversity, adhesion, and protein–protein interactions.

To determine the major B cell epitopes—that is, the regions that a host's immune system recognizes—TRP120 and TRP47 were expressed as recombinant fragments, including the N-terminal portion, the tandem repeat region, and the C-terminal portion. These fragments were probed with serum from a dog or a patient infected with *E. chaffeensis*. Antibodies in the host serum strongly recognized the tandem repeat region, but not the other components, revealing that the major immunogenic epitope are in the tandem repeat region. Similarly, epitopes have been mapped in the tandem repeat region of other TRPs.

By mapping this epitope to the tandem repeat region and using overlapping peptides, a 22-amino-acid peptide in TRP120 that contained the dominant immunogenic epitope was identified. In experiments where antibodies against this peptide were passively transferred into severe combined immunodeficiency (SCID) mice infected with *E. chaffeensis*, a significant reduction in the bacterial load was reported. The spleen weights of the mice treated with antibodies were much less than those of controls, consistent with the findings related to increased bacterial loads in controls. Similar protection was observed after passive transfer of antibodies to TRP32 and TRP47 into SCID mice infected with *E. chaffeensis*. These results suggest that antibodies to these three TRPs induce a measure of protection in the mammalian host.

Microarrays have been used to understand the protein expression levels of TRPs in both mammalian and arthropod hosts. Such studies are important in revealing how a pathogen cycles through the arthropod host and into the mammalian host, for example, and which proteins are actually expressed—and therefore would be good targets for a vaccine. Many TRPs appear to help the pathogen transition into the mammalian host and survive in the macrophage. These proteins are highly upregulated after the pathogen enters the mammalian host. For example, TRP47 is the most highly expressed gene in the *Ehrlichia* genome in the macrophage. Further, one tandem repeat protein—TRP120—is expressed in both the tick and the mammalian host. Two outer membrane proteins are also expressed—one that is expressed in the mammalian and tick hosts—and one, outer membrane protein 1B expressed only in the tick host, which could be considered for a tick-specific vaccine for *E. chaffeensis*. Antibodies directed at outer membrane proteins as well as TRPs have been shown to be protective in mammalian hosts. Some of the earliest antibody responses are directed at these TRPs, which are involved in molecular host–pathogen interactions that may be blocked by antibody. OMP-1 expression is also restricted in the tick, suggesting that vaccines targeting the appropriate outer membrane protein could have bactericidal activity in the tick. Similarly, TRP120 may be a candidate as a vaccine to prevent vector feeding or transmission, or inhibiting infection in the mammalian host. For *A. phagocytophilum*, seven major immunoreactive antigens have been identified, including 44-, 55-, 72-, 100-, and 160 kDa proteins. P44 is an outer membrane protein that recombines and is involved in antigenic variation. Antibodies directed at conserved regions of P44 partially protect a host from a pathogen challenge. Antibodies directed at two cotranscribed surface proteins, *Anaplasma* surface proteins 62 and 55, also partially neutralize *A. phagocytophilum* infection.

*Rickettsia* pathogens differ from *Ehrlichia* and *Anaplasma* in that they lyse the membrane of host cells, and are therefore free in the cytosol. Three mechanisms help define the virulence of *Rickettsia* in a mammalian host. *Rickettsia* enters a cell when adhesins such as OmpA and OmpB and stem cell antigen-1 (Sca-1) and stem cell antigen-2 (Sca-2) interact with Ku70, a surface protein on host cells, and induce them to phagocytose the *Rickettsia*. Second, internalized *Rickettsiae* are initially bound within a phagosome. However, the organism uses four enzymes to quickly lyse the vacuole membrane to escape it. Last, three spotted-fever group *Rickettsiae* use actin-based motility to move inside the cytoplasm and between cells. The actin tail is formed by polymerization of the host actin at one end of the bacterium with the rickettsial protein RickA or Sca-2. Some of the protective immune mechanisms used by the host against *Rickettsia* have been defined. For example, pro-inflammatory cytokines, IFN-$\gamma$ and TNF-$\alpha$, activate endothelial cells to kill intracellular organisms via nitric oxide synthase-dependent mechanisms. Cytotoxic CD8 T cells lyse infected target cells via pathways involving perforin and granzymes and are more important than CD4 T cells in clearing infection against *Rickettsia*. Humoral immunity may be more important in preventing reinfection than in clearing primary infection.

There have been some preliminary experimental vaccines for the rickettsioses. For example, formalin-inactivated vaccines against *Rickettsia rickettsii* have been developed from infected tissue, yolk sacs, and cell culture. These have not been proven to be effective, and subunit vaccines based on outer membrane proteins A and B appear to provide some protection in animals, but their efficacy in humans has not been studied. A newer avenue of vaccine development involves *Rickettsia* gene knockouts of virulence determinants. Two examples, which appear to be avirulent in guinea pigs, are *Rickettsia prowazekii* with the phospholipase D gene removed, and *R. rickettsii* with the *sca-2* gene removed. The *sca-2* gene mutant displays a small-plaque phenotype, but replicates at wild-type levels within Vero cells (Kleba et al., 2010). Furthermore, the *Rickettsia* with the *sca-2* knockout also lacks actin-based motility. A live attenuated vaccine based on that knockout that mimics natural infection would seem promising.

Other efforts have focused on vector proteins that impair tick feeding while also modulating immune responses and coagulation in a mammalian host. Several tick proteins have shown some protective ability, including those involved in iron transport and inflammation regulation, those with antihemostatic and anti-inflammation properties, antioxidants and immune shields, and those involved in IgG binding and secretion. For example, subolesin—a well-conserved protein among tick species—provides protection in mammals against both *Ixodes* and *Amblyomma* tick feeding.

### Knowledge Gaps and Research Opportunities

McBride noted there are a number of avenues for future work on vaccines against tick-borne diseases:

- For *Rickettsia*, live attenuated vaccine mimics the natural infection; thus *Rickettsia* that are genetically attenuated by gene knockouts are promising for future development of vaccines for rickettsial diseases.
- Vector proteins are attractive vaccine candidates. Targeting vector proteins that impair tick feeding, host immune modulating and co-agulation activities, and tick proteins that interact with pathogen are under investigation.
- Vaccines with effective combinations (elements directed against both vector and pathogen) of protective mechanisms are likely to be attractive future approaches to vaccine development.

## DEVELOPING OPPORTUNITIES FOR FUTURE VACCINES

*Wendy Brown, Ph.D., M.P.H., Department of Veterinary Microbiology and Pathology, Washington State University*

Many lessons can be drawn from the study of related organisms in veterinary species, such as cattle, that can inform our understanding of human immunology, pathology, and vaccine development for tick-borne pathogens. From this research, it is known that not all tick-borne pathogens are equal. They consist of a variety of different agents, including viruses, bacteria, and protozoa. Their complexity increases accordingly with their genome size. For example, most viral pathogens have very small genomes, whereas protozoa such as *Babesia bovis, Theileria parva,* or malaria have genomes 1,000-fold larger and considerably more complicated.

Currently, the only vaccines for tick-borne diseases in humans are for viral infections, such as flaviviruses. One of the reasons that existing viral vaccines are effective is that viremia can be controlled by the immune system by increasing titers of IgM and IgG antibodies. Thus, immunizing with an inactivated, live viral vaccine or a killed vaccine can induce a rapid immune response, which can result in the virus being quickly controlled when the animal or human comes in contact with it. The hallmark of these protective vaccines is that they induce a neutralizing antibody response

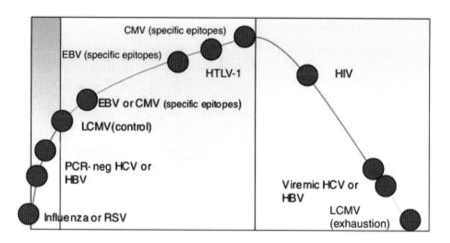

FIGURE 8-1 Pathogens with high antigen load cause immune dysfunction.
SOURCE: Klenerman and Hill, *National Immunology*, 2005.

involving long-lived B lymphocytes and plasma cells, and a long-lived memory B cell and T cell response. This type of protective immune response is the goal of most work on human vaccines against tick-borne pathogens.

Bacterial and protozoal tick-borne pathogens are more complicated than viruses because they involve multiple stages in the host cell, and because they have evolved different strategies to evade the host's immune response. For example, a number of tick-borne pathogens, including *Borrelia burgdorferi*, *B. hermsii*, *Anaplasma. phagocytophilum*, *A. marginale*, and *Babesia bovis* employ antigenic variation to evade a host immune's response. Furthermore, vector-borne pathogens such as *A. marginale*, *B. bovis*, and malarial parasites that cause high levels of pathogen load throughout infection persist in the host and induce a dysfunctional CD4 T lymphocyte response that includes overexpression of inflammatory cytokines and deletion of antigen-specific T cells. Many viruses that induce high viremia also produce severe immune dysfunction that correlates with the load of pathogen in the host (Figure 8-1). Common examples are HIV, hepatitis C virus, and hepatitis B virus, which induce T cell dysfunction leading to T cell exhaustion or deletion.

As research leads to understanding of the molecular characteristics and the cellular pathways involved in pathogenesis, a number of targets have been identified for developing potential vaccines. These include

- Outer membrane or surface proteins produced during the host stage to prevent infection.

- Proteins on the surface of infected cells. For example, one target would be CD8 cytotoxic T cells, which recognize parasite antigens on the surface of infected lymphocytes.
- Tick-stage pathogen antigens (e.g., OspA) that would prevent transmission.
- Antigens produced within the tick, such as those active in its gut to reduce tick feeding and to reduce or prevent transmission of the pathogen.

Vaccines based on outer membrane proteins are of particular interest as they serve as the interface between a pathogen and a host, and are a primary target of the host's immune response. A pathogen uses the outer membrane to adhere to and invade host cells, and often for intracellular survival and growth. The outer membrane of bacterial pathogens expresses complexes of proteins, such as the type III and type IV secretion systems, which serve as virulence factors and send effector molecules into host cells, disrupting their function. Protective vaccines based on purified outer membranes or outer membrane vesicles include *Treponema, Neisseria, Hemophilus influenza, Chlamydia, Francisella,* and *Anaplasma.* Immunizing cattle with outer membranes purified from *A. marginale,* for example, results in complete protection against infection in approximately one-third of the animals. However, vaccines based on individual outer membrane proteins instead of whole membranes induce poor protective immunity. Early efforts on individual outer membrane proteins focused on serologically reactive proteins, which are immunodominant proteins and recognized by serum antibody from an infected individual or an immunized animal. For the five or six immunodominant outer membrane proteins of *A. marginale,* these proteins did not induce protection equivalent to that of whole outer membranes. There are a number of hypotheses to explain why vaccines based on whole outer membranes are protective, while those based on individual outer membrane proteins are not. For example, it is possible that the antigens tested thus far are not the ones that can induce protection, that multiple antigens need to be included in a vaccine, or that the association of proteins within the outer membrane confers ability to induce protective immunity through linked recognition of T cell and B cell epitopes.

Individual outer membrane proteins that stimulate antibodies after infection or immunization have been typically targeted for vaccine development because it is easier to perform than screening antigens to find those that increase production of CD4 T cells. However, the latter is important because those antigens are essential for enabling B cells to switch isotypes to make IgG, the antibody that is important in opsonization. Antigens that effect both IgG antibody and CD4 T cell responses in various hosts are likely to advance our knowledge.

Immunodominant surface proteins have also been typically targeted for vaccine development. For example, *B. bovis* has two major surface antigens, MSA-1 and RAP-1. MSA-1 is abundant and undergoes antigenic variation between strains, and along with RAP-1, it has been shown to provide incomplete or no protection (Brown et al., 2006). Similarly, in *A. marginale*, the two major surface proteins, Msp2 and Msp3, undergo antigenic variation, resulting in numerous antigenic variants in an individual and a population at any given time. These immunodominant proteins conveyed incomplete or no immunoprotection (Palmer et al., 1999). The Waksman Postulate suggests a working hypothesis for why these proteins might be abundant, but not essential. The Postulate noted that "any antigen against which parasites allowed the host to mount an immune response is by definition unimportant for the survival of the organism" (Sher, 1988). It was also noted that "antigens that induce poor or immunosuppressed responses during natural infection should not be ignored since they may be molecules essential for parasite survival" (Sher, 1988). Based on these results, the subdominant, but conserved antigens may be better candidates for vaccines. To begin to understand their role, there is a need to understand how subdominant, conserved antigens associate with other proteins in the outer membrane and how this interaction might affect the generation of immune responses through the linked recognition of T cell and B cell epitopes.

In preliminary studies, proteins were selected based on immunoblots from *A. marginale* that were not immunodominant. Sixty proteins that were recognized by immune sera from three different animals immunized with outer membrane from the pathogen were selected by mass spectrometry. Twenty-one proteins, including three structural proteins of the type IV secretion system, were identified that were mildly reactive with the immune sera. Of these new proteins, 70 percent were recognized by immune serum from all three vaccinated animals with different major MHC class II haplotypes that represent the majority of MHC class II molecules in Holstein cattle. Using a high-throughput *in vitro* transcription and translation system to express those proteins, tags were added to the proteins. The proteins were bound to beads, and then fed to antigen-presenting cells that present antigen to immune T cells. Most of the antigens, including the type IV secretion system proteins, stimulated very strong CD4 T cell responses (Lopez et al., 2008).

Linked recognition of T and B cell epitopes on proteins associated through covalent or non-covalent bonding may be important for these antigens to stimulate antibody to undergo isotype switching. For example, B cells recognize antigen 1, which may or may not be associated with another protein, through their B cell immunoglobulin receptor. If it is associated with antigen 2, then that complex of antigens is taken into the B cell, and those proteins are processed and presented on the cell surface, where they are presented to CD4 T cells that recognize antigen. If the T cells have a receptor for antigen 1 or antigen 2, they can provide help to B cells to make antibody to both antigens 1 and 2. Using MSP1, a heteromer of MSP1-A and MSP1-B surface proteins, to investigate the process in *A. marginale*, some animals have T cell responses to only MSP1-A, but have good antibody responses to both proteins. Thus, MSP1A-specific T cells provide help to B cells to make antibody to both MSP1-A and MSP1-B. There is additional evidence for linked recognition of another outer membrane protein. Several cattle immunized with outer membranes had antibody responses to the type IV secretion system protein VirB9-1, but no T cell response to this outer membrane protein. However, there was a strong T-cell response to VirB9-2 and VirB10. These three proteins are components of a type IV secretion system complex, where the two VirB9 and VirB10 proteins are associated. We hypothesize that in these individuals, VirB10 stimulates T cells that provide help for B cells to make antibody to VirB9-1. The next step is to immunize cattle with these combinations of proteins, either linked or unlinked, to see if they produce protective immunity.

These findings underscore the importance of studying immune responses to tick-borne pathogens in natural hosts. Mouse models have a number of limitations, including the fact that mice cannot be infected with *A. marginale*, for a number of possible reasons. Mice diverged from humans 65 million year ago. Research mice are inbred and have numerous recessive defects that skew immune responses. Finally, there is limited representation of the MHC haplotypes, which present antigens differently among mammalian species. MHC molecules are also highly polygenic and polymorphic within a population. As a result, the T cell epitopes are going to differ between individuals and certainly between species.

### Knowledge Gaps and Research Opportunities

Brown noted that researchers should conduct the following work on vaccines against tick-borne diseases:

- Examine surface-exposed, conserved proteins are priority targets.
- Target the subdominant antigens for persistent pathogens.
- Use naturally associated proteins to increase T cell responses.
- Focus on T cell epitopes recognized by the majority of individuals within a population, as well as by antibodies.
- Study a pathogen in its human host, or an outbred large animal model.
- Develop metrics to measure protective immune responses in these species.

## DISCUSSION

Developing methods to protect humans against tick-borne diseases remains controversial, but many new avenues are being explored. Schutze suggested that researchers put more emphasis on a general vaccine aimed to reduce prolonged tick attachment regardless of the tick genus or species. Another participant questioned whether it was possible to design a vaccine based on salivary proteins from ticks that are conserved among tick populations to prevent prolonged attachment of the tick to humans. McBride noted that vaccines against evolutionary conserved proteins among tick populations such as subolesin, a salivary protein, show promise. Within the vaccine field, there is interest in research on tick salivary proteins and other proteins produced by the tick and pathogens as vaccine candidates. Brown further noted that a few tick genomes have been sequenced so that proteomics are now being applied to identify specific salivary proteins.

Another participant questioned how highly specific bands to *Borrelia*, such as 31-KD OspA and 34-KD OspB, could be used for vaccine development, but not for disease detection. McBride noted that the highly specific bands to *Borrelia* confound diagnosis because despite a demonstrated immune response to those bands, it becomes difficult to differentiate between an infection and a vaccinated individual.

## EDUCATION, BEHAVIOR CHANGE, AND OTHER NON-PHARMACEUTICAL MEASURES AGAINST LYME AND OTHER TICK-BORNE DISEASES

*Paul Mead, M.D., M.P.H., Centers for Disease Control and Prevention*

Although the topic of prevention is often relegated to the end of a meeting or report, this placement does not diminish its importance. For tick-borne diseases, prevention is clearly preferable to treatment, and it should be a foremost concern. Unfortunately, current methods and opportunities for prevention are limited, and there is urgent need for new methods and new approaches.

Personal protective measures—as distinct from community-level measures—represent the final point of intervention for preventing human infection. Familiar personal protective measures include frequent tick checks to remove crawling or attached ticks; use of protective clothing such as long-sleeved shirts, long pants, and light-colored clothes; tucking pants into socks; using repellent; and avoiding tick habitat. These strategies have yielded mixed results in analytic studies.

Some personal protection methods, including some recommended by the Centers for Disease Control and Prevention (CDC), have not been shown to prevent tick-borne diseases. For example, the method of tick removal, tucking pants into one's sock, or wearing light-colored clothing have not been shown to be protective (Smith et al., 1988; Schwartz and Goldstein, 1990; Ley et al., 1995; Orloski et al., 1998; Connally et al., 2009). There is at least one study (Stjernberg and Berglund, 2005) suggesting that individuals are actually more likely to acquire ticks from the environment when wearing light-colored clothing than when wearing dark-colored clothing. To be clear, the CDC does still recommend use of fine-tipped tweezers as a quick and definitive way to remove ticks.

Insect repellent use has been the subject of a number of case-control or cross-sectional observational studies over the past 20 years. The results have been mixed, with some studies showing a protective effect, while others did not (Smith et al., 1988, 2001; Schwartz and Goldstein, 1990; Lane et al., 1992; Ley et al., 1995; Klein et al., 1996; Orloski et al., 1998; Phillips et al., 2001; Vazquez et al., 2008; Connally et al., 2009). The studies have varied as to whether the repellent was applied to the skin or clothing. Other studies focused on whether the repellent was used in the yard, away from the house, at work, or at leisure. Because of this variation in design and the fact that accurate dosage of repellent was not collected, it is difficult to make direct comparisons among these studies.

Tick checks are a potentially important strategy for reducing tick-borne diseases because recognition and removal of ticks before attachment—or even shortly after—can effectively block pathogen transmission. Nevertheless, most studies have failed to demonstrate a protective effect of tick checks. This may be because ticks, especially nymphal ticks, are very small, and there may be practical limitations on people's ability to detect them.

Detailed examination of two studies further illustrates the complexity of evaluating the effectiveness of personal protective measures. During 2000–2003, Vazquez and colleagues conducted a case-control study to evaluate the use of protective clothing, repellents, and tick checks among 700 Connecticut patients with clinically diagnosed Lyme disease and approximately 1,100 matched controls (Vazquez et al., 2008). Participants were divided into those with definite, possible, or unlikely Lyme disease, based on clinical and laboratory evidence. Participants with definite Lyme disease were significantly less likely to report using protective clothing—long-sleeved shirts, long pants, and light-colored clothing—than were controls (46 versus 60 percent). Patients with Lyme disease were also significantly less likely to report using repellent than matched controls. However, about 77 percent of both patients and controls reported checking for ticks.

A second study conducted in Connecticut a few years later examined a wide variety of personal protective behaviors and home landscaping practices among approximately 360 patients with Lyme disease and a similar number of matched controls. Unlike the Vazquez study, these researchers found that protective clothing did not reduce participants' risk of Lyme disease. They did find, however, that performing tick checks within 36 hours of time spent in the yard was protective (with an adjusted odds ratio of 0.55). Furthermore, bathing within 2 hours of spending time in the yard was also protective (with an adjusted odds ratio of 0.4). Wearing repellent trended toward being protective, but this association was not statistically significant.

Bathing within 2 hours of potential tick exposure may be a behavior worthy of further promotion. Bathing allows people a good opportunity to search for attached or engorged ticks, while soap and water may wash off those they miss that are not yet attached. Furthermore, as people typically do not put the same clothes back on after bathing, this may reduce their risk to exposure from tick remaining on their clothing. Finally, bathing is an activity that people perform often. Prevention behavior researchers note that an ideal prevention behavior is one that can be easily incorporated into everyday activities. Making people aware of the protective value of bathing might spur them to time that activity for its greatest effect in preventing tick-borne disease.

A number of caveats are important when considering these observational studies. First, comparisons are difficult to make across studies due to differences in outcome measures. For example, investigators have relied on case-control and cross-sectional studies to evaluate the efficacy of using insect repellent. However, most of these researchers did not collect or did not provide information on the type or dose of repellent that participants actually used. Second, the lack of statistical significance does not mean that an intervention is useless, only that the magnitude of the effect is limited. Third, multiple protective factors may mask or dilute the significance of any one protective behavior. Despite these complexities, personal protective measures are relatively benign even if not always very effective, and there is little downside to encouraging people to use them.

Assuming personal protective measures are effective, questions remain as to whether a sufficient number of individuals can be encouraged to practice these behaviors regularly. General knowledge of disease risk is usually necessary but not sufficient to motivate adoption of new behaviors. Individuals need to have the confidence that they can perform the behavior and need to believe that it is worthwhile (i.e., believing that the disease is a real problem, believing that the behavior is effective in preventing the disease, and believing that the benefits of performing the behavior outweighs the inconvenience of the behavior).

Two studies highlight the range of outcomes for prospective interventional studies. One study randomly assigned passengers on the ferry from Hyannis to Nantucket to watch an entertaining educational demonstration on either bike safety or tick-bite prevention behavior and tick removal

(Daltroy and Phillips, 2007). Two months later, researchers asked participants about recent symptoms of tick-borne disease, and reviewed their medical records when possible. The study enrolled 30,000 participants over a 3-year period.

In the main-effects model, patients who received the educational intervention on tick bites had a lower risk of reporting tick-borne illness, although the finding was not statistically significant. In the more complex intervention-effects model, which accounted for interactions among the variables, there was some evidence that educational intervention was beneficial depending on the visitors' length of stay on the island. The researchers found no difference in risk between intervention and control groups among passengers who stayed on Nantucket for less than 2 weeks. They did find a significantly lower risk, however, among passengers who received the intervention and stayed longer than 2 weeks. Nantucket residents who received the invention also had a slightly lower risk of tick-borne disease, although that finding was not statistically significant.

The interpretation of these results is complicated. The reduced risk of tick-borne disease among passengers staying more than 2 weeks is encouraging. Nevertheless, disease incidence was still very high among passengers staying less than 2 weeks (3 cases per 1,000), and these passengers made up approximately 85 percent of study participants. The lack of a demonstrable effect among this group is surprising and disappointing.

In a second study, intensive, community-wide, multiyear educational programs were evaluated in three health districts in Connecticut (Gould et al., 2008). These programs were developed with input from the communities and provided environmental management and personal protective behavior education to a wide variety of audiences, including schoolchildren, landscapers and gardeners, hikers, and so forth. Approximately 2,800 participating households completed before and after surveys.

During the baseline period, more than 80 percent of respondents said they knew a lot or some about Lyme disease, and more than 70 percent thought Lyme disease was a very serious or somewhat serious problem in their town. More than 50 percent of respondents also thought it was very likely or somewhat likely that someone in their household would contract Lyme disease in the next year. Approximately 5 percent of participants reported a previous diagnosis of Lyme disease.

Given their comprehension of the burden of disease and their personal experience, the study investigated the frequency of performing preventive behaviors. Approximately 99 percent of participants reported that they used some protective behavior some of the time. After the intervention, the proportion of people who reported always checking for ticks rose from around 50 to 57 percent, the proportion who reported using repellent rose from 21 to 28 percent, and the proportion who reported tucking pants into their socks slightly decreased. These findings suggest that—even in a highly motivated population—voluntary behavior change is hard work, and that a portion of the population will not respond to efforts to encourage such change.

In conclusion, there are a few points for state-of-the-science prevention research. First, researchers have repeatedly studied the efficacy of personal protective measures against tick-borne illness. This is not a research gap. Second, these studies show that some behaviors provide some benefit, while others do not. Third, educational campaigns should target behaviors that have some evidence of benefit, such as bathing, and not those that do not, such as tucking pants into socks. Finally, it is important to recognize that the personal protective measures are unlikely to have a major public health benefit for tick-borne diseases. Public health officials have been educating people about Lyme disease for 20 years, for example, but cases have continued to climb, and the disease is spreading to new areas.

Mead noted that these conclusions suggest the need to think more broadly about public health interventions, which can occur at several levels. At one level are interventions targeted toward individuals—behaviors that people must decide to do, and then perform correctly and routinely. At the next level are interventions that involve the individual, but that are enforced legally or through public health policy, such as seat belt laws and vaccination programs. At the third level are interventions implemented at the community level that do not involve the individual, such as municipal water and sewer systems and the pasteurization of milk. The history of public health impact and disease control favors interventions in the third category. In identifying research gaps, future research on preventing Lyme and other tick-borne diseases should focus on interventions implemented at the community level, such as controlling deer populations. Regardless of the method, prevention measures should be judged by their ability to prevent human illness in endemic communities, and not just kill ticks.

## VECTOR- AND HOST-TARGETED STRATEGIES FOR PREVENTION OF TICK-BORNE DISEASES

*José M.C. Ribeiro, M.D., Ph.D., National Institute of Allergy and Infectious Diseases*

As mentioned previously, there are a number of options to develop prevention strategies for tick-borne diseases. Common approaches focus on the vector (tick) directly, their mammalian hosts, or human behavior. This presentation will cover the use of pesticides to control for ticks, targeting the mammalian hosts, and targeting the tick's saliva.

A common approach for controlling vectors is to spray areas where ticks are endemic with acaracides. Given the fact that disease transmission primarily occurs in the forest edge (the first 10 meters), targeted application can be more effective then widespread pesticide application. Pesticide resistance should not be a problem as its development requires that at least 70 percent of the tick population be exposed to a high dose of acaricides. With targeted application, there is the intermixing of the wild-type, insecticide-susceptible ticks that will breed with ticks in the forest edge, thus diluting insecticide resistance genes that may appear.

A second approach to target the vector is to spray an individual's clothing with permanone, an acaricide that kills ticks, or to bathe with soaps containing permethrin soon after potential tick exposure to kill any attached ticks before they can deliver the pathogens, which takes from 12 to 24 hours to occur. However, human toxicity of acaricides is a concern, and some researchers are working on organic or green formulas that could be less toxic.

Vertebrate hosts are needed to sustain the tick population, so targeting mammalian hosts is another prevention strategy. Tick larvae feed mainly on *Peromyscus leucopus*, the white-footed mouse, while adult ticks attach mostly to deer. Those two animals account for the largest mammalian biomass in New England. The biomass decreases by an order of magnitude when other potential hosts are considered. Culling the deer population is often discussed as a strategy for controlling the tick population. With few exceptions, this approach is only successful in the short term. Deer herds need to be significantly reduced or eliminated because if the deer population drops by only half, twice as many ticks will simply attach to each remaining animal (Rand et al., 2004; Jordan et al., 2007).

Another approach is to administer acaricides using a tick's mammalian hosts, such as bait boxes. For the white tail deer, the ticks are concentrated on the deer in late fall and early spring. As mentioned previously, there are self-medicating applicators such as the four-poster to apply insecticides to the host. To be effective, however, researchers need to understand the behavior of the host animal and the interaction with the ticks. Larvae feed on the white foot mouse in August and drop off to molt to a nymphal tick over the winter. Mice are nocturnal animals and sleep during the day, and the tick feeds for a few days and drops off the host in the late afternoon. This means that the ticks are dropping off their host at a time of the day when the mouse is in the burrow. Furthermore, *Permyscus leucopus* makes its nests under the frost line, which means that the ticks are protected during the winter. As the weather becomes colder, it will gather nesting materials to take to the nest. One strategy that has been implemented is permethrin-impregnated cotton that the mice will scavenge to use in their nests. Although rodent-targeted techniques for distributing acaricides are effective in reducing the tick population, they are cumbersome. For example, the impregnated cotton must be distributed every 10 yards because the home range of the mice is 10 to 20 yards. Distribution must also cover a relatively large area to be effective. A single administration on the edge of relatively small area does not work (Deblinger and Rimmer, 1991; Stafford, 1991).

The third approach for vector–host interactions is to target transmission once a tick has attached and begins feeding. During a blood meal, ticks have evolved to be highly adaptive to remain attached to a host's skin for several days and to ingest blood during the entire time. When a tick first attaches to a host, the ticks are coming out of a dormant state. As they start to inject a cementing protein, their metabolism begins to increase. Transcription of various proteins increase, and this new metabolic state likely triggers the pathogen. The feeding phases can be characterized as a slow feeding phase when the metabolic system is increasing followed by a rapid feeding phase. This is the primary reason for targeting tick removal in the first 24 hours.

During the feeding process, a tick faces its host's barrier of the hemostasis, a highly redundant process consisting of blood clotting, platelet aggregation, and vasoconstriction at the site of the attachment. To counter these obstacles, the tick produces a complex salivary potion that neutralizes these host defenses. The site of a tick bite is in an immunosuppressed state as tick saliva contains proteins that will block the activation of histamine, ATP, serotonin, bradykinin, and leukotriene B4, which trigger pain and itching in the hosts, thus the attached tick can go unnoticed unless that person happens to develop an allergy to one or more of its salivary proteins. In brief, tick saliva has antihemostatic, anti-inflammatory, and immunosuppressive properties. Furthermore, the attachment site is high in interleukin 4, for example, and has substances which inhibit the maturation of dendritic cells and the activation of lymphocytes. This environment protects pathogens during transmission.

One prevention strategy is the use of an anti-tick saliva vaccine to prevent disease acquisition. Vaccines traditionally target proteins on the surface of the pathogens, but anti-tick saliva vaccine targets the compounds that aid in the transmission of the pathogen to the new host. For example, rabbits are killed when they are bitten by a tick infected with *Francisella tularensis*. When rabbits were presensitized by exposure to a clean tick, they developed an allergy to the tick bite that triggered a protective response to an infected tick bite (Bell et al., 1979). Furthermore, individual antibodies developed to inhibit a tick protein such as Salp 15, which is known to inhibit the response of mammalian T cells, enabled mice to be protected against *B. burgdorferi*.

Other tick saliva proteins also may be targets for vaccine development. When guinea pigs are exposed to ticks, they develop a large quantity of antibodies that results in rejection of a tick during a second exposure. However, the guinea pigs do not make antibodies against cathepsin inhibitor, a protein that prevents the maturation of dendritic cells, because it is present in very low concentrations in tick saliva. In one experiment, immunity against recombinant cathepsin inhibitor impaired the ability of *Ixodes scapularis* to feed. Thus some antibody responses may be more important than others. The myriad compounds create the redundancy and resiliency of the salivary system, but they also offer a large number of vaccine targets. Future research needs to identify which proteins provide a protective response for the transmission of tick-borne pathogens, including identification of early salivary antigens that might lead to an antibody that trigger a local reaction and alert the vaccinated person to detect and detach the tick soon after attachment. As spirochetes are transmitted 24 hours after exposure, an immediate or even a few hours of a delayed reaction to tick saliva could alert an individual to the need to remove a tick.

Genomics are a promising area of research to aid in identifying these proteins. Ticks have large genomes in comparison to both animals and humans. *I. scapularis* and *I. pacificus* have about two gigabases of genome, more than twice that of the chicken. Another tick, Boophilius microplus, has approximately seven gigabases of genome, which is on the same order of the human genome. It is a large genome with approximately 20 chromosomes, which is a result of genome duplication. With transcriptome analysis, more than 300 proteins in 26 families in tick's salivary glands have been annotated (Ribeiro et al., 2006). For most of these proteins, however, their function is unknown. What is known is that tick proteins have been at a fast pace of evolution. *Ixodes* ticks have protein families that are only expressed in them, so each genus of ticks have evolved independent protein families.

In summary, Ribeiro noted that tick-borne diseases continue to be a problem in the United States. There is a need to use integrated pest management as a strategy to minimize the risk of disease transmission. At the same time, basic research is needed to understand the cellular processes that may aid in developing a vaccine to prevent transmission.

## DISCUSSION

Many non-pharmaceutical methods for prevention exist and range from education to community-level interventions. Awareness is the key for generating community-level action, but action must start at the individual level including the healthcare provider. One participant noted that some cases of Lyme disease are not being diagnosed in a timely fashion. Mead agreed that physician education is important. The CDC has produced some educational materials for physicians, but more work needs to be done. Another participant noted that often the last diagnosis a doctor will consider is Lyme disease, when it should be one of the first.

Another participant noted that everyone needs to be a part of the education process because the entire community needs to consider tick-borne diseases as a serious health concern before protective measures will be effectively employed. To make people more aware of ticks, one participant suggested that the CDC target neighborhoods, present a positive message regarding potential disease risks, and incorporate measures of community risk such as tick drags. Mead noted that awareness is the key, whether for the physicians, the patients, or the community. He noted that community awareness could lead to further adoption of community-level interventions, but there is a need to strategically plan the approach. Another participant noted that prevention is key for reducing the burden of disease and four-posters need to be a part of the strategy for deer. Mead noted that in some states, using four-posters is a problem because wildlife departments are concerned about transmission of chronic wasting disease or the effect of permethrin on hunters. The CDC is starting some research to look at the efficacy of four-posters in various areas. To reach the public, some participants suggested developing public service announcements because many communities are not aware of the importance of tick-borne diseases. Mead noted that the CDC recognizes that Lyme disease is a growing problem and is among the top seven reportable disease in the country. In Northeastern United States, it is among the top two or three. As part of the recognition of the importance of this disease, the CDC has received funding to strengthen their communications activities to more aggressively disseminate effective prevention messages.

A multitude of other preventative strategies beyond promoting awareness have shown promise but require tweaking before they can be implemented. Some participants asked when new vaccines may be developed. McBride noted that vaccines for humans are in the near future. While these vaccines still face numerous obstacles, progress has been made for *Ehrlicia* and *Rickettsia* in particular. A vaccine is currently being tested in Europe and if it is successful, it may be available in the United States in the future.

Finally, another participant questioned why it takes 24 hours for a tick to begin to transmit pathogens. Ribeiro noted that studies using fluorescent spirochetes did not see evidence of pathogen in the salivary glands until 48 hours after attachment (De Silva and Fikrig, 1995; Ribeiro et al., 2006). The pathogen resides in the tick gut, and once the tick attaches to feed, the *Borrelia* begins to multiply. They increase in size and begin to be seen in the hemocele by 24 hours, and then by 48 hours, they are present in the salivary gland.

## CONCLUDING THOUGHTS ON PREVENTION

*Stephen M. Ostroff, M.D., Bureau of Epidemiology,
Pennsylvania Department of Health*

Efforts to develop and implement preventive measures against tick-borne infections—both pharmacological and non-pharmacological—have so far proved disappointing. These measures produce short-term or sustained reductions in the incidence of disease in only limited cases. In no cases have preventive measures halted the geographic spread of disease-carrying ticks or the pathogens they harbor. The incidence of tick-borne infections has therefore grown continuously over the past several decades. That sends an unfortunate—and to a certain degree self-fulfilling—message that these diseases are not preventable.

However, tick-borne diseases should be as amenable to preventive measures as other infections of public health significance. Prevention offers the best opportunity over the long-term to truly reduce the burden and impact of tick-borne infections. Investments in safe, effective, and simple preventive interventions are therefore essential. A combination of these approaches would likely have the greatest success in reducing the overall burden of tick-borne disease.

Among pharmacological interventions, vaccination appears to hold the most promise. Significant efforts are under way to develop vaccines for tick-borne infections, although no human vaccines are now available for any of the major pathogens, and none are close to licensing or even in clinical trials.

Efforts to develop vaccines against Rocky Mountain spotted fever date back to the 1930s, although none has offered significant protection. However, the development and licensing of an outer-surface protein vaccine against Lyme disease in the late 1990s shows that vaccination for tick-borne disease is a viable option. Clinical trials demonstrated that the OspA vaccine was clearly effective in preventing Lyme disease. However, the manufacturer withdrew the vaccine after only 2 years on the market for many other reasons. That setback shows that any future vaccines for tick-borne infections must not only be effective but also easy to administer, cost-effective, and free of concerns about potential short- and long-term side effects.

The two workshop speakers who covered vaccines focused on ehrlichiosis, anaplasmosis, and rickettsial infections. In targeting these infections in both humans and animals, investigators have explored both subunit vaccines and live attenuated vaccines. They are making progress, but must still overcome key challenges. These include better defining immunological responses to infection, understanding mechanisms of immune-based protection, developing the ability to measure protection, and creating animal models to study potential vaccine candidates.

A significant challenge for vaccine development is the sheer diversity of human tick-borne pathogens, along with their antigenic variation. Tick-borne pathogens include rickettsial agents, several bacteria species, and *Babesia* parasites. Each agent has different incidence, geography, epidemiologic features, risk groups, and clinical impact. It is hard to imagine a scenario where vaccines become available for all these agents. Even if they were developed, questions regarding how each vaccine would be used—and whether there is a market large enough to justify their development and licensure—would remain.

An attractive alternative discussed during the workshop is to develop vaccines that generically target the host–tick interaction, rather than pathogen-specific vaccines. Such vaccines could be directed against critical proteins in tick saliva needed for attachment, or they could limit the ability of a tick to take a blood meal if it does attach. Such options are made even more attractive by the fact that the number of tick species responsible for transmitting tick-borne pathogens is quite small. Each species can transmit multiple agents. A single vaccine directed against attachment and feeding of *Ixodes* species, for example, would protect against multiple agents.

Mead explored multiple non-pharmaceutical interventions. The best studied are personal protective measures that involve behavioral change, such as the use of tick checks, long-sleeved clothing, and insecticides, but the results have been variable. Some studies have found a protective effect while others have not. The inconsistencies are likely related to study design or outcome measures, but they highlight the difficulty of implementing and sustaining complex behavioral change. Such interventions need to be simple, used consistently, and reinforced. Mead concluded that despite limited evidence that such interventions work, public officials should still recommend them.

Preliminary data presented by Weber earlier in the workshop showed that the use of permethrin-impregnated clothing by outdoor workers reduced tick bites by 93 percent, and may therefore be an effective strategy to prevent tick-borne infections among people in high-risk occupations. The U.S. military has used such clothing extensively. Although no one has systematically studied such an approach in the general population, it might offer significant protective benefits in high-incidence locations.

Environmental preventive measures, such as the use of acaracides against deer or rodent populations, have been found to be effective. The same applies to targeted deer removal. However, none of these approaches has been widely adopted because of cost, environmental concerns, or difficulties applying them on a large enough scale or over a sustained period of time to have a significant impact on disease occurrence. Ostfeld suggested that approaches to habitat management that promote species diversity would likely be highly effective in reducing the transmission of Lyme disease. Ribiero proposed another innovative approach: identifying endosymbiotic microorganisms that would inhibit or destroy pathogens within the tick vector, or interrupt the tick maturation cycle.

Finally, workshop participants repeatedly emphasized the importance of efforts to educate the public about tick-borne diseases and how to prevent them. Even high-incidence areas have often lacked intense or sustained social marketing campaigns like those designed to combat other diseases. One innovative educational campaign conducted on Massachusetts ferries had a favorable impact on people's knowledge of Lyme disease and efforts to reduce their exposure to ticks. Public health officials should consider similar campaigns—even in lower incidence locations, or targeted to school-children, people in high-risk occupations, and outdoor enthusiasts—as they may improve adherence to prevention measures and reduce the incidence of disease.

# 9

# Closing Panels

The committee invited a panel of stakeholders to listen to the presentations and discussions during the course of the 2-day workshop and to share their observations regarding the research gaps and priorities in the science of tick-borne diseases (TBDs). The panel members were not to come to a consensus, but rather to reflect their own viewpoints. Panelists included a representative from a patient advocacy group, a clinician specializing in Lyme disease, a clinician researcher specializing in *Ehrlichia* and *Anaplasma,* a clinician researcher studying pathogenesis, and a clinician researcher from Europe to provide a global perspective. The member of the patient advocacy group worked with a number of members of his Lyme disease coalition during the workshop, but his perspective does not imply or represent a consensus of all patients or advocacy groups. Similarly, the physicians' and researchers' perspectives do not reflect a consensus of the scientific opinion of their fields, although many panelists had overlapping comments. The committee chose to summarize each panelist's comments individually and to allow these redundancies to emphasize the various viewpoints. To broaden the discussion, the committee invited the general audience to comment following the panel discussion to elicit views or ideas that were not captured during the panel presentations.

After reviewing the presentations and comments in the listening sessions before the workshop and during the workshop, the committee noted that the language and terminology used to describe various facets and manifestations of Lyme disease and coinfecting conditions were inconsistently applied and have likely contributed to misunderstandings and even inaccuracies. Rather than offering its own interpretation of terms and definitions used by the various presenters, the committee presented the terms exactly as transcribed reflecting the use by presenters and other participants. This does not imply that the committee believes that terms such as "post-Lyme disease," "post-treatment Lyme disease," "persistent Lyme disease," and "chronic Lyme disease" are or are not interchangeable, differ in meaning or value, or have differing scientific validity. Similar confusion exists regarding terminology related to recurrent and relapsing Lyme disease with or without reinfection. As highlighted by many presenters, a commonly accepted lexicon of definitions that is consistently applied and understood would improve and advance research efforts regarding Lyme disease and other tick-borne diseases and likely improve patient care. Elucidation of the critical issues of infection and pathogenesis remains to be definitively achieved.

## CRITICAL NEEDS AND GAPS IN UNDERSTANDING TICK-BORNE DISEASES: PRACTICING PHYSICIAN PERSPECTIVE

*John Aucott, M.D., Park Medical Associates*

Most clinicians are aware that an abundant literature exists on classic untreated Lyme disease and its typical early and late manifestations. In contrast, the literature and clinicians' experience with persistent symptoms following antibiotic treatment of Lyme disease are more limited. Regardless of whether one names it chronic Lyme disease or post-Lyme disease syndrome, patients and clinicians are confused about how to proceed when patients report symptoms after a course of antibiotic treatment. A recent survey reported that 48 percent of Connecticut physicians are undecided as to whether chronic Lyme disease exists (Johnson and Feder, 2010). This controversy leaves clinicians uncertain about how to help patients who continue to report symptoms following antibiotic treatment.

The Centers for Disease Control and Prevention (CDC) "definite criteria" for classical signs and symptoms of Lyme disease include: erythema migrans (EM) rash, joint disease with inflammatory synovitis, and neurological disease with objective findings. Even with these straightforward criteria, a gap exists between the textbook descriptions of the disease and clinical practice. Retrospective studies (Aucott et al., 2009) have shown that frequent misdiagnosis occurs in community practices. For example, 23 percent of EM rashes and 54 percent of patients who did not present with a rash were misdiagnosed. Further complicating the clinical practice, as noted throughout the workshop, are the gaps in understanding the serologic response to the disease—how to use the laboratory tests that exist and what the limitations of these tests are.

The CDC has developed a "probable" case definition of Lyme disease that has a viral-like presentation. These patients present with symptoms and a positive serologic test result, but without physical findings or signs of an EM rash. This area of Lyme disease is poorly understood. For example, it is not known whether a subset of late (or chronic) Lyme disease patients may lack physical signs or symptoms and only present with constitutional symptoms such as fatigue. In the recent review by Feder and colleagues (Feder et al., 2007), this scenario would be equivalent to their category 3—"Patients do not have a history of objective clinical findings that are consistent with Lyme disease, but their serum samples contain antibodies against *Borrelia burgdorferi,* as determined by means of standardized assays that were ordered to investigate chronic, subjective symptoms of unknown cause." The question for the clinician is whether this category exists; no studies have been done on the treatment and the outcomes for early or late probable Lyme disease—a research gap.

Another category is patients who experience persistent symptoms following antibiotic treatment of confirmed Lyme disease. It is called different names, but for this discussion, it will be referred to as "post-treatment Lyme disease syndrome." It is known that the visible, physical signs of early Lyme disease respond to appropriate antibiotic treatment, but 10 percent of late Lyme disease patients with Lyme disease arthritis still have joint disease after antibiotic treatment. In fact, in all stages of Lyme disease, persistent symptoms without the classic signs have been observed after antibiotic treatment. For this class of patients (post-treatment Lyme disease syndrome), there are more unknowns than knowns, such as the magnitude of the problem, and the range of severity of the illness.

Some factors that increase the likelihood for poor treatment outcomes and post-treatment Lyme disease syndrome such as delayed diagnosis or treatment with nonideal antibiotics. Whether the combination of high rates of misdiagnosis and nonideal antibiotic therapy result in a population of patients who experience persistent symptoms is unknown. Furthermore, there is a gap in the clinicians' ability to identify patients who have persistent symptoms following antibiotic treatment in part due to the insensitivity of serologic tests, the lack of biomarkers, the lack of pathological material, or the lack of a clinically useful definition. In my community-based clinical practice, when we tried to apply the Infectious Disease Society of America (IDSA) guideline definition for post-Lyme disease syndrome (Wormser et al., 2006) to our patient population, the definition did not match the patients we were seeing. Those patients who were most likely to have post-Lyme disease syndrome based on our clinical history and evaluation ultimately could not meet the IDSA case definition because they were misdiagnosed initially and had not received appropriate initial antibiotic treatment (both of which preclude inclusion in the IDSA case definition).

One gap echoed repeatedly during the workshop is that gap between the existing research on the disease and the knowledge that clinicians need in order to care for patients in the clinical setting. One way to address this gap is to establish a multicenter network for clinical evaluation and treatment of Lyme disease and other TBDs. This network would follow a translational clinical model as a way to link the laboratory study of pathogenesis to community-based patient care. The hallmark of this approach would be the use of a multidisciplinary, coordinated approach to patient evaluation. The goals would include

- Formalizing reproducible case definitions or phenotypes of post-treatment Lyme disease syndrome;
- Performing uniform evaluations of clinical symptoms and signs with validated instruments from a variety of medical disciplines;
- Developing better tests for indentifying biomarkers that can be used for diagnosis, measuring the efficacy of therapy, and establishing prior exposure in patients being evaluated for post-treatment Lyme disease syndrome;
- Establishing a biorepository of blood and tissue from patients with various stages or categories of Lyme disease;
- Analyzing measurement tools and tests for sex-based differences in performance; and
- Developing an evidence-based clinical guideline for post-treatment Lyme disease syndrome that is based on knowledge of the pathophysiology of the illness.

## CRITICAL NEEDS AND GAPS IN UNDERSTANDING TICK-BORNE DISEASES: PATHOGENESIS PERSPECTIVE

*Linda K. Bockenstedt, M.D., Yale University School of Medicine*

The workshop's presentations and discussions underscored the complexity of Lyme disease and the difficulty from an academic and scientific point of view in understanding its various facets. For example, ticks are known to harbor a large number of microbial species, but the relevance of each of these microbes to veterinary and human disease is known only for a few. Scientists do not know the absolute risk for human infection following a tick bite, nor do they understand how coinfection in the tick influences the infectivity and virulence of tick-transmitted pathogens. These unknowns could be answered by applying a systems biology approach to a defined population of ticks.

An ideal scenario for the prevention of tick-borne diseases would be a single vaccine against the tick-borne pathogens that have the greatest potential to cause human disease. This is not likely in the short term given the inherent difficulties with vaccine design, production, and evaluation for safety and efficacy. A vaccine to interrupt tick feeding shows some promise and may be an alternative to pathogen-specific vaccines. All vaccine prevention strategies require continued studies of tick-borne disease pathogenesis to better understand the tick and pathogen life cycles and the response of the mammalian host to the tick and its pathogens. Bockenstedt noted that a demand for better diagnostic tests should not overshadow the need to educate clinicians on the use and limitations of the current diagnostic tests for tick-borne diseases. To meet this need, physicians should be aware of how tick-borne illnesses commonly present. For patients presenting with an acute illness, it is reasonable to consider empiric therapy for the most likely cause(s) of the illness while obtaining appropriate tests to validate or exclude the diagnosis. The approach should weigh risks of treatment against potential benefit. Indiscriminate testing raises clinical conundrums. Borrowing from the field of rheumatology, the prevalence of antinuclear antibodies (ANAs) in healthy people, which in the appropriate clinical setting can be a rheumatic disease marker, ranges from 5 to 30 percent depending on the age group. The clinical significance of this test requires placing results in the context of the patient's symptoms. If the patient does not have an appropriate clinical history compatible with an ANA-related disease, the clinician is faced with deciding how to value the test: Should the clinician monitor the patient or proceed with therapy?

For Lyme disease, Bockenstedt noted that spirochete persistence is another area in need of further research. Without antibiotic treatment, disease manifestations can resolve despite persistence of the spirochete. This area holds a number of unresolved questions in this area: (1) To what degree does the mammal expend immunologic energy when spirochetes are present, but clinically apparent disease is not? (2) Is there a pattern of host gene expression that is a signature of this stage of spirochete infection? (3) What happens to this immune signature with antibiotic treatment? Answering these questions will give us insights into how spirochetes persist in humans and may give us new tools for monitoring response to therapy.

The challenge of "chronic Lyme disease" is that the term means different things to different people. Designing a study to investigate "chronic Lyme disease" is difficult when there is no agreement on the precise definition. Furthermore, there is no animal model has been found that is analogous to patients with "chronic Lyme disease" who do not satisfy the CDC interpretation of Lyme disease serology. All of the animal models, from mice to nonhuman primates, exhibit IgM and IgG antibodies to a broad array of the proteins, even when the animal has been treated with antibiotics and has culture evidence of persistent infection. Clinicians and researchers have not yet explained how a patient with protracted symptoms attributed clinically to "chronic Lyme disease" may fail to develop the expected evolution of antibody responses. Understanding pathogenesis is an important element in explaining some of these clinical disparities. However, it relies heavily on animal models and for some areas (e.g., neuroborreliosis) no animal model exists. There is a strong unmet need for stratifying for study those individuals who have illnesses or disease patterns that are considered "chronic Lyme disease," including those who are being treated for this condition. The creation of a biorepository from well-defined patient populations would be an important first step toward addressing mechanistically their pathobiology.

The ultimate goal of research on disease pathogenesis is to inform us on the ways to ameliorate human disease. A study of the human immune system in normal adults—healthy young adults and healthy elderly—has demonstrated that alterations in immunity occur due to normal aging (van Duin et al., 2007; Panda et al., 2010; Shaw et al., 2011). Other factors, such as infections and comorbid chronic conditions (e.g., obesity), vaccinations, and antibiotic use, also can shape the immune system and immune response (Amar et al., 2007; Didierlaurent et al., 2008). Moreover, studies in animal models suggest that an individual's microbiome contributes to how diseases are expressed (Sekirov et al., 2010). How these factors influence the susceptibility to and clinical expression of tick-borne diseases is an area for further investigation.

## CRITICAL NEEDS AND GAPS IN UNDERSTANDING TICK-BORNE DISEASES: RESEARCHER SPECIALIZING IN *EHRLICHIA* AND *ANAPLASMA*

*J. Stephen Dumler, M.D., Johns Hopkins University School of Medicine*

The workshop presentations and the discussions offered considerable value. One way to approach the research gaps and opportunities is to use the traditional triad of medical science: prevention, identification (including coinfections), and treatments (including disease pathogenesis).

In terms of prevention, many variables that determine the natural burden of disease, tick abundance, pathogen abundance, or pathogen transmission are unknown. More information about these variables may result in prevention strategies that ultimately and substantially reduce the likelihood of transmission and infection. Simultaneously, Dumler noted that surveillance of both human and animal diseases, vectors, and their reservoirs needs to be improved. This research information could improve targeting of habitat or human behavior to reduce the burden of TBDs.

Prevention also can be achieved through vaccines, but questions remain as to whether they are reasonable and practical and, if so, for whom (humans, animals, or ticks). Vaccines are not currently available for tickborne diseases, but they may be more useful with further research and more refined approaches. For example, Dumler noted that scientists need to understand induction of protective immunity versus the induction of immunopathology before moving forward. Furthermore, discussions need to be held to determine the role of technologies, such as high-throughput analyses for facilitating vaccine development and target identification.

Improving diagnosis is crucial, especially for early diagnosis of *Ehrlichia*, *Anaplasma*, and *Rickettsia* infections. This would also facilitate reduction in the number of cases of Lyme disease with persistent manifestations and help curtail serious acute disease and the potential for long-lasting clinical sequelae. More sensitive diagnostics are needed in the earliest stages of disease without sacrificing specificity and increasing false positives. One avenue might be the use of systems biology, but analysis of the data is extremely challenging. A second avenue involves targets from the microbes themselves. Most of the advances in diagnosis have come from basic research, including the VlsE/C6 peptide diagnostics for Lyme disease, polymerase chain reaction (PCR) targets for identification of *Ehrlichia*, *Anaplasma*, and *Rickettsia* infections, and peptide immunoassays for new-generation diagnostics. The presentations underscored a need for research investments to be made on diagnostics.

At the same time that the diagnostic research is continuing, Dumler suggested that the field needs to do a better job of educating physicians in the use of existing and newly developing diagnostic tools. Physician education results in more accurate diagnoses and appropriate treatment. Similarly, there is a need for better corroboration of infection with individual pathogens as well as coinfections.

For treatment, Dumler noted that pathogenetic mechanisms need to be more fully defined so that interventions can be targeted directly at the level of pathophysiology. Animal models are needed to define cellular microbiology and immunology *in vivo*, in a system that will translate to human infection and disease. As noted at different times during the workshop, animal models will show discrepancies. These discrepancies need to be resolved, or researchers need to understand how the results inform understanding of human infection and disease. The question also remains whether the whole-genome survey studies described in the pathogenesis chapter can be translated into human clinical studies that will allow scientists to identify those targeted areas in pathophysiology to create new interventions.

Finally, Dumler noted that large-scale human clinical studies that have sufficient statistical power are needed. As discussed by previous panelists, such studies would allow the acquisition of large numbers of subjects and potentially bring together all of the involved communities—patients, advocate groups, physicians, academicians—to address research uncertainties on a large scale. These clinical trials for tick-borne diseases could easily be assimilated into modern high-throughput methods that may make whole genome surveys feasible. There would need to be some discussion on how many patients would be needed for a single-nucleotide polymorphism (SNP) analysis for neuroborreliosis. A large-scale clinical study would be intense and difficult, but it would rely on the communities coming together. These clinical trial groups could provide critical corroborated subjects and a biorepository of samples for pathogenesis studies. Within the group, one could create and validate the next generation of diagnostics. It would also provide a critical structure for the assessment of the new diagnostics, clinical interventions, and therapeutics.

## CRITICAL NEEDS AND GAPS IN UNDERSTANDING TICK-BORNE DISEASES: THE GLOBAL PERSPECTIVE

*Susan O'Connell, M.D., Southampton University Hospitals Trust*

One of the challenges that has bedeviled this field is the case definition and diagnostic criteria for Lyme disease and other TBDs. The challenge starts with the lack of agreement among stakeholders on the definitions of the various terms, including Lyme borreliosis, disseminated Lyme borreliosis, late Lyme borreliosis, chronic Lyme disease, and post-Lyme disease syndrome and symptoms. Agreeing upon a lexicon is crucial both for the diagnosis and the appropriate management of patients who are suffering now and for the basic research for the future.

From a clinical and a laboratory perspective, improved diagnostic tests are needed for all TBDs. Encouraging progress has been made in the serological tests for Lyme disease, which have improved very significantly since the 1990s. However, now is the time to review the current state of the role of two-tier testing. For example, in-depth discussions are needed on the use of immunoblots versus the modern recombinant and peptide-based tests. Also, high volumes of sera are needed from a large number of well-characterized Lyme borreliosis patients, normal controls, and patients from other disease groups to produce a serum repository that can be used to evaluate new and existing tests. Currently, a relatively small serum panel is available. Scientists also need to review the performance of currently available Lyme borreliosis tests and ensure that maximum information is extracted from them, as exemplified by recent work of American and European groups (Dessau et al., 2010; Porwancher et al., 2011).

IgM tests are problematic (Porwancher et al, 2011). The challenges associated with IgM assays are not unique to tick-borne diseases but occur in other infectious and autoimmune conditions, as IgM antibodies tend to be more polyreactive than other antibody isotypes (Schroeder and Cavacini, 2010). Sera from patients with conditions such as infectious mononucleosis or rheumatoid arthritis can give false-positive reactions in *Borrelia burgdorferi* IgM tests and in many other IgM assays. The use of the IgM tests in the diagnosis of Lyme borreliosis should be limited to appropriate clinical circumstances (i.e., for patients with suspected recently acquired infection) and interpretive laboratory criteria strictly applied, including use of appropriate reaction cut-off controls to minimize overreading of immunoblot reactions. Finally, as many panelists noted, clinician education about appropriate use of diagnostic tests for Lyme borreliosis, appreciation of predictive values, and interpretation of clinical significance of results is needed.

In the clinical arena, a number of questions remain unanswered, such as what proportion of people who get *B. burgdorferi* infections do poorly, and why. Recent prospective and retrospective studies indicated that outcomes were excellent for the great majority of enrolled patients. Early diagnosis and treatment are important factors affecting outcome, requiring increased public and healthcare professional education and awareness for early recognition and management. To assist the effort into finding out why some patients have poor outcomes, scientists need to understand which borrelial strains are associated with infections with poor outcomes and the role that patients' genetic makeup, immune system abnormalities, and other possible conditions (e.g., central pain syndrome) play in the disease manifestations of patients with prolonged symptoms following treatment.

The term "chronic Lyme disease" encompasses several groups of patients, including those with persistent symptoms following treatment; others with active late-stage infections because the diagnosis had been missed at an earlier stage; and some who had been misdiagnosed with Lyme disease but have other conditions. Ultimately, no matter the underlying diagnosis, they are a group of patients who are ill, some seriously incapacitated, who are looking to their clinicians for immediate help. One avenue for investigating some of these issues raised at the workshop is for a large long-term study of these patients to assess accuracy of diagnosis, investigate possible mechanisms of persistent symptoms, examine treatment and management through a multidisciplinary holistic approach, maintain support and assess the long-term outcomes of all recruits, regardless of their eventual diagnostic assignment. A central component of the study would be a biorepository similar to that which other panelists have suggested. Other areas where research is needed include pain research, cognitive studies, and basic pathogenesis studies, including the clearance of infection following treatment.

Finally, O'Connell noted in terms of disease prevention, vaccines are not a viable option in the near future. More immediate options need to be developed to raise awareness among at-risk populations and their healthcare providers. First, more research needs to be done to further our understanding of the complex ecological factors involved, observing geographical changes in the tick range, and translating this information into prevention strategies. Second, there is a need to invest in targeted surveillance. Third, human behavioral factors are the key to prevention. The ideas of following everyday tick bite prevention meausures and removing attached ticks immediately need to be promoted to at-risk populations. Fourth, educational efforts for healthcare professionals and patients need to be increased.

## CRITICAL NEEDS AND GAPS IN UNDERSTANDING TICK-BORNE DISEASES: THE PATIENT PERSPECTIVE

*Greg P. Skall, J.D., National Capital Lyme and*
*Tick-Borne Disease Association*

I would like to begin with an acknowledgment of Representative Frank Wolf (R-VA) for his part in making this workshop a reality. His work, together with his colleagues on the House Appropriations Committee, led to the recognition that we face a serious national Lyme disease and tick-borne disease problem requiring study.

When used by the patient advocate community, the term "Lyme" has become shorthand for all of the diseases that have been discussed at this workshop. So, when referenced in this discussion and going forward, "Lyme" is a label used to encompass all the tick-borne coinfections.

Throughout the 2 days of this workshop, we have heard many important and extraordinary observations and conclusions from the expert presenters. Some of the most salient were

- We have a poor understanding of the true incidence and geographical distribution of Lyme disease. One presenter ventured that, in this regard, we don't have a clue of its magnitude.
- The long-term effects of chronic Lyme disease can last 50–70 years.
- Children cannot be considered little adults in either diagnosis or treatment. Many children have literally lost their childhood to this disease.
- Underpowered studies that purport to demonstrate universal efficacy must be viewed with circumspection.
- Everyone is studying the early stage of this infection; no one is studying the persistent phase of the disease. It is important that those studies occur.
- Current testing and diagnosis is horribly inadequate; some of the declarations heard in this regard were:
  - A person does not require an antibody response to develop the disease!
  - How can you say that after 4 weeks of treatment a patient no longer has Lyme disease? The fact is we don't know!

- o We need direct antigen detection; antibody tests are not sufficiently reliable.
- o Treat the patient, not the test.
- The bitterness of the debate does not serve science or the patient. One presenter stated: All the shouting drowns out all the complexity and the nuance and the work that needs to be done.

A clear direction for future investigation and treatment options emerges from these observations. That direction must not be lost on the scientific and medical community, and the patient community expects it to be pursued. The presentations and discussions we have been privileged to witness in this workshop make it clear that Lyme disease is now recognized as a national epidemic. As a next step, it is crucial that Congress and the medical community recognize the complexity of this disease and the burden it imposes on individuals. That case has been clearly established by these presentations, many of which noted the persistence of the infection in animal models. Unfortunately, these presentations only detailed the work that has been done in mice and do not refer to primate studies. Medical progress depends on bridging this research gap. Furthermore, while this research is being done there must be support for the medical practitioners on the front lines, who are working directly with the patients and the family members burdened with this disease but with inadequate diagnostic tools.

The data clearly demonstrate that the burden of TBDs is enormous on both adults and children. It is so debilitating that it often affects one's livelihood, career, and family, and can wipe out a family's life savings. New research directed to the effects of the disease and treatment of children is a necessity. Children are literally losing their childhood to this disease, and its long-term effects can last many years. Indeed, some patients are losing their lives to it. It is also clear, whether through healthcare costs or the social upheaval that comes from the effect of the disease on an individual's ability to perform and provide for economic well-being, that society bears the final burden.

Multiple presentations clearly demonstrated that Lyme disease is a complex disorder for which there is a critical need for improved diagnostic tools that will allow for better characterization of both the acute and the persistent manifestations of all tick-borne coinfections. The CDC case definition of Lyme disease must be reviewed. That definition, designed specifically and only for surveillance, is often misused as the definitive diagnostic criteria in the clinical setting, so its use is misunderstood in the general medical community. Patients, physicians, and scientists must have a better case definition, expanded to include the entire emerging spectrum of Lyme disease and tick-borne coinfections.

The data presented about Lyme disease clearly indicate it is a grow-ing problem throughout the United States. Therefore, we must discard the often-heard regional biases about the existence and extent of Lyme disease. It is no longer solely a northeast U.S. phenomenon, if it ever was. Our na-tional consciousness must be expanded to include the study and treatment of all tick-borne diseases throughout the United States.

The hallmarks of new studies and research must include

- Developing an automated, standardized report or technique to assist in reporting compliance;
- Developing consistent reporting criteria for all states; and
- Reaching a broadened case definition for surveillance to recog-nize and include advanced late-manifestations of Lyme disease and coinfections.

An enlightened approach to the various manifestations of Lyme disease is urgently needed. Although several presenters did highlight the significance of coinfections and their immune-suppressing properties, most of the sci-ence presented focused only on the acute condition and did not investigate or discuss chronic manifestations. If we are to stem the epidemic, chronic or disseminated Lyme disease must be taken seriously and researched. Physicians should be taught to include it in their differential diagnoses. Symptoms dismissed by some as "subjective" must be studied, quantified, and given clinical weight. They are presented too often and too consistently by too broad a patient population to be ignored.

Finally, "post-Lyme disease syndrome," a derogatory label that subtly suggests a patient no longer has a disease and more likely suffers a psy-chological condition, should be stricken from the diagnostic alternatives unless it can be proven with scientific accuracy that a statistically significant number of patients presenting with chronic Lyme disease symptoms are actually disease free.

Critically important research for the 21st century should include

- Research on the characterization of borrelia genotypes;
- Informatics to create national databases that capture every aspect of the disease in the ecosystem, the vectors, and the patients; and
- Nothing short of a "Manhattan-like project" all-out effort to ad-dress the tick-borne disease burden on patients and on society.

Research for the 21st century should look at other models for guid-ance; one useful reference might be the Alzheimer's Disease Neuro-Imaging Initiative (ADNI) for advancing research on biomarkers and the sharing of data. As suggested above, this research would focus on the complexity of the disease, such as multiple pathogens, the role of mutations, immune system evasion and suppression, subspecies and strain variation, multiple mechanisms for persistence, and patient population heterogeneity.

To accomplish these research goals, new approaches are needed that focus on persistent, post-treatment illness and that employ a broader surveillance case definition than presently used by the CDC study designs. The CDC criteria prejudice the research that relies on it because, by definition, it eliminates the possible inclusion of the vast majority of Lyme disease patients.

Medical progress should no longer be impeded by the polarizing controversy that has characterized Lyme disease research in the past. The dialogue must continue and encourage mutually respectful collaboration across scientific disciplines and among researchers, clinicians, and patients, even when viewpoints differ, if we are to make progress. The National Institute of Health Chronic Fatigue Committee might serve as another example of this type of collaboration.

Finally, a number of state advocacy and support leaders across the country have emphasized areas of concern to them:

- Physicians are not updated on the existence of Lyme disease in their state or the expanded list of symptoms presented by patients. Continuing medical education courses must be designed to recognize and include them.
- When physicians pursue testing, too many rely solely on the enzyme-linked immunosorbent assay (ELISA). The medical community must recognize that the ELISA is not sufficiently accurate to be relied on as the definitive first-stage screen.
- The lack of physician knowledge and poor testing results in incomplete surveillance data, and it leads to a lack of appropriate treatment, all of which must be improved.

Finally, it cannot be overstated that until a highly accurate test is developed and disseminated, Lyme disease is and will remain a clinical diagnosis that relies on the ability of physicians to practice the art of medicine as well as applying the craft of medical technology.

## PANEL DISCUSSION

### Diagnostics

During the workshop, some speakers noted that the IgM Western blot is an unreliable indicator of the disease except for the first two months of illness. One clinician countered by noting that some patients who have a prolonged illness do not have positive ELISAs or their Western blots do not show IgG reactivity. Specimens from these patients may show IgM reactivity with many bands on Western blot; these patients also appear to respond to antibiotic therapy. However, among the panelists there was no consensus on the role and value of IgM tests and the likelihood for false positive IgM Western blots.

## The Role of Collaboration

Collaboration was a major theme throughout the discussion. One participant noted that the various disciplines involved, the clinicians, and the patient advocacy community each have a piece of the puzzle. With more collaboration, the field would have advanced further in the past 30 years. Some participants noted that now is the time for the different factions to come together to focus on the disease and to work to help the patients.

Another participant noted that many individuals echoed the call for partnerships among clinicians, patient advocates, and academics, but the list did not include veterinary colleges and medical entomologists. In addition, community, state, and international collaboration will be essential to moving forward. If the goal is community-based preventive care, the mosquito abatement districts and vector-control programs need to be engaged. Finally, public–private partnerships were not discussed during the workshop. Some participants suggested the need to discuss how to encourage the public and the private entities to work together.

O'Connell raised the question of whether advocates, doctors who see early and late manifestations of Lyme disease, and researchers could design a research project that would meet the needs of the various groups. One participant noted that this workshop demonstrated that everyone could be in the same room and share some common ideas and goals. Instead of working toward one goal, it will be important to work toward two or three goals to meet the needs of various stakeholders. Furthermore, a clinical trial should not be owned by one stakeholder, but by a group of stakeholders. O'Connell expanded on this thought by suggesting that the trial should be a multi-specialty, multidisciplinary effort. It should also have a component that supports the patients within their family and societal structure. The participant further noted that the study should be more prospective and look at people who have a different diagnosis, such as fibromyalgia, chronic fatigue, or multiple sclerosis, and check them for Lyme disease. O'Connell agreed and noted the assertion in her original statement that patients who are found not to have Lyme disease should be kept within the cohort, rather than excluded, so that the long-term outcomes of the whole cohort can be assessed. The findings of such a study could have broader benefits to many patients with medically unexplained illnesses.

## Clinical Management Team

A question was raised about who should comprise a clinical management team to treat patients with long-term symptoms. O'Connell noted that Lyme disease affects a number of different systems, depending to some degree on the borrelial genospecies causing the infection. *Borrelia burgdorferi*, which is the most common strain in the United States and also occurs in Europe, tends to cause Lyme disease arthritis. *Borrelia garinii*, which is strongly associated with neuroborreliosis, and *Borrelia afzelii*, mainly causing skin manifestations, are more common causes of Lyme borreliosis in Europe. To address Lyme disease, O'Connell noted a need for participation by all the major specialties who normally would be involved in addressing the complications of Lyme disease patients. It is important to manage all of patients' symptoms and help them to get their lives back. Rehabilitation is an important part of that process as well, requiring expert input from a variety of specialists working closely with patients and families.

## FINAL SUMMATION AND CLOSING REMARKS

*Lonnie King*

A character in an E. B. White novel said, "I see a great future for complexity." For Lyme disease and other tick-borne diseases, this is certainly true.

Participants need to consider our earlier discussions about looking at tick-borne diseases from 30,000 feet. There is a remarkable dynamic that involves the convergence of people, animals, and ecosystems. More than 7 billion people share space on Earth with rapidly increasing numbers of wildlife and domestic animals. Human–animal interfaces are both being amplified and intensified as our world becomes progressively interconnected. Thus, pathogens and vectors have new opportunities to spread, transmit, and create new niches and survival mechanisms. People live in an unprecedented time regarding new emerging infectious diseases, many of which are vector borne. The pathogens have a favorable environment to become resistant, undergo genetic modification, and move globally as people and products traverse the globe faster than the incubation period for any of these diseases. To address these current and emerging tick-borne diseases, scientists need to refocus their attention to achieve a greater understanding of the convergence of these factors and create greater possibilities for disease control and prevention, including intervention strategies targeted at the vectors, maintenance hosts, and environmental sites.

The ecology of infectious diseases is a field where the available information is imprecise. In addition, significant gaps in knowledge exist that require new studies and research with better integration and the creation of a national research agenda to ensure that there is no duplication of effort and that researchers are properly linked and cohesively working together to leverage limited resources. Perhaps a new portfolio of research and a fresh focus of inquiry may advance the scientific process. A few observations from the presentations can be highlighted:

- The philosopher Nietzsche once stated that "the most common form of ignorance is forgetting what it is that we are trying to do." For Lyme disease and other tick-borne diseases, as noted by Pamela Weintraub, the goals are the reduction in the morbidity and the mortality of this group of diseases, the reduction of the burden of disease, and the creation of better strategies for prevention, control, and amelioration.
- Weintraub noted that perhaps the number one problem that limits progress toward these goals is the polarity that exists between patients and some of the medical community. This can be extended further to the polarization that exists between the medical community and the advocacy groups.
- A number of individuals suggested the need for less hubris and more sensitivity to others' points of view. People are suffering, and there is a need to reframe and refocus the research to generate new ways to reduce disease burden. As one researcher noted, it is about creating a better path forward and not maintaining the status quo.

I believe that science could emerge as the mediator to define a new common ground to reduce the polarity between groups and focus on areas where there is agreement. Scientific research is the key to new knowledge, and the application of this knowledge is the key to reducing the burden of illness. It seems unlikely that any gains in reducing TBD illnesses and impact can occur without filling our gaps in knowledge and better understanding the dynamics and complexities of these diseases through research. A critical review of the state of the science, such as that found in this summary, is an essential first step.

# References

Abbadie, C., J. A. Lindia, A. M. Cumiskey, L. B. Peterson, J. S. Mudgett, E. K. Bayne, J. A. DeMartino, D. E. MacIntyre, and M. J. Forrest. 2003. Impaired neuropathic pain responses in mice lacking the chemokine receptor ccr2. *Proceedings of the National Academy of Sciences of the United States of America* 100(13):7947-7952.

Ablin, J. N., Y. Shoenfeld, and D. Buskila. 2006. Fibromyalgia, infection and vaccination: Two more parts in the etiological puzzle. *Journal of Autoimmunity* 27(3):145-152.

Adamek, B., A. Ksiaiek, A. Szczerba-Sachs, J. Kasperczyk, and A. Wiczkowski. 2006. Tick-borne diseases exposure of forestry workers and preventive methods usage. *Przegl Epidemiology* 60 (Suppl 1):11-15.

Adeyemi, E. O. A., K. D. Desai, M. Towsey, and D. Ghista. 1999. Characterization of autonomic dysfunction in patients with irritable bowel syndrome by means of heart rate variability studies. *American Journal of Gastroenterology* 94(3):816-823.

Adjemian, J. Z., J. Krebs, E. Mandel, and J. McQuiston. 2009. Spatial clustering by disease severity among reported Rocky Mountain spotted fever cases in the United States, 2001-2005. *American Journal of Tropical Medicine and Hygiene* 80(1):72-77.

Aguero-Rosenfeld, M. E., G. Wang, I. Schwartz, and G. P. Wormser. 2005. Diagnosis of Lyme borreliosis. *Clinical Microbiology Reviews* 18(3):484-509.

Ahantarig, A., W. Trinachartvanit, and J. R. Milne. 2008. Tick-borne pathogens and diseases of animals and humans in Thailand. *Southeast Asian Journal of Tropical Medicine & Public Health* 39(6):1015-1032.

Akalin, H., S. Helvaci, and S. Gedikoglu. 2009. Re-emergence of tularemia in Turkey. *International Journal of Infectious Diseases* 13(5):547-551.

Akhtar, J. 2005. Crimean-Congo haemorrhagic fever: An alert for health care workers. *Jcpsp, Journal of the College of Physicians & Surgeons—Pakistan* 15(12):751-752.

Akkoyunlu, M., and E. Fikrig. 2000. Gamma interferon dominates the murine cytokine response to the agent of human granulocytic ehrlichiosis and helps to control the degree of early rickettsemia. *Infection and Immunity* 68:1827-1833.

Alaedini, A., and B. A. Fallon. 2010. *Effect of iv antibiotic therapy on antibody profilein patients with post-treatmentlyme encephalapothy.* Paper presented at 135th Annual Meeting of the American Neurological Association (ANA), San Francisco, CA.

Alexopoulou, L., V. Thomas, M. Schnare, Y. Lobet, J. Anguita, R. T. Schoen, R. Medzhitov, E. Fikrig, and R. A. Flavell. 2002. Hyporesponsiveness to vaccination with *Borrelia burgdorferi* ospa in humans and in tlr1- and tlr2-deficient mice. *Natural Medicine* 8:878-884.

Allan, B. F., F. Keesing, and R. S. Ostfeld. 2003. Effect of forest fragmentation on Lyme disease risk. *Conservation Biology* 17(1):267-272.

Amar, S., Q. Zhou, Y. Shaik-Dasthagirisaheb, and S. Leeman. 2007. Diet-induced obesity in mice causes changes in immune responses and bone loss manifested by bacterial challenge. *Proceedings of the National Academy of Sciences of the United States of America* 104:20466-20471. PMID: 18077329. PMCID: PMC2154454.

Angelakis, E., S. A. Billeter, E. B. Breitschwerdt, B. B. Chomel, and D. Raoult. 2010. Potential for tick-borne bartonelloses. *Emerging Infectious Diseases* 16(3):385-391.

Arnold, L. M., J. I. Hudson, E. V. Hess, A. E. Ware, D. A. Fritz, M. B. Auchenbach, L. O. Starck, and P. E. Keck. 2004. Family study of fibromyalgia. *Arthritis and Rheumatism* 50(3):944-952.

Assous, M. V., and A. Wilamowski. 2009. Relapsing fever borreliosis in Eurasia—forgotten, but certainly not gone! *Clinical Microbiology & Infection* 15(5):407-414.

Aucott, J., C. Morrison, B. Munoz, P. C. Rowe, A. Schwarzwalder, and S. K. West. 2009. Diagnostic challenges of early Lyme disease: Lessons from a community case series. *Bmc Infectious Diseases* 9.

Bacon, R. M., B. J. Biggerstaff, M. E. Schriefer, R. D. Gilmore, M. T. Philipp, A. C. Steere, G. P. Wormser, A. R. Marques, and B. J. B. Johnson. 2003. Serodiagnosis of Lyme disease by kinetic enzyme-linked immunosorbent assay using recombinant vlse1 or peptide antigens of *Borrelia burgdorferi* compared with 2-tiered testing using whole-cell lysates. *Journal of Infectious Diseases* 187(8):1187-1199.

Bacon, R. M., K. J. Kugeler, and P. S. Mead. 2008. Surveillance for Lyme disease—United States, 1992-2006. *Morbidity and Mortality Weekly Report* 57(SS10, Suppl. S):1-9.

Bakken, J. S., J. S. Dumler, S. M. Chen, M. R. Eckman, L. L. Vanetta, and D. H. Walker. 1994. Human granulocytic ehrlichiosis in the upper midwest United-States—a new species emerging. *Journal of the American Medical Association* 272(3):212-218.

Bakken, J. S., P. Goellner, M. Van Etten, D. Z. Boyle, O. L. Swonger, S. Mattson, J. Krueth, R. L. Tilden, K. Asanovich, J. Walls, and J. S. Dumler. 1998. Seroprevalence of human granulocytic ehrlichiosis among permanent residents of northwestern Wisconsin. *Clinical Infectious Diseases* 27(6):1491-1496.

Baldridge, G. D., T. J. Kurtti, N. Burkhardt, A. S. Baldridge, C. M. Nelson, A. S. Oliva, and U. G. Munderloh. 2007. Infection of *Ixodes scapularis* ticks with rickettsia monacensis expressing green fluorescent protein: A model system. *Journal of Invertebrate Pathology* 94(3):163-174.

Ball, R., S. V. Shadomy, A. Meyer, B. T. Huber, M. S. Leffell, A. Zachary, M. Belotto, E. Hilton, M. E. Bryant-Genevier, F. W. Miller, and M. M. Braun. 2009. HLA type and immune response to *Borrelia burgdorferi* outer surface protein a in people in whom arthritis developed after Lyme disease vaccination. *Arthritis and Rheumatism* 60:1179-1186.

Bankhead, T., and G. Chaconas. 2007. The role of vlse antigenic variation in the Lyme disease spirochete: Persistence through a mechanism that differs from other pathogens. *Molecular Biology* 65(6):1547-1558.

Baranton, G., D. Postic, I. Saint Girons, P. Boerlin, J.-C. Piffaretti, M. Assous, and P. A. D. Grimont. 1992. Delineation of *Borrelia burgdorferi* sensu stricto, *Borrelia garinii* sp. Nov., and group vs461 associated with Lyme borreliosis. *International Journal of Systematic Bacteriology* 42(3):378-383.

Barbara, G., and V. Stanghellini. 2009. Biomarkers in ibs: When will they replace symptoms for diagnosis and management? *Gut* 58(12):1571-1575.

Barbet, A. F., P. F. Meeus, M. Belanger, M. V. Bowie, J. Yi, A. M. Lundgren, A. R. Alleman, S. J. Wong, F. K. Chu, U. G. Munderloh, and S. D. Jauron. 2003. Expression of multiple outer membrane protein sequence variants from a single genomic locus of anaplasma phagocytophilum. *Infection and Immunity* 71:1706-1718.

Barbour, A. 2004. Specificity of borrelia-tick vector relationships. In *Microbe-vector interactions in vector-borne diseases*, edited by S. H. Gillespie, G. L. Smith and A. Osbourn. West Nyack, NY: Cambridge University Press. Pp. 75-90.

Barthold, S. W., D. S. Beck, G. M. Hansen, G. A. Terwilliger, and K. D. Moody. 1990. Lyme borreliosis in selected strains and ages of laboratory mice. *Journal of Infectious Diseases* 162:133-138.

Barthold, S. W., C. L. Sidman, and A. L. Smith. 1992. Lyme borreliosis in genetically resistant and susceptible mice with severe combined immunodeficiency. *American Journal of Tropical Medicine and Hygiene* 47:605-613.

Barthold, S. W., E. Hodzic, S. Tunev, and S. L. Feng. 2006. Antibody-mediated disease remission in the mouse model of Lyme borreliosis. *Infection and Immunity* 74(8):4817-4825.

Barthold, S. W., D. Cadavid, and M. T. Philipp. 2010. Animal models of borreliosis. In *Borrelia: Molecular biology, host interaction and pathogenesis*, edited by S. Samuels and J. Radolph. Norfolk, UK: Calister Academic Press.

Batra, H. V. 2007. Spotted fevers & typhus fever in Tamil nadu. *Indian Journal of Medical Research* 126(2):101-103.

Bayless, T. M., and M. L. Harris. 1990. Inflammatory bowel-disease and irritable bowel syndrome. *Medical Clinics of North America* 74(1):21-28.

Beall, M. J., R. Chandrashekar, M. D. Eberts, K. E. Cyr, P. P. V. P. Diniz, C. Mainville, B. C. Hegarty, J. M. Crawford, and E. B. Breitschwerdt. 2008. Serological and molecular prevalence of *Borrelia burgdorferi*, anaplasma phagocytophilum, and ehrlichia species in dogs from Minnesota. *Vector-Borne and Zoonotic Diseases* 8(4):455-464.

Beattie, J. F., M. L. Michelson, and P. J. Holman. 2002. Acute babesiosis caused by babesia divergens in a resident of Kentucky. *New England Journal of Medicine* 347:697-698.

Bechelli, J. R., E. Rydkina, P. M. Colonne, and S. K. Sahni. 2009. *Rickettsia rickettsii* infection protects human microvascular endothelial cells against staurosporine-induced apoptosis by a ciap(2)-independent mechanism. *Journal of Infectious Diseases* 199(9):1389-1398.

Behera, A. K., E. Hildebrand, J. Scagliotti, A. C. Steere, and L. T. Hu. 2005. Induction of host matrix metalloproteinases by *Borrelia burgdorferi* differs in human and murine Lyme arthritis. *Infection and Immunity* 73:126-134.

Behera, A. K., E. Hildebrand, R. T. Bronson, G. Perides, S. Uematsu, S. Akira, and L. T. Hu. 2006a. Myd88 deficiency results in tissue-specific changes in cytokine induction and inflammation in interleukin-18-independent mice infected with *Borrelia burgdorferi*. *Infection and Immunity* 74:1462-1470.

Behera, A. K., E. Hildebrand, S. Uematsu, S. Akira, J. Coburn, and L. T. Hu. 2006b. Identification of a TLR-independent pathway for borrelia burgdorferi-induced expression of matrix metalloproteinases and inflammatory mediators through binding to integrin alpha 3 beta 1. *Journal of Immunology* 177:657-664.

Behera, A. K., E. Durand, C. Cugini, S. Antonara, L. Bourassa, E. Hildebrand, L. T. Hu, and J. Coburn. 2008. *Borrelia burgdorferi* bbb07 interaction with integrin alpha3beta1 stimulates production of pro-inflammatory mediators in primary human chondrocytes. *Cell Microbiology* 10:320-331.

Bell, J. F., S. J. Stewart, and S. K. Wikel. 1979. Resistance to tick-borne francisella-tularensis by tick-sensitized rabbits—allergic klendusity. *American Journal of Tropical Medicine and Hygiene* 28(5):876-880.

Belongia, E. A., K. D. Reed, and P. D. Mitchell. 1999. Clinical and epidemiological features of early Lyme disease and human granulocytic ehrlichiosis in Wisconsin. *Clinical Infectious Diseases* 29:1472-1477.

Benhnia, M. R., D. Wrobleski, M. N. Akhtar, R. A. Patel, W. Lavezzi, S. C. Gangloff, S. M. Goyert, M. N. Caimano, J. D. Radolf, and T. J. Sellati. 2005. Signaling through cd14 attenuates the inflammatory response to *Borrelia burgdorferi*, the agent of Lyme disease. *Journal of Immunology* 174:1539-1548.

Beugnet, F., and J.-L. Marie. 2009. Emerging arthropod-borne diseases of companion animals in Europe. *Veterinary Parasitology* 163(4):298-305.

Bockenstedt, L. K., I. Kang, C. Chang, D. Persing, A. Hayday, and S. W. Barthold. 2001. CD4+ T helper 1 cells facilitate regression of murine Lyme carditis. *Infection and Immunity* 69:5264-5269.

Bockenstedt, L. K., J. Mao, E. Hodzic, S. W. Barthold, and D. Fish. 2002. Detection of attenuated, noninfectious spirochetes in *Borrelia burgdorferi*-infected mice after antibiotic treatment. *Journal of Infectious Diseases* 186:1430-1437.

Bockenstedt, L. K., A. Belperron, D. Gonzalez, and A. Haberman. 2011. Persistent antigenic debris but not viable spirochetes after antibiotic therapy for murine Lyme borreliosis.

Bolz, D. D., R. S. Sundsbak, Y. Ma, S. Akira, C. J. Kirschning, J. F. Zachary, J. H. Weis, and J. J. Weis. 2004. Myd88 plays a unique role in host defense but not arthritis development in Lyme disease. *Journal of Immunology* 173:2003-2010.

Bourdoiseau, G. 2006. Canine babesiosis in France. *Veterinary Parasitology* 138(1-2):118-125.

Bowman, D. D. 2006. Successful and currently ongoing parasite eradication programs. *Veterinary Parasitology* 139(4):293-307.

Bowman, D., S. E. Little, L. Lorentzen, J. Shields, M. P. Sullivan, and E. P. Carlin. 2009. Prevalence and geographic distribution of dirofilaria immitis, *Borrelia burgdorferi*, *Ehrlichia canis*, and *Anaplasma phagocytophilum* in dogs in the United States: Results of a national clinic-based serologic survey. *Veterinary Parasitology* 160(1-2):138-148.

Branda, J. A., M. E. Aguero-Rosenfeld, M. J. Ferraro, B. J. Johnson, G. P. Wormser, and A. C. Steere. 2010. 2-tiered antibody testing for early and late Lyme disease using only an immunoglobulin g blot with the addition of a vlse band as the second-tier test *Clinical Infectious Diseases* 50(1):20-26.

Breitschwerdt, E. B., R. G. Maggi, W. L. Nicholson, N. A. Cherry, and C. W. Woods. 2008. Bartonella sp bacteremia in patients with neurological and neurocognitive dysfunction. *Journal of Clinical Microbiology* 46(9):2856-2861.

Breitschwerdt, E. B., R. G. Maggi, B. B. Chomel, and M. R. Lappin. 2010a. Bartonellosis: An emerging infectious disease of zoonotic importance to animals and human beings. *Journal of Veterinary Emergency and Critical Care* 20(1):8-30.

Breitschwerdt, E. B., R. G. Maggi, P. Farmer, and P. E. Mascarelli. 2010b. Molecular evidence of perinatal transmission of bartonella vinsonii subsp berkhoffii and bartonella henselae to a child. *Journal of Clinical Microbiology* 48(6):2289-2293.

Breitschwerdt, E. B., R. G. Maggi, P. M. Lantos, C. W. Woods, B. C. Hegarty, and J. M. Bradley. 2010c. Bartonella vinsonii subsp berkhoffii and bartonella henselae bacteremia in a father and daughter with neurological disease. *Parasites & Vectors* 3.

Brouqui, P., P. Parola, P. E. Fournier, and D. Raoult. 2007. Spotted fever rickettsioses in southern and eastern Europe. *FEMS Immunology & Medical Microbiology* 49(1):2-12.

Brown, C. R., A. Y. Lai, S. T. Callen, V. A. Blaho, J. M. Hughes, and W. J. Mitchell. 2008. Adenoviral delivery of interleukin-10 fails to attenuate experimental Lyme disease. *Infection and Immunity* 76:5500-5507.

Brown, J. P., J. F. Zachary, C. Teuscher, J. J. Weis, and R. M. Wooten. 1999. Dual role of interleukin-10 in murine Lyme disease: Regulation of arthritis severity and host defense. *Infection and Immunity* 67:5142-5150.

Brown, W. C., D. P. Norimine, D. P. Knowles, and W. L. Goff. 2006. Immune control of babesia bovis infection. *Veterinary Parasitology* 138:2856-2861.

Browne, B. J., B. Edwards, and R. L. Rogers. Dermatologic emergencies. *Primary Care: Clinics in Office Practice* 33(3):685-695.

Bruehl, S., C. R. Carlson, and J. A. McCubbin. 1993. 2 brief interventions for acute pain. *Pain* 54(1):29-36.

Brunner, J. L., and R. S. Ostfeld. 2008. Multiple causes of variable tick burdens on small-mammal hosts. *Ecology* 89(8):2259-2272.

Buckingham, S. C., G. S. Marshall, G. E. Schutze, C. R. Woods, M. A. Jackson, L. E. R. Patterson, and R. F. Jacobs. 2007. Clinical and laboratory features, hospital course, and outcome of Rocky Mountain spotted fever in children. *Journal of Pediatrics* 150(2): 180-184.

Buskila, D., L. Neumann, G. Vaisberg, D. Alkalay, and F. Wolfe. 1997. Increased rates of fibromyalgia following cervical spine injury—A controlled study of 161 cases of traumatic injury. *Arthritis and Rheumatism* 40(3):446-452.

Buskila, D., F. Atzeni, and P. Sarzi-Puttini. 2008. Etiology of fibromyalgia: The possible role of infection and vaccination. *Autoimmunity Reviews* 8(1):41-43.

Butler, C. M., D. J. Houwers, F. Jongejan, and J. H. van der Kolk. 2005. *Borrelia burgdorferi* infections with special reference to horses. A review. *Veterinary Quarterly* 27(4):146-156.

Cabello, F. C., H. P. Godfrey, and S. A. Newman. 2007. Hidden in plain sight: *Borrelia burgdorferi* and the extracellular matrix. *Trends in Microbiology* 15(8):350-354.

Cable, R. G., and D. A. Leiby. 2003. Risk and prevention of transfusion-transmitted babesiosis and other tick-borne diseases. *Current Opinion in Hematology* 10(6):405-411.

Cain, K. C., M. E. Jarrett, R. L. Burr, V. L. Hertig, and M. M. Heitkemper. 2007. Heart rate variability is related to pain severity and predominant bowel pattern in women with irritable bowel syndrome. *Neurogastroenterology and Motility* 19(2):110-118.

Canica, M. M., F. Nato, L. Du Merle, C. Mazie, G. Baranton, and D. Postic. 1993. Monoclonal antibodies for identification of *Borrelia afzelii* sp. Nov. Associated with late cutaneous manifestation of Lyme borreliosis. *Scandinavian Journal of Infectious Diseases* 25(4):441-448.

Cerar, D., T. Cerar, E. Ruzic-Sabljic, G. P. Wormser, and F. Strle. 2010. Subjective symptoms after treatment of early Lyme disease. *American Journal of Medicine* 123(1):79-86.

Chandra, A., G. P. Wormser, M. S. Klempner, R. P. Trevino, M. K. Crow, N. Latov, and A. Alaedini. 2010. Anti-neural antibody reactivity in patients with a history of Lyme borreliosis and persistent symptoms. *Brain Behavior and Immunity* 24(6):1018-1024.

Chapman, A. S., J. S. Bakken, S. M. Folk, C. D. Paddock, K. C. Bloch, A. Krusell, D. J. Sexton, S. C. Buckingham, G. S. Marshall, G. A. Storch, G. A. Dasch, J. H. McQuiston, D. L. Swerdlow, S. J. Dumler, W. L. Nicholson, D. H. Walker, M. E. Eremeeva, and C. A. Ohl. 2006a. Diagnosis and management of tickborne rickettsial diseases: Rocky Mountain spotted fever, ehrlichioses, and anaplasmosis—United States: A practical guide for physicians and other health-care and public health professionals. *MMWR Recommendations and Reports* 55(RR-4):1-27.

Chapman, A. S., S. M. Murphy, L. J. Demma, R. C. Holman, A. T. Curns, J. H. McQuiston, J. W. Krebs, and D. L. Swerdlow. 2006b. Rocky Mountain spotted fever in the United States, 1997-2002. *Vector-Borne and Zoonotic Diseases* 6(2):170-178.

Chen, S., J. S. Dumler, J. S. Baken, and D. Walker. 1994. Identification of granulocytic ehrlichia species as the eitiologic agent of human disease. *Journal of Clinical Microbiology* 32:589-595.

Chomel, B. B., R. W. Kasten, C. Williams, A. C. Wey, J. B. Henn, R. Maggi, S. Carrasco, J. Mazet, H. J. Boulouis, R. Maillard, and E. B. Breitschwerdt. 2009. Bartonella endocarditis: A pathology shared by animal reservoirs and patients. *Annals of the New York Academy of Sciences* 1166:120-126.

Chu, C.-Y., W. Liu, B.-G. Jiang, D.-M. Wang, W.-J. Jiang, Q.-M. Zhao, P.-H. Zhang, Z.-X. Wang, G.-P. Tang, H. Yang, and W.-C. Cao. 2008. Novel genospecies of *Borrelia burgdorferi* sensu lato from rodents and ticks in southwestern China. *Journal of Clinical Microbiology* 46(9):3130-3133.

Cisak, E., J. Sroka, J. Zwolinjski, and J. Chmielewska-Badora. 1999. Risk of tick-borne encephalitis (tbe) virus infection among people occupationally exposed to tick bites. *Wiad Parazytology* 45(3):375-380.

Cisak, E., J. Chmielewska-Badora, J. Zwolinski, A. Wojcik-Fatla, J. Polak, and J. Dutkiewicz. 2005. Risk of tick-borne bacterial diseases among workers of Roztocze National Park (south-eastern Poland). *Annals of Agricultural and Environmental Medicine* 12(1):127-132.

Clark, R. P., and L. T. Hu. Prevention of Lyme disease and other tick-borne infections. *Infectious Disease Clinics of North America* 22(3):381-396.

Clauw, D. J., and P. Katz. 1995. The overlap between fibromyalgia and inflammatory rheumatic disease: When and why does it occur? *Journal of Clinical Rheumatology* 1(6):335-342.

Clauw, D. J., C. C. Engel, R. Aronowitz, E. Jones, H. M. Kipen, K. Kroenke, S. Ratzan, M. Sharpe, and S. Wessely. 2003. Unexplained symptoms after terrorism and war: An expert consensus statement. *Journal of Occupational and Environmental Medicine* 45(10):1040-1048.

Coburn, J., J. R. Fischer, and J. M. Leong. 2005. Solving a sticky problem: New genetic approaches to host cell adhesion by the Lyme disease spirochete. *Molecular Microbiology* 57:1182-1195.

Coleman, J. L., J. A. Gebbia, J. Piesman, J. L. Degen, T. H. Bugge, and J. L. Benach. 1997. Plasminogen is required for efficient dissemination of *B. burgdorferi* in ticks and for enhancement of spirochetemia in mice. *Cell Microbiology* 89:1111-1119.

Conlon, P. J., G. W. Procop, V. Fowler, M. A. Eloubeidi, S. R. Smith, and D. J. Sexton. 1996. Predictors of prognosis and risk of acute renal failure in patients with Rocky Mountain spotted fever. *American Journal of Medicine* 101(6):621-626.

Connally, N. P., A. J. Durante, K. M. Yousey-Hindes, J. I. Meek, R. S. Nelson, and R. Heimer. 2009. Peridomestic Lyme disease prevention results of a population-based case-control study. *American Journal of Preventive Medicine* 37(3):201-206.

Connelly, M., F. J. Keefe, G. Affleck, M. A. Lumley, T. Anderson, and S. Waters. 2007. Effects of day-to-day affect regulation on the pain experience of patients with rheumatoid arthritis. *Pain* 131(1-2):162-170.

Conrad, P. A., A. M. Kjemptrup, and R. A. Carreno. 2006. Description of babesia ducani n.Sp. (apicomplexa: Babesiidae) from humans and its differentiation from other piroplasms. *International Journal for Parasitology* 36:779-789.

Coulter, P., C. Lema, D. Flayhart, A. S. Linhardt, J. N. Aucott, P. G. Auwaerter, and J. S. Dumler. 2005. Two-year evaluation of *Borrelia burgdorferi* culture and supplemental tests for definitive diagnosis of Lyme disease. *Journal of Clinical Microbiology* 43(10):5080-5084.

Coutte, L., D. J. Botkin, L. Gao, and S. J. Norris. 2009. Detailed analysis of sequence changes occurring during vlse antigenic variation in the mouse model of *Borrelia burgdorferi* infection. *PLoS Pathogens* 5(2):e1000293.

Crandall, H., D. M. Dunn, Y. Ma, R. M. Wooten, J. F. Zachary, J. H. Weis, R. B. Weiss, and J. J. Weis. 2006. Gene expression profiling reveals unique pathways associated with differential severity of Lyme arthritis. *Journal of Immunology* 177:7930-7942.

Crofford, L. J., E. A. Young, N. C. Engleberg, A. Korszun, C. B. Brucksch, L. A. McClure, M. B. Brown, and M. A. Demitrack. 2004. Basal circadian and pulsatile acth and cortisol secretion in patients with fibromyalgia and/or chronic fatigue syndrome. *Brain Behavior and Immunity* 18(4):314-325.

Crowder, C. D., H. E. Matthews, S. Schutzer, M. A. Rounds, B. J. Luft, O. Nolte, S. R. Campbell, C. A. Phillipson, F. Li, R. Sampath, D. J. Ecker, and M. W. Eshoo. 2010. Genotypic variation and mixtures of Lyme borrelia in ixodes ticks from North America and Europe. *Plos One* 5(5):e10650, 10651-10659.

Dalton, M. J., M. J. Clarke, R. C. Holman, J. W. Krebs, D. B. Fishbein, J. G. Olson, and J. E. Childs. 1995. National surveillance for Rocky Mountain spotted fever, 1981-1992—epidemiologic summary and evaluation of risk-factors for fatal outcome. *American Journal of Tropical Medicine and Hygiene* 52(5):405-413.

Daltroy, L. H., and C. Phillips. 2007. A controlled trial of a novel primary prevention program for Lyme disease and other tick-borne illnesses. *Health Education & Behavior* 34(3):531-542.

Daniel, M., K. Zitek, V. Danielova, B. Kriz, J. Valter, and I. Kott. 2006. Risk assessment and prediction of *Ixodes ricinus* tick questing activity and human tick-borne encephalitis infection in space and time in the Czech Republic. *International Journal of Medical Microbiology* 296 (Suppl 40):41-47.

Daniels, T. J., D. Fish, and I. Schwartz. 1993. Reduced abundance of *Ixodes scapularis* (acari: Ixodidae) and Lyme disease risk by deer exclusion. *J Med Entomol* 30(6):1043-1049.

Dantzer, R., J. C. O'Connor, G. G. Freund, R. W. Johnson, and K. W. Kelley. 2008. From inflammation to sickness and depression: When the immune system subjugates the brain. *Nature Reviews Neuroscience* 9(1):46-57.

De Silva, A. M., and E. Fikrig. 1995. Growth and migration of *Borrelia burgdorferi* in ixodes ticks during blood feeding. *American Journal of Tropical Medicine and Hygiene* 53(4):397-404.

de Waal, D. T., and M. P. Combrink. 2006. Live vaccines against bovine babesiosis. *Veterinary Parasitology* 138(1-2):88-96.

Deblinger, R. D., and D. W. Rimmer. 1991. Efficacy of a permethrin-based acaricide to reduce the abundance of ixodes dammini (acari: Ixodidae). *Journal of Medical Entomology* 28(5):708-711.

Deblinger, R. D., M. L. Wilson, D. W. Rimmer, and A. Spielman. 1993. Reduced abundance of immature ixodes-dammini (acari, ixodidae) following incremental removal of deer. *Journal of Medical Entomology* 30(1):144-150.

Dedert, E. A., J. L. Studts, I. Weissbecker, P. G. Salmon, P. L. Banis, and S. E. Sephton. 2004. Religiosity may help preserve the cortisol rhythm in women with stress-related illness. *International Journal of Psychiatry in Medicine* 34(1):61-77.

DelaPaz, R., A. Lignelli, K. M. Corbera, H. A. Sackeim, and B. A. Fallon. 2005. *MR imaging in persistent Lyme encephalophathy.* Paper presented at the X International Congress on Lyme Borreliosis, Vienna, Austria.

Demma, L. J., M. E. Eremeeva, W. L. Nicholson, M. Traeger, D. Blau, C. D. Paddock, M. Levin, G. A. Dasch, J. E. Cheek, D. L. Swerdlow, and J. McQuiston. 2006. An outbreak of Rocky Mountain spotted fever associated with a novel tick vector, rhipicephalus sanguineus, in Arizona, 2004: Preliminary report. *Annals of the New York Academy of Sciences* 1078:342-343.

Dessau, R. B., T. Ejlertsen, and J. Hilden. 2010. Simultaneous use of serum IgG and IgM for risk scoring of suspected early Lyme borreliosis: Graphical and bivariate analyses. *Acta Pathologica, Microbiologica et immunologica Scandinavica* 118(4):313-323.

Didierlaurent, A., J. Goulding, S. Patel, R. Snelgrove, L. Low, M. Bebien, T. Laurence, L. S. Van Rijt, B. N. Lambrecht, J. C. Sirard, and T. Hussell. 2008. Sustained desensitization to bacterial toll-like receptor ligands after resolution of respiratory influenza infection. *Journal of Experimental Medicine* 205:323-329.

Dietrich, F., T. Schmidgen, R. G. Maggi, D. Richter, F. R. Matuschka, R. Vonthein, E. B. Breitschwerdt, and V. A. J. Kempf. 2010. Prevalence of *Bartonella henselae* and *Borrelia burgdorferi* sensu lato DNA in *Ixodes ricinus* ticks in Europe. *Applied and Environmental Microbiology* 76(5):1395-1398.

Dolan, M. C., N. S. Zeidner, E. Gabitzsch, G. Dietrich, J. N. Borchert, R. M. Poche, and J. Piesman. 2008. Short report: A doxycycline hyclate rodent bait formulation for prophylaxis and treatment of tick-transmitted *Borrelia burgdorferi*. *American Journal of Tropical Medicine and Hygiene* 78(5):803-805.

Donta, S. 1997. Tetracycline therapy of chronic Lyme disease. *Clinical Infectious Diseases* 25:52-56.

Doudier, B., J. Olano, P. Parola, and P. Brouqui. 2010. Factors contributing to emergence of ehrlichia and anaplasma spp. As human pathogens. *Veterinary Parasitology* 167(2-4):149-154.

Dresser, A. R., P. O. Hardy, and G. Chaconas. 2009. Investigation of the genes involved in antigenic switching at the vlse locus in *Borrelia burgdorferi:* An essential role for the ruvab branch migrase. *PLoS Pathogens* 5(12):e1000680.

Dumler, J. S. 2005. Anaplasma and ehrlichia infection. *Annals of the New York Academy of Sciences* 1063(1):361-373.

Dumler, J. S., and J. S. Bakken. 1995. Ehrlichial diseases of humans: Emerging tick-borne infections. *Clinical Infectious Diseases* 20(5):1102-1110.

Dumler, J. S., A. F. Barbet, C. P. J. Bekker, G. A. Dasch, G. H. Palmer, S. C. Ray, Y. Rikihisa, and F. R. Rurangirwa. 2001. Reorganization of genera in the families rickettsiaceae and anaplasmataceae in the order rickettsiales: Unification of some species of ehrlichia with anaplasma, cowdria with ehrlichia and ehrlichia with neorickettsia, descriptions of six new species combinations and designation of ehrlichia equi and 'hge agent' as subjective synonyms of *Ehrlichia phagocytophila*. *International Journal of Systematic and Evolutionary Microbiology* 51:2145-2165.

Eikeland, R., Å. Mygland, K. Herlofson, and U. Ljøstad. 2011. European neuroborreliosis: Quality of life 30 months after treatment. *Acta Neurologica Scandinavica* 123(6).

Elchos, B. N., and J. Goddard. 2003. Implications of presumptive fatal Rocky Mountain spotted fever in two dogs and their owner. *Journal of the American Veterinary Medical Association* 223(10):1450-1452.

Engin, A., S. Arslan, S. Kizildag, H. Ozturk, N. Elaldi, I. Dokmetas, and M. Bakir. 2010a. Toll-like receptor 8 and 9 polymorphisms in Crimean-Congo hemorrhagic fever. *Microbes and Infection* 12(12-13):1071-1078.

Engin, A., S. Ugurlu, E. Caglar, A. Y. Oztop, D. Inan, N. Elaldi, I. Dokmetas, and M. Bakir. 2010b. Serum levels of mannan-binding lectin in patients with Crimean-Congo hemorrhagic fever. *Vector-Borne and Zoonotic Diseases* 10(10):1037-1041.

Fahrer, H., S. M. Vanderlinden, M. J. Sauvain, L. Gern, E. Zhioua, and A. Aeschlimann. 1991. The prevalence and incidence of clinical and asymptomatic Lyme borreliosis in a population at risk. *Journal of Infectious Diseases* 163(2):305-310.

Fahrer, H., M. J. Sauvain, E. Zhioua, C. Van Hoecke, and L. E. Gern. 1998. Longterm survey (7 years) in a population at risk for Lyme borreliosis: What happens to the seropositive individuals? *European Journal of Epidemiology* 14(2):117-123.

Fallon, B. A., and J. A. Nields. 1994. Lyme disease: A neuropsychiatric illness. *The American Journal of Psychiatry* 151(11):1571-1583.

Fallon, B. A., J. G. Keilp, K. M. Corbera, E. Petkova, C. B. Britton, E. Dwyer, I. Slavov, J. Cheng, J. Dobkin, D. R. Nelson, and H. A. Sackeim. 2008. A randomized, placebo-controlled trial of repeated IV antibiotic therapy for Lyme encephalopathy. *Neurology* 70(13):992-1003.

Fallon, B. A., E. S. Levin, P. J. Schweitzer, and D. Hardesty. 2010. Inflammation and central nervous system Lyme disease. *Neurobiology of Disease* 37(3):534-541.

FDA (Food and Drug Administration). 2008. *Biological product and hematopoietic cell therapy/product (hct/p) deviation report—annual summary for fiscal year 2008.* http://www.fda.gov/BiologicsBloodVaccines/SafetyAvailability/ReportaProblem/BiologicalProductDeviations/ucm12.

Feder, H. M., Jr., B. J. Johnson, S. O'Connell, E. D. Shapiro, A. C. Steere, and G. P. Wormser. 2007a. A critical appraisal of "chronic Lyme disease." *New England Journal of Medicine* 357(14):1422-1430.

Feder, H. M., Jr., B. J. Johnson, S. O'Connell, E. D. Shapiro, A. C. Steere, G. P. Wormser, W. A. Agger, H. Artsob, P. Auwaerter, J. S. Dumler, J. S. Bakken, L. K. Bockenstedt, J. Green, R. J. Dattwyler, J. Munoz, R. B. Nadelman, I. Schwartz, T. Draper, E. McSweegan, J. J. Halperin, M. S. Klempner, P. J. Krause, P. Mead, M. Morshed, R. Porwancher, J. D. Radolf, R. P. Smith, Jr., S. Sood, A. Weinstein, S. J. Wong, and L. Zemel. 2007b. A critical appraisal of "chronic Lyme disease." *New England Journal of Medicine* 357(14):1422-1430.

Feng, H. M., and D. H. Walker. 2004. Mechanisms of immunity to *Ehrlichia muris*: A model of monocytotropic ehrlichiosis. *Infection and Immunity* 72:966-971.

Fish, D., and J. E. Childs. 2009. Community-based prevention of Lyme disease and other tick-borne diseases through topical application of acaricide to white-tailed deer: Background and rationale. *Vector Borne & Zoonotic Diseases* 9(4):357-364.

Fletcher, M. A., X. R. Zeng, K. Maher, S. Levis, B. Hurwitz, M. Antoni, G. Broderick, and N. G. Klimas. 2010. Biomarkers in chronic fatigue syndrome: Evaluation of natural killer cell function and dipeptidyl peptidase IV/CD26. *Plos One* 5(5).

Florin-Christensen, M., L. Schnittger, M. Dominguez, M. Mesplet, A. Rodriguez, L. Ferreri, G. Asenzo, S. Wilkowsky, M. Farber, I. Echaide, and C. Suarez. 2007. Search for babesia bovis vaccine candidates. *Parassitologia* 49 (Suppl 1):9-12.

Fukunaga, M., A. Hamase, K. Okada, and M. Nakao. 1996. *Borrelia tanukii* sp. Nov. and *Borrelia turdae* sp. Nov. Found from ixodid ticks in Japan: Rapid species identification by 16s rna gene-targeted pcr analysis. *Microbiology and Immunology* 40(11):877-881.

Ganta, R. R., M. J. Wilkerson, C. Cheng, A. M. Rokey, and S. K. Chapes. 2002. Persistent *Ehrlichia chaffeensis* infection occurs in the absence of functional major histocompatibility complex class II genes. *Infection and Immunity* 70:380-388

Gebbia, J. A., J. L. Coleman, and J. L. Benach. 2004. Selective induction of matrix metalloproteinases by *Borrelia burgdorferi* via toll-like receptor 2 in monocytes. *Journal of Infectious Diseases* 189:113-119.

Genchi, C. 2007. Human babesiosis, an emerging zoonosis. *Parassitologia* 49 (Suppl 1):29-31.

Gerber, M. A., E. D. Shapiro, P. J. Krause, R. G. Cable, S. J. Badon, and R. W. Ryan. 1994. The risk of acquiring Lyme-disease or babesiosis from a blood-transfusion. *Journal of Infectious Diseases* 170(1):231-234.

Ghosh, S., P. Azhahianambi, and J. de la Fuente. 2006. Control of ticks of ruminants, with special emphasis on livestock farming systems in India: Present and future possibilities for integrated control—a review. *Experimental & Applied Acarology* 40(1):49-66.

Ginsberg, H. S. 1993. Transmission risk of Lyme-disease and implications for tick management. *American Journal of Epidemiology* 138(1):65-73.

Ginsberg, H. S., K. E. Hyland, R. J. Hu, T. J. Daniels, and R. C. Falco. 1998. Tick population trends and forest type. *Science* 281(5375):349-350.

Ginsberg, H. S., P. A. Buckley, M. G. Balmforth, E. Zhioua, S. Mitra, and F. G. Buckley. 2005. Reservoir competence of native North American birds for the Lyme disease spirochete, *Borrelia burgdorferi. Journal of Medical Entomology* 42(3):445-449.

Gockel, M., H. Lindholm, L. Niemisto, and H. Hurri. 2008. Perceived disability but not pain is connected with autonomic nervous function among patients with chronic low back pain. *Journal of Rehabilitation Medicine* 40(5):355-358.

Gomes-Solecki, M. J. C., L. Meirelles, J. Glass, and R. J. Dattwyler. 2007. Epitope length, genospecies dependency, and serum panel effect in the ir6 enzyme-linked immunosorbent assay for detection of antibodies to *Borrelia burgdorferi*. *Clinical and Vaccine Immunology* 14(7):875-879.

Gould, L. H., R. S. Nelson, K. S. Griffith, E. B. Hayes, J. Piesman, P. S. Mead, and M. L. Cartter. 2008. Knowledge, attitudes, and behaviors regarding Lyme disease prevention among Connecticut residents, 1999-2004. *Vector-Borne and Zoonotic Diseases* 8(6):769-776.

Gracely, R. H., F. Petzke, J. M. Wolf, and D. J. Clauw. 2002. Functional magnetic resonance imaging evidence of augmented pain processing in fibromyalgia. *Arthritis and Rheumatism* 46(5):1333-1343.

Granquist, E. G., S. Stuen, L. Crosby, A. M. Lundgren, A. R. Alleman, and A. F. Barbet. 2010. Variant-specific and diminishing immune responses towards the highly variable msp2(p44) outer membrane protein of anaplasma phagocytophilum during persistent infection in lambs. *Veterinary Immunology and Immunopathology* 133:117-124.

Gubernot, D. M., H. L. Nakhasi, P. A. Mied, D. M. Asher, J. S. Epstein, and S. Kumar. 2009. Transfusion-transmitted babesiosis in the United States: Summary of a workshop. *Transfusion* 49(12):2759-2771.

Halperin, J. J., and M. P. Heyes. 1992. Neuroactive kynurenines in Lyme borreliosis. *Neurology* 42(1):43-50.

Hassett, A. L., D. C. Radvanski, S. Buyske, S. V. Savage, and L. H. Sigal. 2009. Psychiatric comorbidity and other psychological factors in patients with "chronic Lyme disease." *American Journal of Medicine* 122(9):843-850.

Hatcher, J. C., P. D. Greenberg, J. Antique, and V. E. Jimenez-Lucho. 2001. Severe babesiosis in Long Island: Review of 34 cases and their complications. *Clinical Infectious Diseases* 32(8):1117-1125.

Hattwick, M. A. W., H. Retailliau, R. J. O'Brien, M. Slutzker, R. E. Fontaine, and B. Hanson. 1978. Fatal Rocky Mountain spotted fever. *Journal of the American Medical Association* 240(14):1499-1503.

Heim, C., U. Ehlert, J. P. Hanker, and D. H. Hellhammer. 1998. Abuse-related posttraumatic stress disorder and alterations of the hypothalamic-pituitary-adrenal axis in women with chronic pelvic pain. *Psychosomatic Medicine* 60(3):309-318.

Herwaldt, B. L., D. Persing, and E. A. Precigout. 1996. A fatal case of babesiosis in Missouri: Identification of another piroplasm that infects humans. *Annals of Internal Medicine* 124:643-650.

Herwaldt, B. L., S. Caccio, and F. Gherlinzoni. 2003. Molecular characterization of a non-babesia divergens organism causing zoonotic babesiosis in Europe. *Emerging Infectious Diseases* 9:942-948.

Hickie, I., T. Davenport, D. Wakefield, U. Vollmer-Conna, B. Cameron, S. D. Vernon, W. C. Reeves, and A. Lloyd. 2006. Post-infective and chronic fatigue syndromes precipitated by viral and non-viral pathogens: Prospective cohort study. *British Medical Journal* 333(7568):575.

Hildebrandt, A., K. P. Hunfeld, M. Baier, A. Krumbholz, S. Sachse, T. Lorenzen, M. Kiehntopf, H. J. Fricke, and E. Straube. 2007. First confirmed autochthonous case of human babesia microti infection in Europe. *European Journal of Clinical Microbiology & Infectious Diseases* 26(8):595-601.

Hilton, E., J. DeVoti, J. L. Benach, M. L. Halluska, D. J. White, H. Paxton, and J. S. Dumler. 1999. Seroprevalence and seroconversion for tick-borne diseases in a high-risk population in the northeast United States. *American Journal of Medicine* 106(4):404-409.

Hirschfeld, M., C. J. Kirschning, R. Schwandner, H. Wesche, J. H. Weis, R. M. Wooten, and J. J. Weis. 1999. Cutting edge: Inflammatory signaling by *Borrelia burgdorferi* lipoproteins is mediated by toll-like receptor 2. *Journal of Immunology* 163:2382-2386.

Hodzic, E., S. Feng, K. Holden, K. J. Freet, and S. W. Barthold. 2008. Persistence of *Borrelia burgdorferi* following antibiotic treatment in mice. *Antimicrobial Agents and Chemotherapy* 52(5):1728-1736.

Holman, R. C., C. D. Paddock, A. T. Curns, J. W. Krebs, J. H. McQuiston, and J. E. Childs. 2001. Analysis of risk factors for fatal Rocky Mountain spotted fever: Evidence for superiority of tetracyclines for therapy. *Journal of Infectious Diseases* 184(11):1437-1444.

Holman, R. C., J. H. McQuiston, D. L. Haberling, and J. E. Cheek. 2009. Increasing incidence of Rocky Mountain spotted fever among the American Indian population in the United States. *American Journal of Tropical Medicine and Hygiene* 80(4):601-605.

Horan, J. J., and J. K. Dellinge. 1974. In vivo emotive imagery—preliminary test. *Perceptual and Motor Skills* 39(1):359-362.

Ismail, N., L. Soong, J. W. McBride, G. Valbuena, J. P. Olano, H. M. Feng, and D. H. Walker. 2004. Overproduction of tnf-alpha by CD8(+) type 1 cells and down-regulation of ifn-gamma production by CD4(+) Th1 cells contribute to toxic shock–like syndrome in an animal model of fatal monocytotropic ehrlichiosis. *Journal of Immunology* 172(3):1786-1800.

Ismail, N., H. L. Stevenson, and D. H. Walker. 2006. Role of tumor necrosis factor alpha (tnf-alpha) and interleukin-10 in the pathogenesis of severe murine monocytotropic ehrlichiosis: Increased resistance of tnf receptor p55-and p75-deficient mice to fatal ehrlichial infection. *Infection and Immunity* 74(3):1846-1856.

Ismail, N., E. C. Crossley, H. L. Stevenson, and D. H. Walker. 2007. Relative importance of T-cell subsets in monocytotropic ehrlichiosis: A novel effector mechanism involved in ehrlichia-induced immunopathology in murine ehrlichiosis. *Infection and Immunity* 75(9):4608-4620.

Ismail, N., K. C. Bloch, and J. W. McBride. 2010. Human ehrlichiosis and anaplasmosis. *Clinics in Laboratory Medicine* 30(1):261-292.

Johnson, M., and H. M. Feder. 2010. Chronic Lyme disease: A survey of Connecticut primary care physicians. *Journal of Pediatrics* 157(6):1025-1029.e1022.

Jones, C. G., R. S. Ostfeld, M. P. Richard, E. M. Schauber, and J. O. Wolff. 1998. Chain reactions linking acorns to gypsy moth outbreaks and Lyme disease risk. *Science* 279(5353):1023-1026.

Jones, K. E., N. G. Patel, M. A. Levy, A. Storeygard, D. Balk, J. L. Gittleman, and P. Daszak. 2008. Global trends in emerging infectious diseases. *Nature* 451(7181):990-U994.

Jordan, R. A., T. L. Schulze, and M. B. Jahn. 2007. Effects of reduced deer density on the abundance of *Ixodes scapularis* (acari: Ixodidae) and Lyme disease incidence in a northern New Jersey endemic area. *Journal of Medical Entomology* 44(5):752-757.

Kalish, R. A., J. M. Leong, and A. C. Steere. 1993. Association of treatment-resistant chronic Lyme arthritis with HLA-dr4 and antibody reactivity to ospa and ospb of *Borrelia-burgdorferi*. *Infection and Immunity* 61(7):2774-2779.

Kato, K., P. F. Sullivan, B. Evengard, and N. L. Pedersen. 2008. A population-based twin study of functional somatic syndromes. *Psychological Medicine* doi:10.1017/S0033291708003784.

Kaufman, W. R., and P. A. Nuttall. 1996. Amblyomma variegatum(acari: Ixodidae): Mechanism and control of arbovirus secretion in tick saliva. *Experimental Parasitology* 82(3):316-323.

Kawabata, H., T. Masuzawa, and Y. Yanagihara. 1993. Genomic analysis of *Borrelia japonica* sp. Nov. Isolated from *Ixodes ovatus* in Japan. *Microbiology and Immunology* 37(11):843-848.

Keesing, F., J. Brunner, S. Duerr, M. Killilea, K. LoGiudice, K. Schmidt, H. Vuong, and R. S. Ostfeld. 2009. Hosts as ecological traps for the vector of Lyme disease. *Proceedings of the Royal Society B—Biological Sciences* 276(1675):3911-3919.

Keirans, J. E., and L. A. Durden. 2005. Tick systematics and identification. In *Tick-borne diseases of humans*, edited by J. L. Goodman, D. T. Dennis, and D. E. Sonenshine. Washington, D.C.: American Society for Microbiology Press. Pp. 123-143.

Kelly, P. J. 2006. *Rickettsia africae* in the West Indies. *Emerging Infectious Diseases* 12(2):224-226.

Killilea, M. E., A. Swei, R. S. Lane, C. J. Briggs, and R. S. Ostfeld. 2008. Spatial dynamics of Lyme disease: A review. *Ecohealth* 5(2):167-195.

Kindberg, E., A. Mickiene, C. Ax, B. Akerlind, S. Vene, L. Lindquist, A. Lundkvist, and L. Svensson. 2008. A deletion in the chemokine receptor 5 (CCR5) gene is associated with tickborne encephalitis. *Journal of Infectious Diseases* 197(2):266-269.

Kinjo, Y., E. Tupin, D. Wu, M. Fujio, R. Garcia-Navarro, M. R. Benhnia, D. M. Zajonc, G. Ben-Menachem, G. D. Ainge, G. F. Painter, A. Khurana, K. Hoebe, S. M. Behar, B. Beutler, I. A. Wilson, M. Tsuji, T. J. Sellati, C. H. Wong, and M. Kronenberg. 2006. Natural killer T cells recognize diacylglycerol antigens from pathogenic bacteria. *Nature Immunology* 7:978-986.

Kirkland, K. B., W. E. Wilkinson, and D. J. Sexton. 1995. Therapeutic delay and mortality in cases of Rocky Mountain spotted fever. *Clinical Infectious Diseases* 20(5):1118-1121.

Kleba, B., T. R. Clark, E. I. Lutter, D. W. Ellison, and T. Hackstadt. 2010. Disruption of the *Rickettsia rickettsii* sca2 autotransporter inhibits actin-based motility. *Infection and Immunity* 78:2240-2247.

Klein, J. D., S. C. Eppes, and P. Hunt. 1996. Environmental and life-style risk factors for Lyme disease in children. *Clinical Pediatrics* 35(7):359-363.

Klempner, M. S., L. T. Hu, J. Evans, C. H. Schmid, G. M. Johnson, R. P. Trevino, D. Norton, L. Levy, D. Wall, J. McCall, M. Kosinski, and A. Weinstein. 2001. Two controlled trials of antibiotic treatment in patients with persistent symptoms and a history of Lyme disease. *New England Journal of Medicine* 345(2):85-92.

Klenerman, P., and A. Hill. 2005. T cells and viral persistence: Lessons from diverse infections. *Nature Immunology* 6(9):873-879.

Klich, M., M. W. Lankester, and K. W. Wu. 1996. Spring migratory birds (aves) extend the northern occurrence of blacklegged tick (acari: Ixodidae). *Journal of Medical Entomology* 33:581-585.

Klompen, H., and D. Grimaldi. 2001. First mesozoic record of a parasitiform mite: A larval argasid tick in cretaceous amber (acari: Ixodida: Argasidae). *Annals of the Entomological Society of America* 94(1):10-15.

Krause, P. J., S. R. Telford, 3rd, A. Spielman, V. Sikand, R. Ryan, D. Christianson, G. Burke, P. Brassard, R. Pollack, J. Peck, and D. H. Persing. 1996. Concurrent Lyme disease and babesiosis. Evidence for increased severity and duration of illness. *Journal of the American Medical Association* 275(21):1657-1660.

Krause, P. J., A. Spielman, S. R. Telford, V. K. Sikand, K. McKay, D. Christianson, R. J. Pollack, P. Brassard, J. Magera, R. Ryan, and D. H. Persing. 1998. Persistent parasitemia after acute babesiosis. *New England Journal of Medicine* 339(3):160-165.

Krause, P. J., K. McKay, C. A. Thompson, V. K. Sikand, R. Lentz, T. Lepore, L. Closter, D. Christianson, S. R. Telford, D. Persing, J. D. Radolf, A. Spielman, and G. Deer-Associated Infect Study. 2002. Disease-specific diagnosis of coinfecting tickborne zoonoses: Babesiosis, human granulocytic ehrlichiosis, and Lyme disease. *Clinical Infectious Diseases* 34(9):1184-1191.

Krause, P. J., K. McKay, J. Gadbaw, D. Christianson, L. Closter, T. Lepore, S. R. Telford, V. Sikand, R. Ryan, D. Persing, J. D. Radolf, A. Spielman. 2003. Increasing health burden of human babesiosis in endemic sites. *American Journal of Tropical Medicine and Hygiene* 68(4):431-436.

Krause, P. J., D. T. Foley, G. S. Burke, D. Christianson, L. Closter, and A. Spielman. 2006. Reinfection and relapse in early Lyme disease. *American Journal of Tropical Medicine and Hygiene* 75(6):1090-1094.

Krause, P. J., J. Daily, S. R. Telford, E. Vannier, P. Lantos, and A. Spielman. 2007. Shared features in the pathobiology of babesiosis and malaria. *Trends in Parasitology* 23(12):605-610.

Krause, P. J., B. E. Gewurz, D. Hill, F. M. Marty, E. Vannier, I. M. Foppa, R. R. Furman, E. Neuhaus, G. Skowron, S. Gupta, C. McCalla, E. L. Pesanti, M. Young, D. Heiman, G. Hsue, J. A. Gelfand, G. P. Wormser, J. Dickason, F. J. Bia, B. Hartman, S. R. Telford, 3rd, D. Christianson, K. Dardick, M. Coleman, J. E. Girotto, and A. Spielman. 2008. Persistent and relapsing babesiosis in immunocompromised patients. *Clinical Infectious Diseases* 46(3):370-376.

Krupp, L. B., L. G. Hyman, R. Grimson, P. K. Coyle, P. Melville, S. Ahnn, R. Dattwyler, and B. Chandler. 2003. Study and treatment of post lyme disease (stop-ld). *Neurology* 60(12):1923-1930.

Kugeler, K. J., K. S. Griffith, L. H. Gould, K. Kochanek, B. J. Delorey, and P. S. Mead. 2011. A review of death certificates listing lyme disease as a cause of death in the United States. *Clinical Infectious Diseases* 52(3):364-367.

Kumaran, D., S. Eswaramoorthy, B. J. Luft, S. Koide, J. J. Dunn, C. L. Lawson, and S. Swaminathan. 2001. Crystal structure of outer surface protein c (ospc) from the lyme disease spirochete, borrelia burgdorferi. *European Molecular Biology Organization Journal* 20(5):971-978.

Lane, R. S., S. A. Manweiler, H. A. Stubbs, E. T. Lennette, J. E. Madigan, and P. E. Lavoie. 1992. Risk-factors for Lyme-disease in a small rural-community in northern California. *American Journal of Epidemiology* 136(11):1358-1368.

Larsson, C., M. Andersson, and S. Bergstrom. 2009. Current issues in relapsing fever. *Current Opinion in Infectious Diseases* 22(5):443-449.

Lashley, F. R. 2007. Lyme disease, ehrlichiosis, anaplasmosis, and babesiosis. In *Emerging infectious diseases: Trends and issues*. 2 ed, edited by F. R. Lashley and J. D. Durham. New York: Springer Publishing Company, Inc. Pp. 255-265.

Le Fleche, A., D. Postic, K. Girardet, O. Peter, and G. Baranton. 1997. Characterization of *Borrelia lusitaniae* sp. Nov. By 16s ribosomal DNA sequence analysis. *International Journal of Systematic Bacteriology* 47(4):921-925.

Lederberg, J., R. E. Shope, S. C. Oaks. 1992. *Emerging infections*. Committee on Emerging Microbial Threats. Washington, DC: National Academy Press.

Leiby, D. A. 2011. Transfusion-transmitted babesia spp.: Bull's-eye on babesia microti. *Clinical Microbiology Reviews* 24(1):14-28.

Levin, M., J. F. Levine, S. Yang, P. Howard, and C. S. Apperson. 1996. Reservoir competence of the Southeastern five-lined skink (eumeces inexpectatus) and the green anole (anolis carolinensis) for *Borrelia burgdorferi*. *American Journal of Tropical Medicine and Hygiene* 54(1):92-97.

Ley, C., E. M. Olshen, and A. L. Reingold. 1995. Case-control study of risk-factors for incident Lyme-disease in California. *American Journal of Epidemiology* 142(9):S39-S47.

Lin, T., L. Gao, D. G. Edmondson, M. B. Jacobs, M. T. Philipp, and S. J. Norris. 2009. Central role of the Holliday junction helicase RuvAB in visE recombination and infectivity of *Borrelia burgdorferi*. *PLoS Pathogens* 5(12):e1000679.

Liu, N., R. R. Montgomery, S. W. Barthold, and L. K. Bockenstedt. 2004. Myeloid differentiation antigen 88 deficiency impairs pathogen clearance but does not alter inflammation in *Borrelia burgdorferi*-infected mice. *Infection and Immunity* 72:3195-3203.

Livengood, J. A., and J. R. D. Gilmore. 2006. Invasion of human neuronal and glial cells by an infectious strain of *Borrelia burgdorferi*. *Microbes and Infection* 8(14-15):2832-2840.

Ljostad, U., and A. Mygland. 2010. Remaining complaints 1 year after treatment for acute Lyme neuroborreliosis. Frequency, pattern and risk factors. *European Journal of Neurology* 17(1):118-123.

Logigian, E. L., K. A. Johnson, M. F. Kijewski, R. F. Kaplan, J. A. Becker, K. J. Jones, B. M. Garada, B. L. Holman, and A. C. Steere. 1997. Reversible cerebral hypoperfusion in Lyme encephalopathy. *Neurology* 49(6):1661-1670.

LoGiudice, K., R. S. Ostfeld, K. A. Schmidt, and F. Keesing. 2003. The ecology of infectious disease: Effects of host diversity and community composition on Lyme disease risk. *Proceedings of the National Academy of Sciences of the United States of America* 100(2):567-571.

Lopez, J. E., P. A. Beare, R. A. Heinzen, J. Normine, K. K. Lahmers, G. H. Palmer, and W. C. Brown. 2008. High-throughput identification of t-lymphocyte antigens from anaplasma marginale expressed using in vitro transcription and translation. *Journal of Immunological Methods* 332((1-2)):129-141.

Lu, Z., M. Broker, and G. Liang. 2008. Tick-borne encephalitis in mainland China. *Vector Borne & Zoonotic Diseases* 8(5):713-720.

Ma, Y., K. P. Seiler, E. J. Eichwald, J. H. Weis, C. Teuscher, and J. J. Weis. 1998. Distinct characteristics of resistance to *Borrelia burgdorferi*-induced arthritis in c57bl/6n mice. *Infection and Immunity* 66:161-168.

Ma, Y., J. C. Miller, H. Crandall, E. T. Larsen, D. M. Dunn, R. B. Weiss, M. Subramanian, J. H. Weis, J. F. Zachary, C. Teuscher, and J. J. Weis. 2009. Interval-specific congenic lines reveal quantitative trait Loci with penetrant Lyme arthritis phenotypes on chromosomes 5,11,12. *Infection and Immunity*.

Maggi, R. G., M. P. B. J., B.C. Hegarty, E. B. Breitschwerdt. 2010. Enhanced molecular detection and isolation of bartonella species from human blood samples using the bartonella alpha proteobacteria growth medium (bapgm) platform. Paper read at 24th Meeting of the American Society of Rickettsiology, July 31-August 3, 2010, Stevenson, Washington.

Marconi, R., D. Liveris, and I. Schwartz. 1995. Identification of novel insertion elements, restriction fragment length polymorphism patterns, and discontinuous 23s rrna in Lyme disease spirochetes: Phylogenetic analyses of rrna genes and their intergenic spacers in *Borrelia japonica* sp. Nov. and genomic group 21038 (*Borrelia andersonii* sp. Nov.) isolates. *Journal of Clinical Microbiology* 33(9):2427-2434.

Margos, G., S. A. Vollmer, M. Cornet, M. Garnier, V. Fingerle, B. Wilske, A. Bormane, L. Vitorino, M. Collares-Pereira, M. Drancourt, and K. Kurtenbach. 2009. A new borrelia species defined by multilocus sequence analysis of housekeeping genes. *Applied Environtal Microbiology* 75(16):5410-5416.

Markowski, D., H. S. Ginsberg, K. E. Hyland, and R. J. Hu. 1998. Reservoir competence of the meadow vole (rodentia : Cricetidae) for the Lyme disease spirochete *Borrelia burgdorferi*. *Journal of Medical Entomology* 35(5):804-808.

Marques, A., M. R. Brown, and T. A. Fleisher. 2009. Natural killer cell counts are not different between patients with post-Lyme disease syndrome and controls. *Clinical and Vaccine Immunology* 16(8):1249-1250.

Martin, M. E., K. Caspersen, and J. S. Dumler. 2001. Immunopathology and ehrlichial propagation are regulated by interferon-gamma and interleukin-10 in a murine model of human granulocytic ehrlichiosis. *American Journal of Pathology* 158(5):1881-1888.

Martinez-Medina, M. A., G. Alvarez-Hernandez, J. G. Padilla-Zamudioa, and M. G. Rojas-Guerra. 2007. Rocky Mountain spotted fever in children: Clinical and epidemiological features. *Gaceta Medicina De Mexico* 143(2):137-140.

Mast, W. E., and W. M. Burrows. 1976. Erythema chronicum migrans and Lyme arthritis. *Journal of the American Medical Association* 236(21):2392-2392.

Masuzawa, T., N. Takada, M. Kudeken, T. Fukui, Y. Yano, F. Ishiguro, Y. Kawamura, Y. Imai, and T. Ezaki. 2001. Borrelia sinica sp. Nov., a Lyme disease-related borrelia species isolated in China. *IInternational Journal of Systematic and Evolutionary Microbiology* 51(5):1817-1824.

Mattner, J., K. L. DeBord, N. Ismail, R. D. Goff, C. Cantu, D. P. Zhou, P. Saint-Mezard, V. Wang, Y. Gao, N. Yin, K. Hoebe, O. Schneewind, D. Walker, B. Beutler, L. Teyton, P. B. Savage, and A. Bendelac. 2005. Exogenous and endogenous glycolipid antigens activate NKT cells during microbial infections. *Nature* 434(7032):525-529.

McBeth, J., Y. H. Chiu, A. J. Silman, D. Ray, R. Morriss, C. Dickens, A. Gupta, and G. J. Macfarlane. 2005. Hypothalamic-pituitary-adrenal stress axis function and the relationship with chronic widespread pain and its antecedents. *Arthritis Research & Therapy* 7(5):R992-R1000.

McCabe, G. J., and J. E. Bunnell. 2004. Precipitation and the occurrence of Lyme disease in the northeastern United States. *Vector-Borne and Zoonotic Diseases* 4(2):143-148.

McKisic, M. D., W. L. Redmond, and S. W. Barthold. 2000. Cutting edge: T cell-mediated pathology in murine Lyme borreliosis. *Journal of Immunology* 164:6096-6099.

McLean, S. A., D. A. Williams, R. E. Harris, W. J. Kop, K. H. Groner, K. Ambrose, A. K. Lyden, R. H. Gracely, L. J. Crofford, M. E. Geisser, A. Sen, P. Biswas, and D. J. Clauw. 2005. Momentary relationship between cortisol secretion and symptoms in patients with fibromyalgia. *Arthritis and Rheumatism* 52(11):3660-3669.

McQuiston, J. H. 2011. *Rickettsia diseases: spectrum of disease, spatial, clustering, at-risk populations, and research needs.* Presented to the IOM Committee on Lyme Disease and Other Tick-borne Diseases: The State of the Science. Washington, DC.

McQuiston, J. H., R. C. Holman, A. V. Groom, S. F. Kaufman, J. E. Cheek, and J. E. Childs. 2000. Incidence of Rocky Mountain spotted fever among American Indians in Oklahoma. *Public Health Reports* 115(5):469-475.

Medical News. 1976. What may be new form of arthritis is discovered in New England area. *Journal of the American Medical Association* 236: 241-242.

Miller, J. C., Y. Ma, J. Bian, K. C. Sheehan, J. F. Zachary, J. H. Weis, R. D. Schreiber, and J. J. Weis. 2008. A critical role for type I ifn in arthritis development following *Borrelia burgdorferi* infection of mice. *Journal of Immunology* 181:8492-8503.

Miller, J. C., H. Maylor-Hagen, Y. Ma, J. H. Weis, and J. J. Weis. 2010. The Lyme disease spirochete borrelia burgdorferi utilizes multiple ligands, including RNA, for interferon regulatory factor 3-dependent induction of type I interferon-responsive genes. *Infection and Immunity* 78:3144-3153.

Miranda, H., L. Kaila-Kangas, M. Heliovaara, P. Leino-Arjas, J. Haukka, J. Liira, and E. Viikari-Juntura. 2010. Musculoskeletal pain at multiple sites and its effects on work ability in a general working population. *Occupational and Environmental Medicine* 67(7):449-455.

Mixson, T. R., S. R. Campbell, J. S. Gill, H. S. Ginsberg, M. V. Reichard, T. L. Schulze, and G. A. Dasch. 2006. Prevalence of ehrlichia, borrelia, and rickettsial agents in amblyomma americanum (acari : Ixodidae) collected from nine states. *Journal of Medical Entomology* 43(6):1261-1268.

Morgen, K., R. Martin, R. D. Stone, J. Grafman, N. Kadom, H. F. McFarland, and A. Marques. 2001. Flair and magnetization transfer imaging of patients with post-treatment lyme disease syndrome. *Neurology* 57(11):1980-1985.

Morrison, T. B., Y. Ma, J. H. Weis, and J. J. Weis. 1999. Rapid and sensitive quantification of borrelia burgdorferi-infected mouse tissues by continuous fluorescent monitoring of pcr. *Journal of Clinical Microbiology* 37:987-992.

Munderloh, U. G., and T. J. Kurtti. 1995. Cellular and molecular interrelationships between ticks and prokaryotic tick-borne pathogens. *Annual Review of Entomology* 40:221-243.

Mygland, A., U. Ljostad, V. Fingerle, T. Rupprecht, E. Schmutzhard, and I. Steiner. 2010. Efns guidelines on the diagnosis and management of European Lyme neuroborreliosis. *European Journal of Neurology* 1:8-16.

Nau, R., H.-J. Christen, and H. Eiffert. 2009. Lyme disease—current state of knowledge. *Deutsches Arzteblatt International* 106(5):72-81; quiz 82.

Niebylski, M. L., and M. G. Peacock. 1999. Lethal effect of *Rickettsia rickettsii* on its tick vector (dermacentor andersoni). *Applied & Environmental Microbiology* 65(2):773.

Nigrovic, L. E., and S. L. Wingerter. Tularemia. *Infectious Disease Clinics of North America* 22(3):489-504.

Norris, S. J., J. Coburn, J. M. Leong, L. T. Hu, and M. Höök. 2010. Pathobiology of Lyme disease *borrelia*. In *Borrelia: Molecular biology, host interaction and pathogenesis*, edited by D. S. Scott and J. D. Radolf. Hethersett, Norwich, UK: Caister Academic Press. Pp. 299-331.

Nowakowski, J., R. B. Nadelman, R. Sell, D. McKenna, L. F. Cavaliere, D. Holmgren, A. Gaidici, and G. P. Wormser. 2003. Long-term follow-up of patients with culture-confirmed Lyme disease. *American Journal of Medicine* 115(2):91-96.

O'Garra, A., and K. M. Murphy. 2009. How pathogens and their products stimulate apcs to induce T (h) 1 development. *Nature Immunology* 10:929-932.

Ogata, H., P. Renesto, S. Audic, C. Robert, G. Blanc, P. E. Fournier, H. Parinello, J. M. Claverie, and D. Raoult. 2005. The genome sequence of *Rickettsia felis* identifies the first putative conjugative plasmid in an obligate intracellular parasite. *Plos Biology* 3(8):1391-1402.

Olano, J. R., E. Masters, W. Hogrefe, and D. H. Walker. 2003. Human monocytotropic ehrlichiosis, Missouri. *Emerging Infectious Diseases* 9(12):1579-1586.

Oliveira, A. M., R. G. Maggi, C. W. Woods, and E. B. Breitschwerdt. 2010. Suspected needle stick transmission of bartonella vinsonii subspecies berkhoffii to a veterinarian. *Journal of Veterinary Internal Medicine* 24(5):1229-1232.

Olson, S. H., and J. A. Patz. 2010. *Global environmental change and tick-borne disease incidence*. Paper presented at Institute of Medicine Committee on Lyme Disease and Other Tick-Borne Diseases: The State of the Science, Washington, DC.

Olson, Jr., C. M., T. C. Bates, H. Izadi, J. D. Radolf, S. A. Huber, J. E. Boyson, and J. Anguita. 2009. Local production of ifn-gamma by invariant NKT cells modulates acute Lyme carditis. *Journal of Immunology* 182:3728-3734.

One Health Initiative. *One Health Initiative—One World One Medicine One Health*. http://www.onehealthinitiative.com/mission.php.

Oosting, M., A. Berende, P. Sturm, H. J. Ter Hofstede, D. J. de Jong, T. D. Kanneganti, J. W. van der Meer, B. J. Kullberg, M. G. Netea, and L. A. Joosten. 2010. Recognition of *Borrelia burgdorferi* by nod2 is central for the induction of an inflammatory reaction. *Journal of Infectious Diseases* 201:1849-1858.

Openshaw, J. J. 2010. Rocky mountain spotted fever in the United States, 2000-2007: Interpreting contemporary increases in incidence (vol 83, pg 174, 2010). *American Journal of Tropical Medicine and Hygiene* 83(3):729-730.

Orloski, K. A., G. L. Campbell, C. A. Genese, J. W. Beckley, M. E. Schriefer, K. C. Spitalny, and D. T. Dennis. 1998. Emergence of Lyme disease in Hunterdon County, New Jersey, 1993: A case-control study of risk factors and evaluation of reporting patterns. *American Journal of Epidemiology* 147(4):391-397.

Ostfeld, R. S. 2009. Biodiversity loss and the rise of zoonotic pathogens. *Clinical Microbiology & Infection* 15 (Suppl 1):40-43.

Ostfeld, R. S., C. G. Jones, and J. O. Wolff. 1996. Of mice and mast. *Bioscience* 46(5):323-330.

Ostfeld, R. S., C. D. Canham, K. Oggenfuss, R. J. Winchcombe, and F. Keesing. 2006. Climate, deer, rodents, and acorns as determinants of variation in Lyme-disease risk. *Plos Biology* 4:1058-1068.

Paddock, C. D., and S. R. Telford III. 2010. *Through a glass, darkly: The global incidence of tick-borne diseases.* Paper presented at Institute of Medicine Committe on Lyme Disease and Other Tick-Borne Diseases: The State of the Science, Washington, DC.

Paddock, C. D., and M. J. Yabsley. 2007. Ecological havoc, the rise of white-tailed deer, and the emergence of amblyomma americanum-associated zoonoses in the United States. *Current Topics in Microbiology & Immunology* 315:289-324.

Palmer, G. H., F. R. Rurangirwa, K. M. Kocan, and W. C. Brown. 1999a. Molecular basis for vaccine development against the ehrlichial pathogen anaplasma marginale. *Parasitology Today* 15(7):281-286.

Palmer, M. V., D. L. Whipple, and S. C. Olsen. 1999b. Development of a model of natural infection with mycobacterium bovis in white-tailed deer. *Journal of Wildlife Diseases* 35:450-457.

Panda, A., F. Qian, S. Mohanty, D. Van Duin, F. K. Newman, L. Zhang, S. Chen, V. Towle, R. Belshe, and E. Fikrig. 2010. A generalized, age-associated defect in toll-like receptor function in primary human dendritic cells. *Journal of Immunology* 184:2518-2527.

Persing, D. H., B. L. Herwaldt, C. Glaser, R. S. Lane, J. W. Thomford, D. Mathiesen, P. J. Krause, D. F. Phillip, and P. A. Conrad. 1995. Infection with a babesia-like organism in northern california. *New England Journal of Medicine* 332(5):298-303.

Petzke, M. M., A. Brooks, M. A. Krupna, D. Mordue, and I. Schwartz. 2009. Recognition of *Borrelia burgdorferi*, the Lyme disease spirochete, by tlr7 and tlr9 induces a type I ifn response by human immune cells. *Journal of Immunology* 183:5279-5292.

Phillips, C. B., M. H. Liang, O. Sangha, E. A. Wright, A. H. Fossel, R. A. Lew, K. K. Fossel, and N. A. Shadick. 2001. Lyme disease and preventive behaviors in residents of Nantucket Island, Massachusetts. *American Journal of Preventive Medicine* 20(3):219-224.

Piesman, J., J. G. Donahue, T. N. Mather, and A. Spielman. 1986. Transovarially acquired Lyme-disease spirochetes (*Borrelia-burgdorferi*) in field-collected larval ixodes-dammini (acari, ixodidae). *Journal of Medical Entomology* 23(2):219-219.

Porwancher, R., C. G. Hagerty, J. Fan, L. Landsberg, B. J. Johnson, M. Kopnitsky, A. C. Steere, K. Kulas, and S. J. Wong. 2011. Multiplex immunoassay for Lyme disease using vlse1-IgG and pepc10-IgM antibodies: Improving test performance through bioinformatics. *Clinical and Vaccine Immunology* doi:10.1128/CVI.00409-10.

Postic, D., N. M. Ras, R. S. Lane, M. Hendson, and G. Baranton. 1998. Expanded diversity among californian borrelia isolates and description of *Borrelia bissettii* sp. Nov. (formerly borrelia group dn127). *Journal of Clinical Microbiology* 36(12):3497-3504.

Qiu, W.-G., D. E. Dykhuizen, M. S. Acosta, and B. J. Luft. 2002. Geographic uniformity of the Lyme disease spirochete (*Borrelia burgdorferi*) and its shared history with tick vector (*Ixodes scapularis*) in the northeastern United States. *Genetics* 160(3):833-849.

Qiu, W. G., J. F. Bruno, W. D. McCaig, Y. Xu, I. Livey, M. E. Schriefer, and B. J. Luft. 2008. Wide distribution of a high-virulence *Borrelia burgdorferi* clone in Europe and North America. *Emerging Infectious Diseases* 14(7):1097-1104.

Ramsey, A. H., E. A. Belongia, C. M. Gale, and J. P. Davis. 2002. Outcomes of treated human granulocytic ehrlichiosis cases. *Emerging Infectious Diseases* 8(4):398-401.

Rand, P. W., C. Lubelczyk, G. R. Lavigne, S. Elias, M. S. Holman, E. H. Lacombe, and R. P. Smith, Jr. 2003. Deer density and the abundance of *Ixodes scapularis* (acari: Ixodidae). *Journal of Medical Entomology* 40(2):179-184.

Rand, P. W., C. Lubelczyk, M. S. Holman, E. H. Lacombe, and R. P. Smith. 2004. Abundance of *Ixodes scapularis* (acari : Ixodidae) after the complete removal of deer from an isolated offshore island, endemic for Lyme disease. *Journal of Medical Entomology* 41(4):779-784.

Ribeiro, J. M., T. N. Mather, J. Piesman, and A. Spielman. 1987. Dissemination and salivary delivery of Lyme disease spirochetes in vector ticks (acari: Ixodidae). *Journal of Medical Entomology* 24(2):201-205.

Ribeiro, J. M., F. Alarcon-Chaidez, I. M. Francischetti, B. J. Mans, T. N. Mather, J. G. Valenzuela, and S. K. Wikel. 2005. An annotated catalog of salivary gland transcripts from ixodes scapularis ticks. *Insect Biochemistry and Molecular Biology* 36(2):111-129.

Richter, D., A. Spielman, N. Komar, and F. R. Matuschka. 2000. Competence of American robins as reservoir hosts for Lyme disease spirochetes. *Emerging Infectious Diseases* 6(2):133-138.

Richter, D., D. Postic, N. Sertour, I. Livey, F.-R. Matuschka, and G. Baranton. 2006. Delineation of *Borrelia burgdorferi* sensu lato species by multilocus sequence analysis and confirmation of the delineation of *Borrelia spielmanii* sp. Nov. *International Journal of Systematic and Evolutionary Microbiology* 56(4):873-881.

Rodgers, S. E., C. P. Zolnik, and T. N. Mather. 2007. Duration of exposure to suboptimal atmospheric moisture affects nymphal blacklegged tick survival. *Journal of Medical Entomology* 44:372-375.

Rodriguez, S. D., M. A. Garcia Ortiz, R. Jimenez Ocampo, and C. A. Vega y Murguia. 2009. Molecular epidemiology of bovine anaplasmosis with a particular focus in Mexico. *Infection, Genetics & Evolution* 9(6):1092-1101.

Romero, J. R., and K. A. Simonsen. Powassan encephalitis and Colorado tick fever. *Infectious Disease Clinics of North America* 22(3):545-559.

Rosa, P. A., K. Tilly, and P. E. Stewart. 2005. The burgeoning molecular genetics of the Lyme disease spirochaete. *National Review of Microbiology* 3:129-143.

Rosner, F., M. H. Zarrabi, J. L. Benach, and G. S. Habicht. 1984. Babesiosis in splenectomized adults—review of 22 reported cases. *American Journal of Medicine* 76(4):696-701.

Rovery, C., and D. Raoult. Mediterranean spotted fever. *Infectious Disease Clinics of North America* 22(3):515-530.

Rudenko, N., M. Golovchenko, T. Lin, L. Gao, L. Grubhoffer, and J. H. Oliver, Jr. 2009. Delineation of a new species of the *Borrelia burgdorferi* sensu lato complex, *Borrelia americana* sp. Nov. *Journal of Clinical Microbiology* 47(12):3875-3880.

Ruderman, E. M., J. S. Kerr, S. R. Telford III, A. Spielman, L. H. Glimcher, and E. M. Gravellese. 1995. Early murine Lyme carditis has a macrophage predominance and is independent of major histocompatibility complex class II-CD4+ T cell interactions. *Journal of Infectious Diseases* 171:362-370.

Ruebush Ii, T. K., D. D. Juranek, and A. Spielman. 1981. Epidemiology of human babesiosis on Nantucket Island. *American Journal of Tropical Medicine and Hygiene* 30(5):937-941.

Rupprecht, T. A., H. W. Pfister, B. Angele, S. Kastenbauer, B. Wilske, and U. Koedel. 2005. The chemokine cxcl13 (blc): A putative diagnostic marker for neuroborreliosis. *Neurology* 65(3):448-450.

Rydkina, E., S. K. Sahni, L. A. Santucci, L. C. Turpin, R. B. Baggs, and D. J. Silverman. 2004. Selective modulation of antioxidant enzyme activities in host tissues during *Rickettsia conorii* infection. *Microbiology and Pathology* 36(6):293-301.

Rydkina, E., L. C. Turpin, and S. K. Sahni. 2010. *Rickettsia rickettsii* infection of human macrovascular and microvascular endothelial cells reveals activation of both common and cell type-specific host response mechanisms. *Infection and Immunity* 78(6):2599-2606.

Sahni, S. K., D. J. Van Antwerp, M. E. Eremeeva, D. J. Silverman, V. J. Marder, and L. A. Sporn. 1998. Proteasome-independent activation of nuclear factor kappab in cytoplasmic extracts from human endothelial cells by *Rickettsia rickettsii*. *Infection and Immunity* 66(5):1827-1833.

Saito, Y. A., P. Schoenfeld, and G. R. Locke. 2002. The epidemiology of irritable bowel syndrome in North America: A systematic review. *American Journal of Gastroenterology* 97(8):1910-1915.

Salgo, M. P., E. E. Telzak, B. Currie, D. C. Perlman, N. Litman, M. Levi, G. Nathenson, J. L. Benach, R. Alhafidh, and J. Casey. 1988. A focus of Rocky Mountain spotted fever within New York City. *New England Journal of Medicine* 318(21):1345-1348.

Samuels, S. D., and J. D. Radolf. 2010. *Borrelia: Molecular biology, host interaction, and pathogenesis*. Norfolk, England: Caister Academic Press.

Schroder, N. W. J., I. Diterich, A. Zinke, J. Eckert, C. Draing, V. von Baehr, D. Hassler, S. Priem, K. Hahn, K. S. Michelsen, T. Hartung, G. R. Burmester, U. B. Gobel, C. Hermann, and R. R. Schumann. 2005. Heterozygous arg753gln polymorphism of human TLR-2 impairs immune activation by *Borrelia burgdorferi* and protects from late stage Lyme disease. *Journal of Immunology* 175(4):2534-2540.

Schroeder, H. W., and L. Cavacini. 2010. Structure and function of immunoglobulins. *Journal of Allergy and Clinical Immunology* 125(2):S41-S52.

Schuijt, T. J., J. W. Hovius, T. van der Poll, A. P. van Dam, and E. Fikrig. 2011. Lyme borreliosis vaccination: The facts, the challenge, the future. *Trends in Parasitology* 27:40-47.

Schulze, T. L., R. A. Jordan, and R. W. Hung. 1995. Suppression of subadult *Ixodes-scapularis* (acari, ixodidae) following removal of leaf-litter. *Journal of Medical Entomology* 32(5):730-733.

Schutze, G. E., and R. F. Jacobs. 1997. Human monocytic ehrlichiosis in children. *Pediatrics* 100(1):e10.

Schwartz, B. S., and M. D. Goldstein. 1990. Lyme-disease in outdoor workers—risk-factors, preventive measures, and tick removal methods. *American Journal of Epidemiology* 131(5):877-885.

Schwartz, B. S., M. D. Goldstein, and J. E. Childs. 1994. Longitudinal study of *Borrelia-burgdorferi* infection in New Jersey outdoor workers, 1988-1991. *American Journal of Epidemiology* 139(5):504-512.

Scorpio, D. G., J. S. Dumler, N. C. Barat, J. A. Cook, C. E. Barat, B. A. Stillman, K. C. Debisceglie, M. J. Beall, and R. Chandrashekar. 2010. Comparative strain analysis of anaplasma phagocytophilum infection and clinical outcomes in a canine model of granulocytic anaplasmosis. *Vector Borne & Zoonotic Diseases* 11(3):223-229.

Seinost, G., D. E. Dykhuizen, R. J. Dattwyler, W. T. Golde, J. J. Dunn, I. N. Wang, G. P. Wormser, M. E. Schriefer, and B. J. Luft. 1999. Four clones of *Borrelia burgdorferi* sensu stricto cause invasive infection in humans. *Infection and Immunity* 67(7):3518-3524.

Sekirov, I., S. L. Russell, L. C. M. Antunes, and B. B. Finlay. 2010. Gut microbiota in health and disease. *Physiology Review* 90:859-904.

Shadick, N. A., C. B. Phillips, E. L. Logigian, A. C. Steere, R. F. Kaplan, V. P. Berardi, P. H. Duray, M. G. Larson, E. A. Wright, K. S. Ginsburg, J. N. Katz, and M. H. Liang. 1994. The long-term clinical outcomes of Lyme disease. A population-based retrospective cohort study. *Annals of Internal Medicine* 121(8):560-567.

Shaw, A. C., A. Panda, S. Joshi, F. Qian, H. G. Allore, and R. R. Montgomery. 2010. Dysregulation of human toll-like receptor function in aging. *Ageing Research Review*.

Sher, A. 1988. Vaccination against parasites: Special problems imposed by the adaptation of parasitic organisms to the host immune response. In *The biology of parasitism*, edited by P. T. Englund and A. Sher. New York: Alan R. Liss. Pp. 169-182.

Shih, C. M., L. P. Liu, W. C. Chung, S. J. Ong, and C. C. Wang. 1997. Human babesiosis in Taiwan: Asymptomatic infection with a babesia microti-like organism in a Taiwanese woman. *Journal of Clinical Microbiology* 35(2):450-454.

Shin, O. S., R. R. Isberg, S. Akira, S. Uematsu, A. K. Behera, and L. T. Hu. 2008. Distinct roles for myd88 and toll-like receptors 2,5, and 9 in phagocytosis of *Borrelia burgdorferi* and cytokine induction. *Infection and Immunity* 76:2341-2351.

Sigal, L. H., and S. Williams. 1997. A monoclonal antibody to *Borrelia burgdorferi* flagellin modifies neuroblastoma cell neuritogenesis in vitro: A possible role for autoimmunity in the neuropathy of Lyme disease. *Infection and Immunity* 65(5):1722-1728.

Sillanpaa, H., P. Lahdenne, and H. Sarvas. 2007. Immune responses to borrelial vlse ir6 peptide variants. *International Journal of Medicinal Microbiology* 297:45-52.

Silverman, D. J. 1984. *Rickettsia rickettsii*-induced cellular injury of human vascular endothelium in vitro. *Infection and Immunity* 44(3):545-553.

Silverman, M. N., C. M. Heim, U. M. Nater, A. H. Marques, and E. M. Sternberg. 2010. Neuroendocrine and immune contributors to fatigue. *PM & R : the Journal of Injury, Function, and Rehabilitation* 2(5):338-346.

Smith, G., E. P. Wileyto, R. B. Hopkins, B. R. Cherry, and J. P. Maher. 2001. Risk factors for Lyme disease in Chester County, Pennsylvania. *Public Health Reports* 116:146-156.

Smith, P. F., J. L. Benach, D. J. White, D. F. Stroup, and D. L. Morse. 1988. Occupational risk of Lyme disease in endemic areas of New York State. *Annals of the New York Academy of Sciences* 539:289-301.

Smith, R. P., P. W. Rand, E. H. Lacombe, S. R. Morris, D. W. Holmes, and D. A. Caporale. 1996. Role of bird migration in the long-distance dispersal of *Ixodes dammini*, the vector of Lyme disease. *Journal of Infectious Diseases* 174(1):221-224.

Smith, T., and F. L. Kilborne. 1893. Investigations into the nature, causation and prevention of Texas or southern cattle fever. *Government Print Off, Bureau of Animal Industry Bulletin* 1.

Solomon, S. P., E. Hilton, B. S. Weinschel, S. Pollack, and E. Grolnick. 1998. Psychological factors in the prediction of Lyme disease course. *Arthritis Care and Research* 11(5):419-426.

Stafford, K. C. 1991. Effectiveness of host-targeted permethrin in the control of *Ixodes dammini* (acari: Ixodidae). *Journal of Medical Entomology* 28(5):611-617.

Stafford, K. C., A. J. Denicola, and H. J. Kilpatrick. 2003. Reduced abundance of *Ixodes scapularis* (acari : Ixodidae) and the tick parasitoid *Ixodiphagus hookeri* (hymenoptera : Encyrtidae) with reduction of white-tailed deer. *Journal of Medical Entomology* 40(5):642-652.

Standaert, S. M., J. E. Dawson, W. Schaffner, J. E. Childs, K. L. Biggie, B. S. Singleton, R. R. Gerhardt, M. L. Knight, and R. H. Hutcheson. 1995. Ehrlichiosis in a golf-oriented retirement community. *New England Journal of Medicine* 333(7):420-425.

Steere, A. C., and L. Glickstein. 2004. Elucidation of Lyme arthritis. *Nature Reviews Microbiology* 4:143-152.

Steere, A. C., and V. K. Sikand. 2003. The presenting manifestations of Lyme disease and the outcomes of treatment. *New England Journal of Medicine* 348(24):2472-2474.

Steere, A. C., S. E. Malawista, and D. R. Snydman. 1977. Lyme arthritis: An epidemic of oligoarticular arthritis in children and adults in three Connecticut communities. *Arthritis and Rheumatism* 20(1):7-17.

Steere, A. C., R. T. Schoen, and E. Taylor. 1987. The clinical evolution of Lyme arthritis. *Annals of Internal Medicine* 107(5):725-731.

Steere, A. C., E. Dwyer, and R. Winchester. 1990. Association of chronic Lyme arthritis with HLA-dr4 and HLA-dr2 alleles. *New England Journal of Medicine* 323(4):219-223.

Steere, A. C., V. K. Sikand, F. Meurice, D. L. Parenti, E. Fikrig, R. T. Schoen, J. Nowakowski, C. H. Schmid, S. Laukamp, C. Buscarino, D. S. Krause, and G. Lyme Dis Vaccine Study.

1998. Vaccination against Lyme disease with recombinant *Borrelia burgdorferi* outer-surface lipoprotein A with adjuvant. *New England Journal of Medicine* 339(4):209-215.

Steere, A. C., D. Gross, A. L. Meyer, and B. T. Huber. 2001. Autoimmune mechanisms in antibiotic treatment-resistant Lyme arthritis. *Journal of Autoimmunity* 16:263-268.

Steere, A. C., G. McHugh, C. Suarez, J. Hoitt, N. Damle, and V. K. Sikand. 2003. Prospective study of coinfection in patients with erythema migrans. *Clinical Infectious Diseases* 36(8):1078-1081.

Steere, A. C., G. McHugh, N. Damle, and V. K. Sikand. 2008. Prospective study of serologic tests for Lyme disease. *Clinical Infectious Diseases* 47(2):188-195.

Stevenson, H. L., J. A. Jordan, Z. Peerwani, H. Q. Wang, D. H. Walker, and N. Ismail. 2006. An intradermal environment promotes a protective type-1 response against lethal systemic monocytotropic ehrlichial infection. *Infection and Immunity* 74(8):4856-4864.

Stevenson, H. L., M. D. Estes, N. R. Thirumalapura, D. H. Walker, and N. Ismail. 2010. Natural killer cells promote tissue injury and systemic inflammatory responses during fatal ehrlichia-induced toxic shock–like syndrome. *American Journal of Pathology* 177(2):766-776.

Stjernberg, L., and J. Berglund. 2005. Detecting ticks on light versus dark clothing. *Scandinavian Journal of Infectious Diseases* 37(5):361-364.

Stjernberg, L., K. Holmkvist, and J. Berglund. 2008. A newly detected tick-borne encephalitis (tbe) focus in south-east Sweden: A follow-up study of tbe virus (tbev) seroprevalence. *Scandinavian Journal of Infectious Diseases* 40(1):4-10.

Straubinger, R. K., B. A. Summers, Y. F. Chang, and M. J. Appel. 1997. Persistence of *Borrelia burgdorferi* in experimentally infected dogs after antibiotic treatment. *Journal of Clinical Microbiology* 35:111-116.

Stricker, R. B., and E. E. Winger. 2001. Decreased cd57 lymphocyte subset in patients with chronic Lyme disease. *Immunology Letters* 76(1):43-48.

———. 2003. Musical hallucinations in patients with Lyme disease. *Southern Medical Journal* 96(7):711-715.

Stricker, R. B., J. J. Burrascano, and E. E. Winger. 2002. Longterm decrease in the cd57 lymphocyte subset in a patient with chronic Lyme disease. *Annals of Agricultural and Environmental Medicine* 9(1):111-113.

Sun, T., M. J. Tenenbaum, J. Greenspan, S. Teichberg, R. T. Wang, T. Degnan, and M. H. Kaplan. 1983. Morphologic and clinical observations in human infection with babesia-microti. *Journal of Infectious Diseases* 148(2):239-248.

Sun, W., J. W. Ijdo, S. R. Telford III, E. Hodzic, Y. Zhang, S. W. Barthold, and E. Fikrig. 1997. Immunization against the agent of human granulocytic ehrlichiosis in a murine model. *Journal of Clinical Investigation* 100:3014-3018.

Suss, J. 2008. Tick-borne encephalitis in Europe and beyond—the epidemiological situation as of 2007. *Euro Surveillance: Bulletin Europeen sur les Maladies Transmissibles = European Communicable Disease Bulletin* 13(26):26.

Suss, J., C. Klaus, F.-W. Gerstengarbe, and P. C. Werner. 2008. What makes ticks tick? Climate change, ticks, and tick-borne diseases. *Journal of Travel Medicine* 15(1):39-45.

Swanson, S. J., D. Neitzel, K. D. Reed, and E. A. Belongia. 2006. Coinfections acquired from ixodes ticks. *Clinical Microbiology Reviews* 19(4):708-727.

Sykes, J. E., L. L. Lindsay, R. G. Maggi, and E. B. Breitschwerdt. 2010. Human coinfection with bartonella henselae and two hemotropic mycoplasma variants resembling mycoplasma ovis. *Journal of Clinical Microbiology* 48(10):3782-3785.

Tektonidou, M. G., and M. M. Ward. 2010. Validity of clinical associations of biomarkers in translational research studies: The case of systemic autoimmune diseases. *Arthritis Research & Therapy* 12:R179.

Thabane, M., and J. K. Marshall. 2009. Post-infectious irritable bowel syndrome. *World Journal of Gastroenterology* 15(29):3591-3596.

Tjernberg, I., M. Carlsson, J. Ernerudh, I. Eliasson, and P. Forsberg. 2010. Mapping of hormones and cortisol responses in patients after Lyme neuroborreliosis. *Bmc Infectious Diseases* 10.

Tokarz, R., K. Jain, A. Bennett, T. Briese, and W. I. Lipkin. 2010. Assessment of polymicrobial infections in ticks in New York State. *Vector-Borne and Zoonotic Diseases* 10(3):217-221.

Tonnetti, L., A. F. Eder, B. Dy, J. Kennedy, P. Pisciotto, R. J. Benjamin, and D. A. Leiby. 2009. Transfusion complications: Transfusion-transmitted babesia microti identified through hemovigilance. *Transfusion* 49(12):2557-2563.

Tupin, E., M. R. Benhnia, Y. Kinjo, R. Patsey, C. J. Lena, M. C. Haller, M. J. Caimano, M. Imamura, C. H. Wong, S. Crotty, J. D. Radolf, T. J. Sellati, and M. Kronenberg. 2008. NKT cells prevent chronic joint inflammation after infection with *Borrelia burgdorferi. Proceedings of the National Academy of Sciences of the United States of America* 105(50):19863-19868.

U.S. Congress, House, 2009. Departments of Labor, Health and Human Services, and Education, and Related Agencies Appropriations Bill, 2010. Report of the Committee in Appropriations together with Minority Views to accompany H.R. 3293. 111th Cong., 1st sess., pp. 81.

Valbuena, G., and D. H. Walker. 2009. Infection of the endothelium by members of the order rickettsiales. *Thromb Haemost* 102(6):1071-1079.

Vallings, R. 2010. A case of chronic fatigue syndrome triggered by influenza h1n1 (swine influenza). *Journal of Clinical Pathology* 63:184-185.

Van Den Eede, F., G. Moorkens, B. Van Houdenhove, P. Cosyns, and S. J. Claes. 2007. Hypothalamic-pituitary-adrenal axis function in chronic fatigue syndrome. *Neuropsychobiology* 55(2):112-120.

van Duin, D., V. Thomas, S. Mohanty, R. R. Montgomery, S. Ginter, E. Fikrig, H. G. Allore, R. Medzhitov, and A. C. Shaw. 2007. Age-associated defect in human tlr1 function and expression. *Journal of Immunology* 178:970-975.

Vannier, E., I. Borggraefe, S. R. Telford, S. Menon, T. Brauns, A. Spielman, J. A. Gelfand, and H. H. Wortis. 2004. Age-associated decline in resistance to *Babesia microti* is genetically determined. *Journal of Infectious Diseases* 189(9):1721-1728.

Vannier, E., B. E. Gewurz, and P. J. Krause. 2008. Human babesiosis. *Infectious Disease Clinics of North America* 22(3):469-488.

Vaughn, M. F., and S. R. Meshnick. 2011. Pilot study assessing the effectiveness of long-lasting permethrin-impregnated clothing for the prevention of tick bites. *Vector-Borne and Zoonotic Diseases*, ahead of print.

Vazquez, M., S. S. Sparrow, and E. D. Shapiro. 2003. Long-term neuropsychologic and health outcomes of children with facial nerve palsy attributable to Lyme disease. *Pediatrics* 112(2):e93-e97.

Vazquez, M., C. Muehlenbein, M. Cartterj, E. B. Hayes, S. Ertel, and E. D. Shapiro. 2008. Effectiveness of personal protective measures to prevent Lyme disease. *Emerging Infectious Diseases* 14(2):210-216.

von Loewenich, F. D., D. G. Scorpio, U. Reischl, J. S. Dumler, and C. Bogdan. 2004. Frontline: Control of anaplasma phagocytophilum, an obligate intracellular pathogen, in the absence of inducible nitric oxide synthase, phagocyte nadph oxidase, tumor necrosis factor, toll-like receptor (TLR)2 and tlr4, or the TLR adaptor molecule myd88. *European Journal of Immunology* 34:1789-1797.

Vrethem, M., L. Hellblom, and M. Widlund. 2002. Chronic symptoms are common in patients with neuroborreliosis – a questionnaire follow-up study. *Acta Neurologica Scandinavica* 106:205-208.

Walker, D. H., and H. N. Kirkman. 1980. Rocky mountain spotted fever and deficiency in glucose-6-phosphate dehydrogenase. *Journal of Infectious Diseases* 142(5):771.

Walker, D. H., H. K. Hawkins, and P. Hudson. 1983. Fulminant Rocky Mountain spotted fever—its pathologic characteristics associated with glucose-6-phosphate-dehydrogenase deficiency. *Archives of Pathology & Laboratory Medicine* 107(3):121-125.

Walker, D. H., C. D. Paddock, and J. S. Dumler. 2008. Emerging and re-emerging tick-transmitted rickettsial and ehrlichial infections. *Medical Clinics of North America* 92(6):1345-1361.

Wang, G., A. P. van Dam, A. Le Fleche, D. Postic, O. Peter, G. Baranton, R. de Boer, L. Spanjaard, and J. Dankert. 1997. Genetic and phenotypic analysis of *Borrelia valaisiana* sp. Nov. (borrelia genomic groups vs116 and m19). *International Journal of Systematic Bacteriology* 47(4):926-932.

Wang, G., C. Ojaima, H. Wu, V. Saksenberg, R. Iyer, D. Liveris, S. A. McClain, G. P. Wormser, and I. Schwartz. 2002. Disease severity in a murine model of Lyme borreliosis is associated with the genotype of the infecting *Borrelia burgdorferi* sensu stricto strain. *Journal of Infectious Diseases* 186:782-791.

Wang, H. L., M. Moser, M. Schiltenwolf, and M. Buchner. 2008. Circulating cytokine levels compared to pain in patients with fibromyalgia—A prospective longitudinal study over 6 months. *Journal of Rheumatology* 35(7):1366-1370.

Wang, I.-N., D. E. Dykhuizen, W. Qiu, J. J. Dunn, E. M. Bosler, and B. J. Luft. 1999. Genetic diversity of ospc in a local population of borrelia burgdorferi sensu stricto. *Genetics* 151(1):15-30.

Wang, T. M., M. Akkoyunlu, R. Banerjee, and E. Fikrig. 2004. Interferon-gamma deficiency reveals that 129sv mice are inherently more susceptible to anaplasma phagocytophilum than c57bl/6 mice. *FEMS Immunology & Medical Microbiology* 42:299-305.

Warren, J. W., V. Brown, S. Jacobs, L. Horne, P. Langenberg, and P. Greenberg. 2008. Urinary tract infection and inflammation at onset of interstitial cystitis/painful bladder syndrome. *Urology* 71(6):1085-1090.

Wei, Q., M. Tsuji, A. Zamoto, M. Kohsaki, T. Matsui, T. Shiota, S. R. Telford, and C. Ishihara. 2001. Human babesiosis in Japan: Isolation of babesia microti-like parasites from an asymptomatic transfusion donor and from a rodent from an area where babesiosis is endemic. *Journal of Clinical Microbiology* 39(6):2178-2183.

Weintraub, P. 2008. *Cure unknown: Inside the Lyme Epidemic.* New York: St. Martin's Press.

Weiss, E. 1973. Growth and physiology of rickettsiae. *Bacteriology Review* 37(3):259-283.

Weissbecker, I., A. Floyd, E. Dedert, R. Salmon, and S. Sephton. 2006. Childhood trauma and diurnal cortisol disruption in fibromyalgia syndrome. *Psychoneuroendocrinology* 31(3):312-324.

Weller, M., A. Stevens, N. Sommer, H. Wietholter, and J. Dichgans. 1991. Cerebrospinal fluid interleukins, immunoglobulins, and fibronectin in neuroborreliosis. *Archives of Neurology* 48(8):837-841.

White, D. J., J. Talarico, H. G. Chang, G. S. Birkhead, T. Heimberger, and D. L. Morse. 1998. Human babesiosis in New York State—review of 139 hospitalized cases and analysis of prognostic factors. *Archives of Internal Medicine* 158(19):2149-2154.

Widhe, M., S. Jarefors, C. Ekerfelt, M. Vrethem, S. Bergstrom, P. Forsberg, and J. Ernerudh. 2004. "Borrelia"-specific interferon-γ and interleukin-4 secretion in cerebrospinal fluid and blood during lyme borreuosis in humans: Association with clinical outcome. *The Journal of Infectious Diseases* 189(10):1881-1891.

Willadsen, P. 2006. Tick control: Thoughts on a research agenda. *Veterinary Parasitology* 138(1-2):161-168.

Williams, C. V., J. L. Van Steenhouse, J. M. Bradley, S. I. Hancock, B. C. Hegarty, and E. B. Breitschwerdt. 2002. Naturally occurring *Ehrlichia chaffeensis* infection in two prosimian primate species: Ring-tailed lemurs (lemur catta) and ruffed lemurs (varecia variegata). *Emerging Infectious Diseases* 8(12):1497-1500.

Williams, J. V., R. Martino, N. Rabella, M. Otegui, R. Parody, J. M. Heck, and J. J. E. Crowe. 2005. A prospective study comparing human metapneumovirus with other respiratory viruses in adults with hematologic malignancies and respiratory tract infections. *Journal of Infectious Diseases* 192(6):1061-1065.

Wilson, M. L., S. R. Telford, 3rd, J. Piesman, and A. Spielman. 1988. Reduced abundance of immature *Ixodes dammini* (acari: Ixodidae) following elimination of deer. *Journal of Medical Entomology* 25(4):224-228.

Wingenfeld, K., C. Heim, I. Schmidt, D. Wagner, G. Meinlschmidt, and D. H. Hellhammer. 2008. Hpa axis reactivity and lymphocyte glucocorticoid sensitivity in fibromyalgia syndrome and chronic pelvic pain. *Psychosomatic Medicine* 70(1):65-72.

Winslow, G. M., E. Yager, K. Shilo, E. Volk, A. Reilly, and F. K. Chu. 2000. Antibody-mediated elimination of the obligate intracellular bacterial pathogen *Ehrlichia chaffeensis* during active infection. *Infection and Immunity* 68:2187-2195.

Woldehiwet, Z. 2006. Anaplasma phagocytophilum in ruminants in Europe. *Annals of the New York Academy of Sciences* 1078:446-460.

Wooten, R. M., Y. Ma, R. A. Yoder, J. P. Brown, J. H. Weis, J. F. Zachary, C. J. Kirschning, and J. J. Weis. 2002. Toll-like receptor 2 is required for innate, but not acquired, host defense to Borrelia burgdorferi. *The Journal of Immunology* 168:348-355.

Wormser, G. P., D. McKenna, J. Carlin, R. B. Nadelman, L. F. Cavaliere, D. Holmgren, D. W. Byrne, and J. Nowakowski. 2005. Brief communication: Hematogenous dissemination in early Lyme disease. *Annals of Internal Medicine* 142(9):751-755.

Wormser, G. P., R. J. Dattwyler, E. D. Shapiro, J. J. Halperin, A. C. Steere, M. S. Klempner, P. J. Krause, J. S. Bakken, F. Strle, G. Stanek, L. K. Bockenstedt, D. Fish, J. S. Dumler, and R. B. Nadelman. 2006. The clinical assessment, treatment, and prevention of Lyme disease, human granulocytic anaplasmosis, and babesiosis: Clinical practice guidelines by the Infectious Diseases Society of America *Clinical Infectious Diseases* 43(9):1089-1134.

Wormser, G. P., D. Brisson, D. Liveris, K. Hanincova, S. Sandigursky, J. Nowakowski, R. B. Nadelman, S. Ludin, and I. Schwartz. 2008a. *Borrelia burgdorferi* genotype predicts the capacity for hematogenous dissemination during early Lyme disease. *Journal of Infectious Diseases* 198(9):1358-1364.

Wormser, G. P., J. Nowakowski, R. B. Nadelman, P. Visintainer, A. Levin, and M. E. Aguero-Rosenfeld. 2008b. Impact of clinical variables on *Borrelia burgdorferi*-specific antibody seropositivity in acute-phase sera from patients in North America with culture-confirmed early Lyme disease. *Clinical and Vaccine Immunology* 15(10):1519-1522.

Wormser, G. P., A. Prasad, E. Neuhaus, S. Joshi, J. Nowakowski, J. Nelson, A. Mittleman, M. Aguero-Rosenfeld, J. Topal, and P. J. Krause. 2010. Emergence of resistance to azithromycin-atovaquone in immunocompromised patients with *Babesia microti* infection. *Clinical Infectious Diseases* 50(3):381-386.

Wozniak, E. J., L. J. Lowenstine, R. Hemmer, T. Robinson, and P. A. Conrad. 1996. Comparative pathogenesis of human wa-1 and *Babesia microti* isolates in Syrian hamster model. *American Association for Laboratory Animal Science* 50(3):507-515.

Yager, J. A., S. J. Best, R. G. Maggi, M. Varanat, N. Znajda, and E. B. Breitschwerdt. 2010. Bacillary angiomatosis in an immunosuppressed dog. *Veterinary Dermatology* 21(4):420-428.

Young, C., and P. J. Krause. 2009. The problem of transfusion-transmitted babesiosis. *Transfusion* 2548-2550.

Zambrano, M. C., A. A. Beklemisheva, A. V. Bryksin, S. A. Newman, and F. C. Cabello. 2004. *Borrelia burgdorferi* binds to, invades, and colonizes native type I collagen lattices. *Infection and Immunity* 72(6):3138-3146.

Zautra, A. J., L. M. Johnson, and M. C. Davis. 2005. Positive affect as a source of resilience for women in chronic pain. *Journal of Consulting and Clinical Psychology* 73(2):212-220.

Zent, O., and M. Broker. 2005. Tick-borne encephalitis vaccines: Past and present. *Expert Review of Vaccines* 4(5):747-755.

Zhang, J. R., and S. J. Norris. 1998. Kinetics and in vivo induction of genetic variation of vlse in *Borrelia burgdorferi*. *Infection and Immunity* 66(8):3689-3697.

Zhang, J. R., J. M. Hardham, A. G. Barbour, and S. J. Norris. 1997. Antigenic variation in Lyme disease borreliae by promiscuous recombination of vmp-like sequence cassettes. *Cell* 89(2):275-285.

Zhioua, E., L. Gern, A. Aeschlimann, M. J. Sauvain, S. Van der Linden, and H. Fahrer. 1998. Longitudinal study of Lyme borreliosis in a high risk population in Switzerland. *Parasite-Journal De La Societe Francaise De Parasitologie* 5(4):383-386.

Zintl, A., G. Mulcahy, H. E. Skerrett, S. M. Taylor, and J. S. Gray. 2003. *Babesia divergens*, a bovine blood parasite of veterinary and zoonotic importance. *Clinical Microbiology Reviews* 16(4):622-636.

# A

# Commissioned Papers

The Committee on Lyme Disease and Other Tick-Borne Diseases: The State of the Science commissioned 10 papers on range of topics that were not covered in depth at the workshop. The committee felt these papers were necessary for the discussion at the workshop. These papers are reproduced in their entirety in this appendix.

# A1
# THROUGH A GLASS, DARKLY:
# THE GLOBAL INCIDENCE OF TICK-BORNE DISEASES

*Christopher D. Paddock, M.D., M.P.H.T.M.,*
*and Sam R. Telford III, Sc.D.*

Infectious Diseases Pathology Branch, National Center for Emerging and
  Zoonotic Infectious Diseases, Centers for Disease Control and Preven-
  tion, Atlanta, GA
Division of Infectious Diseases, Department of Biomedical Sciences, Tufts
  University Cummings School of Veterinary Medicine

*Corresponding author:*
*Christopher D. Paddock*

Infectious Diseases Pathology Branch, Bldg 18, Rm. SB 109, Mailstop
  G-32, Centers for Disease Control and Prevention

The findings and conclusions in this report are those of the authors and
do not necessarily represent the official position of the Centers for Disease
Control and Prevention.

## Introduction

Several events that occurred during the final decades of the 20th Century, and at the cusp of the 21st Century, suggest that increases in the scope
and magnitude of tick-borne infections have occurred worldwide. These
include recent national and regional epidemics of historically recognized
diseases, including tick-borne encephalitis (TBE) in Central and Eastern Europe, Kyasanur forest disease (KFD) in Karnataka state in India, Crimean-
Congo hemorrhagic fever (CCHF) in northern Turkey and the southwestern
regions of the Russian Federation, and Rocky Mountain spotted fever
(RMSF) in Arizona and Baja California (Randolph, 2008; Pattnaik, 2006;
Maltezou et al., 2010; McQuiston et al., 2010; Bustamente Moreno and
Pon Méndez, 2010a). Globally, the recognized number of distinct and
epidemiologically important diseases transmitted by ticks has increased
considerably during the last 30 years. By example, >10 newly recognized
spotted fever rickettsioses have been identified since 1984 (Raoult et al.,
1996; Parola et al., 2005; Paddock et al., 2008; Shapiro et al., 2010). In
the United States, only 2 tick-borne diseases, RMSF and tularemia, were
nationally notifiable in 1990; by 1998, this list included 3 newly recognized

infections: Lyme disease, human granulocytic ehrlichiosis [anaplasmosis] (*Anaplasma phagocytophilum* infection), and human monocytic ehrlichiosis (*Ehrlichia chaffeensis* infection), each of which has increased steadily in average annual incidence. Lyme disease is now the most commonly reported vector-borne illness in the United States, with the number of reported cases increasing 101% (from 9,908 to 19,931) during 1992-2006. (Bacon et al., 2008). During 2000-2008, the annual reported incidence of RMSF in the United States also increased dramatically, from 1.7 to 9.4 cases per million persons (Figure A1-1), representing the steepest rise to the highest rate ever recorded (Openshaw et al., 2010). From 2000-2007, the incidence of infections caused by *A. phagocytophilum* and *E. chaffeensis* also increased linearly, from 0.80 to 3.0, and 1.4 to 3.0, cases per million population, respectively (Dahlgren et al., in press).

Against this background of rapidly expanding pathogen recognition and escalating incidence have been concerns about the accuracy of case counts that form the basis for these statistics (Mantke et al., 2008; Raoult and Parola, 2008; Paddock, 2009). Many of these agents were catapulted into the realm of human recognition by extraordinary advances in molecular technology; however, epidemiologic tools for capturing cases and calculating incidence have not undergone similar transformative changes. Paradoxically, the discoveries of new pathogens made possible by contemporary diagnostic methods have cast suspicion on certain aspects of the

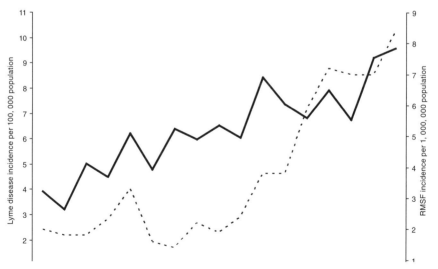

**FIGURE A1-1** Average annual incidence of Rocky Mountain spotted fever and Lyme disease in the United States, 1992-2008 (Bacon et al., 2008; Openshaw et al., 2010).

distribution, frequency, and clinical heterogeneity of some older, historically recognized, tick-borne diseases. In essence, the pace of pathogen discovery has eclipsed fundamental epidemiologic knowledge of many of the diseases caused by these agents.

Incidence rates of tick-borne infections pale in comparison with those of many other arthropod-borne diseases, including malaria, dengue, Chagas' disease, onchocerciasis, and leishmaniasis. Only Lyme disease, with tens of thousands of new cases each year, distributed across several continents, can be considered as prevalent across a wide distribution (Table A1-1). Lyme

**TABLE A1-1** Estimated Global Incidence and Distribution of Major Tick-Borne Infections

| Global Incidence and Distribution of Major Tick-Transmitted Infections |
| --- |
| Very common (>10,000 new cases each year) |
|     Lyme disease – Holarctic |
|         (Bacon et al., 2008) |
| Common (1000-10,000 new cases each year) |
|     Tick-borne encephalitis – Holarctic |
|         (www.isw-tbe.info/upload/medialibrary/12th_ISW-TBE_Newsletter.pdf) |
|     Tick-borne relapsing fever – tropical Africa; western United States |
|         (Felsenfeld, 1971; Trape et al., 1996; Vial et al., 2006) |
|     Tick-borne spotted fever group rickettsioses – global |
|         (Rovery et al. 2008; Openshaw et al., 2010) |
|     Ehrlichiosis and anaplasmosis – global |
|         (Demma et al., 2005b) |
|     Masters' disease – eastern, central, and south-central United States |
|         (CDC, 1990) |
|     Crimean-Congo hemorrhagic fever– southern Europe, Africa, western and central Russian Federation, North Asia |
|         (www.ecdc.europa.eu/en/Publications/0809_MER_Crimean_Congo_Haemorrhagic_Fever_Prevention_and_Control.pdf) |
| Moderately common (100-1,000 new cases each year) |
|     Colorado tick fever and other other coltivirus infections– western United States; central Europe |
|         (http://www.cdphe.state.co.us/dc/zoonosis/tick/Colorado_tick_diseases.pdf) |
|     Babesiosis – northeastern United States; Europe |
|         (Telford et al., in press) |
|     Omsk hemorrhagic fever – eastern Russia and Siberia |
|         (Lvov, 1988) |
|     Tick-borne tularemia – eastern and central United States; central Europe; Russian Federation |
|         (CDC, 2002) |
|     Kyasanur forest disease – Karnataka and adjacent states in India; Saudi Arabia; Egypt |
|         (Dandawate et al., 1994; Pattnaik, 2006; Carletti et al., 2010) |
| Rare (sporadic cases) |
|     Powassan/deer tick virus – Canada; northeastern and north central United States |
|         (Ebel, 2010) |

disease is still less common, by an order of magnitude, than leishmaniasis, represented by 1 million new cases a year among a population at risk of 350 million persons (Anonymous, 1994). Nonetheless, in some regions of the world, such as Europe, tick-borne diseases are the most widespread and medically important of all vector-borne infectious diseases (Randolph, 2010). In addition, some tick-borne diseases are associated with high case-fatality rates or long-term morbidity, and frequently generate considerable fear among the population who reside in areas where these pathogens are endemic; in this context, public health concerns may far exceed actual disease burden. By example, the average annual incidence of Brazilian spotted fever in São Paulo State, Brazil, during 2000-2008 ranged from 0.2 to 1.1 cases per million population, comprising only 285 total cases; however, 89 of these resulted in death, for an average case-fatality rate of 31% (www.cve.saude.sp.gov.br/htm/zoo/fm_i8503.htm). Other tick-borne diseases, including CCHF and KFD, are associated with high case-fatality rates that rival or exceed those of many of the most severe infectious diseases (Hoogstraal, 1979; Swanepoel et al., 1987; Pattnaik, 2006).

This discussion compares the perceived and actual burden of various tick-borne infections suggested by existing surveillance data, evaluates some of the strengths and limitations of current systems that measure incidence, and suggests several approaches for improving the accuracy of incidence determinations for these diseases. While tick-borne infections also pose important veterinary health problems around the world, this synopsis focuses on the occurrence of these diseases in human populations. Although this discussion also incorporates some information that is anecdotal, inferred, or derived from non-controlled circumstances, we hope that a contemporary synthesis of all observations may serve as a guide for subsequent epidemiologic approaches to this remarkably diverse and important collection of zoonotic diseases.

### Case Counts, Reporting, and Incidence of Tick-Borne Diseases

Are the global rises in incidence reflective of true events or greater levels of reporting? Simplistically, increased reporting is indeed responsible for these trends; however, this question is somewhat circular, because incidence statistics are obtained principally from reported cases of disease. Incidence rates are dependent directly on the size of the population at risk during a specific interval of time and the number of identified cases of disease; however, from most of the scientific literature, it is difficult to determine whether a change in incidence reflects increased transmission, better reporting, or a change in the population at risk. Ideally, surveillance systems for tick-borne diseases accurately identify rises or declines of the disease in question; however, any of a number of variables may change over time, including ecologic, climatologic, or social variables, case definitions, diagnostic assays, or the appearance or emigration of cognizant and enthusiastic clinicians who actively search for cases and specifically pursue confirmatory tests.

## Incidence and Regional Context

Incidence statistics of tick-borne infections, when interpreted flatly as national rates, characteristically lose impact and meaning. These zoonoses are influenced profoundly by a complex mixture of predictable and unpredictable factors that include landscape, climate, wildlife hosts, and tick distributions that coalesce to create regional pockets of intensified risk (Pavlovskey, 1966); in this context, incidence rates for these diseases assume far greater impact when viewed regionally. Because of marked differences in population sizes across regions, it is axiomatic that high incidence does necessarily equate to a large number of reported cases. By example, sparsely populated Cameron County, Pennsylvania, reported only 14 cases of Lyme disease during 2002-2006; however, the county's average annual incidence rate was greater than the incidence of the more populous Windham County, Connecticut, where approximately 18 × as many cases were reported during the same interval (Bacon et al., 2008). Nantucket County in Massachusetts, reported 151 cases of Lyme disease during 1992-2006, representing only 0.061% of 248,074 total reports received by CDC during this interval; however, it ranked highest in incidence of all U.S. counties during 1992-2001, and third during 2002-2006, with rates of 361 to 755 per 100,000 population (Figure A1-2A). By comparison, the average annual rate of Lyme disease in the entire state of Massachusetts was 14.5 per 100,000 population during the same study period (Bacon et al., 2008).

During 1989-2000, Portugal reported the highest country-wide incidence of Mediterranean spotted fever (MSF) in the Mediterranean basin (9.8 per 100,000 persons); however, the regional incidence in this country ranged markedly, from 3.1 per 100,000 in Lisboa and Vale do Teja, to 31 per 100,000 in the nearby region of Alentejo (de Sousa et al., 2003). During 2000-2007, 11,531 cases of RMSF were reported from 46 states and the District of Colombia; however, approximately two-thirds of these cases originated from only 5 states (Arkansas, Missouri, North Carolina, Oklahoma, and Tennessee), where the incidence ranged from 20.3 to 52.6 per million persons (Figure A1-2B). By comparison, the national incidence of RMSF during the study period was 4.9 per million (Openshaw et al., 2010). These statistics are magnified further when foci of infected ticks overlap rural or undeveloped regions with relatively low population density. During 2003-2009, 88 cases of RMSF were reported from 3 Apache Indian communities in Eastern Arizona that resulted in an average annual incidence of

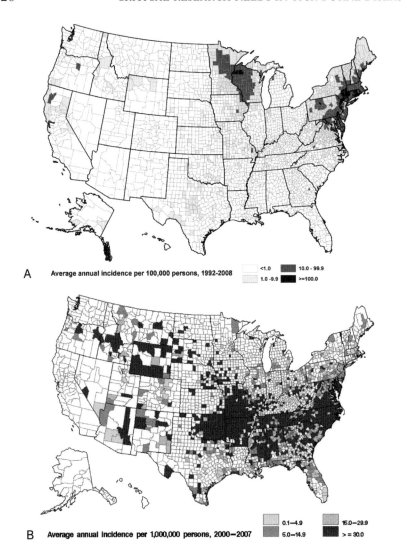

A    Average annual incidence per 100,000 persons, 1992-2008

<1.0       10.0 - 99.9
1.0 -9.9   >=100.0

B    Average annual incidence per 1,000,000 persons, 2000—2007

0.1—4.9    15.0—29.9
5.0—14.9   > = 30.0

FIGURE A1-2 Average annual incidence, by county of residence, of reported cases of Lyme disease, 1992-2008 (a) and Rocky Mountain spotted fever, 2000-2007 (b), in the United States (Bacon et al., 2008; Openshaw et al., 2010).

437 /million persons for this 5,000 square mile region, more than 62 times greater than the national average (McQuiston et al., 2010). In some circumstances, regional variation develops when cultural, racial or socioeconomic homogeneity exists among the population at risk. By example, the incidence of RMSF among American Indians has risen dramatically (Figure A1-3), when compared with other racial groups in the United States: during 2001-2005, the average annual incidence among American Indians was 16.8 per 1,000,000 population, compared with rates of 4.2 and 2.6 among white and black racial groups, respectively (Holman et al., 2009).

*Trends in Drequency and Distribution*

Dramatic shifts in numbers of reported cases of tick-borne diseases over time and space are well-recognized; indeed, such shifts are epidemiologic hallmarks of many of these infections. National or regional trends are best characterized by surveillance systems with sufficient maturity and camber to accommodate for input that might otherwise immediately confound interpretation. The incidence of TBE in the Czech Republic has exhibited at least 4 cycles of rising and declining incidence since 1971, with the greatest upsurge occurring during 1990-1995, when the incidence climbed steadily from approximately 1.7 to 7.2 /100,000 population (Kriz et al., 2004). Similar increases were witnessed in several other eastern European countries

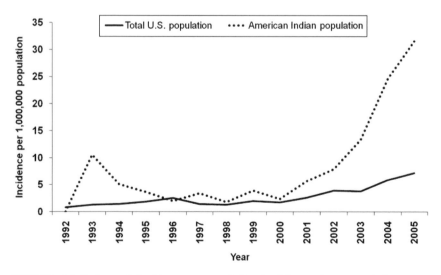

FIGURE A1-3 Annual incidence rates of Rocky Mountain spotted fever, per 1 million population, among American Indians, and the total U.S. population, 1992-2005 (Holman et al., 2009).

during this same interval (Figure A1-4) (Šumilo et al., 2007; Randolph, 2008) and more recently, has extended across several countries of Western Europe, including Italy, Germany, and Switzerland, where the incidence of TBE in 2006 exceeded average levels for the previous decade by as much as 183% (Zimmerman, 2005; Randolph et al., 2008; Rizzoli et al., 2009).

In the United States, the annual incidence of RMSF has undergone 3 major shifts (Figure A1-5) since national surveillance for this disease was initiated in 1920 (Childs and Paddock, 2003; Openshaw et al., 2010). While average annual incidence rates of Lyme disease in the United States increased steadily during 1992-2006 (Figure A1-1), at least 88% of all U.S. cases reported in any given year, and 229,782 (92.6%) of the 248,074 cases reported cumulatively during this interval, originated consistently from the 10 states in which Lyme disease is highly endemic (Bacon et al., 2008). During the mid-1970s through the early 1980s, increases in the case numbers

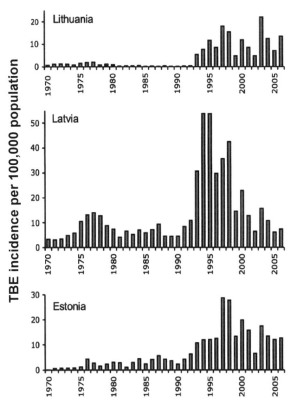

FIGURE A1-4 Incidence of tick-borne encephalitis, per 100,000 population, in Lithuania, Latvia, and Estonia, 1970-2006 (Šumilo et al., 2007).

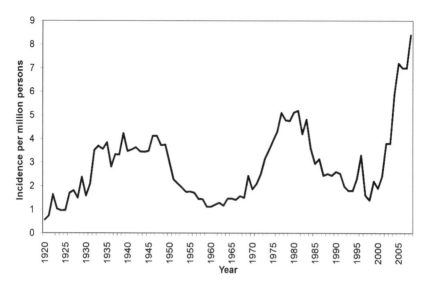

**FIGURE A1-5** Average annual incidence of Rocky Mountain spotted fever, per 1 million population in the United States, 1920-2008 (Childs and Paddock, 2002; Openshaw et al., 2010).

of reported spotted fever group rickettsioses were documented in several countries bordering the Mediterranean Sea, including Israel, Italy, and Spain (Piras et al., 1982; Segura and Font, 1982; Otero et al., 1982; Gross et al., 1982; Mansueto et al. 1986). Approximately 30 cases of MSF were reported in Italy each year during 1962-1973; however, during the next 6 years, the number of cases identified rose dramatically, to >800 annually by 1979 (Scaffidi, 1981). In the area of the Vallés Occidental near Barcelona, Spain, the incidence of MSF, per 100,000 persons, rose from 3.28 cases in 1979 to 19.05 cases in 1984 (Espejo Arenas et al., 1986). During the mid-1980s through the early 1990s, <20 cases of Japanese spotted fever were reported annually; during the subsequent 15 years, reports climbed steadily to 129 cases in 2009 (Anonymous, 1999; Anonymous, 2006; Anonymous, 2010).

## Drivers of Incidence

Unfortunately, the reasons suggested for major periods of increased or diminished incidence of tick-borne diseases have, with few exceptions, been difficult to investigate and even more difficult to corroborate. These infections have circulated dynamically in nature for many thousands of years, and biological equilibria among the pathogen, tick, and vertebrate hosts parasitized by the tick or infected by the pathogen characteristically exist in the absence of humans. Nonetheless, the emergence and flux of tick-borne diseases can most often be traced to specific human activities and behaviours that create disequilibrium in these cycles and position greater numbers of persons into disrupted ecosystems. Outbreaks of tick-borne disease are often linked to ecologic and social upheavals, resulting directly from human influence, that create circumstances advantageous for large numbers of ticks and reservoir hosts. During World War II, following the occupation of Crimea by Axis forces, there was abandonment of agricultural lands and diminished hunting of European hares (*Lepus europaeus*) because of combat activities. When Soviet troops reoccupied the Crimean steppes in 1944, pastures and farms had become overgrown by weeds, and hares had become extremely abundant and were heavily parasitized with *Hyalomma* ticks. The combination of these factors is believed to have contributed to an epidemic of CCHF among military personnel during 1944-1945, involving especially signalmen and surveyors, who frequented brushy areas (Hoogstraal, 1979).

A careful analysis of climatic and vegetation features with georeferenced cases of CCHF in Turkey during 2003-2008 identified a recent expansion of extensively fragmented habitats in the Anatolia region as the most important factor for the CCHF epidemic in this region. This process resulted from the loss of mature forests to farming activities, and the reversion of farms to dense undergrowth and subsequent to second growth forest with the emigration of persons from rural to urban areas (Estrada-Peña et al., 2010). In a similar manner, whole-scale clearing of primary old-growth forests by inhabitants in the northeastern United States in the late 18th and early 19th Centuries, followed by the abandonment of farms during the westward expansion of the late 19th Century, and subsequent deciduous successional growth that provided ideal habitats for white-tailed deer (*Odocoileus virginianus*) and deer ticks (*Ixodes scapularis* (*dammini*), fueled the emergence of Lyme disease in the second half of the 20th Century (Spielman et al., 1985). In Italy, changes in forest management practices during the last several decades of the 20th Century transitioned a greater percentage of coppice cover (small areas of broad-leaved forest harvested regularly for firewood) to high-stand forests and improving habitat suitability for small reservoir hosts of *Ixodes ricinus* ticks. This manipulation of forest structure is believed to have contributed to the steadily increasing incidence of TBE observed in 17 northern alpine provinces since the early 1990s (Rizzoli et al., 2009).

## Tick Abundance and Distribution

Environmental disturbance is a frequent trigger for outbreaks of tick-borne infection. The most extensively studied example, Lyme disease in the northeastern United States, resulted from reforestation, increased deer density, and increased development and use of forested sites by humans (Spielman et al., 1985). It is likely that the deer tick vector and its microbial guild survived in relict sites during and after glaciation and through Colonial times (Telford et al., 1993; Hoen et al., 2009). Infestations of the deer tick were first recognized from the terminal moraine areas of southern New England and Long Island as well as northwest Wisconsin; these were also the sites where the first cases of Lyme disease or babesiosis were identified in the United States (Spielman et al., 1985; Scrimenti, 1970; Western et al., 1970). In the mid-1980s, Ipswich, Massachusetts represented the northernmost established infestation in the Northeast (Lastavica et al., 1989). Within a decade, the distribution of the deer tick expanded on a north-south axis to the Bar Harbor region in Maine and the coastal peninsula of Delaware, Maryland, and Virginia (Rand et al., 1998). Infestation of migratory birds by deer tick larvae and nymphs served as the primary mode of introduction (Battaly et al., 1993; Ginsberg, 1993). Transport of adult ticks by deer along major waterways also contributed to a rapid spread, particularly in the Hudson River Valley (Chen et al., 2005).

Other recent examples of range expansions of medically important tick species include the establishment of *Amblyomma americanum* (a vector of *E. chaffeensis* and *Ehrlichia ewingii*) in the northeastern United States (Paddock and Yabsley, 2007) *Amblyomma maculatum* (a vector of *Rickettsia parkeri*) throughout Arkansas (Trout et al., 2010), *I. scapularis* across the lower peninsula of Michigan (Hamer et al., 2010), and *Dermacentor reticularis* (a vector of *Rickettsia raoultii*) in western Germany and the Netherlands (Dautel et al., 2006; Nijhof et al., 2007).

Conversely, loss of habitat or a host species may reduce the abundance of a historically dominant tick species. From a tick surveillance program in Ohio during 1984-1989 *D. variabilis* ticks accounted for 13,351 (97%) of 13,764 ticks submitted to the Vector-Borne Disease Unit of the Ohio Department of Health by the general public, physicians, and local health departments from every county in the state; fewer than 1% of the ticks submitted during this period were *A. americanum* (Pretzman et al., 1990). However, during 1994-1999, only 3,841 (62%) of 6,234 of the submitted ticks were *D. variabilis*, with 1,351 (22%) now comprising *A. americanum* (Scott Odee, Richard Gary, pers. comm.). From 1978-1981, 1,342 adult *D. variabilis* ticks were collected during a mark-and-release survey of ticks at Panola Mountain State Park in Georgia (Newhouse, 1983); however, *D. variabilis* was only rarely encountered when extensive tick surveys were conducted at this same park approximately 20 years later (Michael Levin, pers. comm.). The causes of these apparent shifts remain speculative; however, a hypothesis to explore is the effect of periodic scarcity of keystone hosts for *D. variabilis*, i.e., skunks and raccoons, from repeated rabies epizootics in certain areas of the eastern United States (Anthony et al., 1990; Guerra et al., 2003).

*Changes in Vertebrate Host Abundance and Distribution*

The anthropogenic nature of tick-borne infections is considerable and sustained human activities that deplete or amplify the vertebrate host populations can manifest as surges of disease incidence in human populations. In Brazil, capybara (*Hydochoerus hydrochaeris*) are important hosts to the tick *Amblyomma cajennense*, a vector of RMSF, and an effective amplifying host for *R. rickettsii* (Souza et al., 2009). The resurgence of RMSF in many areas of São Paulo State in Brazil during 1998-2007 coincides with explosive increases in the numbers of capybara, and a broadening distribution of these rodents into urban areas of this region (Verdade and Ferraz, 2006). Collectively, these data suggest that dramatic increases in the numbers of RMSF in São Paulo State (www.cve.saude.sp.gov.br/htm/zoo/fm i8503. htm), and other areas of southeastern Brazil, may be linked closely to a rapidly expanding population of a tick host species that is well adapted to anthropogenic habitats (Labruna et al., 2004; Angerami et al., 2006).

Several arguments document the role of white-tailed deer in the emergence and expansion of Lyme disease, babesiosis, ehrlichiosis, and anaplasmosis (Piesman et al., 1979; Spielman et al., 1993; Paddock and Yabsley, 2007). These 4 diseases were identified and characterized during the last 3 decades of the 20th century, following a period of near-exponential growth of white-tailed deer populations in multiple regions of the eastern United States. At the end of the 19th Century, following several decades of overhunting and habitat loss, an estimated 300,000-500,000 deer existed in the United States. Intensive conservation efforts, coupled with expansive environmental changes that inadvertently provided ideal habitats for these animals to proliferate, caused an eruptive increase of the numbers of deer to approximately 18 million animals by 1992. Because these animals serve as keystone hosts for I. scapularis and *A. americanum* ticks, the extraordinary increase in range and numbers of white-tailed deer also contributed to increases in these vector tick populations. Because *O. virginianus* is also an important reservoir host for *E. chaffeensis* and *E. ewingii,* this remarkable increase in numbers also expanded considerably the reservoir pool of these pathogens (Paddock and Yabsley, 2007). In a similar manner, roe deer (*Capreolus capreolus*) were nearly extirpated from the Italian Alps by the end of World War II; however, changes in wildlife practices during the last 50 years enabled a dramatic rebound of this species, by as much as 2000% in some provinces. Because roe deer are also considered crucial in maintaining and amplifying *I. ricinus* tick populations, an upsurge in deer denisty in northern Italy is likely to have contributed to the rapid and steady rise in TBE incidence witnessed in this same region since the early 1990s (Rizzoli et al., 2009).

Mediterranean spotted fever all but disappeared from the Côte Varoise of France during 1952-1966, a period that closely approximated the disappearance wild rabbits (*Oryctolagus cuniculus*) following an epizootic of myxomatosis along the Mediterranean coast. In 1967, a dramatic resurgence of MSF in the region occurred simultaneously with the recovery of the wild rabbit population, suggesting to some investigators that these two events were linked ecologically and epidemiologically (Le Gac et al., 1969). Disequilibrium among domesticated animals may create drastic changes as well. More than 90 cases of RMSF, including 11 deaths, have been reported from several small communities in the White Mountain area of eastern Arizona since 2003. This outbreak appears to be linked directly to enormous numbers of *R. rickettsii*-infected *R. sanguineus* ticks in the peridomestic environment that resulted from unchecked populations of stray and free-ranging dogs in the community (Demma et al., 2005; Nicholson et al., 2006). During the 1940s, investigators in Mexico reported a similar occurrence in states of Sonora, Coahuila, Durango, Nuevo León, and San Luis Potosí (Bustamente and Varela, 1947).

*Climate Change*

Direct effects of climate change on the incidence of tick-borne infections remain largely speculative; (Šumilo et al., 2007; Rizzoli et al. 2009; Randolph, 2009a; Randolph, 2010; Randolph et al., 2008). Many transmission models have been developed, but the lacuna in virtually all of these systems is a quantitative assessment of the "zoonotic bridge," i.e, biological events that introduce the pathogen from the natural enzootic cycle into the realm of human health (Spielman and Rossignol, 1984). Risk factors for human exposure to vectors, and human-associated factors that modify this risk, including activity patterns and the use of personal protection, remain poorly studied. In addition, incidence data of sufficient duration and at the appropriate temporal and spatial scales are often not available to validate existing quantitative models. Accordingly, if one cannot accurately predict incidence for a site over a short interval of time, despite readily measured surveillance variables, then any long-term prediction for the results of climate change remain conjectural. Nonetheless, climate change has been implicated frequently as an important driver of incidence. The spread of tick-borne borreliosis in West Africa is possibly linked to a sub-Saharan drought that allowed the tick vector, *Alectorobius sonrai*, to colonize new savannah areas (Trape et al., 1996). It has been suggested that warmer weather increases the frequency with which *R. sanguineus* will bite humans and thereby transmit its associated pathogens (Parola et al., 2008).

Of the tick-borne diseases, TBE perhaps has the best incidence data across a range of scales, as well as ecological data, that permit detailed examination for causality. For several years, rising incidence of TBE throughout central Europe was attributed by many investigators to climate change (http://www.ecologyandsociety.org/vol2/iss1/art5/). During the mid-1980s, the incidence of TBE in Sweden increased from 2 to 5 per 100,000 population, and two opposing factors confounded epidemiologic analyses: an increase in roe deer density, to suggest a greater abundance of *I. ricinus* ticks and increased transmission, and the introduction of a TBE vaccine, suggesting greatly diminished risk. Even with confounding, a multiple regression analysis of meteorological data and TBE incidence suggested that a milder winter in the previous year, with 2 consecutive mild spring and fall seasons, predicted increased incidence.

However, climate change alone does not adequately explain the remarkably rapid increase in the incidence of TBE across much of Europe during the last few decades, particularly in the Baltic States (Figure A1-4); the factors that influence changes in TBE transmission, and ultimately human risk, appear to be more numerous and complex. What is known is that the risk of TBE in humans is dependent on the frequency of exposure to bites by infected ticks, which is dependent on human behaviour and on various biotic and abiotic factors, including climate (Rizzoli et al., 2009). Starting in 1989, mean springtime temperatures increased across the Baltics; however, the change in TBE incidence among these counties was spatiotemporally heterogeneous and inconsistent with regional weather phenomena (Sumilo et al., 2007). Simultaneously, a decline of collective farming in the post-communism Baltic States conceivably induced successional growth that promoted landscape changes, altering the fauna associated with *I. ricinus* ticks. In addition, berry picking, mushroom gathering, and other socioeconomically related food-seeking activities placing individuals in more frequent contact with tick-infested habitats are believed to have increased during this same period, as a result of economic changes associated with the fall of the Soviet Union. In this context, short-term climate changes that provided optimal growing conditions for mushrooms and berries in Baltic forests may indeed have been a driver for risk, but only in direct association with human behaviors that resulted in increased exposure to tick-infested habitats (Figure A1-6) (Randolph, 2008; Randolph et al., 2010).

*Changes in Funding and Scientific Interest*

Scientific, medical, or veterinary interest in a particular pathogen, or changes in the epidemiologic programs or organizational frameworks used to survey for a particular disease, may have enormous impact on the recorded incidence. By example, only 27 cases of Powassan encephalitis were

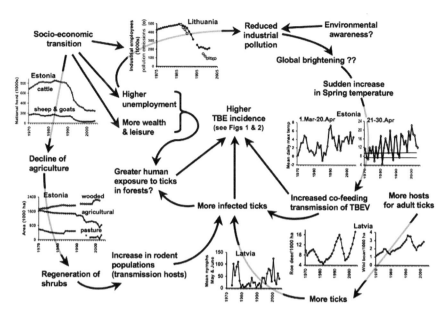

**FIGURE A1-6** Hypothetical explanation for the upsurge in cases of tick-borne encephalitis in Estonia, Latvia, and Lithuania, following the end of Soviet rule (Šumilo et al., 2007)

reported in North America during the 3 decades after its discovery in 1958; however, the introduction of West Nile virus to the continent in the late 1990s stimulated enhanced surveillance for arthropod-borne encephalitis by state and local health departments, and is believed to be the major factor in the recognition of 20 U.S. cases of this disease during 1999-2009, including identifications from 4 northeastern and upper Midwestern states that had never previously reported the disease (Hinten et al., 2008; Hoang Johnson et al., 2010).

Prior to the early 1980s, research in tick-borne infections focused largely on RMSF, TBE, and diseases associated directly with animal health, such as babesiosis and theileriosis. The emergence of Lyme disease in the northeastern United States during the late 1970s, particularly at sites where an affluent population lived or vacationed, stimulated a renaissance in tick biology and ecology that was driven, in part, by increased availability of state and federal funds for Lyme disease research. A single individual with interest in a specific disease, particularly one that is otherwise infrequently diagnosed and seldom reported, can have tremendous impact on the incidence of that disease. By example, no cases of MSF from Algeria were documented in the medical literature until 1 clinician identified 93 cases during a 4-month interval in 2004 (Mouffok et al., 2006). Austria and Slovenia have among the highest reported rates of Lyme disease in Europe, with an average annual incidence of 135 and 206 per 100,000 population, respectively (Smith and Takkinen, 2006); however, reporting in these countries is likely enhanced because of particularly energetic Lyme disease researchers who work in this region (Stanek and Strle, 2009). Conversely, it has been suggested that the precipitous drop in reported cases of RMSF witnessed in the United States during the 1950s might be attributable, in part, to the death in 1949 of R. R. Parker, who had been the driving force behind U.S. RMSF surveillance activities for more than 3 decades (Burgdorfer, 1975).

## Active and Passive Surveillance

In the United States, surveillance data for tick-borne diseases are acquired voluntarily through separate but complementary reporting instruments that collectively comprise a national system of passive surveillance. The National Electronic Disease Surveillance System (NEDSS), (formerly the National Electronic Telecommunications System for Surveillance [NETSS]) represents the primary reporting instrument. Incidence statistics for all U.S. tick-borne diseases are calculated from electronically reported data; however, these systems acquire relatively limited supplemental information, so that detailed clinical data must be gathered by using other collection instruments, including an extended NEDSS record for Lyme disease, and a standardized case report form (CRF) for RMSF, ehrlichiosis, and anaplasmosis. State or local health departments are responsible for ensuring that cases reported to CDC through NEDSS meet the case definition for these diseases, while CRF data are generally screened at CDC for accuracy and consistency. Understandably, compliance with requests to physicians and state and local health department staff to provide supplemental data is problematic. By example, only 61% of Lyme disease cases reported to CDC during 1992-2006 contained data for reported signs and symptoms (Bacon et al., 2008). During 2000-2007, the number of CRFs submitted for RMSF was approximately 68% of the 11,531 cases reported through NETSS (Openshaw et al., 2010). Submitted CRFs often lack requested information necessary to confirm the diagnosis approved by the Council of State and Territorial Epidemiologists (CSTE) and CDC. Indeed, only 6% of RMSF CRF cases could be classified as confirmed during 2000-2007 (Openshaw et al., 2010). The non-submission of CRFs and the incompleteness of supplementary data collection suggest that a considerable percentage of cases tick-borne disease in the United States are unavailable for detailed analyses, including analysis of risk factors that determine severity (Childs and Paddock, 2002).

*Case Definitions*

Establishing an accurate and specific case definition that couples well-defined clinical characteristics with specific laboratory confirmation is fundamentally important in all forms of surveillance and provides the foundation from which subsequent epidemiologic parameters are derived. The absence of standardized case definitions for tick-borne diseases that cross regional or national borders remains a crucial problem in the accumulation of broad scale incidence data for many of these infections. Despite a system of mandatory reporting for TBE in Poland since 1970, no standardized case classification for this disease existed until 2005, creating a mix of confirmed, probable, or possible cases that were defined by clinical or laboratory criteria that differed among the county's multiple provinces. When a national working group created a uniform case definition and retrospectively evaluated data from 1999-2002, they determined that only 25% of cases reported during this interval had sufficient laboratory testing to be classified as confirmed (Stefanoff et al., 2005).

Case definitions are not immutable, and as clinical knowledge about a particular disease expands and evolves, the case definition may be remodeled to include clinical or laboratory data specific to the disease. Because so many tick-borne infections are relatively new to science and medicine, it is not surprising that case definitions and surveillance systems for several of these diseases have required years or decades of refinement (Table A1-2). In this context, incidence statistics, particularly early in the evolution of these systems, should be interpreted cautiously, and comparisons of data from year-to-year, or even decade-to-decade, may be misleading. While passive surveillance requires a reasonably high level of stability to maintain its effectiveness, it must also remain malleable, and responsive to new information gained about a particular disease. By example, the nationally notifiable disease category of "Rocky Mountain spotted fever" was modified in 2010 to a less specific, but more inclusive and more accurate designation of "Spotted fever rickettsiosis, including Rocky Mountain spotted fever," to adjust to recent data identifying causes of spotted fever group rickettsioses in the United States other than *R. rickettsii* (Council of State and Territorial Epidemiologists, 2009a).

A well-crafted case definition provides more robust surveillance for the recognized disease and better positions investigators to detect clinically or epidemiologically similar diseases that otherwise might be embedded in data gathered by using a non-specific case definition. Erythema migrans rashes were noted on many patients in the southern and southcentral United States during the late 1980s (Masters et al., 1998), and in 1989, 715 cases of 'Lyme disease' were reported from Georgia (CDC, 1990), placing this state among the top 7 in the country for reporting Lyme disease. In the

**TABLE A1-2** Changes in Case Definitions of Selected Nationally Notifiable Tick-Borne Diseases in the United States, 1996-2008

| Disease (year of first case definition) | Year of change(s) in case definition | Change(s) | Reference |
|---|---|---|---|
| Lyme disease (1990) | 1996 | Recommendation of 2-tiered approach for serologic confirmation. | CDC, 1996a |
| | 2008 | Inclusion of western blot testing as a single confirmatory assay; addition of probable and suspect categories to case classification. | CDC, 2008a |
| Ehrlichiosis (1996) | 2000 | Inclusion of *Ehrlichia ewingii* as an agent of ehrlichiosis; distinction between laboratory assays for *Ehrlichia chaffeensis* and *Ehrlichia phagocytophila* (*Anaplasma phagocytophilum*); formation of new reporting category, ehrlichiosis/anaplasmosis, human, undetermined. | CDC, 2000 |
| | 2008 | Nomenclature change from human monocytic ehrlichiosis to *E. chaffeensis* infection; from ehrlichiosis (unspecified, or other agent) to *E. ewingii* infection; from human granulocytic ehrlichiosis to *Anaplasma phagocytophilum* infection; inclusion of ELISA format as laboratory criterion for diagnosis of probable infection. | CSTE, 2009a |
| Rocky Mountain spotted fever (1990) | 1996 | Inclusion of PCR testing for laboratory confirmation; single titer of greater than or equal to 64 defined as laboratory criterion for a probable case. | CDC, 1996b |
| | 2004 | Inclusion of ELISA format as laboratory criterion for diagnosis of confirmed or probable case; inclusion of immunohistochemical staining of tissue specimen as confirmatory laboratory criterion; cutoff titers used to determine probable cases defined by individual laboratories; elimination of *Proteus* OX-2 and OX-19 agglutinin titers as supportive laboratory criteria for a probable case. | CDC, 2004 |
| | 2008 | Confirmation by serologic testing defined as fourfold change in IgG antibody titer; single elevated IgG or IgM titer sufficient for a probable case; ELISA format sufficient only to determine probable cases; inclusion of suspect case classification. | CDC, 2008b |
| | 2010 | Change of disease category from "Rocky Mountain spotted fever" to "Spotted fever rickettsiosis"; inclusion of an eschar as clinical evidence of disease; requirement of PCR or cell culture isolation as laboratory confirmation of Rocky Mountain spotted fever. | CSTE, 2009b |

following year, however, only 161 cases were reported from Georgia (CDC, 1991), and even fewer cases in subsequent years. The decline in reported cases reflected the adoption of the CDC surveillance case definition in 1990 by the Georgia Department of Public Health. The abundance of cases reported during 1989 most likely reflected a Lyme disease mimic, associated with bites of lone star ticks, now recognized as Masters' disease, or southern tick-associated rash illness (Felz et al., 1999; Wormser et al., 2005).

In a similar scenario, investigators in southern Spain identified several patients with atypical 'Lyme borreliosis,' who were serologically reactive with *Borrelia burgdoreferi* antigens, but who lacked classical erythema migrans skin lesions and who originated from a region of the country where the recognized tick vector of Lyme borreliosis was distributed sparsely. Indeed, blood cultures subsequently revealed a relapsing fever *Borrelia* sp., genetically distinct from *B. burgdorferi* and transmitted by an entirely different tick species. In this case, discovery of a novel disease agent occurred because these patients did not meet the established case definition for Lyme borreliosis (Anda, et al., 1996; Guy, 1996). Recent discoveries of novel rickettsioses in the United States caused by *R. parkeri* and *Rickettsia* sp. 364D were precipitated by reports of atypical 'RMSF,' associated prominently with eschars, which are characteristically absent in the great majority of cases of classical RMSF (Paddock, 2008; Shapiro et al., 2010).

The efforts required to verify that reported data comply with an established case definition are considerable and are magnified further when clinical data and exposure history are uncoupled from laboratory results. Electronic laboratory reporting, used increasingly by states to expand case identification of Lyme disease, captures positive test results, but does not provide supportive information about clinical findings or exposure history. Instead, these data must be collected by public health personnel, creating added burden to surveillance endeavors that often exceeds investigative capacity (Kudish et al., 2007; CDC, 2008c). In response, CSTE Epidemiologists modified the national surveillance case definition for Lyme disease in 2007 to allow reporting of probable cases, i.e., those diagnosed by a health care provider and supported with laboratory evidence of infection (CDC, 2008a).

## Strengths and Limitations of Passive and Active Surveillance

The most accurate incidence rates are obtained through active surveillance, but these apply to relatively small catchment areas defined for the investigation, and typically provide a snapshot of incidence in a specified region during a relatively short interval of time. This process allows greater control in the selection of clinical specimens and data collected, but is labor-intensive and requires a level of funding that is prohibitive to sustain indefinitely. Indeed, most contemporary active surveillance endeavors are supported by federal grants and have a defined period of patient enrollment that spans, at most, only a few years (IJdo et al., 2000; Olano et al., 2003). In contrast, passive surveillance systems provide data that define endemicity and provide long-term trends over larger geographic regions; however, there is generally less control over the quality and quantity of the acquired data, and this activity requires sustained commitment and appropriate infrastructure at local, state, and national levels to collect, collate, and analyze data collected over broad intervals of time and space.

Inherent differences between these systems preclude direct comparisons of the data generated by each method. By example, prospective active surveillance for ehrlichiosis in southeast Missouri identified 29 confirmed and probable cases from 1997-1999, for a calculated average annual incidence of 3.2 cases per 100,000 population during this 3-year interval (Olano et al., 2003). By comparison, the average annual incidence of ehrlichiosis for the entire state of Missouri, determined by passive surveillance, was only 0.52 cases per 100,000 during 1997-2001 (Gardner et al., 2003), and 0.68 cases per 100,000 during 2001-2002 (Demma et al., 2005b). The nature of active and passive surveillance explains these marked differences in incidence rates. Catchment areas for active surveillance are not chosen at random; rather, these are selected by investigators using passive surveillance estimates that indicate the disease exists in relative abundance in that region (Wilfert et al., 1984; IJdo et al., 2000). In the case of the Missouri investigation, patient ascertainment was facilitated by a motivated clinician who was skilled at identifying potential cases of ehrlichiosis. Additionally, national surveillance for ehrlichiosis was initiated only in 1997, and several years of maturation may be required before passive surveillance systems reach a level of familiarity and frequent use by clinicians and epidemiologists.

Underreporting of true cases is a problem inherent to all passive surveillance systems and can be substantive: in the Marshfield Clinic Epidemiologic Research Study Area, only 34% of the identified Lyme disease cases were reported to the Wisconsin Department of Public Health during 1992-1998 (Naleway et al., 2002). Even for epidemiological statistics that document outcomes as important as death, there is considerable underreporting to public health authorities. From a capture-recapture study evaluating deaths caused by RMSF in the United States during 1983-1998, approximately 64% of fatal RMSF cases identified by death certificate data were not reported to state health departments or to CDC (Paddock et al., 2002)

Prospective cohort studies provide the best estimates of incidence but the resources that are needed to undertake such research preclude their use over larger scales. A good example of the value of a prospective study is that of the clinical trials for SmithKline Beecham's Lymerix Lyme disease vaccine during 1994-1998. Phase II dose-ranging studies were done during

1994-1995 in coastal New England with 353 enrolled subjects. A conservative case definition was adopted, with definite Lyme disease comprising compatible clinical manifestations and laboratory confirmation. Cases of suspected symptomatic Lyme disease comprised erythema migrans without laboratory confirmation and compatible clinical manifestations without other plausible explanation. Such active case finding demonstrated an incidence of 3.4% (95% CI, 1.2-9.5) for either confirmed or suspected Lyme disease among the placebo subjects. This study cost $250,000 (Telford et al., unpublished). Starting in 1995, 10,936 subjects were enrolled in a controlled, double-blind, multicenter Phase III trial in 31 sites in 10 northeastern and mid-Atlantic states from Maine to Maryland (Steere et al., 1998). In the placebo group, the incidence of Lyme disease was 1.5% (95% CI, 1.2-1.9) during the first year, and 2.0% (1.6-2.4) in the second year. Of particular interest were the percentages of asymptomatic seroconversion (16% and 14%, respectively) (Smith et al., 2002). This expensive (>$5,000,000) trial provided our best estimates for Lyme disease incidence, as well as data on the asymptomatic to symptomatic ratio, a critical statistic to help define burden of disease.

### Accuracy of Surveillance Data

Underreporting is invariably cited as a limitation to surveillance activities, but over-reporting may be even more damaging to epidemiologic assessments. One of the greatest obstacles to surveillance is ensuring that the data collected represent the disease under consideration. Blended data arise when a single common diagnosis is used to identify multiple related diseases caused by distinct pathogens. This process ultimately creates epidemiological havoc by producing incorrect distributions, hospitalization rates, and case-fatality rates, based erroneously on amalgamated characteristics of several individual diseases.

Most diagnoses of tick-borne infections are diagnosed, and subsequently categorized as 'confirmed cases' for epidemiologic analyses, by detecting antibodies in the serum of patients in whom the disease was suspected. Unfortunately, the antibodies generated by humans to specific pathogens often react with other closely related agents that are similar antigenically, but may cause illnesses that differ considerably in disease severity and clinical outcome. Overreliance on serologic methods is also the basis for many non-confirmed cases of tick-borne diseases. It has been demonstrated repeatedly that antibody responses for many of these diseases, including ehrlichiosis and RMSF, often require 7-10 days before a diagnostic titer is detected. Most patients may appear for care during the first few days of the illness, and may never return for subsequent evaluation. From 1 study, approximately two-thirds of culture-confirmed patients infected with

*E. chaffeensis* lacked diagnostic IgG titers, as measured by IFA, when they initially presented for care (Childs et al., 1999). Because diagnostic levels of IgG and IgM antibodies are frequently absent from the serum of patients who die from RMSF, fatal cases of this disease are often not confirmed if appropriate samples are not collected for immunohistochemical, molecular, or culture-based diagnotics (Paddock et al., 1999).

Diagnostically relevant levels of antibodies reactive with *R. rickettsii* have been detected in approximately 5%-10% of the U.S. population (Wilfert et al., 1985; Graf et al., 2008; Marshall et al., 2003; Taylor et al., 1985; Hilton et al., 1999). Even more troubling are the frequent descriptions of seroconversions to spotted fever group (SFG) *Rickettsia* and *Ehrlichia* spp. antigens that occur among as many as a 33% of healthy asymptomatic individuals following exposure to tick bites and tick-infected habitats. (Sanchez et al., 1992; Yevich et al., 1995; Hilton et al., 1999; McCall et al., 2001). Nonetheless, serology is used increasingly to diagnose cases of RMSF; as a result, fewer cases are confirmed and a far greater percentage of cases are considered probable (Figure A1-7). The impact of diagnostic inaccuracy upon epidemiologic observations may be considerable. During 2000-2007, the reported case fatality rate for RMSF in the United States was 0.5%, based on CRF denominator data comprising 7,796 cases, or approximately 1000 cases each year (Openshaw, 2010). The validity of this statistic is unreasonable when considered with historical U.S. case-fatality rates of RMSF that typically approach 10%. One explanation

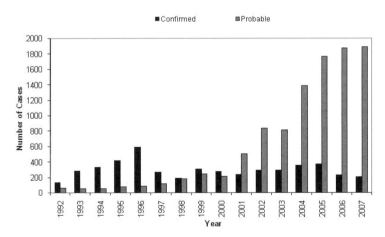

**FIGURE A1-7** Reported cases of Rocky Mountain spotted fever in the United States, by case classification status, 1992-2007 (Openshaw et al., 2010).

for this estimate lies in the composition of the denominator, which is likely populated with patients with milder infections, caused by SFG *Rickettsia* species other than *Rickettsia rickettsii* (Paddock, 2009).

Under some circumstances, serological methods may produce results that divert attention from the true arthropod vector, creating a false portrait of the disease ecology. In this situation, a 'tick-borne' disease may in fact be something altogether different. By example, patients infected with *Rickettsia felis*, a flea-borne pathogen, generate antibodies that react with various SFG Rickettsia species. Because R. *felis* has a cosmopolitan distribution and commonly infects multiple species of wild and commensal human-biting fleas, (Reif and Macaluso, 2009), the potential for human infections is enormous. Recent studies in Kenya and Senegal revealed a prevalence of infection with R. *felis* in approximately 4% of 297 febrile patients from rural areas of these countries; only 1 patient from either series was infected with a tick-borne *Rickettsia* sp. (Socolovschi et al., 2010; Richards et al., 2010). To place these results in context, it is important to recognize that at least 7 pathogenic, tick-borne SFG *Rickettsia* species have been detected in ticks or human patients from the immense and ecologically diverse continent of Africa (Cazorla et al., 2008). If these researchers had not used molecular techniques to correctly identify R. *felis* as the causative agent, and relied only on serologic methods (as many investigators have done for >50 years), the etiology of the disease in these patients could have been ascribed erroneously to any of multiple tick-borne SFG rickettsial pathogens endemic to this continent. Broader use of similar techniques around the world might change considerably existing notions about the ecology, epidemiology, and clinical presentations of tick-borne rickettsioses.

### Network Approaches for Detecting Shifts in Incidence and Disease Severity: Challenges, Prospects, and New Rubrics for Surveillance

Any form of surveillance requires sustained and coordinated efforts to provide meaningful data. As with all regional and national services, these programs require continuous funding and prospective governmental commitment, based on public health priorities defined by that state or country. Coordinated national efforts that track these diseases are notably absent in many developed countries. In Germany, an estimated 60,000 new cases of Lyme borreliosis occur each year; however, Lyme borreliosis is not a nationally notifiable disease in this country and precise incidence data do not exist (Mehnert and Krause, 2005). Many countries with active, internationally recognized research programs in rickettsioses, including Australia and France, lack formal national surveillance for tick-borne rickettsioses (Stephen Graves and Philippe Parola, pers. comms). Even in countries where national surveillance exists for one or more of these diseases, the systems are often porous or lack the discriminatory power needed to epidemiologically characterize individual infections. In Italy, tick-borne rickettsioses are lumped in the general category of "rickettsiosis," without respect to specific disease or arthropod vector species (Ciceroni et al., 2006). In Norway, only cases of disseminated or chronic Lyme borreliosis are notifiable to the Norwegian Institute of Public Health; the majority of infections, represented by erythema migrans, are not tabulated (Nygård et al., 2005).

Not surprisingly, tick-borne diseases are seldom included as nationally notifiable conditions in developing countries with considerable and diverse infectious disease burdens. In the southern Indian state of Karnataka, approximately 400-900 cases of KFD were reported annually during 2001-2004 (Pattnaik, 2006); however, the lack of national surveillance for this potentially lethal hemorrhagic fever has contributed to a belief that this disease is confined to a few small districts of a single state in this vast country. This seems highly improbable, considering that the virus as been isolated from or transmitted experimentally by at least 16 species of hard and soft ticks (Boshell, 1969; Pattnaik, 2006), and strains of the flavivirus responsible for the disease have been isolated from patients as far away as Saudi Arabia and Egypt (Mehla et al., 2009; Carletti et al., 2010), suggesting that variants of KFD might be found in other parts of India or other countries.

*Expanding and Unifying Epidemiologic Coverage*

More countries need to adopt national surveillance for tick-borne infections, and work to better harmonize and coordinate case definitions of diseases that cross national borders. Meaningful comparisons of incidence across broad geographical expanses are compromised when a melange of independent and varied case definitions exist for the same disease. Currently there are no standardized case definitions for CCHF notification or contact tracing in European countries, despite a vector tick (*Hyalomma marginatum*) that is distributed broadly across southern and southeastern Europe, and epidemic disease occurring in neighboring parts of Turkey (Figure A1-8), and in several Territories and Republics of the Russian Federation (Maltezou et al., 2010). From a recent survey of 21 European countries that compared national surveillance efforts for TBE, it was determined that case definitions differed widely across these countries, and for 6 countries where the disease is endemic, there was no officially or clearly formulated case definition (Mantke et al., 2008).

The European Union Concerted Action on Lyme Borreliosis (EUCALB) was established in 1997 to provide information on all aspects of Lyme disease, obtained from peer-reviewed literature and edited by a committee of experienced researchers and clinicians. Despite the intent to provide

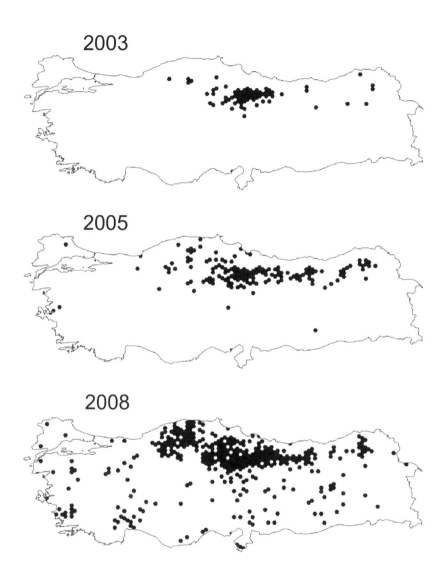

**FIGURE A1-8** Spatial distribution of reported cases of Crimean-Congo hemorrhagic fever in Turkey, 2003-2008 (Estrada-Peña et al., 2010).

guidance for obtaining and disseminating the highest standard of information, EUCALB has not been able to standardize surveillance across
the European Union, and the compilation of European Union case definitions (http://eur-lex.europa.eu/LexUriServ/LexUriServ.do?uri=OJ:L:2008
:159:0046:0090:EN:PDF) does not have an entry for Lyme borreliosis.
Few European countries have made Lyme disease a compulsorily notifiable condition. Estimates of incidence for this and other tick-borne
diseases in many countries are derived from laboratory-based reporting
which typically lacks sufficient clinical information to integrate into a
robust case definition. Accordingly, many of the same problems for Lyme
disease surveillance in the United States are also seen for the European
Union as a whole and for most of the member states.

*Applying Species-Specific Diagnostics*

Robust and predictive epidemiology is predicated on the use of sensitive
and specific diagnostic assays. Currently, molecular techniques represent
the most widely available standard for species-specific diagnosis. Whenever possible, culture isolation, the microbiological reference standard of
diagnosis, should also be attempted to compliment molecular assays. Repeatedly, these methods have leveraged the discovery of novel tick-borne
infections and clarified long-standing epidemiologic concerns regarding
atypical clinical manifestations, unusual geographic distributions, or exag-
gerated or diminished severity of diseases that were incorrectly diagnosed.
Diligent use of molecular and culture-based diagnostics during a study of
140 Portuguese patients with MSF enabled investigators to identify specifically a strain of *R. conorii* that was more frequently associated with severe
disease in this patient population (de Sousa et al., 2008). The case-fatality
rate in this series, determined by using accurate and specific diagnostic assays, was 21%, more than 8 times greater than the previously recognized
lethality of this disease (Parola et al., 2005). Molecular techniques were
used recently to identify infections with *E. ewingii* and *E. chaffeensis* in
dogs and *R. sanguineus* ticks in Cameroon (Ndip et al., 2005: Ndip et al.,
2010). These findings provided impetus to search for cases of ehrlichiosis
in humans; surprisingly, 12 (10%) of 118 Cameroonian patients with undifferentiated febrile illnesses in whom malaria and typhoid were excluded
showed PCR evidence of infection with *E. chaffeensis* (Ndip et al., 2009).

In Missouri, investigators used molecular methods to discriminate infections caused by *E. ewingii* from those caused by *E. chaffeensis* (Buller
et al., 1999). Their discovery unveiled a second, clinically and ecologically
similar illness, the identity of which was previously obscured because of
sufficient overlap of disease manifestations and a shared tick vector. Indeed,
surveys examining the relative prevalence of *Ehrlichia* spp. in reservoir

hosts and lone star ticks in the United States suggest that *E. ewingii* occurs in these species at frequencies similar to, or in some cases greater than, infection with *E. chaffeensis* (Paddock et al., 2005). However, *E. ewingii* appears to cause a milder illness, and most commonly causes disease in immunosuppressed patients. Without molecular methods, these infections would have remained submerged among those caused by *E. chaffeensis*, contributing to a falsely heterogeneous portrait of *E. chaffeensis* ehrlichiosis. More recently, an *Ehrlichia muris*-like agent, identified by molecular methods from the blood of 4 patients in Minnesota and Wisconsin, is likely responsible for many other serologically diagnosed cases of ehrlichiosis in the upper Midwestern United States, where neither *E. chaffeensis* nor *E. ewingii* are endemic (McFadden et al., 2010).

Repeatedly, patients with antibodies reactive to multiple SFG *Rickettsia* spp. are found ultimately to be infected with unexpected agents when PCR and cell culture methods are used. In these circumstances, the diagnosis sheds light on clinical or epidemiologic characteristics not conventionally associated with the presumed pathogen, including occurrence of disease in a different geographical region, greater or lesser severity of illness, or presence or absence of prominent cutaneous manifestations. Just a few of the recent discoveries that exemplify the utility of these assays include *Rickettsia heilongjiangensis* in Japan, *R. parkeri* in the southeastern United States, *Rickettsia* sp. 364D in California, *Rickettsia massiliae* in Argentina, and *Rickettsia sibirica mongolotimonae* in southern France (Raoult et al., 1996; Paddock, 2009; Shapiro et al., 2010; Ando et al., 2010; Garciá-Garciá et al., 2010). Each of these diagnoses provides a foundation to explain more accurately the epidemiology of the historically recognized SFG rickettsioses for which these were initially confused.

### Improved Integration of Entomologic and Veterinary Sciences

For decades, epidemiologists have integrated surveillance of non-human sources, such as mosquitoes, birds, and domesticated animals, in the detection of arboviruses. Similar efforts must be considered with tick-borne infections. Entomologic expertise ensures correct species identification of tick vectors, defines appropriate ecologic associations, and most importantly, provides data otherwise missing that establish the zoonotic bridge and better define incidence.

### Epidemiological Entomology

Robust programs in medical entomology at state and national levels are essential to predict and respond to issues relating to tick-borne infections. In 2003, investigators in Mexicali, Mexico, conducted an entomologic survey to determine the prevalence of *R. sanguineus* among 94 stray and privately owned dogs in the city, and determined that 60% of these animals were infested with *R. sanguineus*, a prevalence far greater than reported in other areas of Mexico and other parts of the world (Tinoco-Gracia et al., 2009). In retrospect, these results served as a tocsin to an epidemic of RMSF that occurred in Mexicali and other areas of Baja California during 2009, resulting in 275 confirmed and 734 probable infections (Bustamente Moreno and Pon Méndez, 2010a). In 2009, surveys for *R. sanguineus* identified these ticks in all 14 districts of Mexicali, where 96% of the cases occurred (Sanchez et al., 2009; Bustamente Moreno and Pon Méndez, 2010b). A survey for ticks on dogs from a small community in São Paulo, Brazil, in 2005, identified *R. sanguineus*-infested animals at approximately one-third of the households, including specimens infected with *R. rickettsii*. A canine serosurvey conducted in the same community one year later revealed that 70% of the sampled dogs showed high levels of antibodies reactive with *R. rickettsii*, and that human cases were also occurring (Morares-Filho et al., 2008).

Even in the absence of accurate incidence data, entomologic studies can provide objective and quantifiable data to reconcile a real or perceived public health burden. By example, a coastal Maryland community determined by questionnaire that Lyme disease afflicted more than 15% of their residents each year, creating apprehension among residents and local public health officials. Entomologic surveillance, in conjunction with a cross-sectional epidemiologic study, provided objective evidence that Lyme disease was actually rare, and disproportional to the perceived risk. In fact, the community did not know that it was plagued by an infestation of *A. americanum* ticks, that accounted for >90% of all ticks saved by residents, and the majority of ticks collected from vegetation (Armstrong et al., 2001).

Tick-borne infections may be thought of as guilds, or a group of species, not necessarily related, that utilize a common resource. The best example of a tick microbial guild may be found within deer ticks, comprising *B. burgdorferi*, *Babesia microti*, *A. phagocytophilum*, and deer tick virus (Telford et al. 1997). Globally, wherever there are related ticks from the *Ixodes persulcatus* complex, Lyme disease spirochetes, babesiae, *Anaplasma* sp., and a TBE- group virus may be found. Indeed, detecting one member of the guild is cause for search for all of the others (Telford and Goethert, 2008). Because concurrent or sequential infection with more than one agent is not infrequent (Krause et al., 1996) the guild model has epidemiologic implications. Accordingly, when a patient is diagnosed with Lyme disease, evidence of babesiosis and anaplasmosis should also be sought. When Nantucket Cottage Hospital started using a clinical laboratory that automatically tested for direct molecular evidence of infection with *B. burgdorferi*, *B. microti*, and *A. phagocytophilum* of all patients with a suspected tick-borne illness, the number of confirmed cases of babesiosis and anaplasmosis immediately doubled (T. J. Lepore, pers. comm.).

Natural cycles of known pathogens do not necessarily imply a zoonotic risk to humans. By example, *Ixodes dentatus* feeds primarily on rabbits, and only rarely bites humans, yet maintains a diverse guild of pathogens and potential pathogens comprising *Borrelia andersoni*, *B. microti*, a *Babesia divergens*-like parasite, *A. phagocytophilum*, *Anaplasma bovis*, and a Kemerovo-group orbivirus in northeastern U.S. sites (Telford and Spielman 1989; Goethert and Telford, 2003 a, b, c). However, this guild has minimal epidemiological importance, even when sympatric with human-biting deer ticks, because deer ticks rarely feed on rabbits. Ticks, similar to all multicellular organisms, harbor a diverse array of microbes, and novel high-throughput DNA amplification and sequencing techniques are unveiling the complex microbiome of ticks (Benson et al., 2004; Clay et al., 2008); however, and public health relevance of an agent detected in a tick should never be assumed a priori.

Currently applied entomological risk indices include only the prevalence of infection in host-seeking ticks and the number of ticks collected in an hour (Piesman et al., 1987). However, an epidemiologically predictive risk index will require information on the species of ticks infesting humans, how frequently these attach, and the actual duration of attachment. Although *B. burgdorferi* typically infects 20% of host-seeking nymphal deer ticks in northeastern United States, the median annual incidence of Lyme disease from 9 prospective studies in the most intensely enzootic communities is only 2% (range, 0.4%-4.0%) (Hanrahan et al., 1984; Steere et al., 1986; Lastavica et al., 1989; Alpert et al., 1992; Shapiro et al., 1992; Krause and Telford, unpublished; Wormser et al., 1998; Steere et al., 1998; Sigal et al., 1998). In addition, fewer than 10% of all Lyme disease cases in the northeastern United States are reported during the fall or winter months when adult deer ticks are most active, even though as many as 50%-75% of host-seeking adult ticks contain spirochetes (Piesman et al., 1986). These apparent paradoxes can be answered by entomology: most tick-borne bacterial pathogens require a period of 'reactivation' before they attain infectivity (Spencer and Parker, 1923; Piesman et al. 1987; Katavolos et al., 1997). The probability of infection is directly proportional to the duration of feeding and may differ by life stage of the tick, so that 24-48 hours of attachment are generally required for *B. burgdorferi* to be transmitted by nymphal deer ticks; in contrast, adult deer ticks require approximately 3-5 days of attachment to transmit *B. burgdorferi* to a susceptible host (Telford, unpublished).

*Sentinel Species for Tick-Borne Disease*

Despite repeated successes using wildlife and domesticated animals as sentinel species for tick-borne infections, these resources remains under-utilized in formal surveillance programs around the world. Because domestic dogs are frequently parasitized by human-biting ticks, develop robust antibody titers to most agents, are closely associated with human habitation, and are easily sampled, these animals represent exceptional sentinel species for tick-borne pathogens. This technique has been used effectively to predict or corroborate the occurrence, or in some cases, relative absence, of disease burden in human populations, including spotted fever group rickettsiosis in southeastern Australia (Sexton et al., 1991), and Lyme disease and anaplasmosis in the United States (Guerra et al., 2001; Hinrichsen et al., 2001; Duncan et al., 2004; Bowman et al., 2009).

With respect to infections caused by SFG rickettsiae, canine antibodies typically show greater specificity to the infecting agent than to other, antigenically related *Rickettsia* spp. (Nicholson et al., 2006; Demma et al., 2006; Piranda et al., 2008), and may provide greater accuracy than results of human antibody assessments in serologic surveys. Retrospective analysis of 329 archival canine serum specimens, collected from dogs in a community in the White Mountain region of eastern Arizona during 1996, revealed epidemiologically relevant titers of antibodies reactive with *R. rickettsii* in only 2 (0.6%). When dogs were tested 7 years later, following recognition of an RMSF epidemic in this community, 70 (72%) of 97 animals demonstrated epidemiologically relevant antibody titers, and the geometric mean titer was > 84 times higher than observed in 1996 (Demma et al., 2006). Of even greater interest, high antibody titers were also detected in 8 (57%) of 14 dogs sampled at a second community, 60 miles distant, where no cases of RMSF had been reported; however, the following year, an outbreak of RMSF occurred in the second community, involving 9 residents and causing 2 deaths. This approach was later applied to serosurvey of dogs in counties adjacent to the outbreak communities, where approximately 6% of animals demonstrated antibodies to *R. rickettsii*, primarily among *R. sanguineus*-infected dogs, suggesting future cases of human disease outside of the recognized boundaries established during the initial outbreak (McQuiston et al., 2009).

Because white-tailed deer are important hosts for several species of ticks that transmit infectious agents to humans, these animals have been used effectively in the United States as sentinels for multiple tick-borne infections, including *E. chaffeensis* ehrlichiosis and Lyme disease. Among the advantages cited for this species include an extensive and inclusive distribution throughout the range of these diseases, the relatively sedentary nature of deer, rates of exposure to ticks that far exceed those of human exposures, and regulated harvests in all states that facilitates collection of samples from hunter-killed animals (Yabsley et al., 2003; Gill et al., 1994).

*Prospecting Other Databases*

Tick-borne infections can mimic many other infectious diseases, including meningococcemia, leptospirosis, hantavirus pulmonary syndrome, dengue, and malaria. Recent investigations in Senegal and Togo suggest that tick-borne relapsing fever may be a common cause of fever in many parts of West Africa; however, the diagnosis is seldom considered, because many cases are misdiagnosed with malaria. Indeed, several studies have identified infections with *Borrelia* spp. in as many as 10% of febrile patients (Vial et al., 2006; Nordstrand et al., 2007).

From a 1993 study of dengue fever in Yucatan and Jalisco states of Mexico, 50 patients with a recent compatible illness had no serologic evidence of infection with dengue virus. Of these, 20 had high levels of antibody reactive to SFG rickettsiae (Zavala-Velazquez et al., 1996). A similar approach was used for a study in Colombia, when 158 serum samples collected from febrile patients during 2000-2004 as part of national or regional surveillance for malaria, dengue, or yellow fever were evaluated for SFG rickettsiae and 21% showed antibodies suggesting recent infection with a Rickettsia species (Hildago et al., 2007).

Evaluations of databases comprising those patients negative for a particular tick-borne disease of interest may be especially fruitful, as many of these patients have been bitten by ticks, reside in tick-infested areas, or present during periods of peak tick activity. From a study conducted by investigators at CDC, paired serum samples collected from 3 (10%) of 29 patients for whom RMSF was suspected, but subsequently showed no serologic evidence of acute disease, were determined retrospectively to have seroconversions to *Ehrlichia* antigens, and corroborative clinical evidence of ehrlichiosis (Fishbein et al., 1987). A novel bunyavirus, transmitted by Haemaphysalis longicornis ticks, was recently identified as the cause of a life-threatening disease (severe fever with thrombocytopenia syndrome), confirmed in 171 patients from six provinces in Central and Northeast China. Clinical similarities with human anaplasmosis, and an asssociation with tick bites, focused initial investigations on A. phagocytophilum as the suspect pathogen; however, when molecular and serologic assays failed to identify this agent with the outbreak, culture of clinical specimens in multiple permissive cell lines, eventually yielded isolates of a previously undescribed phlebovirus (Yu et al., 2011).

Every year, spider bite statistics are collected by poison control centers across the United States; however, the accuracy of these data have been questioned by prominent arachnologists, who argue that hundreds of reports of necrotic arachnidism attributed to the brown recluse spider (*Loxosceles reclusa*) originate from areas where these spiders are absent (Vetter and Furbee, 2006), including much of Georgia, Florida, and South Carolina (Vetter et al., 2004; Vetter et al. 2009). Because necrotic arachnidism is occasionally considered by physicians as a diagnosis for patients with eschar-associated rickettsioses (Paddock et al., 2008) and Lyme disease (Rosenstein and Kramer, 1987; Osteroudt et al., 2002), closer inspection of these databases could uncover many previously undiagnosed and uncounted cases of tick-borne disease. This approach could also yield interesting results in other parts of the world, including Australia and Brazil, where necrotic skin lesions are also often attributed to bites from spiders that do not exist in the reporting area (Ibister, 2004).

*Extracting New Data from Existing Surveillance Systems*

Increasingly, physicians and scientists are identifying specific genetic characteristics and co-morbid or infectious conditions in patients that predispose these individuals to particularly severe forms of certain tick-borne infection. These include life-threatening disease in HIV-infected patients who become co-infected with *E. chaffeensis*, fulminant *R. rickettsii* and *R. conorii* infections in patients with glucose-6-phosphate dehydrogenase deficiency, fatal MSF in alcoholics, and increased severity of TBE in patients with a specific deletion in the chemokine receptor CCR5 (Walker et al., 1983; Raoult et al., 1986; Paddock et al., 2001; Kindberg et al., 2008; de Sousa et al., 2008). These observations have been identified in relatively small cohorts of patients who have been evaluated by relatively few clinicians who become cognizant of a specific characteristic that places these patients at increased risk for more severe infection; to identify similar characteristics among the total number of counted cases in a state or country poses a great challenge for future surveillance efforts (Childs and Paddock, 2002).

Age-specific incidence data gained from the first several years of national surveillance (Demma et al., 2005b; CDC, unpublished data) for ehrlichiosis and anaplasmosis show a striking age-related increase in frequency of these infections among older persons (Figure A1-9). One plausible hypothesis for this observation suggests that cholesterol dependence by *E. chaffeensis* and *A. phagocytophilum* may correlate with greater disease severity in older patients, because cholesterol levels typically rise with increasing age, and these bacteria lack all of the genes necessary for the biosynthesis of lipid A (Lin and Rikihisa, 2003). A direct association between cholesterol levels and the clinical severity of other forms of gram-negative sepsis add support to this hypothesis (Ayyadurai et al., 2010); in this context, serum cholesterol levels, collected as supplemental data on CRFs, could ultimately provide important clues to the pathogenesis of these diseases.

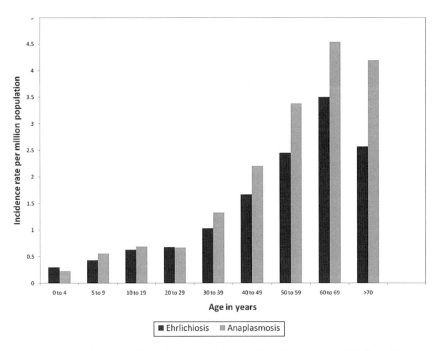

**FIGURE A1-9** Age-specific incidence of human ehrlichiosis (n = 3,104) and human anaplasmosis (n = 4,134) in the United States, 2000-2007 (Dahlgren et al., in press).

## In Silico Analytic Methods

Molecular phylogenetic tools have refined our understanding of the etiology of tick-borne infections. Advances in data analysis, made possible by tremendous computing power, should provide similar refinement of our understanding of transmission dynamics and environmental correlates of risk. Predictive models for guiding intervention and proactively studying new zoonotic sites are currently untenable. Validation of these models would require incidence data at the same scale as that for enzootic parameters; it is not axiomatic that the case counts for an entire state would be predicted by regressors, such as an entomological risk index, estimated from solely one town in that state. Although some analyses demonstrate correlations between measured tick density and Lyme disease case reports (Stafford et al., 1998; Mather et al., 1996), a priori predictions are not currently possible.

Vector-borne infections are complex to model. Sir Ronald Ross initiated mathematical modeling for malaria risk in 1909, but it was not until coordinated efforts in the 1950s (MacDonald, 1957) promoted enough quantitative understanding of malaria epidemiology that the effects of interventions such as vaccination could be predicted (Molineaux, 1985). In this respect, considerably more attention needs to be directed toward studies that provide data for quantitative models of tick-borne diseases. These efforts could also help develop testable hypotheses on critical aspects of tick life cycles or pathogen transmission cycles. Given the difficulty of finding study sites for longitudinal ecology study of *R. rickettsii*, for example, the role of transovarial transmission in perpetuating this agent in nature could be explored by modeling (Telford, 2009).

Great advances in remote sensing of environmental parameters and data analysis algorithms such as Geographic Information Systems (GIS) may allow prediction of the distribution of infection, or even incidence. However, given the extremely focal nature of transmission for most tick-borne infections, the utility of GIS would be a function of the scale of the analyses, which would depend on the availability of satellite data of a useful scale. For GIS analyses, as with mathematical models, the bridge from nature to human risk requires the filter of human behaviors; in the absence of this filter, associations of environmental variables with incidence data, even when available at the correct scale and duration, are less robust. In this context, GIS analyses are potentially powerful tools, whose practical utility are currently limited by our understanding of the basis for and measurement of human risk.

## Summary and Perspective

Tick-borne diseases are the Cinderella of vector-borne disease (VBD) systems: always beautiful, but for so long over-shadowed by the big ugly sisters of insect-borne malaria, trypanosomiasis, dengue, etc. In traditional happy-ending style, they are now emerging as the princess of VBDs, their full significance appreciated: as important in temperate as tropical regions, as much a veterinary as a medical problem to fit neatly into the 'one world, one health' maxim, and with an exquisite complexity to keep many a scientist fully occupied over a lifetime.

S. E. Randolph, 2009b

Predicting the future is an imprecise science; nonetheless, a clear association exists between human disturbance of natural habitats and the emergence and expansion of tick-borne diseases, and it is precisely this link that portends important increases in the scope and range of these zoonoses in the years to come. Remarkable scientific and medical discoveries during the last several decades have expanded considerably the known spectrum of tick-borne infections. Fundamental surveillance efforts for these infections, curiously, have not made similar strides. There are many practical reasons to explain the paucity of effective surveillance systems for tick-borne diseases around the world, including perceived need, long-term interest, and monetary commitments necessary to sustain these programs. These factors affect the longevity necessary for fine-tuning of case definitions and collection instruments, and ultimately, meaningful interpretations of the collected data; however, as more unique pathogens are identified, distinctions among the diseases caused by these agents may become increasingly subtle. In the end, the effort required to discover a new disease is generally far less than the subsequent endeavors required to establish and maintain long-lasting and accurate surveillance for that disease.

The measurement of incidence is important because it can be used to quantify and rank the causes of ill health so that scarce resources may be allocated. Incidence is critical to refine and validate predictive or explanatory models, which help develop new testable hypotheses or identify critical breakpoints. Changes in incidence may point to fundamental alterations of ecology or human behavior. Measuring incidence accurately, however, can be prohibitively expensive, as seen with the Lymerix Phase III trials. Indeed, surveillance will become increasingly important in the places that have the least existent infrastructure and the fewest resources to devote to establishing such programs. In Africa, scientific and medical concerns for tick-borne diseases are vastly overshadowed by other arthropod-borne infections; nonetheless, the unrecognized burden of these infections could be considerable. By example, the incidence of tick-borne relapsing fever in Senegal has been estimated at 5.1% (Trape et al., 1996), and the spread of infections with *Ehrlichia* spp. among an expanding and highly vulnerable HIV-infected cohort on this continent could have devastating consequences (Ndip et al., 2009).

Our challenge is to improve the measurement of incidence within the limits of available resources and capacities. With technological advances, global disparities in the capacity to collect this information may lessen; today, even the poorest countries are rapidly gaining access to thermal cyclers and the Internet, and the coverage of such critical technology will only increase. In the interim, our use of the currently available data—a dark glass—can be enhanced if we understand its limitations and frame our interpretations accordingly.

*Acknowledgments*

We thank the following individuals who generously provided data and input to this work: Marcelo Labruna (Cidade Universitária São Paulo, São Paulo, Brazil); Elba de Lemos (Instituto Oswaldo Cruz, Rio de Janeiro, Brazil); Rita de Sousa (Instituto Nacional de Saúde Dr Ricardo Jorge, Lisboa, Portugal); José Oteo (Hospital San Pedro, Logroño, Spain); Shuji

Ando (National Institute of Infectious Diseases, Tokyo, Japan); Agustín Estrada-Pena (University of Zaragoza, Zaragoza, Spain); Claudia Colomba (Universita di Palermo, Palermo, Italy); Philippe Parola (Université de la Mediterannée, Marseille, France); Robert Swanepoel (National Institute for Communicable Diseases, Sandringham, South Africa); Stephen Graves (Hunter Area Pathology Service, New South Wales, Australia); Scott O'Dee and Richard Gary (Zoonotic Disease Program, Ohio Department of Health), and; Scott Dahlgren and Robert Holman (Division of High Consequence Pathogens and Pathology, CDC). We are indebted to Paul Mead and Jennifer McQuiston (Division of Vector-borne Diseases, CDC) for their thoughtful review and invaluable comments to the manuscript. SRT is supported by NIH R01 AI 064218.

# References

Alpert, B., J. Esin, S. L. Sivak, and G. P. Wormser. 1992. Incidence and prevalence of Lyme disease in a suburban Westchester County community. *New York State Journal of Medicine* 92: 5-8.

Anda, P., W. Sánchez-Yebra, M. del Mar Vitutia, et al. 1996. A new *Borrelia* species isolated from patients with relapsing fever in Spain. *Lancet* 348: 162-141.

Ando, S., M. Kurosawa, A. Sakata, et al. 2010. Human *Rickettsia heilongjiangensis* infection, Japan. *Emerging Infectious Diseases* 16: 1306-1308.

Angerami, R. N., M. R. Resende, A. F. C. Feltran, et al. 2006. Brazilian spotted fever: a case series from an endemic area in southeastern Brazil. Epidemiologic aspects. *Annals of the New York Academy of Sciences* 1078: 170-172.

Anonymous. 1994. Leishmaniasis. *Pan American Health Organization Epidemiological Bulletin* 15: 8-11.

Anonymous. 1999. Japanese spotted fever. *Infectious Agents Surveillance Report* 20: 211-212.

Anonymous. 2006. Scrub typhus and Japanese spotted fever in Japan, as of December 2005. *Infectious Agents Surveillance Report* 27: 27-29.

Anonymous. 2010. Scrub typhus and Japanese spotted fever in Japan 2006-2009. *Infectious Agents Surveillance Report* 31: 120-122.

Anthony, J. A., J. E. Childs, G. E. Glass, G. W. Korch, L. Ross, and J. K. Grigor. 1990. Land use associations and changes in population indices of urban raccoons during a rabies epizootic. *Journal of Wildlife Diseases* 26: 170-179.

Armstrong, P. M., L. R. Brunet, A. Spielman, and S.R. Telford III. 2001. Risk of Lyme disease: perceptions of residents of a lone star tick-infected community. *Bulletin of the World Health Organization* 79: 916-925.

Ayyadurai, S., H. Lepidi, C. Nappez, D. Raoult, and M. Drancourt. 2010. Lovastatin protects against experimental plague in mice. *PLoS One* 5: e10926.

Bacon, R. M., K. J. Kugler, and P. S. Mead. 2008. Surveillance for Lyme disease—United States, 1992-2006. *MMWR* 57(No. SS-10): 1-9.

Battaly, G. R. and D. Fish. 1993. Relative importance of bird species as hosts for immature Ixodes dammini (Acari: Ixodidae) in a suburban residential landscape of southern New York. *Journal of Medical Entomology* 30: 740-747.

Benson, M. J., J. D. Gawronski, D. E. Eveleigh, and D. R. Benson. 2004. Intracellular symbionts and other bacteria associated with deer ticks (*Ixodes scapularis*) from Nantucket and Wellfleet, Cape Cod, Massachusetts. *Applied and Environmental Microbiology* 70: 616-620.

Boshell, J. M. 1969. Kyasanur forest disease: ecologic considerations. *American Journal of Tropical Medicine and Hygiene* 18: 67-80.

Bowman, D., S. E. Little, L. Lorentzen, J. Shields, M. P. Sullivan, and E. P. Carlin. 2009. Prevalence and geographic distribution of *Dirofilaria immitis, Borrelia burgdorferi, Ehrlichia canis*, and *Anaplasma phagocytophilum* in dogs in the United States: results of a national clinic-based serologic survey. *Veterinary Parasitology* 160: 138-148.

Buller, R. S., M. Arens, S. P. Himmel, et al. 1999. *Ehrlichia ewingii*, a newly recognized agent of human ehrlichiosis. *New England Journal of Medicine* 341: 148-155.

Burgdorfer, W. 1975. A review of Rocky Mountain spotted fever (tick-borne typhus), its agent, and its tick vectors in the United States. *Journal of Medical Entomology* 12: 269-278.

Bustamente, M. E., and G. Varela. 1947. IV. Estudios de fiebre manchada en Mexico. Papel del *Rhipicephalus sanguineus* en la transmisión de la fiebre manchada en la República Mexicana. *Revista del Instituto de Salubridad y Enfermadades Tropicales* 8: 138-141.

Bustamente Moreno, J. G., and A. Pon Méndez. 2010a. Actualización en la vigilancia epidemiológica de "rickettsiosis". Part I. *Epidemiológia Boletin* 6: 1-4.

Bustamente Moreno, J. G., and A. Pon Méndez. 2010b. Actualización en la vigilancia epidemiológica de "rickettsiosis". Part II. *Epidemiológia Boletin* 7: 1-3.

Carletti, F., C. Castilletti, A. Di Caro, et al. 2010. Alkhurma hemorrhagic fever in travelers returning from Egypt, 2010. *Emerging Infectious Diseases* 16: 1979-1982.

Cazorla, C., C. Socolovschi, M. Jensenius, and P. Parola. 2008. Tick-borne diseases: tick-borne spotted fever rickettsioses in Africa. *Infectious Disease Clinics of North America* 22: 531-544.

Centers for Disease Control and Prevention. 1990. Lyme disease surveillance—United States, 1989-1990. MMWR 39:397-399.

Centers for Disease Control and Prevention. 1991. Lyme disease surveillance—United States, 1990-1991. MMWR 40: 417-421.

Centers for Disease Control and Prevention. 1996a. Lyme disease (*Borrelia burgdorferi*) 1996 case definition. http://www.cdc.gov/ncphi/disss/nndss/casedef/lyme_disease_1996.htm.

Centers for Disease Control and Prevention. 1996b. Rocky Mountain spotted fever (*Rickettsia rickettsii*) (RMSF) 1996 case definition. http://www.cdc.gov/ncphi/disss/nndss/casedef/rocky_mountain_spotted_fever_1996.htm.

Centers for Disease Control and Prevention. 2000. Ehrlichiosis (HGE, HME, other or unspecified) 2000 case definition. http://www.cdc.gov/ncphi/disss/nndss/casedef/ehrlichiosis_2000.htm.

Centers for Disease Control and Prevention. 2002. Tularemia—United States, 1990-2002. MMWR 51:182-184.

Centers for Disease Control and Prevention. 2004. Rocky Mountain spotted fever (*Rickettsia rickettsii*) (RMSF) 2004 case definition. http://www.cdc.gov/ncphi/disss/nndss/casedef/rocky_mountain_spotted_fever_2004.htm.

Centers for Disease Control and Prevention. 2008a. Lyme disease (*Borrelia burgdorferi*) 2008 case definition http://www.cdc.gov/ncphi/disss/nndss/casedef/lyme_disease_2008.htm.

Centers for Disease Control and Prevention. 2008b. Rocky Mountain spotted fever (RMSF) (*Rickettsia rickettsii*) 2008 case definition. http://www.cdc.gov/ncphi/disss/nndss/casedef/rocky_mountain_spotted_fever_2008.htm.

Centers for Disease Control and Prevention. 2008c. Effect of electronic reporting on the burden of Lyme disease surveillance—New Jersey, 2001-2006. *MMWR* 57: 42-45.

Charrel, R. N., H. Attoui, and A. M. Butenko. 2004. Tick borne virus diseases of human interest in Europe. *Clinical Microbiology and Infection* 10: 1040-1055.

Chen, H., D. J. White J, T. B. Caraco, and H. H. Stratton . 2005. Epidemic and spatial dynamics of Lyme disease in New York State, 1990-2000. *Journal of Medical Entomology* 42:899-908.

Childs, J. E., and C. D. Paddock. 2002. Passive surveillance for Rocky Mountain spotted fever: is there more to learn? *American Journal of Tropical Medicine and Hygiene* 66: 450-457.

Childs, J. E., J. W. Sumner, W. L. Nicholson, R. F. Massung, S. M. Standaert, and C. D. Paddock. 1999. Outcome of diagnostic tests using samples from patients with culture-proven human monocytic ehrlichiosis: implications for surveillance. *Journal of Clinical Microbiology* 37: 2997-3000.

Ciceroni, L., A. Pinto, S. Ciarrochi, and A. Ciervo. 2006. Current knowledge of rickettsial diseases in Italy. *Annals of the New York Academy of Sciences* 1078: 143-149.

Clay, K., N. Klyachko, D. Grindle, et al. 2008. Microbial communities and interactions in the lone star tick, *Amblyomma americanum*. *Molecular Ecology* 17: 4371-4381.

Council of State and Territorial Epidemiologists. 2009a. Position statement 09-ID-15. Public health reporting and national notification for human ehrlichioses and anaplasmosis. http://www.cste.org/ps2009/09-id-15.pdf.

Council of State and Territorial Epidemiologists. 2009b. Position statement 09-ID-16. Public health reporting and national notification for spotted fever rickettsiosis (including Rocky Mountain spotted fever). http://www.cste.org/ps2009/09-id-16.pdf.

Dahlgren, F. S., E. Mandel, J. Krebs, R. Massung, and J. H. McQuiston. Surveillance for infections with *Ehrlichia chaffeensis* and *Anaplasma phagocyophilum* in the United States, 2000-2007. In press. *American Journal of Tropical Medicine and Hygiene*.

Dandawate, C. N., G. B. Desai, T. R. Achar, and K. Banerjee. 1994. Field evaluation of formalin inactivated Kyasanur forest disease virus tissue culture vaccine in three districts of Karnataka state. *Indian Journal of Medical Research* 99: 152-158.

Dautel, H., C. Dippel, R. Oehme, K. Hartlet, and E. Schettler. 2006. Evidence for an increased geographical distribution of *Dermacentor reticularis* in Germany and detection of *Rickettsia* sp. RpA4. *International Journal of Medical Microbiology* 296: 149-156.

de Sousa, R., S. Dória Nóbrega, F. Bacellar, and J. Torgal. 2003. Sobre a realidade da febre escaro-nodular em Portugal. *Acta Médica Portuguesa* 16: 429-436.

de Sousa, R., A. França, S. D. Nòbrega, et al. 2008. Host- and microbe-related risk factors for and pathophysiology of fatal *Rickettsia conorii* infection in Portuguese patients. *Journal of Infectious Diseases* 198: 576-585.

Demma, L. J., M. S. Traeger, W. L. Nicholson, et al. 2005a. Rocky Mountain spotted fever from an unexpected vector in Arizona. *New England Journal of Medicine* 353: 587-594.

Demma, L. J., R. C. Holman, J. H. McQuiston, J. W. Krebs, and D. L. Swerdlow. 2005b. Epidemiology of human ehrlichiosis and anaplasmosis in the United States, 2001-2002. *American Journal of Tropical Medicine and Hygiene* 73: 400-409.

Demma, L. J., M. Traeger, D. Blau, et al. 2006. Serologic evidence for exposure to *Rickettsia rickettsii* in eastern Arizona and recent emergence of Rocky Mountain spotted fever in this region. *Vector-Borne and Zoonotic Diseases* 6: 423-429.

Duncan, A. W., M. T. Correa, J. F. Levine, and E. B. Breitschwerdt. 2004. The dog as a sentinel for human infection: prevalence of *Borrelia burgdorferi* C6 antibodies in dogs from the southeastern and mid-Atlantic states. *Vector-Borne and Zoonotic Diseases* 4: 221-229.

Ebel, G. 2010. Update on Powassan virus: emergence of a North American tick-borne flavivirus. *Annual Review of Entomology* 55: 95-110.

Espejo Arenas, E., B. Font Creus, F. Bella Cueto, and F. Segura Porta. 1986. Climatic factors in resurgence of Mediterranean spotted fever. *Lancet* 1: 1333.

Estrada-Peña, A., Z. Vatansever, A. Gargili, and Ö. Ergönul. 2010. The trend towards habitat fragmentation is the key factor driving the spread of Crimean-Congo haemorrhagic fever. *Epidemiology and Infection* 138: 1194-1203.

Felsenfeld, O. 1971. *Borrelia*: strains, vectors, human and animal borreliosis. W. H. Green, St. Louis, MO.

Felz, M. W., F. W. Chandler Jr, J. H. Oliver Jr. 1999. Solitary erythema migrans in Georgia and South Carolina. *Archives of Dermatology* 135: 1317-1326.

Fishbein, D. B., L. A. Sawyer, C. J. Holland, et al. 1987. Unexplained febrile illnesses after exposure to ticks: infection with an *Ehrlichia*? *Journal of the American Medical Association* 257: 3100-3104.

Garciá-Garciá, J. C., A. Portillo, M. J. Núñez, et al. 2010. Case report: a patient from Argentina infected with *Rickettsia massiliae*. *American Journal of Tropical Medicine and Hygiene* 82: 691-692.

Gardner, S. L., R. C. Holman, J. W. Krebs, R. Berkelman, and J. E. Childs. 2003. National surveillance for the human ehrlichioses in the United States, 1997-2001, and proposed methods for evaluation of data quality. *Annals of the New York Academy of Sciences* 990: 80-89.

Gill, J. S., R. G. McLean, R. B. Shriner and R. C. Johnson. 1994. Serologic surveillance for the Lyme disease spirochete, *Borrelia burgdorferi*, in Minnesota by using white-tailed deer as sentinel animals. *Journal of Clinical Microbiology* 32: 444-451.

Ginsberg, H. S. 1993. Geographical spread of *Ixodes dammini* and *Borrelia burgdorferi*. In Ginsberg, H.S. (ed.) *Ecology and environmental management of Lyme disease*. Rutgers University Press, New Brunswick, NJ. pp. 63-82.

Goethert, H. K., and S. R. Telford III. 2003a. Enzootic transmission of the agent of human granulocytic ehrlichiosis among cottontail rabbits. *American Journal of Tropical Medicine and Hygiene* 68: 633-637.

Goethert, H. K., and S. R. Telford III. 2003b. Enzootic transmission of *Babesia divergens* among cottontail rabbits on Nantucket Island, Massachusetts. *American Journal of Tropical Medicine and Hygiene* 69: 455-460.

Goethert, H. K., and S. R. Telford III. 2003c. Enzootic transmission of *Anaplasma bovis* in Nantucket cottontail rabbits. *Journal of Clinical Microbiology* 41: 3744-3747.

Graf, P. C. F., J. P. Chretien, L. Ung, J. C. Gaydos, and A. L. Richards. 2008. Prevalence of seropositivity to spotted fever group rickettsiae and *Anaplasma phagocytophilum* in a large, demographically diverse U.S. sample. *Clinical Infectious Diseases* 46: 70-77.

Gross, E. M., P. Yagupsky, V. Torok, and R. A. Goldwasser. 1982. Resurgence of Mediterranean spotted fever. *Lancet* 2: 1107.

Guerra, M. A., E. D. Walker, and U. Kitron. 2001. Canine surveillance system for Lyme borreliosis in Wisconsin and northern Illinois: geographic distribution and risk factor analysis. *American Journal of Tropical Medicine and Hygiene* 65: 546-552.

Guerra, M. A., A. T. Curns, C. E. Rupprecht, C. A. Hanlon, J. W. Krebs, and J. E. Childs. 2003. Skunk and raccoon rabies in the eastern United States: temporal and spatial analysis. *Emerging Infectious Diseases* 9: 1143-1150.

Guy, E. 1996. Epidemiological surveillance for detecting atypical Lyme disease. *Lancet* 348: 141-142.

Hamer, S. A., J. I. Tsiao, E. D. Walker, and G. J. Hickling. 2010. Invasion of the Lyme disease vector *Ixodes scapularis*: implications for *Borrelia burgdorferi* endemicty. *EcoHealth* doi: 10.1007/s10393-010-0287-0.

Hanrahan, J. P., J. L. Benach, J.L. Coleman, et al. 1984. Incidence and cumulative frequency of endemic Lyme disease in a community. *Journal of Infectious Diseases* 150: 489-496.

Hildago, M., L. Orejuela , P. Fuya, et al. 2007. Rocky Mountain spotted fever, Colombia. *Emerging Infectious Diseases* 13: 1058-1060.

Hilton, E., J. DeVoti, J. L. Benach, et al. 1999. Seroprevalence and seroconversion for tick-borne diseases in a high-risk population in the Northeast United States. *American Journal of Medicine* 106: 404-409.

Hinrichsen, V. L., U. G. Whitworth, E. B. Breitschwerdt, B. C. Hegarty, and T. N. Mather. 2001. Assessing the association between the geographic distribution of deer ticks and seropositivity rates to various tick-transmitted disease organisms in dogs. *Journal of the American Veterinary Medicine Association* 218: 1092-1097.

Hinten, S. R., G. A. Beckett, K. F. Gensheimer, et al. 2008. Increased recognition of Powassan encephalitis in the United States, 1999-2005. *Vector-borne and Zoonotic Diseases* 8: 733-740.

Hoang Johnson, D. K., J. E. Staples, M. J. Sotir, D. M. Warshauer, and J. P. Davis. 2010. Tickborne Powassan virus infections among Wisconsin residents. *Wisconsin Medical Journal* 109: 91-97.

Hoen, A. G., G. Margos, S. J. Bent, et al. 2009. Phylogeography of *Borrelia burgdorferi* in the eastern United Staes reflects multiple independent Lyme disease emergence events. *Proceedings of the National Academy of Sciences U.S.A.* 106: 15013-15018.

Holman, R. C., J. H. McQuiston, D. L. Haberling, and J. E. Cheek. 2009. Increasing incidence of Rocky Mountain spotted fever among the American Indian population of the United States. *American Journal of Tropical Medicine and Hygiene* 80: 601-605.

Hoogstraal, H. 1979. The epidemiology of tick-borne Crimean-Congo hemorrhagic fever in Asia, Europe, and Africa. *Journal of Medical Entomology* 15: 307-417.

Ibister, G. K. 2004. Necrotic arachnidism: the mythology of a modern plague. *Lancet* 364: 549-553.

IJdo, J. W., J. I. Meek, M. L. Carter, et al. 2000. The emergence of another tickborne infection in the 12-town area around Lyme, Connecticut: human granulocytic ehrlichiosis. *Journal of Infectious Diseases* 181: 1388-1393.

Katavolos, P., P. M. Armstrong, J. E. Dawson, and S. R. Telford III. 1998. Duration of tick attachment required for transmission of human granulocytic ehrlichiosis. *Journal of Infectious Diseases* 177: 1422-1425.

Kindberg, E., A. Mickienė, C. Ax., et al. 2008. A deletion in the chemokine receptor 5 (*CCR5*) gene is associated with tickborne encephalitis. *Journal of Infectious Diseases* 197: 266-269.

Krause, P. J., S. R. Telford III, A. Spielman, et al. 1996. Concurrent Lyme disease and babesiosis. Evidence for increased severity and duration of illness. *Journal of the American Medical Association* 275: 1657-1660.

Kudish, K., W. Sleavin, and L. Hathcock. 2007. Lyme disease trends: Delaware, 2000-2004. *Delaware Medical Journal* 79: 51-58.

Labruna, M. B., T. Whitworth, M. C. Horta, et al. 2004. *Rickettsia* species infecting *Amblyomma cooperi* ticks from an area in the State of São Paulo, Brazil, where Brazilian spotted fever is endemic. *Journal of Clinical Microbiology* 42: 90-98.

Lastavica, C. C., M. L. Wilson, V. P. Berardi, et al. 1989. Rapid emergence of a focal epidemic of Lyme disease in coastal Massachusetts. *New England Journal of Medicine* 320: 133-137.

Le Gac, P., E. Gouyer, and P. Barisain-Monrose. 1969. Réapparition de la fiévre exanthématique boutonneuse sur le littoral méditerranéen. *Comps Rendues de l'Academie de Sciences Paris* 269 : 1723-1725.

Lin, M., and Y. Rikihisa. 2003. *Ehrlichia chaffeensis* and *Anaplasma phagocytophilum* lack genes for lipid A biosynthesis and incorporate cholesterol for their survival. *Infection and Immunity* 71: 5324-5331.

Lvov, D. K. 1988. Omsk hemorrhagic fever. In Monath, T. P. (ed). The arboviruses: epidemiology and ecology. Volume III. CRC Press, Boca Raton, FL. pp 205-216.

MacDonald, G. 1957. *The epidemiology and control of malaria*. Oxford University Press, Cambridge. 201 pp.

Maltezou, H. C., L. Andonova, R. Andraghetti, et al. 2010. Crimean-Congo hemorrhagic fever in Europe: current situation calls for preparedness. *Eurosurveillance* 15: pii=19504.

Mansueto, S., G. Tringali and D. H. Walker. 1986. Widespread, simultaneous increase in the incidence of spotted fever rickettsioses. *Journal of Infectious Diseases* 154: 539-540.

Mantke, O. D., R. Schädler, and M. Niedrig. 2008. A survey on cases of tick-borne encephalitis in European countries. *Eurosurveillance* 13: pii=18848.

Marshall, G. S., G. G. Stout, R. F. Jacobs, et al. 2003. Antibodies reactive to *Rickettsia rickettsii* among children living in the southeast and south central regions of the United States. *Archives of Pediatric and Adolescent Medicine* 157: 443-448.

Masters, E., S. Granter, P. Duray, and P. Cordes. 1998 . Physician-diagnosed erythema migrans and erythema migrans-like rashes following lone star tick bites. *Archives of Dermatology* 134: 955-960.

Mather, T. N., M. C. Nicholson, E. F. Donnelly, and B. T. Matyas. 1996. Entomologic index for human risk of Lyme disease. *American Journal of Epidemiology* 144:1066-1069.

McCall, C. L., A. T. Curns, L. D. Rotz, et al. 2001. Fort Chaffee revisited: the epidemiology of tick-borne rickettsial and ehrlichial diseases at a natural focus. *Vector-Borne and Zoonotic Diseases* 1: 119-127.

McFadden, J. D., K. M. McElroy, D. K. Hoang, et al. 2010. *Ehrlichia* infection previously unidentified in North America—Wisconsin and Minnesota, 2009. Paper presented at the 2010 International Conference on Emerging Infectious Diseases, Atlanta, Georgia.

McQuiston, J. H., R. C. Holman, A. V. groom, S. F. Kaufman, J. E. Cheek, and J. E. Childs. 2000. Incidence of Rocky Mountain spotted fever among American Indians in Oklahoma. *Public Health Reports* 115: 469-475.

McQuiston, J. H., M. A. Guerra, M.R. Watts, et al. 2009. Evidence of exposure to spotted fever group rickettsiae among Arizona dogs outside of a previously documented outbreak area. *Zoonoses and Public Health* doi: 10.1111/j.1863-2378.2009.01300.x.

McQuiston, J., C. Levy, M. Traeger, et al. 2010. Rocky Mountain spotted fever associated with *Rhipicephalus sanguineus* ticks: from emergence to establishment of an enzootic focus in the United States. Paper presented at the 2010 International Conference on Emerging Infectious Diseases, Atlanta, Georgia.

Mehla, R., S. R. P. Kumar, P. Yadav, et al. 2009. Recent ancestry of Kyasanur forest disease virus. *Emerging Infectious Diseases* 15: 1431-1437.

Mehnert, W. H., and G. Krause. 2005. Surveillance of Lyme borreliosis in Germany, 2002 and 2003. *Eurosurveillance* 10: pii=531.

Molineaux, L. 1985. The pros and cons of modeling malaria transmission. *Transactions of the Royal Society of Tropical Medicine and Hygiene* 79: 743-747.

Moraes-Filho, M., A. Pinter, R. C. Pacheco, et al. 2009. New epidemiological data on Brazilian spotted fever in an endemic area in the state of São Paulo, Brazil. *Vector-Borne and Zoonotic Diseases* 9: 73-78.

Mouffok, N., A. Benabdellah, H. Richet, et al. 2006. Reemergence of rickettsiosis in Oran, Algeria. *Annals of New York Academy of Sciences* 1078: 180-184.

Naleway, A. L., E. A. Belongia, J. J. Kazmierczak, et al. 2002. Lyme disease incidence in Wisconsin: a comparison of state-reported rates and rates from a population-based cohort. *American Journal of Epidemiology* 155: 1120-1127.

Ndip, L. M., R. N. Ndip, S. N. Esemu, et al. 2005. Ehrlichial infection in Cameroonian canines by *Ehrlichia canis* and *Ehrlichia ewingii*. *Veterinary Microbiology* 111: 59-66.

Ndip, L. M., M. Labruna, R. N. Ndip, D. H. Walker, and J. W. McBride. 2009. Molecular and clinical evidence of *Ehrlichia chaffeensis* infection in Cameroonian patients with undifferentiated febrile illness. *Annals of Tropical Medicine and Parasitology* 103: 719-725.

Ndip, L. M., R. N. Ndip, S. N. Esemu, D. H. Walker, and J. W. McBride. 2010. Predominance of *Ehrlichia chaffeensis* in *Rhipicephalus sanguineus* ticks from kennel-confined dogs in Limbe, Cameroon. *Experimental and Applied Acarology* 50: 163-168.

Newhouse, V. F. 1983. Variations in population density, movement, and rickettsial infection rates in a local population of *Dermacentor variabilis* (Acarina: Ixodidae) ticks in the Piedmont of Georgia. *Environmental Entomology* 12: 1737-1746.

Nicholson, W. L., C. D. Paddock, L. Demma, et al. 2006. Rocky Mountain spotted fever in Arizona: documentation of heavy environmental infestations of *Rhipicephalus sanguineus* at an endemic site. *Annals of the New York Academy of Sciences* 1078: 338-341.

Nijhof, A. M., C. Bodaan, M. Postigo, et al. 2007. Ticks and associated pathogens collected from domestic animals in the Netherlands. *Vector-Borne and Zoonotic Diseases* 7: 585-595.

Nordstrand, A., I. Bunilis, C. Larsson, et al. 2007. Tickborne relapsing fever diagnosis obscured by malaria, Togo. *Emerging Infectious Diseases* 13: 117-123.

Nygård, K., A. Broch Branstæter, and R. Mehl. 2005. Disseminated and chronic Lyme borreliosis in Norway, 1995-2004. *Eurosurveillance* 10: pii=568.

Olano, J. P., E. Masters, W. Hogerfe, and D. H. Walker. 2003. Human monocytotropic ehrlichiosis, Missouri. *Emerging Infectious Diseases* 9: 1579-1586.

Openshaw, J. J., D. L. Swerdlow, J. W. Krebs, et al. 2010. Rocky Mountain spotted fever in the United States: interpreting contemporary increases in incidence. *American Journal of Tropical Medicine and Hygiene* 83: 174-182.

Osterhoudt, K. C., T. Zaoutis, and J. J. Zorc. 2002. Lyme disease masquerading as brown recluse spider bite. *Annals of Emergency Medicine* 39: 558-561.

Otero, R., A. Fenoll, and J. Casal. 1982. Resurgence of Mediterranean spotted fever. *Lancet* 2: 1107.

Paddock, C. D. 2009. The science and fiction of emerging rickettsioses. *Annals of the New York Academy of Sciences* 1166: 133-143.

Paddock, C. D., and M. J. Yabsley. 2007. Ecological havoc, the rise of white-tailed deer, and the emergence of *Amblyomma americanum*-associated zoonoses in the United States. *Current Topics in Microbiology and Immunology* 315: 289-324.

Paddock, C. D., P. W. Greer, T. L. Ferebee, et al. 1999. Hidden mortality attributable to Rocky Mountain spotted fever: immunohistochemical detection of fatal, serologically unconfirmed disease. *Journal of Infectious Diseases* 179: 1469-1476.

Paddock, C. D., S. M. Folk, G. M. Shore, et al. 2001. Infections with *Ehrlichia chaffeensis* and *Ehrlichia ewingii* in persons coinfected with human immunodeficiency virus. *Clinical Infectious Diseases* 33: 1586-1594.

Paddock, C. D., R. C. Holman, J. W. Krebs, and J. E. Childs. 2002. Assessing the magnitude of fatal Rocky Mountain spotted fever in the United States: comparison of two national data sources. *American Journal of Tropical Medicine and Hygiene* 67: 349-354.

Paddock, C. D., A. M. Liddell, and G. A. Storch. 2005. Other causes of tick-borne ehrlichioses, including *Ehrlichia ewingii*. In *Tick-borne diseases of humans*, edited by J. L. Goodman, D. T. Dennis, and D. E. Sonenshine. Washington, D.C.: ASM Press. Pp. 258-267.

Paddock, C. D., R. W. Finley, C. S. Wright, et al. 2008. *Rickettsia parkeri* rickettsiosis and its clinical distinction from Rocky Mountain spotted fever. *Clinical Infectious Diseases* 47: 1188-1196.

Parola, P., C. D. Paddock, and D. Raoult. 2005. Tick-borne rickettsioses around the world: emerging diseases challenging old concepts. *Clinical Microbiology Reviews* 18: 719-756.

Parola, P., C. Socolovschi, L. Jeanjean, et al. 2008. Warmer weather linked to tick attack and emergence of severe rickettsioses. *PLoS Neglected Tropical Diseases* 2: e338.

Pattnaik, P. 2006. Kyasanur forest disease: an epidemiological view in India. *Reviews in Medical Virology* 16: 151-165.

Pavlovsky, E. N. 1966. *Natural nidality of transmissible diseases*. University of Illinois Press, Urbana, IL.

Philip, R. N. 2000. *Rocky Mountain spotted fever in Western Montana. Anatomy of a pestilence*. Bitter Root Valley Historical Society. Hamilton, MT.

Piesman, J., A. Spielman, P. Etkind, T. K. Ruebush, and D. D. Juranek. 1979. Role of deer in the epizootiology of *Babesia microti* in Massachusetts USA. *Journal of Medical Entomology* 15: 537-540.

Piesman, J., T. N. Mather, J. G. Donahue, et al. 1986. Comparative prevalence of *Babesia microti* and *Borrelia burgdorferi* in four populations of *Ixodes dammini* in eastern Massachusetts. Acta Tropica 43: 263-70.

Piesman, J., T. N. Mather, G. J. Dammin, et al. 1987. Seasonal variation of transmission risk of Lyme disease and human babesiosis. *American Journal of Epidemiology* 126: 1187-1189.

Piesman, J., T. N. Mather, R. J. Sinsky, and A. Spielman. 1987. Duration of tick attachment and *Borrelia burgdorferi* transmission. *Journal of Clinical Microbiology* 25: 557-558.

Piranda, E. M., J. L. H. Faccini, A. Pinter, et al. 2008. Experimental infection of dogs with a Brazilian strain of *Rickettsia rickettsii*: clinical and laboratory findings. *Memorias de Intstituto de Oswaldo Cruz, Rio de Janeiro* 103: 696-701.

Pretorius, A. M., and R. J. Birtles. 2002. *Rickettsia aeschlimannii*: a new pathogenic spotted fever group rickettsia, South Africa. *Emerging Infectious Diseases* 8: 874.

Pretzman, C., N. Daugerty, K. Poetter , and D. Ralph. 1990 The distribution and dynamics of rickettsia in the tick population of Ohio. *Annals of the New York Academy of Sciences* 590: 227-236.

Rand, P. W., E. H. LaCombe, R. P. Smith, and J. Ficker. 1998. Participation of birds (Aves) in the emergence of Lyme disease in southern Maine. *Journal of Medical Entomology* 35: 270–276.

Randolph, S. E. 2008. Tick-borne encephalitis in Central and Eastern Europe: consequences of political transition. *Microbes and Infection* 10: 209-216.

Randolph, S. E. 2009a. Perspectives on climate change impacts on infectious diseases. *Ecology* 90: 927-931.

Randolph, S. E. 2009b. Tick-borne disease systems emerge from the shadows: the beauty lies in molecular detail, the messsage in epidemiology. *Parasitology* 136: 1403-1413.

Randolph, S. E. 2010. To what extent has climate change contributed to the recent epidemiology of tick-borne diseases? *Veterinary Parasitology* 167: 92-94.

Randolph, S. E., and D. J. Rogers. 2000. Fragile transmission cycles of tick-borne encephalitis virus may be disrupted by predicted climate change. *Proceedings of the Royal Society of London B* 267: 1741-1744.

Randolph, S. E., L. Asokliene, T. Avsic-Zupanc, et al. 2008. Variable spikes in tick-borne encephalitis incidence in 2006 independent of variable tick abundance but related to weather. *Parasites and Vectors* 1: 44.

Randolph, S. E., on behalf of the EDEN-TBD sub-project team. 2010. Human activities predominate in determining changing incidence of tick-borne encephalitis in Europe. *Eurosurveillance* 15: pii=19606.

Raoult, D., D. Lena, H. Perrimont, H. Gallais, D. H. Walker, and P. Cassanova. 1986. Haemolysis with Mediterranean spotted fever and glucose-6-phosphate dehydrogenase deficiency. *Transactions of the Royal Society of Tropical Medicine and Hygiene* 80: 961-962.

Raoult, D., and P. Parola. 2008. Rocky Mountain spotted fever in the USA: a benign disease or a common diagnostic error? *Lancet* 8: 587-589.

Raoult, D., P. Broqui, and V. Roux. 1996. A new spotted fever group rickettsiosis. *Lancet* 348: 412.

Reif, K. E., and K. R. Macaluso. 2009. Ecology of *Rickettsia felis*: a review. *Journal of Medical Entomology* 46: 723-736.

Richards, A. L., J. Jiang, S. Omulo, et al. 2010. Human infection with *Rickettsia felis*, Kenya. *Emerging Infectious Diseases* 16: 1081-1086.

Rizzoli, A., H. C. Hauffe, V. Tagliapietra, M. Neteler, and R. Rosa. 2009. Forest structure and roe deer density abundance predict tick-borne encephalitis risk in Italy. *PLoS ONE* 4: e4336.

Rosenstein, E. D., and N. Kramer. 1987. Lyme disease misdiagnosed as a brown recluse spider bite. *Annals of Internal Medicine* 107: 782.

Rovery, C., P. Brouqui, and D. Raoult. 2008. Questions on Mediterranean spotted fever a century after its discovery. *Emerging Infectious Diseases* 14:1360-1367

Sanchez, J. L., W. H. Candler, D. B. Fishbein, et al. 1992. A cluster of tick-borne infections: association with military training and asymptomatic infections due to *Rickettsia rickettsii*. *Transactions of the Royal Society of Tropical Medicine and Hygiene* 86: 321-325.

Sanchez, R., C. Alpuche, H. Lopez-Gatell, et al. 2009. *Rhipicephalus sanguineus*–associated Rocky Mountain spotted fever in Mexicali, Mexico: observations from an outbreak in 2008-2009. Paper presented at the 23rd Annual meeting of the American Society for Rickettsiology, Hilton Head, SC (abstract # 75).

Scaffidi, V. 1981. Attuale espansione endemo-epidemica della febbre bottonosa in Italia. *Minerva Medica* 72:2063-2070.

Scrimenti, R. J. 1970. Erythema chronicum migrans. *Archives of Dermatology* 102: 104-105.

Segura, F., and B. Font. 1982. Resurgence of Mediterranean spotted fever in Spain. *Lancet* 2: 280.

Sexton, D. J., J. Banks, S. Graves, K. Hughes, and B. Dwyer. 1991. Prevalence of antibodies to spotted fever group rickettsiae in dogs from southeastern Australia. *American Journal of Tropical Medicine and Hygiene* 45: 243-248.

Shapiro, E. D., M. A. Gerber, N. B. Holabird, et al. 1992. A controlled trial of antimicrobial prophylaxis for Lyme disease after deer-tick bites. *New England Journal of Medicine* 327: 1769-1773

Shapiro, M. R., C. L. Fritz, K. Tait, et al. 2010. *Rickettsia* 364D : a newly recognized cause of eschar-associated illness in California. *Clinical Infectious Diseases* 50: 541-8.

Sigal, L. H., J. M. Zahradnik, P. Lavin, et al. 1998. A vaccine consisting of recombinant *Borrelia burgdorferi* outer-surface protein A to prevent Lyme disease. *New England Journal of Medicine.* 339: 216-222.

Smith, R. P., R. T. Schoen, D. W. Rahn, et al. 2002. Clinical characteristics and treatment outcome of early Lyme disease in patients with microbiologically confirmed erythema migrans. *Annals of Internal Medicine* 136: 421-428.

Smith, R., and J. Takkinen, and the Editorial team. 2006. Lyme borreliosis: Europe-wide coordinated surveillance and action needed? *Eurosurveillance* 11: pii=2977.

Socolovschi, C., Mediannikov O., Sokhna C., et al. 2010. *Rickettsia felis*-associated uneruptive fever, Senegal. *Emerging Infectious Diseases* 16: 1140-1142.

Souza, C. E., J. Morares-Filho, M. Ogrzewalska, et al. 2009. Experimental infection of capybaras *Hydrochoerus hydrochaeris* by *Rickettsia rickettsii* and evaluation of the tranmission of the infection to ticks *Amblyomma cajennense*. *Veterinary Parasitology* 161: 116-121.

Spencer, R. R., and R. R. Parker. 1923. Rocky Mountain spotted fever: infectivity of fasting and recently fed ticks. *Public Health Reports* 38:333-339.

Spielman, A., C. M. Clifford, J. Piesman, et al. 1979. Human babesiosis on Nantucket Island, USA: description of the vector, *Ixodes (Ixodes) dammini*, n.sp. (Acarina:Ixodidae). *Journal of Medical Entomology* 15: 218-234.

Spielman, A., and P. Rossignol. 1984. Insect vectors and scalars. In *Tropical and geographic medicine*, edited by K. S Warren and A. A. F. Mahmoud. McGraw Hill, New York. Pp. 167-183.

Spielman, A., M. L. Wilson, J. F. Levine, and J. Piesman. 1985. Ecology of *Ixodes dammini*-borne human babesiosis and Lyme disease. *Annual Review of Entomology* 30: 439-460.

Spielman, A., S. R. Telford III, and R. J. Pollak. 1993. The origins and course of the present outbreak of Lyme disease. In *Ecology and environmental management of Lyme disease*, edited by H. S. Ginsberg. New Brunswick, NJ: Rutgers University Press. Pp. 83-96.

Stafford III, K. C., M. L. Cartter, L. A. Magnarelli, et al. 1998. Temporal correlations between tick abundance and prevalence of ticks infected with *Borrelia burgdorferi* and increasing incidence of Lyme disease. *Journal of Clinical Microbiology* 36: 1240-1244.

Stanek, G., and F. Strle. 2009. Lyme borreliosis: a European perspective on diagnosis and clinical management. *Current Opinions in Infectious Diseases* 22: 450-454.

Steere, A. C., E. Taylor, M. L. Wilson, et al. 1986. Longitudinal assessment of the clinical and epidemiological features of Lyme disease in a defined population. *Journal of Infectious Diseases* 154: 295-300.

Steere, A. C, V. K. Sikand, F. Meurice, et al. 1998. Vaccination against Lyme disease withrecombinant *Borrelia burgdorferi* outer surface lipoprotein A with adjuvant. *New England Journal of Medicine* 339: 209-215.

Stefanoff, P., M. Eidson, D. L. Morse, and Z. Zielinski. 2005. Evaluation of tickborne encephalitis case classification in Poland. *Eurosurveillance* 10: pii=514.

Šumilo, D., L. Asokliene, A. Bormane, et al. 2007. Climate change cannot explain the upsurge of tick-borne encephalitis in the Baltics. *PLoS One* 2: e500.

Swanepoel, R., A. J. Shepherd, P. A. Leman, et al. 1987. Epidemiologic and clinical features of Crimean-Congo hemorrhagic fever in Southern Africa. *American Journal of Tropical Medicine and Hygiene* 36: 120-132.

Taylor, J. P., W. B. Tanner, J. A. Rawlings, et al. 1985. Serological evidence of subclinical Rocky Mountain spotted fever infections in Texas. *Journal of Infectious Diseases* 151: 367-369.

Telford, S. R. III, and A. Spielman. 1989. Enzootic transmission of the agent of Lyme disease in rabbits. *American Journal of Tropical Medicine and Hygiene* 41: 482-490.

Telford, S. R. III., A. Gorenflot, P. Brasseur, and A. Spielman. 1993. Babesial infections in humans and wildlife. In *Parasitic protozoa,* Vol. 5, edited by J. P. Kreier. San Diego Academic Press. Pp. 1-47.

Telford, S. R. III, P. M. Armstrong, P. Katavolos, et al. 1997. A new tick-borne encephalitis-like virus infecting deer ticks, *Ixodes dammini. Emerging Infectious Diseases* 3: 165-170.

Telford, S. R. III, and H. K. Goethert. 2008. Emerging and emergent tickborne infections. In *Ticks: biology, disease, and control*, edited by L. H Chappell, A. S. Bowman, and P. A. Nuttall. Cambridge University Press. Pp. 344-376.

Telford, S. R. 2009. Status of the "East side hypothesis" (transovarial interference) 25 years later. *Annals of the New York Academy of Sciences* 1166: 144-150.

Telford, S. R. III, P.F. Weller, and J.H. Maguire. In press. Babesiosis. In *Tropical infectious diseases: principles, pathogens, practice*, 3rd edition, edited by R. Guerrant, D. H. Walker, and P. F. Weller. Churchill Livingstone.

Tinoco-Gracia, L., H. Quiroz-Romero, M. T. Quintero-Martínez, et al. 2009. Prevalence of *Rhipicephalus sanguineus* ticks on dogs in a region on the Mexico-USA border. *Veterinary Record* 164: 59-61.

Trape, J. F., B. Godeluck, G. Diatta, et al. 1996. The spread of tick-borne borreliosis in West Africa and its relationship to sub-Saharan drought. *American Journal of Tropical Medicine and Hygiene* 54: 289-293.

Trout, R. T., C. D. Steelman, A. L. Szalanski, and K. Loftin. 2010. Establishment of *Amblyomma maculatum* (Gulf Coast tick) in Arkansas, U.S.A. *Florida Entomologist* 93: 120-122.

Verdade, L. M., and K. M. P. M. B. Ferraz. 2006. Capybaras in an anthropogenic habitat in southeastern Brazil. *Brazilian Journal of Biology* 66: 371-378.

Vetter, R. S., G. B. Edwards, and L. F. James. 2004. Reports of envenomization by brown recluse spiders (Araneae: Sicariidae) outnumber verifications of *Loxosceles* spiders in Florida. *Journal of Medical Entomology* 41: 593-597.

Vetter, R. S., and R. B. Furbee. 2006. Caveats in interpreting poison control centre data in spider bite epidemiology studies. *Public Health* 120: 179-181.

Vetter, R. S., N. C. Hinckle, and L. M. Ames. 2009. Distribution of the brown recluse spider (Araneae: Sicariidae) in Georgia with comparison to poison center reports of envenomations. *Journal of Medical Entomology* 46: 15-20.

Vial, L., G. Diatta, A. Tall, et al. 2006. Incidence of tick-borne relapsing fever in West Africa: longitudinal study. *Lancet* 368: 37-43.

Walker, D. H., H. K. Hawkins, and P. Hudson. 1983. Fulminant Rocky Mountain spotted fever. Its pathologic characteristics associated with glucose-6-phosphatate dehydrogenase deficiency. *Archives of Pathology and Laboratory Medicine* 107: 121-125.

Western, K. A., G. D. Benson, N. N. Gleason, et al. 1970. Babesiosis in a Massachusetts resident. *New England Journal of Medicine* 283: 854-856.

Wilfert, C. M., J. N. MacCormack, K. Kleeman, et al. 1984. Epidemiology of Rocky Mountain spotted fever as determined by active surveillance. *Journal of Infectious Diseases* 150: 469-479.

Wilfert, C. M., J. N. MacCormack, K. Kleeman, et al. 1985. The prevalence of antibodies to *Rickettsia rickettsii* in an endemic area for Rocky Mountain spotted fever. *Journal of Infectious Diseases* 151: 823-831.

Wormser, G. P., J. Nowakowski, R. B. Nadelman, et al. 1998. Efficacy of an OspA vaccine preparation for prevention of Lyme disease in New York State. *Infection* 26: 208-212.

Wormser, G. P., E. Masters, J. Nowakowski, et al. 2005. Prospective clinical evaluation of patients from Missouri and New York with erythema migrans-like skin lesions. *Clinical Infectious Diseases* 41:958-965.

Yabsley, M. J., V. G. Dugan, D. E. Stallknecht, et al. 2003. Evaluation of a prototype *Ehrlichia chaffeensis* surveillance system using white-tailed deer (*Odocoileus virginianus*) as natural sentinels. *Vector-Borne and Zoonotic Diseases* 3: 195-207.

Yevich, S. J., J. L. Sánchez, R. F. DeFraites, et al. 1995. Seroepidemiology of infections due to spotted fever group rickettsiae and *Ehrlichia* species in military personnel exposed in areas of the United States where such infections are endemic. *Journal of Infectious Diseases* 171: 1266-1273.

Yilmaz, G. R., T. Buzgan, H. Irmak, et al. 2009. The epidemiology of Crimean-Congo hemorrhagic fever in Turkey, 2002-2007. *International Journal of Infectious Diseases* 13: 380-386.

Yu, X. J., M. F. Liang, S. Y. Zhang, et al. 2011. Fever with thrombocytopenia associated with a novel bunyavirus in China. New England Journal of Medicine 10.1056/NEJMoa1010095.

Zavala-Velazquez, J. E., X. J. Yu, P. D. Teel, and D. H. Walker. 1996. Unrecognized spotted fever group rickettsiosis masquerading as dengue fever in Mexico. *American Journal of Tropical Medicine and Hygiene* 55: 157-159.

Zimmerman, H. 2005, Tickborne encephalitis in Switzerland: significant increase in notified cases, 2005. *Eurosurveillance* 10: pii=2806.

## A2
## GLOBAL ENVIRONMENTAL CHANGE AND TICK-BORNE DISEASE INCIDENCE

*Sarah H. Olson, Ph.D., and Jonathan A. Patz, M.D., M.P.H.*

### Introduction

The diverse and complex ecology of tick-borne diseases (TBDs) is exceptional among vector-borne diseases. Today it is estimated that tick species exceed 850 and inhabit every continent (Dennis and Piesman 2005, Benoit et al 2007). Their resilience and persistence in the environment can be traced back in the fossil record, which suggests that they originated 65-146 million years ago (Fuente 2003). The Swiss Army knife of disease vectors, ticks generate a neurotoxin and they can host bacterial, viral, and protozoan pathogens as well, a greater variety of disease agents than any other arthropod vector (Sonnenshine 1991).

Grouped into Ixodidæ and Argasidæ families, or hard- and soft-bodied ticks respectively, all ticks are obligate blood-suckers and undergo three stages of development: larval, nymphal, and adult. The life cycle of ticks starts when, "larvæ seek hosts, attach, feed, detach, and develop in sheltered microenvironments where they molt to nymphs; nymphs follow the same pattern and molt to adults (except argasids, which first molt into further nymphal stages); adults seek hosts, mate, feed, and in the case of engorged females, drop off to deposit eggs" (Dennis and Piesman 2005). Tick hosts are terrestrial vertebrates, and host-seeking activity is called questing. Ticks may have vastly different host preferences, among species and at different developmental stages, as well as seasonal questing that depends on climate and environmental conditions (Dennis and Piesman 2005). See Table A2-1 for an overview of major tick-borne diseases, their vectors, endemic areas, and studies relevant to global environmental change.

Global environmental change is the cumulative effect of climate change, the changing built environment and landscape, and evolving biodiversity (MEA 2005). This review will emphasize these three elements. In the context of disease ecology, climate change encompasses abiotic risk factors of temperature, precipitation, and the intensity and frequency of extreme weather events. Globally these events are shifting climatic zones and influencing seasonality. Landscape risk factors include observations of the amount and arrangement of land cover types and uses, from native land cover to urban development. Landscapes provide both the habitat for host and tick vector populations and set the stage for human behavioral risk factors. The presence of host and vector populations are key biodiversity risk factors in TBD ecology, but a less obvious risk factor is the biodiversity of

**TABLE A2-1** Major Tick-Borne Diseases, Their Vectors, Endemic Areas, and Studies Relevant to Global Environmental Change

| Disease | Vector | Research | Effects |
|---|---|---|---|
| Tick-borne paths | [Anaplasma phagocytophilum, Ehrlichia caffeensis | Wimberly et al 2008 | Climate: Habitat (bkwrds finding) biodiversity |
| TBE | Ixodes ricinus | Perkins et al 2006 | Biodiversity |
| TBE | Ixodes ricinus | Gilbert et al 2010 | Climate: habitat |
| TBE | Ixodes ricinus | Ogden et al 2008 | Climate: Habitat |
| TBE | Ixodes ricinus | Randolph and Rogers 2000 | Climate: Habitat |
| TBE | Ixodes ricinus | Lindgren and Gustafson 2001 | Climate: Seasonality |
| TBE | Ixodes ricinus | Lindgren et al 2000 | Climate: Seasonality |
| TBE | Ixodes ricinus | Carpi et al 2008 | Climate: Seasonality and habitat |
| TBE | Ixodes ricinus | Estrada-Peña et al 2003 | Habitat |
| TBE | Ixodes ricinus | Halos et al 2010 | No climate habitat/built enviro |
| TBE | Ixodes ricinus | Vanwambeke et al 2009 | No climate habitat/built enviro |
| Lyme | Ixodes ricinus TBEV B. burgdorferi sensu lato | Danielová et al 2010 | Climate: Habitat |
| Lyme | Ixodes scapularis | Brisson et al 2008 | Biodiversity |
| Lyme | Ixodes scapularis | Brunner et al 2008 | Biodiversity |
| Lyme | Ixodes scapularis | Giardina et al 2000 | Biodiversity |
| Lyme | Ixodes scapularis | Keesing et al 2009 | Biodiversity |
| Lyme | Ixodes scapularis | Ostfeld and Keesing 2000 | Biodiversity |
| Lyme | Ixodes scapularis | Ostfeld and Keesing 2000 | Biodiversity |
| Lyme | Ixodes scapularis | Ostfeld and Keesing 2006 | Biodiversity |
| Lyme | Ixodes scapularis | Schauber et al 2005 | Biodiversity/Climate-weather mice acorns |
| Lyme | Ixodes scapularis | Brownstein et al 2003 | Climate: Habitat |
| Lyme | Ixodes scapularis | Ogden et al 2005 | Climate: Habitat |
| Lyme | Ixodes scapularis | Jones and Kitron 2000 | Climate: Seasonality |
| Lyme | Ixodes scapularis | Kitrone and Kazmierczak 1997 | Climate: Seasonality |
| Lyme | Ixodes scapularis | Prusinski et al 2006 | Habitat |
| Lyme | Ixodes scapularis | Wilder and Meikle 2004 | Habitat (bkwrds finding)/ biodiversity |
| Lyme | Ixodes scapularis | Bunnell et al 2003 | No climate habitat |
| Lyme | Ixodes scapularis | Allan et al 2003 | No climate habitat/built enviro |

| Disease | Vector | Research | Effects |
|---------|--------|----------|---------|
| Lyme | *Ixodes scapularis* | Brownstein et al 2005 | No climate habitat/built enviro |
| Lyme | *Ixodes scapularis* | Cromley et al 1998 | No climate habitat/built enviro |
| Lyme | *Ixodes scapularis* | Das et al 2002 | No climate habitat/built enviro |
| Lyme | *Ixodes scapularis* | Frante et al 1998 | No climate habitat/built enviro |
| Lyme | *Ixodes scapularis* | Horobik et al 2006 | No climate habitat/built enviro |
| | Mix | Cumming and Van Vuuren 2006 | Climate: Habitat |
| | Multiple | Altizer et al 2006 | Climate: Seasonality |
| Rickettsioses | *Rhipicephalus sanguineus* | Parola et al 2008 | Climate: Seasonality |
| | *Dermacentor andersoni, Ixodes ricinus* | Eisen et al 2008 | Climate: Seasonality |

other vertebrate species in the community. Predation and competition may affect host densities, depending on the species composition of biodiversity changes. Lastly, just as the elements of global environmental change range from local to worldwide (Patz and Olson 2006, Patz et al 2008), temporal and spatial scale effects of global environmental change on vector-borne diseases are anticipated (Kovats et al 2001, Patz et al 2005, Plowright et al 2008).

Tick vector species are often vectors for multiple disease-causing micro-organisms (Table A2-1), so our approach allows generalization of changing environmental effects on pathogens not yet studied. Other important elements of disease emergence, including genetic, biological, social, political and economic factors, are included when available, but in-depth analysis of these risk factors is beyond the scope of this paper (IOM 2003).

## Climate Change

Research on climate change and TBD is directed toward three areas of investigation. First, the fundamental question is *how* climate change will impact the tick vector and microbial agent. In vitro observations allow us to understand precisely how temperature and humidity affect tick and pathogen development, behavior, and survival. The second question is *where* will climate change affect the transmission of TBD. Use of information from in-vitro studies can be used (directly or in simulation models) to identify current and future projected climate-based geographic ranges (Ogden et al

2005, 2006). Alternatively (and particularly useful where detailed information on climate effects on vector biology are not available) correlations between observed current distributions of vectors and climate (accounting for other important variable such as habitat) are generalized to large areas using simulations of projected climate change. Finally, *when* may TBD be altered under future climate change scenarios, or more specifically changes to transmission intensity and duration, including patterns of tick, host, and microbe seasonality and synchrony? For this question, data-rich longitudinal field studies are particularly useful to sort out the integrated impact of climate change on disease ecology.

Methodological approaches are implicit to the framing of each question and the different approaches provide varied perspectives of climate change impacts on TBD. A severe lack of long-term data on coupled disease and environmental systems restricts integrated assessment of all three questions (Pascual and Bouma 2009). So uncertainty grows between the research gaps, but taken together, a mosaic is slowly taking shape of how, where and when TBD will be modulated by climate change.

## How Will Climate Affect Tick-Borne Diseases?

Many dimensions of tick development and behavior and TBD transmission are directly linked to climate cues. Higher temperatures yield faster development rates of larvae, nymphs, and adults, with the precise rate of development varying between stages and species. Diapause, or a period of rest between stages, has latitudinal relationships corresponding to photoperiod (tropical species) and temperature-linked physiological aging (temperate species). Together photoperiod and temperature also influence host questing. "At the end of each year, decreasing day length reduces the probability of questing and low temperatures may inhibit activity altogether while at the start of each year, increasing day length is permissive, but only if temperatures are high enough" (Randolph 2004). Of particular note are species and stage specific temperature thresholds for tick activity (3.9–9.8°C), coordinating host seeking activity (7.2–13.9°C), and cold temperature survival (-18.5 – -11.6°C) (Clark 1995, Vandyk et al 1996, Schulze et al 2001). Slight temperature changes around thresholds can have a large impact on tick survival and host-seeking behavior. Beyond temperature in the tropics, *Rhipicephalus appendiculatus* female to larvae survival drops under conditions of high rainfall but low humidity (Randolph 1994, 1997). At local scales, there are exceptions to these climate maxims (Schulze et al 2009, Hubalek et al 2003). Lastly, there is some evidence for direct effects of climate on the pathogen. The rate of parva transmission to cattle increases at higher temperatures but the development of *Theileria parva requires* a specific temperature range (18–28°C) (Ochanda et al 1988, 2003; Young and Leitch 1981).

Dichotomous habitat and host-seeking behavior define two distinct groups of ticks. Exophilic or nonnidicolous species live in the open environment, whereas nidicolous ticks live in the nests and burrows of host species. Since non-nidiculous ticks spend nearly 90% of the life off the host, they are consequently sensitive to external conditions caused by climate change. In contrast, nidiculous ticks are dependent on the presence of host-related microhabitats (e.g., nests, burrows) and are thus sensitive to species distributions, which may change as a result of climate change.

"Nidicolous ticks exhibit behavioral patterns that restrict their distribution to these cryptic microhabitats, avoiding bright sunlight and low humidity. Under these conditions nidicolous ticks can wait for months or even years until hosts arrive and take up residence in these shelters. For the nonnidicolous ticks, survival in the open environment depends upon many factors, among the most important of which is tolerance to desiccation. Ticks adapted to the cool, humid arboreal and deciduous forests of northern Europe and North America typically have only limited tolerance of desiccation. After brief periods of questing on vegetation for passing hosts where they are exposed to subsaturated air, the loss of body water overwhelms their hunger and induces them to retreat to saturated atmospheres in the rotting meadow vegetation or damp leaf litter on the forest floor." (Sonenshine 2005)

Climate, along with other biotic factors such as host availability, is strongly connected to the population density of nonnidicoulous ticks, which transmit the majority of human TBDs. Primarily, this is because climate factors, such as cumulative degree-days and humidity, affect tick survival and longevity (McEnroe 1977, McEnroe 1984, Lindsay et al 1995). In Illinois, Jones and Kitron report severe drought in the previous year significantly lowers *Ixodes scapularis* larval density on *Peromyscus leucopus* mice. There are also positive correlations between larval density and cumulative rainfall and degree-days (2000). In fact, climate is thought to be the major factor controlling Lyme disease occurrence, stronger even than host factors (Randolph 2000). And the importance of climate extends from macro down to micro scale, as survival strongly depends on narrow microclimatic conditions found on the ground, which may be very different even from local ambient conditions (Daniel and Dusbabek 1994, Bertrand and Wilson 1996). When ambient air temperature (measured 50cm above ground) is substituted for ground air temperature, a model of *I. ricinus* development erroneously predicts nymphs emerge 2–3 weeks earlier than observed in southern UK (Randolph 2004). Sensitivity analyses of a population-based land use and land cover physiological tick model of the cattle-tick species *Boophilus* spp confirmed bi-hourly temperature and relative humidity strongly affect tick population dynamics (Corson et al 2004). Landscape and soil conditions will need to be integrated with high-resolution climate projections in order to model tick emergence effectively.

Altitudinal gradients are useful to study the specific mechanisms of climate change on TBDs (Eisen 2008). An altitude gradient creates a linear temperature gradient that represents different climate scenarios while holding other environmental factors relatively constant. Across a difference of 380m and a temperature loss of 0.72°C per 100m gained in elevation, Jouda and colleagues show annual questing nymph and adult *I. ricinus* density and the spring onset of questing is negatively associated with changes in elevation or positively associated with warmer temperatures (2004). A follow-up study between earlier years and more recent times on these same slopes attributed a significant increase in tick density and phenology at higher elevations to recent warmer summers and falls in the higher elevations as measured by saturation deficit (the drying ability of the atmosphere). They also observed an increase in the density of nymphs infected with *Borrelia* at the highest elevation, but overall *Borrelia* infection prevalence dropped with altitude (Cadenas et al 2007, Burri et al 2007). While this study was not able to adjust for differences in host populations across the elevation gradient, another study in Scotland showed *Ixodes ricinus* tick abundance decreases with altitude, again as higher elevations are cooler, even after controlling host (deer) abundance. The authors conclude, "It could be inferred that ticks may become more abundant at higher altitudes in response to climate warming. This has potential implications for pathogen prevalence such as louping ill virus if tick numbers increase at elevations where competent transmission hosts (red grouse *Lagopus lagopus scoticus* and mountain hares *Lepus timidus*) occur in higher numbers" (Gilbert 2010). However, the authors fail to consider how climate change may shift the abundance of grouse and hare hosts at the higher elevations. In Colorado, Eisen observed *Dermacentor andersoni* (Stiles) along an altitudinal gradient and projected a 1 to 2°C increase in mean maximum April-September temperature would generate the same peak tick abundances at 2390 to 2480m that currently occur at 2290m (2008). Adaptation to specific local conditions may also influence future patterns of TBD, as Eisen also observed a site-specific positive correlation between daily maximum temperatures during peak tick host-seeking activity and mean daily maximum temperatures (2007). In sum, the literature consistently shows warmer temperatures increase tick abundance but cautions against assumptions that host distributions will remain relatively constant.

Just as climate influences overall tick population dynamics, evidence suggests biting rates of ticks also are affected by climate. A fascinating epidemiological detective story began in May 2007 when two patients presented with *Rickettsia massiliae and R. conorii* infections in southern France. In April, both patients had visited the residence of a mutual friend. An entomological survey of the residence in July found 218 adult *Rhipicephalus sanguineus* ticks in just one hour, of which roughly one-fourth were positive for rickettsia. The authors point out that April 2007 was the warmest since 1950, and they also performed a healthy volunteer human biting study with pathogen-free *Rh. sanguineus* to test affiliations between aggressive tick biting behavior and temperature. Surprisingly, between 27-67 percent of larvae incubated at 40°C attached to the skin where only 0-6 percent of larvae incubated at 25°C attached successfully. Known commonly as the dog tick, *Rh. sanguineus* transmits dog pathogens but also vectors important and emerging human rickettsioses (Parola et al 2008). Few studies have investigated temperature and *I. scapularis* biting affinity, but McCabe and Bunnell attribute greater numbers of Lyme disease cases to increased survival and tick activity in the northeastern United States brought about by above average rainfall in May and June (2004).

How climate change will impact TBDs is further complicated by the way it alters host diversity, abundance, dispersal, the development cycle of the pathogen, and the suitability of habitat for both tick and hosts (Schulze and Jordan 1996, Gubler et al 2001). Using structural equation modeling, Cumming and Guegan show climate will have a greater direct influence on community richness of the tick vectors than on the pathogens themselves, but that alterations in tick biodiversity will then affect pathogen diversity (2006). In addition to direct effects of climate change on tick and pathogen populations, routes and species of migratory birds transporting Crimean-Congo haemorrhagic fever virus (CCHFV) may change under future climate scenarios. In fact, climate is interwoven into multiple elements of CCHFV zoonotic transmission, from the risk of dispersal by changing migration patterns and bird species to shifting livestock and small vertebrate reservoirs (Gale et al 2009). There may be complicated interactions between temperature, host behavior, and tick population dynamics (Craine et al 1995). A study found when temperatures exceeded 40°C, radio-tracked Australian lizards were more likely to seek out microhabitats or dens where they became infested with high numbers of ticks (Kerr and Bull 2006). Researchers anticipate weather will also affect human behavior in TBD transmission. Randolph et al point to climate influences on cultural practices and socioeconomic conditions as a more critical pathway than climate influences on tick abundance for a tick-borne encephalitis (TBE) epidemic in Europe in 2006. "An alternative explanation, supported by qualitative reports and some data, involves human behavioural responses to weather favourable for outdoor recreational activities, including wild mushroom and berry harvest, differentially influenced by national cultural practices and economic constraints" (Randolf 2008).

*Where Might Climate Change Affect Tick-Borne Diseases?*

Just as there are multiple factors that contribute to TBD risk, there may be more than one factor that limits the geographic range of a tick-borne disease. At regional and national scales the spatial area of Lyme disease risk has been documented to correlate with annual precipitation, temperature, and drought events (Estrada-Peña 2002; McCabe and Bunnell 2004; Jones and Kitron 2000). Therefore, why is Lyme disease not more prevalent in the southern United States where ideal climate conditions already occur? Ostfeld and Keesing suggest that higher species richness, and especially those of ground-dwelling birds, reduces transmission probabilities, or in other words, creates a protective dilution effect (2000a). Therefore, in the south Lyme disease is restricted by biodiversity and species assemblages that limit its ability to spread. Other tick-borne pathogens reveal similar limitations from other factors. The joint distribution of *Ehrlichia chaffeensis* and *Anaplasma phagocytophilum*, the agents of human monocytotropic ehrlichiosis and human granulocytic anaplasmosis, respectively, is bounded in range by climate in the southeastern United States and by the forest fragmentation and cover of the Great Plains (Wimberly et al 2007). While the likelihood of whether climate or land use has a greater effect on tick abundance is an interesting question, it overlooks the dynamic balance of joined climate *and* land use systems. Land use may be a dominant factor in one year and one location, followed by climate the next. More likely both may limit the geographic extent of TBDs.

The relative dominance of climate or land use on the tick vector of Lyme disease, *Ixodes scapularis*, will depend on the location, the rate of change of climate, the rate of change of land-use conditions, and scale. To forecast tick distribution 40 years hence requires an understanding of both current and projected trends of land use and climate. Climate projections for 2050 from B1-low and A2-high scenarios estimate 1.0-3.7°C warming for mean temperatures in Dec/Jan/Feb and June/July/Aug over the present range of Lyme disease transmission (Hulme and Sheard 1999). Generally, earlier spring and warmer winters are positively associated with tick abundance and Lyme disease incidence. Land-use patterns in the last 50 years in the United States reveal exurban development leading to habitat fragmentation changed 20-60 percent for much of the range of Lyme disease (Brown et al 2005) (see Figure A2-1).

Recent research shows that at present climate is limiting the migration of *Ixodes* ticks into eastern Canada and that under several climate change scenarios this migration is anticipated to spread to the southeastern corner of Alberta and across to the eastern tip of Newfoundland by 2050 or 2080 (Ogden et al 2005; Ogden et al 2006) (see Figure A2-2). The rate of climate change is relatively assured, compared to the rate of land-use change, which

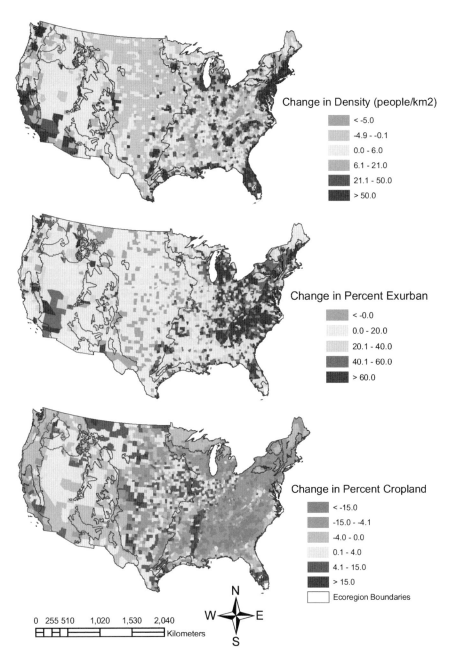

**FIGURE A2-1** Land-use patterns in the last 50 years in the United States.

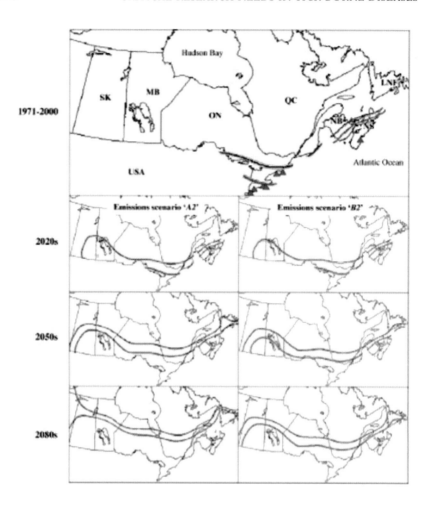

**FIGURE A2-2** Land-use change in rural America.

varies with economic, social, and political institutions. As *Ixodes* is new
to this environment all predictions are uncertain. Knowledge of land use
and tick habitat suitability is still emerging. Unlike climate, land use is not
readily quantifiable. For example, it is difficult to state that 10 ha of type A
landcover relates to a given degree of risk. Over the next century, climate is
a good bet to be the dominant driver that spreads Lyme disease into Canada
(Ogden et al 2010). Land-use change may influence the intensity of the initial epidemic and persistence of endemicity that follows this expansion. In
the Northeast, to the extent that climate and forests are linked ecosystems,

there may be synergistic effects of climate and land-use change. Deforested and fragmented lands may not be able to support historical tick densities under different climate regimes. We are only beginning to quantify the consequences of land-use and climate patterns on biodiversity, vector-borne diseases and human health (Hansen 2005).

The complex dynamics of climate and land use patterns are underscored by a debate on the rising incidence of tick-borne encephalitis (TBE) in Central Europe that began in the mid-1990s. A survey of dogs carrying ticks and tick collections were performed in 2001 and 2002 and compared to a 1957 survey of small terrestrial vertebrates. The authors conclude *I. ricinus* tick habitat encroached up to around 1000m from 700m in elevation as a result of climate change since the 1950s (Daniel et al 2003, 2006). Another research group that included landscape in a more comprehensive analysis of risk factors found that "there was little evidence for the role of climate change in the increase in infections . . . in northern Italy from 1996 to 2006. However, support was found for the influence on TBE increases due to changing forest landscapes and that both red and roe deer, essential hosts in maintaining and amplifying tick populations, had increased 10% from 1996 to 2000 in the region and over 300% in the last 50 years" (Rizzoli et al 2009). The large influence of the host population in this case study underscores the importance of gestalt in disease ecology systems.

Despite this cautionary tale, geographic areas of TBD risk are projected to change globally. An expert panel concluded climate change would have the greatest impact on the distribution of ticks that transmit two of the top three vector-borne viruses in the EU, African horse sickness virus (AHSV) and Crimean-Congo haemorrhagic fever virus (CCHFV) (Gale et al 2010). Increases in the density and geographic range of *I. ricinus* in the mid-1990s is attributed to milder winters compared to the early 1980s (Lindgren 2000). Further research in Sweden found a correlation between increased TBE, transmitted by *I. ricinus* ticks and global warming trends that led to earlier onset of spring and milder winters (Lindgren and Gustafson 2001). It remains unclear why the UK is experiencing a large increase in the distribution and abundance of this tick (Kirby et al 2004; Scharlemann et al 2008). A rising number of TBE cases reported in Slovakia since 1980 appears to reflect a migration of the disease to submountainous habitat as a response to a warming climate (Lukan et al 2010). Yet this relationship may not directly translate to entomological risk (Zeman and Bene 2004, Danielová et al 2010). Scientists using a global habitat suitability model for 73 African tick species predict that over the next 100 years the habitat area will increase 1-9 million square kilometers. "If this is also typical of other invertebrates, then climate change will disrupt not only the geographic location of [their] communities but also their structure. Changes in tick communities are also likely to influence tick-borne pathogens" (Cumming and Van Vuuren 2006).

### When Will Climate Change Affect Tick-Borne Diseases?

The significance of climate change on TBDs goes beyond the debate of shifting distributions of ticks (Pascual and Bouma 2009). "Seasonal patterns are one major pathway for the subtle but potentially drastic effects of climate change on disease dynamics" (Pascual and Dobson 2005). Further, "empirical evidence points to several biologically distinct mechanisms by which seasonality can impact host-pathogen interactions, including seasonal changes in host social behaviour and contact rates, variation in encounters with infective stages in the environment, annual pulses of host births and deaths and changes in host immune defenses" (Alitzer et al 2006). Seasonal patterns of host pathogen prevalence also need to be considered. Sero prevalence of *Anaplasma phagocytophilum*, an emerging pathogen in roe deer in Denmark, was nearly two times higher in the summer versus the fall hunting season (Skarphédinsson et al 2005). The challenge of monitoring these dynamics is further complicated by adaptation and evolution (Tabachnick 2010). Simulations done by Ogden and colleagues demonstrate different seasonal patterns predicted by climate change will select for *I. scapularis*-borne pathogens that are "shorter-lived, less efficiently transmitted, and more pathogenic to their natural hosts, i.e. altered frequency distribution and evolution trajectories" (Ogden et al 2008a).

### Climate Caveats

The narrow focus of this section on climate change (or the focus of the following section) should not dismiss the critical role of human behavioral factors along with social and political changes (Randolph 2008, 2010; Vanwambeke et al 2010).

### Biodiversity, the Landscape, and Built Environment

> "Epidemiological models should consider not only the demographic structure of the host population, but its spatial structure as well, and this can in some cases be effectively inferred from landscape structure." (Langlois et al 2001)

The complex interwoven ties between disease ecology and biodiversity, landscape, and the built environment were first elucidated for Lyme borreliosis in the northeastern United States. It was observed that small mammal reservoir competency, or the ability of a species to infect a biting larva, varies from species to species. In the northeast, white-footed mice (*Peromyscus leucopus*), eastern chipmunks (*Tamias striatus*), and short-tailed or masked shrews (*Blarina brevicauda* or *Sorex cinereus*) are the reservoir for 80-90 percent of infected nymphs (Brisson et al 2008). Because the tick is a nonspecific feeder, diverse community assemblages effectively decrease disease spread by reducing the number of blood meals taken from more competent reservoirs. So in high biodiversity settings, this phenomenon, called the "dilution effect," decreases the likelihood that larval blood meals are taken from mice, an animal with high reservoir competence, while increasing the likelihood that larval blood meals are taken from species with lower reservoir competence, such as raccoons or squirrels (Norman et al 1999; Schmidt and Ostfeld 2001; LoGuidice et al 2003; Brisson et al 2008).

Research suggests the dilution effect is an ecological disease process related to forest fragmentation and that landscape metrics can detect this process. Landscape metrics quantify the amount and arrangement of landscape components. Following the theory, in smaller forest patches the population density of white-footed mice, a highly competent reservoir of Lyme disease, nymphal infection prevalence (NIP), and density of infected nymphs increase exponentially (Nupp and Swihart 1998; Allan et al 2003). Diverse communities of small mammals and birds (lacking in small forest fragments) limit disease spread by reducing the number of blood meals taken from mice, which have the highest reservoir competency (Ostfeld and Keesing 2000a, b). Landscape patterning is important because the disease-buffering ability of an ecosystem may decline with reduced species richness, which often results from decreasing habitat patch size.

Notably, the universality of the dilution effect is being challenged. Recent modeling suggests changing host abundance may also amplify pathogen transmission, "with the outcome depending precisely on mechanisms of competition, host contact rates with ticks, and acquired host resistance to ticks" (Ogden and Tsao 2009; Salkeld et al 2010). Further, the emerging infectious disease, enzootic granulocytic anaplasmosis seroprevalence was greatest in habitats with high biodiversity (ticks, rodents and vegetation) (Foley et al 2009). Bottom line, depending on locality, biodiversity can increase or decrease TBD transmission.

In addition to the dilution effect, other environmental and ecological processes may relate Lyme disease to specific landscapes. Habitat fragmentation can alter host movements and disease transmission dynamics. Micro-infestations or dense patches of *I. ricinus* in a habitat mosaic landscape are critical nodes in a host movement network that sustain the permanent tick population on 1,400 km$^2$ in northern Spain (Estrada-Peña et al 2003). Lyme disease is linked to numerous environmental and ecological systems. Soil characteristics (including order and texture), bedrock, land cover and forest type, sandy soil, low elevation, and deciduous forests have all been implicated (Bunnell et al 2003; Jones and Kitron 2000; McCabe and Bunnell 2004). Deciduous forests have edaphic characteristics that support higher levels of ticks than coniferous forests (Guerra et al 2001; Bunnell et al 2003). In townships surrounding Lyme, Connecticut, landscape metrics of fragmentation are positively associated with tick density and NIP (Brownstein et al 2005). Smaller deer exclosures (less than 2.5 ha) had greater tick densities and within those exclosures, greater densities in the center (Perkins et al 2006). These varied findings suggest that there may be multiple forest fragmentation-linked ecological processes related to Lyme disease.

Tick habitat suitability, a common surrogate estimate of Lyme borrelosis risk, is defined by landscape characteristics across spatial scales. In the North Central United States, Guerra et al (2002) demonstrate tick presence or absence depends on soil order and texture, bedrock, land cover and forest type. In Maryland, agricultural land use has lower tick abundance than forested land cover (Das et al 2002). And along the East Coast, climate, sandy soil, low elevation, deciduous forests, soil characteristics and water availability are all related to elevated abundance of adult ticks (Bunnell et al 2003). In Wisconsin, vegetation detected by satellite—the spring and autumn normalized difference vegetation index (NDVI)—helped distinguish agricultural from forested areas and was significantly associated with human disease cases and tick distributions (Kitron and Kazmierczak 1997). In between this patchwork of regional scale analyses, a lack of uniform surveillance and environmental data limit the understanding of landscape characteristics and tick habitat suitability. Even the fine scale structure of understory vegetation may drive tick density and infection prevalence (Prusinski et al 2006).

Landscape ecology studies provide a powerful reminder that in addition to landscape composition, its configuration plays an important roll in biodiversity and TBD risk. Indices of landscape configuration suggest underlying biological relationships depend on the arrangement of the natural and built environments (Turner 2005). Fragmentation, edge and patch landscape metrics can help describe risks in the built environment, host abundance and distribution, vector abundance, and pathogen prevalence. Jackson et al show high incidence rates of Lyme borrelosis in Maryland are best explained by the amount of edge between forest and herbaceous land cover (2006). The configuration of the built environment, specifically the density and size of residential settings, defines the greatest variation of Lyme cases in a hyperendemic community in Connecticut (Cromley et al 1998). The dilution effect, noted above, is directly connected to the arrangement of the forest; the density of a highly competent Lyme reservoir, the white-footed mouse, is closely associated with the size of forest fragments (Nupp and Swihart 1998). Yet, fragmentation-related entomological risk may or may not necessarily translate into human risk (Brownstein et al 2005, Wilder and Meikle 2004, Horobik et al 2006).

The survivability and stability of ticks in a world of declining biodiversity is not well understood. Biodiversity loss is a silent endpoint of global environmental change. "For the past 300 years, recorded extinctions for a few groups of organisms reveal rates of extinction at least several hundred times the rate expected on the basis of the geological record. The loss of biodiversity is the only truly irreversible global environmental change the Earth faces today" (Dirzo and Raven 2003). Studies of the dilution effect show higher rates of TBD transmission occur when vertebrate biodiversity that effectively buffers pathogen prevalence is reduced (Schmidt and Ostfeld 2001, LoGuidice et al 2003). However, TBD transmission may decline if just the highly competent pathogen reservoirs are absent (Giardina et al 2000). Kessing et al recently proposed another perspective on biodiversity in an ecological disease system. They find hosts, by killing ticks, can act as "ecological traps," and the removal of these hosts may elevate TBD risk, "by increasing both vector numbers and vector infection rates with a zoonotic pathogen" (2009).

Biodiversity plays an important but unassuming role in controlling ticks. There are numerous "natural enemies" of ticks, including mammals and birds, parasitoid wasps, nematodes, bacteria, and fungi proposed to be used as bio-control agents (Ostfeld et al 2006a, Samish et al 2004). For instance, "fire ants" (*Solenopsis invecta)* are thought to have reduced populations of the tick *Amblyomma americanum* in southern US, while spiders are thought to have reduced populations of the tick *Rhipicephalus sanguineus* in Corsica (Wilson 1994). Another biodiversity-linked method of tick control is the exploitation of host pheromones and immunology. These natural organic compounds stimulate tick assembly, dispersal, attraction, attachment and mating behavior (Sonenshine 2006). Micro-infestations of ticks can emerge from pheromonal feedback loops (Yoder et al 2008). And natural systems of biodiversity are critical in identification of pheromones that may support future tick control. For instance, recently penguins in the Antarctic Peninsula were found to provide an assembly pheromone (via guano) of the seabird tick, *Ixodes uriae* (Benoit et al 2008). Another discovery shows the blood of a lizard host of *I. pacificus* blood contains an anti-bacterial agent that effectively eliminates *Borrelia burgdorferi s.l.* from its blood stream (Lane and Quistad 1998).

Given the historical resilience and persistence of ticks through the millennium, their expanding geographic range at the very least introduces a powerful vector of infectious disease and the impact of that introduction depends on local biodiversity. Tick distributions and tick-borne disease transmission potential have localized dependencies on biotic diversity (Ogden and Tsao 2009). In alpine regions in Italy the increased abundance of roe deer is a strong predictor of resurgent TBE, along with changes in forest structure (Rizzoli et al 2009). But locally in the same region deer exclosures were found to have greater nymphal tick abundance on rodents (Perkins et al 2006). As another example, when deer density in a New Jersey township with endemic Lyme borrelosis was reduced, transmission appeared to increase the population of host-seeking ticks (Jordan et al 2007). Anticipating future transmission risk is challenging in a static environment, and even more so under scenarios of tick migration, as the spatial habitats of key reservoir species, which may also vary by locality, are also shifting (Jannette et al 2007, Brisson et al 2009, Surgeoner et al 1997, Sutherst et al 2007). The gross impact of tick expansion into new areas will be mitigated by local relationships of species richness and diversity and new adaptations within the community (Ogden et al 2008b, Frank et al 1998).

*Integration on Environmental Determinants*

The study of TBDs is uncovering dynamic ecological disease processes. One classic and elegant study tells the story of how Lyme disease risk in Dutchess County, New York, is embedded in an oak forest system, and connected to masting and rodent, deer, and gypsy moth abundance (Ostfeld et al 1996). But ecological disease processes cannot always be isolated from anthropogenic processes. Vanwambeke et al tracked TBE incidence in Latvia from 1999–2003, and found it was related to land cover, but also patterns of land use and ownership (2009). Further, at a regional scale the TBE increase in Central and Eastern Europe is attributed in part to "human behaviour determined by socio-economic conditions" that followed the collapse of the Soviet Union (Randolph 2007).

Scientists continue to move ahead with studies of global environmental change and the complex disease ecology of TBDs turning research gaps into challenges:

> "The emerging research field focusing on climate-driven change in spatial and temporal patterns of arthropod vectors, vector-borne pathogens, or incidence of vector-borne diseases is characterized by a plethora of models based on empirical data of variable quality and a disturbing lack of empirical long-term studies that will allow us to demonstrate that future change was in fact driven by climate factors." (Eisen 2008)

> "[There is] a need for a more standardized and comprehensive approach to studying the spatial dynamics of the Lyme disease (LD) system. . . . Significant progress in identifying the determinants of spatial variation in LD risk and incidence requires that: (1) existing knowledge of the biology of the individual components of each LD system is utilized in the development of spatial models; (2) spatial data are collected over longer periods of time;

(3) data collection and analysis among regions are more standardized; and (4) the effect of the same environmental variables is tested at multiple spatial scales." (Killilea et al 2008)

"Improved methods for collection and presentation of spatial epidemiologic data are needed for vectorborne diseases in the United States. Lack of reliable data for probable pathogen exposure sites has emerged as a major obstacle to the development of predictive spatial risk models. . . . New methods are urgently needed to determine probable pathogen exposure sites that will yield reliable results while taking into account economic and time constraints of the public health system and attending physicians. Recent data demonstrate the need for a change from use of the county spatial unit for presentation of incidence of vectorborne diseases to more precise ZIP code or census tract scales." (Eisen and Eisen 2007)

Added to these challenges is the need for comprehensive transdisciplinary approaches to risk assessment, disease surveillance, and treatments (Patz et al 2004). This need requires collaboration among academics and practitioners of public health to join epidemiological, environmental and social determinants, and it must cross political boundaries (Aagaard-Hansen et al 2009, Ahmed et al 2009, Hui 2006). The best science on global environmental change TBD ecology will need to reflect the complex and dynamic ecological connections driving them.

## Acknowledgements

The authors greatly appreciate the comments and feedback from Dr. Nicholas Odgen and Dr. Jack Teng, as well as editing by George Allez. We also thank the Robert Wood Johnson Working Group on Interdisciplinary Perspectives on Health and Society (based at the University of Wisconsin) for a Graduate Research Award to Dr. Olson to address land-use change and Lyme disease risk.

## References

Aagaard-Hansen, J., B. H. Sorensen, and C. L. Chaignat. 2009. A comprehensive approach to risk assessment and surveillance guiding public health interventions. *Tropical Medicine & International Health* 14(9): 1034-1039.

Ahmed, J., M. Bouloy, O. Ergonul, A. R. Fooks, J. Paweska, V. Chevalier, C. Drosten, and R. Moormannet. 2009. International network for capacity building for the control of emerging viral vector-borne zoonotic diseases: Arbo-zoonet. *Eurosurveillance* 14(12): 12-15.

Allan, B.F., F. Keesing and R.S. Ostfeld. 2003. Effect of forest fragmentation on lyme disease risk. *Conservation Biology* 17(1): 267-272. doi:10.1046/j.1523-1739.2003.01260.x.

Altizer, S., A. Dobson, P. Hosseini, P. Hudson, M. Pascual and P. Rohani. 2006. Seasonality and the dynamics of infectious diseases. *Ecology Letters* 9(4): 467-484. doi:10.1111/j.1461-0248.2005.00879.x.

Benoit, J.B., J. A. Yoder, G. Lopez-Martinez, M. A. Elnitsky, R. E. Lee and D. L. Denlinger. 2007. Habitat requirements of the seabird tick, *Ixodes uriae* (Acari: Ixodidae), from the Antarctic Peninsula in relation to water balance characteristics of eggs, nonfed and engorged stages. *Journal of Comparative Physiology B: Biochemical, Systemic, and Environmental Physiology* 177(2): 205-215, DOI: 10.1007/s00360-006-0122-7.

Benoit, J.B., G. Lopez-Martinez, S.A. Philips, M. A. Elnitsky, J. A. Yoder, R.E. Lee and D.L. Denlinger. 2008. The seabird tick, *Ixodes uriae,* uses uric acid in penguin guano as a kairomone and guanine in tick feces as an assembly pheromone on the Antarctic Peninsula. *Polar Biology* 31(12): 1445-1451. doi:10.1007/s00300-008-0485-1. http://www.springerlink.com/index/10.1007/s00300-008-0485-1.

Brisson, D., D. E. Dykhuizen and R. S. Ostfeld. 2008. Conspicuous impacts of inconspicuous hosts on the Lyme disease epidemic. *Proceedings Of The Royal Society B-Biological Sciences* 275(1631): 227-235.

Brown, D.G., K.M. Johnson, T.R. Loveland and D.M. Theobald. 2005. Rural land-use trends in the conterminous United States, 1950-2000. *Ecological Applications* 15(6): 1851-1863.

Brown, R.N., R.S. Lane and D.T. Dennis. 2005. Geographic distributions of tick-borne diseases and their vectors. In tick-borne diseases of humans, J.L. Goodman, D.T. Dennis, and D.E. Sonenshine, 363-391. ASM Press.

Brownstein, J. S., D. K. Skelly, T. R. Holford and D. Fish. 2005. Forest fragmentation predicts local scale heterogeneity of Lyme disease risk. *Oecologia* 146: 469-475.

Bunnell, J.E., S.D. Price, A. Das, T.M. Shields and G E Glass.. 2003. Geographic Information Systems and spatial analysis of adult *Ixodes scapularis* (Acari : Ixodidae) in the Middle Atlantic region of the USA. *Journal of Medical Entomology* 40(4): 570-576.

Burri, C., F.M. Cadenas, V. Douet, J. Moret and L. Gern. 2007. *Ixodes ricinus* density and infection prevalence of *Borrelia burgdorferi* sensu lato along a North-facing altitudinal gradient in the Rhône Valley (Switzerland). *Vector Borne and Zoonotic Diseases* (Larchmont, N.Y.) 7(1): 50-58. doi:10.1089/vbz.2006.0569. http://www.ncbi.nlm.nih.gov/pubmed/17417957.

Cadenas, F.M., O. Rais, F. Jouda, V. Douet, P.F. Humair, J. Moret and L. Gern. 2007. Phenology of *Ixodes ricinus* and infection with *Borrelia burgdorferi* sensu lato along a north- and south-facing altitudinal gradient on Chaumont Mountain, Switzerland. *Journal of Medical Entomology* 44(4): 683-693. http://www.ncbi.nlm.nih.gov/pubmed/17695026.

Carey, J.R. 2001. Insect biodemography. *Ann. Rev. Entomol* 46: 79-110.

Clark, D.D. 1995. Lower temperature limits for activity of several Ixodid ticks (Acari: Ixodidae): effects of body size and rate of temperature change. *Journal of Medical Entomology* 32, no. 4: 449-452. http://www.ncbi.nlm.nih.gov/pubmed/7650705.

Corson, M.S., P.D. Teel and W.E. Grant 2004. Microclimate influence in a physiological model of cattle-fever tick (*Boophilus* spp.) population dynamics. *Ecological Modeling* 180(4): 487-514. doi:10.1016/j.ecolmodel.2004.04.034.

Craine, N.G., S.E. Randolph and P.A. Nuttall. 1995. Seasonal variation in the role of grey squirrels as hosts of *Ixodes ricinus*, the tick vector of the Lyme disease spirochaete, in a British woodland. *Folia Parasitologica* 42: 73-80.

Cromley, E.K., M.L. Cartter, R.D. Mrozinski and S.H. Ertel. 1998. Residential setting as a risk factor for Lyme disease in a hyperendemic region. *American Journal of Epidemiology* 147(5): 472-477.

Cumming, G.S. and D.P. Van Vuuren. 2006. Will climate change affect ectoparasite species ranges?. *Global Ecology and Biogeography* 15(5): 486-497.

Cumming, G.S. and J.F. Guegan. 2006. Food webs and disease: is pathogen diversity limited by vector diversity? *EcoHealth* 3:163-170.

Daniel, M. and F. Dusbabek. 1994. Micrometeorological and micro-habitat factors affecting maintenance and dissemination of tick-borne diseases in the environment. In: Sonenshine, DE, Mather, TN, eds. *Ecological Dynamics of Tick-borne Zoonoses*. Oxford, UK: Oxford University Press; 91-138.

Danielová, V., M. Daniel, L. Schwarzová, J. Materna, N. Rudenko, M. Golovchenko, J. Holubová, L. Grubhoffer and P. Kilián 2010. Integration of a tick-borne encephalitis virus and *Borrelia burgdorferi* sensu lato into mountain ecosystems, following a shift in the altitudinal limit of distribution of their vector, *Ixodes ricinus* (Krkonoše Mountains, Czech Republic). *Vector-borne and Zoonotic Diseases* 10(3): 223-230.

Das, A., S.R. Lele, G.E. Glass, T. Shields and J. Patz. 2002. Modeling a discrete spatial response using generalized linear mixed models: application to lyme disease vectors. *International Journal of Geographical Information Science* 16(2): 151-166.

Dennis, D.T. and J.E. Piesman. 2005. Overview of tick-borne infections of humans. In tick-borne diseases of humans, Jesse L. Goodman, David Tappen Dennis, and Daniel E. Sonenshine, 3-11. ASM Press.

Dirzo, R. and P.H. Raven. 2003. Global State of Biodiversity and Loss. Annual Review of Environment and Resources 28(1): 137-167. doi:10.1146/annurev.energy.28.050302.105532. http://arjournals.annualreviews.org/doi/abs/10.1146/annurev.energy.28.050302.105532.

Eisen, L. and R.J. Eisen. 2007. Need for improved methods to collect and present spatial epidemiologic data for vectorborne diseases. *Emerging Infectious Diseases* 13(12): 1816-1820.

Eisen, L. 2008. Climate change and tick-borne diseases: A research field in need of long-term empirical field studies. *International Journal of Medical Microbiology* 298: 12-18. doi:10.1016/j.ijmm.2007.10.004.

Estrada-Peña, A. 2002. Increasing habitat suitability in the United States for the tick that transmits Lyme disease: A remote sensing approach. *Environmental Health Perspectives* 110(7): 635-640.

Estrada-Peña, A. 2003. The relationships between habitat topology, critical scales of connectivity and tick abundance *Ixodes ricinus* in a heterogeneous landscape in northern Spain. *Ecography* 26(5): 661-671. doi:10.1034/j.1600-0587.2003.03530.x.

Foley, J.E., N.C. Nieto and P. Foley. 2009. Emergence of tick-borne granulocytic anaplasmosis associated with habitat type and forest change in northern California. *The American Journal of Tropical Medicine and Hygiene* 81(6): 1132-1140. doi:10.4269/ajtmh.2009.09-0372. http://www.ncbi.nlm.nih.gov/pubmed/19996448.

Frank, C., A.D. Fix, C.A. Pena and G.T. Strickland.. 2002. Mapping Lyme disease incidence for diagnostic and preventive decisions, Maryland. *Emerging Infectious Diseases* 8(4): 427-429.

Fuente, J.D.L. 2003. The fossil record and the origin of ticks (Acari: Parasitiformes: Ixodida). *Vector-borne and Zoonotic Diseases* 29: 331-344.

Gale, P., A. Estrada-Peña, M. Martinez, R.G. Ulrich, A. Wilson, G. Capelli and P. Phipps. 2009. The feasibility of developing a risk assessment for the impact of climate change on the emergence of Crimean-Congo hemorrhagic fever in livestock in Europe: a Review. *Journal of Applied Microbiology* 108: 1859-1870. doi:10.1111/j.1365-2672.2009.04638.x.

Gale, P., A. Brouwer, V. Ramnial, L. Kelly, R. Kosmider, A.R. Fooks and E.L. Snary. 2010. Assessing the impact of climate change on vector-borne viruses in the EU through the elicitation of expert opinion. *Epidemiology and Infection* 138(2): 214-225. doi:10.1017/S0950268809990367.

Giardina, A.R., K.A. Schmidt, E.M. Schauber and R.S. Ostfeld. 2000. Modeling the role of songbirds and rodents in the ecology of Lyme disease. *Canadian Journal of Zoology* 78(12): 2184-2197. doi:10.1139/cjz-78-12-2184.

Gilbert, L. 2010. Altitudinal patterns of tick and host abundance: a potential role for climate change in regulating tick-borne diseases?. *Oecologia* 162(1): 217-225. doi:10.1007/s00442-009-1430-x. http://www.ncbi.nlm.nih.gov/pubmed/19685082.

Gubler, D., J. Reiter and Ebi, K.L. 2001. Climate variability and change in the United States: potential impacts on vector- and rodent-borne diseases. *Environmental Health Perspectives*, 109: 223-233.

Guerra, M.A., E.D. Walker and U. Kitron. 2001. Canine surveillance system for Lyme borreliosis in Wisconsin and northern Illinois: Geographic distribution and risk factor analysis. *The American Journal of Tropical Medicine and Hygiene* 65(5): 546-552.

Guerra, M., E. Walker, C. Jones, S. Paskewitz, M.R. Cortinas and A. Stancil. 2002. Predicting the risk of Lyme disease: Habitat suitability for *Ixodes scapularis* in the north central United States. *Emerging Infectious Diseases* 8(3): 289-297.

Hansen, A.J., R.L. Knight, J.M. Marzluff, S. Powell, K. Brown and P.H. Gude, 2005. Effects of exurban development on biodiversity: patterns, mechanisms, and research needs. *Ecological Applications* 15(6): 1893-1905.

Horobik, V., F. Keesing and R.S. Ostfeld. 2006. Abundance and *Borrelia burgdorferi*-infection prevalence of nymphal *Ixodes scapularis* ticks along forest–field edges. *EcoHealth* 3(4): 262-268. doi:10.1007/s10393-006-0065-1.

Hubalek, Z., J. Halouzka and Z. Juricova. 2003. Host-seeking activity of Ixodid ticks in relation to weather variables. *Journal of Vector Ecology* 28(2): 159-165.

Hui, E.K.W. 2006. Reasons for the increase in emerging and re-emerging viral infectious diseases. *Microbes and Infection* 8(3): 905-916.

Hulme, M. and N. Sheard. 1999. Climate change scenarios for the United States of America. Norwich, UK: Climatic Research Unit.

IOM (Institute of Medicine). 2003. Microbial threats to health: emergence, detection, and response. By Mark S. Smolinski, Margaret A. Hamburg, Joshua Lederberg, Institute of Medicine (U.S.). Committee on Emerging Microbial Threats to Health in the 21st Century. The National Academies Press, Washington, DC.

Jackson, L.E., E.D. Hilborn and J.C. Thomas. 2006. Towards landscape design guidelines for reducing Lyme disease risk. *International Journal of Epidemiology* 35(2): 315-322. doi:10.1093/ije/dyi284.

Jannett, F.J., M.R. Broschart, L.H. Grim and J.P. Schaberl. 2007. Northerly range extensions of mammalian species in Minnesota. *The American Midland Naturalist* 158(1): 168-176. doi:10.1674/0003-0031.

Jones, C.J. and U.D. Kitron. 2000. Populations of *Ixodes scapularis* (Acari: Ixodidae) are modulated by drought at a Lyme disease focus in Illinois. *Journal of Medical Entomology* 37(3): 408-415. http://www.ncbi.nlm.nih.gov/pubmed/15535585.

Jordan, R.A., T.L. Schulze and M.B. Jahn. 2007. Effects of reduced deer density on the abundance of *Ixodes scapularis* (Acari: Ixodidae) and Lyme disease incidence in a northern New Jersey endemic area. *Journal of Medical Entomology* 44(5): 752-757. http://www.ncbi.nlm.nih.gov/pubmed/17915504.

Jouda, F., J.L. Perret and L. Gern 2004. *Ixodes ricinus* density, and distribution and prevalence of *Borrelia burgdorferi* sensu lato infection along an altitudinal gradient. *Journal of Medical Entomology* 41(2): 162-169. http://www.ncbi.nlm.nih.gov/pubmed/15061274.

Keesing, F., J. Brunner, S. Duerr, M. Killilea, K. Logiudice, K. Schmidt, H. Vuong and R.S. Ostfeld. 2009. Hosts as ecological traps for the vector of Lyme disease. *Proceedings of the Royal Society B: Biological Sciences* 276(1675): 3911-3919. doi:10.1098/rspb.2009.1159. http://www.ncbi.nlm.nih.gov/pubmed/19692412.

Kerr, G.D. and C.M. Bull. 2006. Interactions between climate, host refuge use, and tick population dynamics. *Parasitology Research* 99(3): 214-222. doi:10.1007/s00436-005-0110-y. http://www.ncbi.nlm.nih.gov/pubmed/16541265.

Killilea, M.E., A. Swei, R.S. Lane, C.J. Briggs and R.S. Ostfeld. 2008. Spatial dynamics of Lyme disease: a review. *EcoHealth* 5(2): 167-195. doi:10.1007/s10393-008-0171-3. http://www.ncbi.nlm.nih.gov/pubmed/18787920.

Kirby, A.D., A.A. Smith, T.G. Benton and P.J. Hudson. 2004. Rising burden of immature sheep ticks (*Ixodes ricinus*) on red grouse (*Lagopus lagopus* scoticus) chicks in the Scottish uplands. *Medecal Veterinary Entomology* 18: 67-70.

Kitron, U. and J.J. Kazmierczak. 1997. Spatial analysis of the distribution of Lyme disease in Wisconsin. *American Journal of Epidemiology* 145(6): 558-566. http://www.ncbi.nlm.nih.gov/pubmed/9063347.

Kovats, R.S., D. H. Campbell-Lendrum, A.J. McMichel, A.Woodward and J.S.H. Cox. 2001. Early effects of climate change: do they include changes in vector-borne disease?. *Philosophical Transactions of the Royal Society B: Biological Sciences* 356(1411): 1057-1068. doi:10.1098/rstb.2001.0894.

Langlois, J.P., L. Fahrig, G. Merriam and H. Artsob. 2001. Landscape structure influences continental distribution of hantavirus in deer mice. *Landscape Ecology* 16(3): 255-266.

Lindgren, E., L. Talleklint and T. Polfeldt. 2000. Impact of climatic change on the northern latitude limit and population density of the disease-transmitting European tick *Ixodes ricinus*. *Environmental Health Perspective.* 108(2): 119-123. http://www.jstor.org/stable/3454509.

Lindgren, E. and R. Gustafson. 2001. Tick-borne encephalitis in Sweden and climate change. *Lancet* 358(9275): 16-18.

Lindsay, L.R., I.K. Barker, G.A. Surgeoner, S.A. McEwen, T.J. Gillespie and J.T. Robinson. 1995. Survival and development of *Ixodes scapularis* (Acari: Ixodidae) under various climatic conditions in Ontario, Canada. *Journal of Medical Entomology* 32(2): 143-152. http://www.ncbi.nlm.nih.gov/pubmed/7608920.

LoGiudice, K., R.S. Ostfeld, K.A. Schmidt and F. Keesing. 2003. The ecology of infectious disease: Effects of host diversity and community composition on Lyme disease risk. *Proceedings of the National Academy of Sciences of the United States of America* 100(2): 567-571.

Lukan, M., E. Bullova and B. Petko. 2010. Climate warming and tick-borne encephalitis, Slovakia. *Emerging Infectious Diseases* 16(3): 524-526. http://www.ncbi.nlm.nih.gov/pubmed/20202437.

McCabe, G.J. and J.E. Bunnell. 2004. Precipitation and the occurrence of Lyme disease in the northeastern United States. *Vector-borne and Zoonotic Diseases* 4(2): 143-148.

McEnroe, W.D. 1997. The restriction of the species range of *Ixodes scapularis*, say, in Massachusetts by fall and winter temperature. *Acarologia* (18): 618-625.

McEnroe, W.D. 1984. Winter survival and spring breeding by the fall tick, *Ixodes dammini*, in Massachusetts (Acarina: Ixodidae). *Acarologia* (25): 233-229.

MEA (Millennium Ecosystem Assessment). 2005. Ecosystems and human well-being: Synthesis. Washington, DC: World Resources Institute.

Norman, R., R.G. Bowers, M. Begon and P.J. Hudson. 1999. Persistence of tick-borne virus in the presence of multiple host species: tick reservoirs and parasite-mediated competition. *J. Theoretical. Biology.* 200: 111-118.

Nupp, T.E. and R.K. Swihart. 1998. Effects of forest fragmentation on population attributes of white-footed mice and eastern chipmunks. *Journal of Mammalogy* 79(4): 1234-1243.

Ochanda, H., A.S. Young, J.J. Mutugi, J. Mumo, P.L. Omwoyo. 1998. The effect of temperature on the rate of transmission of *Theileria parva* parva infection to cattle by its tick vector, *Rhipicephalus appendiculatus*. *Parasitology* 97(2): 239-245.

Ochanda, H., A.S. Young and M. Graham. 2003. Survival of *Theileria parva* in its nymphal tick vector *Rhipicephalus appendiculatus* under laboratory and quasi natural conditions. *Parasitology* 126(6): 571-576.

Ogden, N.H., M. Bigras-Poulin, C.J. O'Callaghan, I.K. Barker, L.R. Lindsay, A. Maarouf, K.E. Smoyer-Tomic, D. Waltner-Toews and D. Charron. 2005. A dynamic population model to investigate effects of climate on geographic range and seasonality of the tick *Ixodes scapularis*. *International Journal for Parasitology* 35(4): 375-389.

Ogden, N.H., H.A. Maarouf, I.K. Barker, M. Bigras-Poulin, L.R. Lindsay, M.G. Morshed, C.J. O'Callaghan, F. Ramay, D. Waltner-Toews and D.F. Charron. 2006. Climate change and the potential for range expansion of the Lyme disease vector *Ixodes scapularis* in Canada. *International Journal for Parasitology* 36(1): 63-70. http://www.ncbi.nlm.nih. gov/pubmed/16229849.

Ogden, N.H., M. Bigras-Poulin, K. Hanincová, A. Maarouf, C.J. O'Callaghan and K. Kurtenbach. 2008a. Projected effects of climate change on tick phenology and fitness of pathogens transmitted by the North American tick *Ixodes scapularis*. *Journal of Theoretical Biology* 254(3): 621-632. http://www.ncbi.nlm.nih.gov/pubmed/18634803.

Ogden, N.H., L.R. Lindsay, K. Hanincová, I.K. Barker, M. Bigras-Poulin, D.F. Charron and A. Heagy. 2008b. Role of migratory birds in introduction and range expansion of *Ixodes scapularis* ticks and of *Borrelia burgdorferi* and *Anaplasma phagocytophilum* in Canada. *Applied and Environmental Microbiology* 74(6): 1780-1790. doi:10.1128/AEM.01982-07. http://www.pubmedcentral.nih.gov/articlerender.fcgi?artid=2268299&tool=pmcentrez&rendertype=abstract.

Ogden, N.H. and J.I. Tsao. 2009. Biodiversity and Lyme disease: Dilution or amplification?. *Epidemics* 1(3): 196-206. doi:10.1016/j.epidem.2009.06.002. http://linkinghub.elsevier. com/retrieve/pii/S1755436509000322.

Ostfeld, R.S. and C.G. May 1996. Of mice and mast. *Bioscience* 46(5).

Ostfeld, R.S. and F. Keesing. 2000a. Biodiversity and disease risk: The case of Lyme disease. *Conservation Biology* 14(3): 722-728.

Ostfeld, R. and F. Keesing. 2000b. The function of biodiversity in the ecology of vector-borne zoonotic diseases. *Canadian Journal of Zoology-Revue Canadienne De Zoologie* 78(12): 2061-2078. ://000165450400002 .

Ostfeld, R.S., A. Price, V.L. Hornbostel, M.A. Benjamin and F. Keesing. 2006. Ticks controlling and tick-borne and zoonoses with biological chemical agents. *Sciences-New York* 56(5): 383-394.

Parola, P., C. Socolovschi, L. Jeanjean, I. Bitam, P.E. Fournier, A. Sotto, P. Labauge and D. Raoult. 2008. Warmer weather linked to tick attack and emergence of severe rickettsioses. *PLoS neglected tropical diseases* 2(11): e338. doi:10.1371/journal.pntd.0000338. http://www.pubmedcentral.nih.gov/articlerender.fcgi?artid=2581602&tool=pmcentrez& rendertype=abstract.

Pascual, M. and A. Dobson. 2005. Seasonal patterns of infectious diseases. *PLoS Medicine* 2(1): 18-20.

Pascual, M. and M.J. Bouma. 2009. Do rising temperatures matter?. *Ecology* 90(4): 906-912. http://www.ncbi.nlm.nih.gov/pubmed/19449684.

Patz, J.A., P. Daszak, G.M. Tabor, A.A. Aguirre, M. Pearl, J. Epstein, N.D. Wolfe, A.M. Kilpatrick, J. Foufopoulos, D. Molyneux, D.J. Bradley and Members of the Working Group on Land Use Change and Disease Emergence. 2004. Unhealthy Landscapes: Policy Recommendations on Land Use Change and Infectious Disease Emergence. *Environ Health Perspect* 101: 1092-1098.

Patz, J.A., D. Campbell-Lendrum, T. Holloway and J.A. Foley. 2005. Impact of regional climate change on human health. *Nature* 438: 310-317.

Patz, J.A. and S.H. Olson. 2006. Climate change and health: global to local influences on disease risk. *Annals of Tropical Medicine and Parasitology* 100(5-6): 535-549.

Patz, J.A., S.H. Olson, C.K. Uejio and H.K. Gibbs. 2008. Disease emergence from climate and land use change. *Medical Clinics of North America* 92: 1473-1491.

Perkins, S.E., I.M. Cattadori, V. Tagliapietra, A.P. Rizzoli and P.J. Hudson. 2006. Localized deer absence leads to tick amplification. *Ecology* 87(8): 1981-1986. http://www.ncbi.nlm .nih.gov/pubmed/16937637.

Plowright, R.K., S.H. Sokolow, M.E. Gorman, P. Daszak and J.E. Foley. 2008. Causal inference in disease ecology: investigating ecological drivers of disease emergence. *Frontiers in Ecology and the Environment* 6(8): 420-429. doi:10.1890/070086. http://www.esajournals.org/doi/abs/10.1890/070086.

Prusinski, M.A., H.Y. Chen, J.M. Drobnack, S.J. Kogut, R.G. Means, J.J. Howard, J. Oliver, G. Lukacik, P.B. Backenson and D.J. White. 2006. Habitat structure associated with *Borrelia burgdorferi* prevalence in small mammals in New York State. *Environmental Entomology* 35(2): 308-319. ://000236865500016.

Randolph, S.E. 1994. Population dynamics and density-dependent seasonal mortality indices of the tick *Rhipicephalus appendiculatus* in east and southern Africa. *Medical and Veterinary Entomology* 8: 351-368.

Randolph, S.E. 1997. Abiotic and biotic determinants of the seasonal dynamics of the tick *Rhipicephalus appendiculatus* in South Africa. *Medical and Veterinary Entomology* 11: 25-37.

Randolph, S.E. and D.J. Rogers. 2000. Fragile transmission cycles of tick-borne encephalitis virus may be disrupted by predicted climate change. *Proceedings Of The Royal Society B-Biological Sciences* 267(1454): 1741-1744. doi:10.1098/rspb.2000.1204. http://www.pubmedcentral.nih.gov/ articlerender.fcgi?artid=1690733&tool=pmcentrez&rendertype =abstract.

Randolph, S.E. 2004. Tick ecology: processes and patterns behind the epidemiological risk posed by ixodid ticks as vectors. *Parasitology* 129(7): S37-S65. doi:10.1017/S0031182004004925.

Randolph, S.E., L. Asokliene, T. Avsic-Zupanc, A. Bormane, C. Burri, L. Gern and I. Golovljova. 2008. Variable spikes in tick-borne encephalitis incidence in 2006 independent of variable tick abundance but related to weather. *Parasites & Vectors* 1(1): 44. doi:10.1186/1756-3305-1-44.

Randolph, S.E. 2008. Tick-borne encephalitis incidence in Central and Eastern Europe: consequences of political transition. *Microbes and Infection / Institut Pasteur* 10(3): 209-216. doi:10.1016/j.micinf.2007.12.005. http://www.ncbi.nlm.nih.gov/pubmed/18316221.

Randolph, S.E. 2010. To what extent has climate change contributed to the recent epidemiology of tick-borne diseases?. *Veterinary parasitology* 167(2-4): 92-94. doi:10.1016/j.vetpar.2009.09.011. http://www.ncbi.nlm.nih.gov/pubmed/19833440.

Rizzoli, A., H.C. Hauffe, V. Tagliapietra, M. Neteler and R. Rosa. 2009. Forest structure and roe deer abundance predict tick-borne encephalitis risk in Italy. *PLoS ONE* 4, e4336. doi:10.1371/journal.pone.0004336.

Salkeld, D.J. and R.S. Lane. 2010. Community ecology and disease risk: lizards, squirrels, and the Lyme disease spirochete in California, USA. *Ecology* 91(1): 293-298. http://www.ncbi.nlm.nih.gov/pubmed/20380218.

Samish, M., H. Ginsberg and I. Glazer. 2004. Biological control of ticks. *Parasitology* 129: S389-S403.

Scharlemann, J.P.W., P.J. Johnson, A.A. Smith, D.W. Macdonald and S.E. Randolph. 2008. Trends in ixodid tick abundance and distribution in Great Britain. *Medical Veterinary Entomology* 22: 238-247.

Schmidt, K.A. and R.S. Ostfeld. 2001. Biodiversity and the dilution effect in disease ecology. *Ecological Society of America* 82(3): 609-619.

Schulze, A.L. and R.A. Jordan. 1996. Seasonal and long-term variations in abundance of adult *Ixodes scapularis* (Acari: Ixodidae) in different coastal plain habitats of New Jersey. *Journal of Medical Entomology* 33: 963-970.

Schulze, T.L., R.A. Jordan and R.W. Hung. 2001. Effects of Selected Meteorological Factors on Diurnal Questing of *Ixodes scapularis* and *Amblyomma americanum* (Acari :Ixodidae). *Journal of Medical Entomology* 38(2): 318-324.

Schulze, T.L., R.A. Jordan, C.J. Schulze and R.W. Hung. 2009. Precipitation and temperature as predictors of the local abundance of *Ixodes scapularis* (Acari: Ixodidae) nymphs. *Journal of Medical Entomology* 46(5): 1025-9. http://www.ncbi.nlm.nih.gov/pubmed/19769032.

Skarphédinsson, S., P.M. Jensen and K. Kristiansen. 2005. *Infectious Diseases* 11(7): 1055-1061.

Sonenshine, D. 1991. *Biology of Ticks*. Vol. 1. Oxford: Oxford University Press.

Sonenshine, D. 2005. The Biology of Tick Vectors of Human Disease. In *Tick-Borne Diseases of Humans*, by Jesse L. Goodman, David Tappen Dennis, and Daniel E. Sonenshine, 12-36. ASM Press.

Sonenshine, D.E. 2006. Tick pheromones and their use in tick control. *Annual Review of Entomology* 51(21): 557-580. doi:10.1146/annurev.ento.51.110104.151150. http://www.ncbi.nlm.nih.gov/pubmed/16332223.

Surgeoner, A., A. McEwen and I.K. Barker. 1997. Duration of *Borrelia burgdorferi* infectivity in white-footed mice for the tick vector *Ixodes scapularis* under laboratory and field conditions in Ontario. *Journal of Wildlife Diseases* 33(4): 766-775.

Sutherst, R. W., G. F. Maywald and A. S. Bourne. 2007. Including species interactions in risk assessments for global change. *Global Change Biology* 13(9): 1843-1859. doi:10.1111/j.1365-2486.2007.01396.x. http://www.blackwell-synergy.com/doi/abs/10.1111/j.1365 2486.2007.01396.x.

Tabachnick, W.J. 2010. Challenges in predicting climate and environmental effects on vector-borne disease episystems in a changing world. *Journal of Experimental Biology* 213(6): 946-954. ://000275002600016.

Turner, M.G. 2005. Landscape ecology: What is the state of the science? *Annual Review of Ecology, Evoution, and Systematics* 36: 319-344.

Vandyk, J.K., D.M. Bartholomew, W.A. Rowley and K.B. Platt. 1996. Survival of *Ixodes scapularis* (Acari: Ixodidae) exposed to cold. *Journal of Medical Entomology* 33(1): 6-10. http://www.ncbi.nlm.nih.gov/pubmed/8906898.

Vanwambeke, S.O., D. Sumilo, A. Bormane, E.F. Lambin and S.E. Randolph. 2010. Landscape predictors of tick-borne encephalitis in Latvia: land cover, land use, and land ownership. *Vector Borne and Zoonotic Diseases* 10(5): 497-506. doi:10.1089/vbz.2009.0116. http://www.ncbi.nlm.nih.gov/pubmed/19877818.

Wilder, S.M. and D.B. Meikle. 2004. Prevalence of deer ticks (Ixodes Scapularis) on white-footed mice (*Peromyscus Leucopus*) in forest fragments. *Journal of Mammalogy* 85(5): 1015-1018. doi:10.1644/020. http://www.bioone.org/doi/abs/10.1644/020.

Wilson, M.L. 1994. Population ecology of tick vectors: Interaction, measurement, and analysis. In *Ecological Dynamics of Tick-Borne Zoonoses*, ed. T.N. Sonenshine and D.E. Mather, pp. 20-44. Oxford: Oxford University Press.

Wimberly, M.C., M.J. Yabsley, A.D. Baer, V.G. Dugan and W.R. Davidson. 2007. Spatial heterogeneity of climate and land-cover constraints on distributions of tick-borne pathogens. *Global Ecology and Biogeography*. http://www.blackwell-synergy.com/doi/abs/10.1111/j.1466-8238.2007.00353.x.

Yoder, J.A., J.T. Ark and A.C. Farrell. 2008. Failure by engorged stages of the lone star tick, *Amblyomma americanum*, to react to assembly pheromone, guanine and uric acid. *Medical and Veterinary Entomology* 22(2): 135-139. doi:10.1111/j.1365-2915.2008.00729.x. http://www.ncbi.nlm.nih.gov/pubmed/18498612.

Young, A.S. and B.L. Leitch. 1981. Epidemiology of East Coast fever: some effects of temperature on the development of *Theileria parva* in the tick vector, *Rhipicephalus appendiculatus*. *Parasitology* 83(1): 199-211. http://www.ncbi.nlm.nih.gov/pubmed/6791119.

Zeman, P. and C. Bene. 2004. A tick-borne encephalitis ceiling in central Europe has moved upwards during the last 30 years: possible impact of global warming? *International Journal of Medical Microbiology* 293: 48.

## A3
# THE HUMAN DIMENSION OF LYME AND OTHER
# TICK-BORNE DISEASES: THE PATIENT PERSPECTIVE

*Submitted by: The National Capital Lyme &*
*Tick-Borne Disease Association*

"Courage is what it takes to stand up and speak; courage is what it takes
to sit down and listen."

Winston Churchill

When one family member is infected with *Borrelia burgdorferi (Bb)*,
the entire family is affected. Life as previously lived comes to a screeching
halt. The focus of the family turns to survival of a disease that drains the
energy, ability and hope from the patient and replaces it with pain, weakness and helplessness.

The unfortunate patients who fail the 2-4 week course of antibiotics
are often reassured by their doctor they need no further treatment. They
fall further into the progressive illness that includes facial paralysis, cognitive processing delays, difficulty walking, slurred speech, pain, and the loss
of their former life and self. Prescription bottles and IV poles become the
norm in the home. The roles of parent and spouse disappear as the victim of
the disease can no longer fulfill responsibilities that once had been second-
nature. Child patients often require individualized education plans, accommodations and special education. Some children must be home-schooled
because they cannot get out of bed to participate in a regular classroom
curriculum.

Months and years of illness march on and the patient grows wearier of
any possibility of recovery. While the medical community spends its time
arguing over whether to provide promising additional treatment, the patient
faces a daily battle alone with the medical safety net stretched thin. Doctors,
family and friends, who long since have had no viable answers, continue to
be at a loss to know how to help and stop communicating. The fortunate
patients who respond to aggressive antibiotic treatment face a slow climb
back to their former life and health. Extensive treatment, however, comes
with a price tag that for most patients means the obliteration of their retirement plans and, for some, becoming a financial burden to their children.
When the IV pole has been moved from the bedroom to the garage, the
question remains: "Do we give it away, or might we need it again?" Tick
populations and their related illnesses are increasingly creating epidemics in
neighborhood after neighborhood. Each year, more and more new cases are
tabulated, documented and stored somewhere . . . *and the band plays on.*

## Overview

Lyme borreliosis, commonly referred to as Lyme disease, alone or concurrent with other tick-borne infections, can be a debilitating illness that severely diminishes a person's health and quality of life. The more inclusive term "Lyme borreliosis" is used in this paper, rather than Lyme disease, to include patients with persistent and relapsing infections of the *Borrelia burgdorferi* bacterium after initial therapy. This paper documents the impact of tick-borne infections on patients and their families. It draws on survey data, patient testimonies, and scientific research to examine symptom manifestation, chronicity of illness, and the human and economic costs of tick-borne infections. Children account for a significant number of Lyme borreliosis cases, and this paper examines how tick-borne infections disrupt their development into productive adults. Despite years of research on Lyme borreliosis, understanding of this infection and its impact on patients remains inadequate. This paper identifies gaps in research and medical care. The overwhelming consensus of Lyme patients and their families is that neither the government research community nor the medical community gives sufficient credibility to this disease or devotes adequate resources to combating it. The paper concludes with recommendations that include future research and policy changes needed to combat the serious and growing problem of tick-borne diseases in the United States.

## Onset of Illness and Problems of Diagnosis

The beginning of patients' struggle with Lyme borreliosis can be confusing and frightening. Misperception about tick bites, tick-related rashes, and the variety of symptoms leaves the patient feeling bewildered with a medical system that does not produce answers. As the mother of a 15-year-old patient from New Jersey described the situation, "The most worrisome thing was not knowing what was afflicting my daughter—not knowing who the enemy was for lack of a diagnosis." Worry returns when doctors offer no explanation for the recurrence of symptoms after a short course of treatment.

Patients are fortunate if they observe the telltale erythema migrans (EM) or bull's-eye rash at the time of their tick bite, which alerts them to seek immediate antibiotic treatment. As few as 44 percent of Lyme patients with chronic illness recall seeing a rash and only 29 percent recall seeing a tick bite (Donta, 1997). Unfortunately, many of those patients who do seek care for a rash do not always receive accurate or appropriate medical advice. Physicians unfamiliar with the many variations of EM rashes may miss the diagnosis of Lyme disease. Only 19 percent of rashes resemble a classic bull's-eye rash (Tibbles and Edlow, 2007), and as many as 15 percent of EM rashes were misdiagnosed, most often as spider bites but also as cellulitis and shingles (Aucott et al, 2009).

*Sister of Patient A from Virginia, ill for 6 years:*[1]

"She told the doctor of her fear of Lyme and showed him the bull's-eye rash and she was ignored. We went to doctors located in Virginia where my sister resides and was bitten who said, 'Lyme doesn't exist here. We will not treat.' My beloved twin began a horrible spiral that has gone downhill ever since. She, a woman who worked in healthcare 17 years helping people with HIV, became a victim of a system she used to believe in."

One of the most common patient experiences is the misuse of the Centers for Disease Control and Prevention's (CDC) Lyme disease surveillance case definition for diagnostic purposes. Many doctors are not aware that the CDC's case definition opens with the warning, "This surveillance case definition was developed for national reporting of Lyme disease; it is not intended to be used in clinical diagnosis" (CDC, 2010a). Despite such admonitions, many doctors refuse to diagnose and treat unless the patient meets the CDC's recommended two-tier testing criterion which requires a positive enzyme-linked immunosorbent assay (ELISA) or IFA before use of the Western blot. When the ELISA is negative, patients are routinely refused the more specific Western blot test. As a patient from New Hampshire reports, "All of my five Elisa tests were negative. I was sick with fatigue, headaches, and cognitive issues for a year and a half and missed a whole year of school. When a Western blot was finally done it was CDC positive for Lyme disease."

Moreover, the tests for Lyme disease are notoriously unreliable due to the lack of sensitivity and specificity. Studies have found the sensitivity of the ELISA test for *Bb* infection to vary from 59 to 95 percent (Depietropaolo et al, 2005), meaning that tests can miss up to two-in-five of all cases. The authors found that two-tier testing further decreases test sensitivity, resulting in more missed diagnoses. Unreliable testing hampers both surveillance and patient care when the CDC criteria, designed for patient surveillance purposes, are being misused to deny treatment to patients.

The two-tier testing for *Bb* infection is not recommended since testing is unreliable until several weeks after the onset of illness as the test reflects antibodies in the blood that are not produced until that time (Aguero-Rosenfeld et al, 2005; Depietropaolo et al, 2005). Many patients report that they are tested prior to 4-6 weeks; and when their ELISA comes back

---

[1] Patient testimonies were obtained from various sources, including email requests from various Lyme support patient groups, stories collected by Lyme advocates, and published sources. To ensure patient anonymity, patients are identified only by their state of residence and years of illness.

negative, they are not re-tested, and their infection goes undiagnosed. Since early diagnosis and treatment greatly improve outcomes, it is a tragedy that so many patients do not receive a timely diagnosis.

*Patient B from North Carolina, sick for unknown years:*

"I continue to deteriorate, now so weak I couldn't go any real distance without a wheelchair . . . I experienced violent muscle jerks that left me sore afterwards, as if I had been beaten up. I went into long coma-like sleep lasting 20 hours a day, waking up lethargic, as if I never slept. I started to have impaired short term memory loss, difficulty multitasking or concentrating and forgetting how to do the simplest tasks, like how to take off my seatbelt. As I'm knee deep in this hell, my dogs start to get sick one right after the other. Their tick titers came back positive for ehrlichiosis, Lyme, and Rocky Mountain spotted fever. It was then I researched Lyme for myself and found all my seemingly unrelated symptoms. Excited I had found the answer, I went back to my doctor and told him to test me for Lyme. We did the Elisa which was negative, so he confidently proclaimed, 'You do not have Lyme. We do not have it in North Carolina.'"

Even positive test results are sometimes dismissed by doctors as irrelevant without additional investigation into the cause of their illness. As one Virginia patient states, "Even with a positive ELISA and Western Blot and 23 symptoms I am being told by Infectious Disease [doctor] I am negative. I am being told we are not sure what you have had for 7 years but it is not Lyme." This common experience indicates a perception of unreliability of *Bb* tests in the medical community, and therefore Lyme borreliosis should remain a clinical diagnosis. Far too many patients never hear about the possibility of Lyme borreliosis. A Johns Hopkins study found that 54 percent of patients were misdiagnosed when they did not present with a rash (Aucott et al, 2009). Other patients see a number of specialists who are unable to determine the proper diagnosis.

*Mother on behalf of Patient C from Illinois, sick for 10 years:*

"He saw 21 doctors who ran numerous tests. He was getting sicker, missing school and no one was putting it all together . . . the contact with friends diminished. At times he wondered what he has to live for."

Lyme borreliosis is often not considered in the differential diagnosis of a patient's worsening symptoms. Rather, patients are offered a diagnosis such as chronic fatigue syndrome or fibromyalgia, conditions for which there is no known cause or cure. Eventually, depression may also be diagnosed and antidepressants prescribed. Rarely do antidepressants relieve symptoms that Lyme patients experience.

*Patient D, sick for more than 5 years:*

"Sometimes I wonder if things would have been different had I been diagnosed earlier and received treatment at a younger age. This illness has destroyed my quality of life. Before my illness, I was a very active person capable of working long hours, jogging, tennis, running a household, and active in my church and community activities. It destroyed 2 marriages and I was not able to have children. It is not only costly, it is demoralizing to not be able to take care of yourself on a daily basis."

Some patients with enough observable signs and symptoms are diagnosed with multiple sclerosis, lupus, or amyotrophic lateral sclerosis (ALS). Steroids are prescribed, which have the effect of worsening the Lyme patient's infection through immune suppression, a finding reflected in rhesus monkey studies (Pachner et al, 2001). While the possibility of Lyme borreliosis is overlooked or outright rejected, patients are given seemingly unrelated diagnoses as varied as postural orthostatic tachycardia syndrome (POTS), gastroparesis, autonomic dysfunction disorder, hypoadrenalism, sleep apnea, obsessive compulsive disorder, Aspergers, Tourette syndrome, blood clotting disorders or cyclic vomiting syndrome.

*Patient E from California, sick for 7 years:*

"My father had unknowingly contracted Lyme, Babesia, and Bartonella. Six years later, he began to lose strength and felt like he was losing muscle. His HMO doctor ignored his complaint for over a year. A neurologist diagnosed him with ALS. My brother urged our father to pursue Lyme testing and a Western blot came back positive. The HMO agreed to put him on IV antibiotics for one month. After thirty days, Dad could stand up again but [the HMO] refused to continue IV antibiotics citing IDSA treatment guidelines. The HMO insisted Dad had ALS not Lyme Disease, ignoring the fact Dad gained back the use of his legs. [The HMO] also insisted that he had tongue atrophy and put him on a feeding tube. We were told to take Dad home to die and call Hospice. We chose to take our father out of [the HMO hospital] and put him in a nursing home under the care of a physician who would treat him for advanced Lyme Disease. An occupational therapist found that our father did not have tongue atrophy and he began to eat three meals a day. In the next eight months, my father was walking, off the ventilator, and off the feeding tube."

Reaching the correct diagnosis of Lyme borreliosis can be a long and arduous process. A survey of patients conducted by the California Lyme Disease Association (CALDA) in 2009 found that 35 percent of patients consulted 10 or more doctors before receiving the diagnosis of Lyme borreliosis and 36 percent reported a delay of six years or more between onset of illness and diagnosis. Lack of public and physician awareness leads to significant diagnostic delays. Like the correct diagnosis itself, the search for a knowledgeable physician proves *extremely difficult* for 58 percent of patients surveyed.

*Mother on behalf of Patient F from Virginia, sick for 13 years:*

"My son was diagnosed with chronic Lyme at age 18 after being misdiagnosed with chronic sinus infections and Chronic Fatigue Syndrome. He started having chronic headaches, fatigue and low fevers at age 9, and would improve on antibiotics, but then relapse a couple months after discontinuing them. He saw a CFS/FM specialist and was treated symptomatically for 5 years. He had to be home schooled the whole time due to his severe fatigue. He also acquired a severe sleep disorder, severe POTS, tremors, sound and light sensitivity, and severe cognitive issues (primarily brain fog, concentration problems and word retrieval difficulty.) He lost 35 lbs. At age 18, he was diagnosed with chronic Lyme disease. At age 22 after long-term Lyme treatment, he is improved enough to attend college part-time."

## Other Tick-Borne Infections

Joseph Piesman, who oversees the tick-borne disease program at the CDC, notes that, "The more people study ticks, the more new pathogens are discovered" (Landro, 2010). More than a dozen tick-borne diseases have been documented to cause serious illness in humans. "Ticks can be infected with bacteria, viruses, or parasites. Some of the most common tick-borne diseases in the United States include: Lyme disease, babesiosis, ehrlichiosis, Rocky Mountain Spotted Fever, anaplasmosis, Southern Tick-Associated Rash Illness, Tick-Borne Relapsing Fever, and tularemia. Other tick-borne diseases in the United States include Colorado tick fever, Powassan encephalitis, and Q-fever" (CDC, 2010b). A tick study from southern Connecticut found that 20 percent of the 230 *Ixodes scapularis* ticks collected were infected with *Bb*, and of these ticks 68 percent were co-infected with one or more additional pathogens (Sapi et al, 2009). Consequently, a person bitten by a tick is at risk for being infected with multiple tick-borne diseases.

The National Capital Lyme and Tick-borne Disease Association (NatCapLyme) conducted an online survey in July 2010 on Lyme disease for 10 days.[2] A total of 1,438 subjects, elicited via e-mail from patient

---

[2] The survey was an Internet survey, conducted from July 9 to July 19, 2010. Subjects from the United States, Canada and Europe were recruited by email. Announcements about the survey were posted on Lyme patient support websites. The reported data are for the United States only (1,438 respondents). Respondents who reported that they were infected outside the United States were not included in the analysis (121 respondents). Duplicate response entries were also excluded.

support groups across the country, participated in the survey. Such a large response in so short a time demonstrates that those affected with tick-borne infections want serious consideration and recognition of the impact of the disease.

The NatCapLyme survey found that 46 percent of the respondents had been diagnosed with two or more tick-borne infections. Babesiosis is the most common co-infection, with 41 percent of respondents afflicted. Patients who are co-infected with Lyme borreliosis and other tick-borne infections experience more symptoms and more persistent illness than those with only *Bb* infection (Krause et al, 1996). Because symptoms for other tick-borne infections can be similar to those of Lyme borreliosis, these infections may go undiagnosed, contributing to ongoing illness despite treatment.

*Patient G from Virginia, sick for 13 years:*

"After my initial two and a half years of 'lyme' treatment, it was believed the lyme was 'cured.' Unfortunately, after a couple months, not only did all my symptoms come back, but, I had developed cardiac issues. Sadly, at this time, I was also diagnosed with Babesia and Bartonella by a specialty lab which verified IgG and IgM for Babesia. The physician believed the initial regional test he had performed earlier for Babesia did not include the strain I had, which was WA-1. If the co-infection testing had been accurate back in early 2004, I may not have had the struggle I still face with cardiac issues due to years of infection with Babesia and Bartonella."

Lyme patients frequently suffer from other infections. The NatCapLyme survey found that fully 39 percent of respondents had been diagnosed with bartonellosis in addition to Lyme borreliosis. The tick study from southern Connecticut found the *Bartonella henselae* bacterium to be present in 30 percent of ticks, suggesting an association with ticks as a vector.

The exact role that other tick-borne diseases and opportunistic illnesses play in the disease course is poorly understood, suggesting the need for more research. Researchers have found that spirochete DNA remains in the circulation longer in subjects co-infected with both Lyme disease and babesiosis, compared to patients with Lyme disease alone, leading them to speculate that "babesial infection may impair human host defense mechanisms, as it does in cattle and mice" (Krause et al, 1996). Tick-borne infections can overwhelm the immune system, making the patient vulnerable to other infections, such as mycoplasma, Epstein Barr virus, yeast, H. pylori and Chlamydia pneumoniae, etc. Consequently, a downward spiral of health problems may consume the patient's life and resources.

## Ongoing Illness

Some patients report a full or nearly complete recovery following a month or less of antibiotic treatment for Lyme borreliosis. Receiving early treatment is critical, because left untreated, Lyme borreliosis can become a debilitating disease. "When ticks transmit B. burgdorferi to humans, a rash develops where the spirochetes enter the skin. Several days to weeks later, there may be symptoms elsewhere in the body, where the spirochetes have spread. The symptoms are more likely to appear in the joints, the nervous system, and the heart than anywhere else in the body. When the symptoms of Lyme disease appear in these parts of the body, the person may be considerably disabled. It is this potential for disability that, understandably, makes people so afraid of the disease" (Barbour, 1996).

Early treatment often fails when medication is discontinued prior to full recovery. Some patients experience a slow, insidious deterioration, while others report an abrupt return of former symptoms as well as new, disturbing ones. A literature review on treatment failure of antibiotic therapy found that after a 2-4 week course of treatment, 10 to 61 percent of patients relapse with debilitating symptoms that are indistinguishable from those of late Lyme borreliosis (Green, 2009). Further delay in treatment comes when patients wait to call their doctors during the initial relapse because they do not want to complain after being treated with what they have been told should be sufficient treatment. They are naturally bewildered that the therapy ceases before they feel better, since it is common for doctors to repeat a course of antibiotics when a throat or ear infection persists. In the case of Lyme disease, the end of treatment is often dictated by treatment guidelines rather than the resolution of symptoms.

It is well-documented that *Bb* can infect most parts of the body, producing different symptoms at different times (Steere, 1989; Duray, 1989). Early symptoms are easily mistaken as aches and pains attributable to the common flu, stress at work, over-exercising, or simply the natural aging process. The initial dismissal of possible *Bb* infection allows an otherwise more easily treated infection to develop into a full-blown central nervous system infection which is difficult to treat.

One of the more perplexing dimensions of untreated or under-treated infection is the multiplicity of symptoms that seem to change, appear and disappear suddenly, only to reappear. In patients with Lyme meningitis, Pachner (1995) notes that, "Symptoms can be surprisingly variable, so that days of near normality can alternate with days of profound debility." Symptoms can include, but are not limited to, fever, chills, fatigue, body aches, headaches, rash, swollen lymph nodes, stiff neck, pain, meningitis, neurological problems, poor motor coordination, cognitive impairment, heart problems, eye inflammation, skin disorders, gastrointestinal issues, and general weakness. The great range of symptoms can make disease recognition difficult.

*Mother of Patient H from Florida, sick for 15 years:*

"One of her doctors told us that if one doesn't want to be bored in the medical profession, one should focus on Lyme disease since every organ in the body is affected. Our daughter has had brain encephalitis, arthritis, vision problems, sporadic rashes, extreme fatigue, a headache that has lasted 11 years, photosensitivity, hyperacusis, tinnitus, skin sensitivity, carditis, autonomic nervous system dysautonomia and much, much more."

Patients choosing to continue their search for a treating physician often report great difficulties finding a doctor who has experience in treating persisting infection. Many patients report that the specialists they consult are focused on their chosen field of medicine and miss the multi-system nature of the disease. When this multi-system concept is understood and patients receive long-term antibiotic therapy, they report benefits. A patient survey found that between 72 and 78 percent of respondents experienced improvement in neuropathy, joint pain, concentration difficulties and fatigue with additional treatment beyond 2-4 weeks (CALDA, 2009).[3] Also, two NIH-funded studies on re-treatment of patients with persistent Lyme borreliosis found a statistically significant improvement in symptoms. A study found that 64 percent of patients in the treatment group, versus 19 percent in the placebo group, showed substantial and sustained improvement in fatigue (Krupp et al, 2003). Another study found that patients with more severe symptoms who received an additional 10 weeks of antibiotics reported sustained improvement in pain and physical functioning (Fallon et al, 2008). Although there are treatment failures, long-term, combination antibiotic therapies do return many patients to functional and rewarding lives.

*Patient I:*

"After 10 weeks of Rocephin therapy, I had regained about 80% of my previous health, and most significantly, the return of my intellect and termination of my depression. . . . Now after 6 weeks on oral antibiotics, I'm approximately at 90% recovered. . . . And the big question: will my improvement hold with the eventual ending of antibiotics?"

A common theme in the patient stories we collected was that patients asked for more effective treatment. More research is needed regarding treatment failures in order to meet the needs of those Lyme borreliosis patients who continue to be ill. Lyme borreliosis can lower the quality of

---

[3] The percentages were determined from the survey subsample with the given symptom.

life dramatically. Chronic Lyme borreliosis patients experience deficits in health status of someone with congestive heart failure or osteoarthritis and suffer more impairment than someone living with type 2 diabetes or a recent heart attack (Klempner et al, 2001). A more recent study found the fatigue level in patients with chronic Lyme disease equals that of multiple sclerosis (Fallon et al, 2008).

## Impact on Work

Quality of life for adults with Lyme borreliosis is marked by major declines in vocational, social and recreational functioning, as well as overall deterioration in cognitive and neuropsychiatric impairment. Persistent Lyme borreliosis severely impacts patients' abilities to function in the workplace. A James Madison University survey (Wilcox and Uram, 2009) on the impact of persistent Lyme disease on workplace performance found that patients experience difficulties working. Prior to their illness, all the respondents had been working full-time (a selection criterion), whereas only 28 percent were still working full-time at the time of the survey.

Cognitive impairment, memory, attention deficiencies, and lack of word fluency interfere with Lyme disease patients' work performance. Eighty-nine percent of the 315 respondents said that their symptoms had either a "moderate impact" or a "severe impact" on their ability to remember facts and details. Moreover, 75 percent said that Lyme disease impacted their ability to understand complex concepts and analyze information. More than half of the respondents reported an adverse impact on their basic skills of reading, writing, and math. Such impaired employees are not the only ones affected. When they cannot fulfill their duties, their colleagues are forced to pick up the slack, which has a complex, negative impact on the workplace itself.

Fatigue, pain and dizziness also negatively affect Lyme patients' ability to work. A study of Lyme patients with persistent symptoms found that 90 percent suffered from fatigue and malaise (Klempner et al, 2001); and nearly all of the respondents (95%) in the work performance survey reported that fatigue made it difficult, and in many cases impossible, to maintain a full-time workload (Wilcox and Uram, 2009). Connecticut biologist Joe Dowhan conducted tick research and brought the first *Ixodes scapularis* ticks to Dr. Allen Steere in 1976. Dowhan struggled to keep up with his work as he developed chronic Lyme disease:

"By the beginning of July (of 1976), I was crawling up the stairs to get home. The other biologists were finally telling me to just stay in the car because it was slowing everyone down. I was incapacitated with the disease. . . . In 1990, I started feeling a generalized malaise, a real fatigue, headaches, neck aches . . . I just had overwhelming fatigue, unrelated to exercise. I would find myself at two in the afternoon absolutely needing to drop my head on the desk. I just couldn't move. I'd come home. My pockets would be stuffed with notes (to myself); I was having a difficult time remembering things and getting dinged by my bosses for not following through with things, not even remembering phone conversations with them" (Edlow, 2003).

Dowhan's story is repeated in workplaces across the country. Many Lyme patients struggle to adequately fulfill the requirements and responsibilities of their jobs. More than half (52%) of the respondents in the work performance survey changed jobs, usually for a less challenging and less stressful job (Wilcox and Uram, 2009). Many Lyme patients eventually became too disabled to work as their health deteriorated. Half (51%) of the respondents had left the workforce, and 55 percent of those who stopped working were receiving disability benefits.

*Patient J from Maryland, sick for 6 years:*

"In 2004, I developed severe left-sided head pain and pressure, and eventually migraine headaches. In November 2006 I collapsed at my job where I was working as a surgical nurse in open heart surgery. I had no feeling from the neck down. I have been on disability since. I had a constant 'buzzing' or ringing in my ears, with occasional loud blasts of sounds. Extreme fatigue, blurred vision, floaters in my eyes were next. Tingling and numbness in my legs and eventually my arms. Balance problems were next, stumbling and falling also. I eventually walked with a cane. . . . I could have avoided all of this if I had been treated with oral Doxycyline for 28 days. I would still be working as a registered nurse, a job that I loved. I have been disabled since I was 52. . . . After 3 years of treatment for Lyme Disease, I am better, but very different from a high functioning nurse that I was. I am mentally challenged and every day is a struggle, but I am thankful that I am alive."

### Functionality at Home

Many Lyme patients have to cut back on usual everyday activities. Cooking, cleaning, and other household tasks become arduous, if not impossible, to perform due to cognitive problems, pain and fatigue. Fifty-six percent of respondents to the NatCapLyme survey said that their ability to cook a meal was "moderately impacted" or "severely impacted" by their illness, and 70 percent said that cleaning the house was nearly impossible.

*Patient K from Maryland, sick for more than 10 years:*

"Despite [my husband's] long work days, he was now in charge of meals and most everything else. I was rarely able to do the shopping. I no longer cooked. One morning I decided I wanted scrambled eggs for breakfast. I remember standing at the stove, spatula in hand, looking down at these yellow things in a pan, and very clearly thinking: I DON'T KNOW WHAT THESE ARE."

Many patients have to curtail driving due to dizziness, vision problems and/or cognitive problems. Forty-six percent of the respondents in NatCapLyme's survey said that their driving was impaired. Lyme patients have reported that they have become lost just blocks from their own home, as they are unable to recognize familiar landmarks. One Lyme patient from Maryland wrote, "Cognitive function declined rapidly . . . I would get lost less than a mile from my home that I lived at for thirty years." Consequently, patients become dependent on family and friends for transportation or otherwise find themselves homebound and isolated.

## Social Impact

Interpersonal relationships are strained to the breaking point by the challenges of Lyme borreliosis. Sometimes family and friends are sympathetic to the initial illness, assuming that it will pass like the flu. Patience wears thin, however, when a patient cannot resume normal vocational and recreational activities. Being part of a school, work, sports or social event requires accommodations for the patient. Only the immediate family members, who witness the planning required to get ready for simple daily activities, understand the extent of the efforts required to maintain some normalcy. Everyday grooming requires effort. Acting normal requires stamina. Showing up requires mobility. Patients must adopt a "one day at a time" philosophy and have to cancel vacations and other important events at the last minute due to flaring symptoms. Patients feel that repeated comments from family and friends ranging from "You look fine" and "Do you still have Lyme?" to "Why don't you take some energy pills and get back into life?" invalidate their illness.

*Patient L from Virginia, sick for unknown years:*

"At first my children told me that I didn't have Lyme disease, that it was all in my head, and then they began to make fun of me, and finally, now that I have a doctor and have been under treatment, they tell me I spend too much time focusing on my Lyme disease, that I need to stop thinking about it. . . . I have learned, over the years, to keep it hidden as much as possible, to say nothing, to never ask for help, because when and if I try to talk to them about it, I am quickly silenced or humiliated. Their lack of compassion and understanding is what hurts the most."

The patients' testimonies frequently speak about broken engagements, divorces and abandonment by loved ones who have difficulty accepting that the person they once knew has unnaturally changed. Meanwhile, patients suffer a loss of self-esteem due to the burden of their illness being imposed on the family. Marriages are understandably strained. Spouses may be frustrated by their partner's sudden inability or unwillingness to have children. Disagreements erupt over the patient's inability to work and care for their children as well as the drain of life savings to pay for treatment. Parents may differ about how to treat an ailing child, and adult children can underestimate the depth of their parents' suffering.

*Mother on behalf of Patient M from Virginia, sick for 8 years:*

"It's rough on a marriage to have a child sick without a diagnosis for a long period of time. And, it's even more difficult once there's a controversial diagnosis that is very expensive to treat. Add to that a sick spouse and the opportunities for implosion are everywhere. Our life turned from activities, work, vacations, individual pursuits, hobbies and pleasures to pain, isolation, pressure to make treatment decisions based on limited understanding, and total exhaustion."

Many times Lyme borreliosis infects multiple family members. If one or both parents are affected, children reverse roles and become caretakers to their parents at the expense of their own social lives and with undue stress on their personal development. The focus of the entire family is redirected toward daily survival of new and variable symptoms, the reduction of pain, and the potential for emergency room visits. The healthy family members feel the full weight of being the caregivers. Some have to start working multiple jobs to compensate for the patient's lost income and the added financial burden.

The patient's personality may undergo significant changes due to the illness. Previously vibrant people become confused, scared, and angry. A mother from New Jersey wrote: "In his teen years his health and personality changed. He was having problems with anger that were uncharacteristic for him. Over several years he became homicidal, suicidal, and was in jail." Patients who were independent before their illness become dependent on family and friends for everything. Friendships are hard to maintain, and many patients feel isolated and alone. Feeling they are a burden to their loved ones makes it difficult to face another day of suffering. Seven percent of the respondents in the NatCapLyme survey said they had attempted suicide after contracting Lyme disease and 42 percent had suicidal thoughts.

*Patient N from Kansas, sick for 9 years:*

"Last September, I tried to commit suicide. I ended up in the hospital due to my wounds for two weeks. Everyone thought I just had a bad case of post-partum depression. But I knew the truth, I wasn't depressed, I was absolutely terrified about how lyme was destroying my body, and I just could not take the pain anymore. Slowly I have gotten better on antibiotics. It has almost been a year . . . I have come a long way from where I was, and I am able to function as wife and mother again."

As patients seek understanding on how to deal with the multi-faceted issues related to having Lyme disease, support groups can play an important role in helping patients regain their health. Struggling with bewildered family members and the lack of support from physicians and insurance companies, they turn to Lyme disease support groups to learn more about their illness and how to cope. Support groups provide life skills in how to deal with daily challenges, illness-related social problems, and disability and insurance issues. As former U.S. Surgeon General, C. Everett Koop, MD, explained: "I believe in self-help as an effective way of dealing with problems, stress, hardship and pain. . . . Mending people . . . is no longer enough; it is only part of the total health care that most people require."

## Financial Impact

As the illness stretches into months and then years, health care costs accumulate. NatCapLyme's survey asked respondents for their "best estimate" of the total costs of their Lyme-related treatments. Forty-six percent said that they and their insurance company paid $50,000 or more for treatment. Many patients find their insurance coverage is inadequate to cover their growing health care needs (Jorgensen, 2010). Patients also report that their health insurance company has denied coverage of antibiotic therapy for persistent Lyme borreliosis based on the Infectious Diseases Society of America's (IDSA) 2006 treatment guidelines on Lyme disease. A patient from Virginia, sick for over a year, explains, "Not only do Lyme patients have to battle the medical community for a proper diagnosis, but they are forced to battle the insurance companies for treatment." Treatment that falls outside the guidelines is deemed "to exceed the standard of care" or is considered "experimental" and therefore is not covered. Thirty-five percent in the NatCapLyme survey responded that they were denied either insurance coverage or treatment due to IDSA treatment guidelines. A husband of a patient from Virginia who has been sick for 3 years states, "I have paid medical insurance premiums for more than 50 years but today's medical system allows my insurance carrier to deny coverage of lyme treatment. Big insurance is allowed to practice medicine without a license." Insurance denial leaves Lyme patients with the choice of either paying for treatment out of pocket or being condemned to a life of persistent illness.

*Patient O from Iowa, sick for 6 years:*

"Our insurance company to this date refuses to pay for the treatment and antibiotics citing them to be experimental and not medically necessary. We exhausted all appeals with the insurance company, put a mortgage on our home and cashed out our retirement funds to pay for the medical bills. We currently have a case pending before the Supreme Court of Iowa pertaining to medical coverage denied by our health insurer."

Most health care costs could be avoided if the infection were diagnosed in a timely manner and treated aggressively. According to a CDC study on the economic impact of Lyme disease, the estimated average annual costs, both medical and non-medical, per patient with late-stage Lyme disease are $18,880 (in 2009 dollars). That amount is 10 times higher than the per patient costs for early-stage Lyme disease (Zhang et al, 2006).

Lyme borreliosis poses a serious financial strain on families. Numerous patients with persistent Lyme borreliosis are forced to cut back on work, modify their career goals, or stop working altogether. Parents may have to curtail work hours to care for a sick child. According to the JMU work performance survey, 37 percent of the respondents had lost $100,000 or more in income and wages from onset of illness to the time of the survey. Job loss usually means health insurance coverage is lost as well. Families often deplete savings accounts, run out of personal resources, and lose their homes to pay for medical care. Many patients must depend on government assistance. Twenty-five percent of respondents in the CALDA survey had been on public support or received disability benefits for their illness.

The loss of income has a staggering effect on Lyme patients and represents a burden on our economy. The CDC estimates the national annual economic impact of Lyme disease to be $295 million (in 2009 dollars) (Zhang et al, 2006).[4] This figure underestimates the true economic impact for several reasons. First, the CDC acknowledges significant underreporting (by a factor of 6 to 12) in the number of Lyme disease cases under their case definition (CDC, 2004). This means that the actual number of new Lyme disease cases could be over 300,000 per year. Secondly, the CDC's economic impact study looked at a narrow set of economic variables. It excluded the costs of loss in productivity resulting from spouses and parents taking time

---

[4] The total economic costs figure was based on the CDC's estimate of $203 million (in 2002 dollars) by Zhang et al, converted into 2009 dollars, using the Consumer Price Index (CPI-U) and adjusted for the increase in the number of reported cases from 23,763 in 2002 to 28,921 in 2008.

off from work to care for a family member. Other economic costs, such as those associated with childcare services and adults needing in-home or assisted living services also were not included. A 2007 study on the economic burden of persistent disease found that caregivers' lost productivity can add fully 7 percent to economic costs (DeVol and Bedroussian, 2007). Not only does the disease affect patients' financial stability, it has the potential to impact the financial security of generations to come.

*Patient P from Maryland, sick for more than 20 years:*

"If the doctors had met their most basic obligations, or cared at all, I would have been cured decades ago. . . . They have decided I do not have value as a human being and am not worthy of a healthy, happy life."

### Youth

According to the CDC, children 5 to 14 years of age face one of the highest risks of *Bb* infection (CDC, 2006). This risk is likely due to the amount of time children spend playing outdoors, and a lack of awareness of the importance of finding and removing ticks. While children experience the same range of symptoms as adults, they often do not have the capacity to express and understand what they are feeling. Parents and doctors often dismiss non-specific symptoms of headaches, fatigue, gastrointestinal issues, and behavioral changes as a part of growing up. Such dismissal often results in delayed diagnosis, thereby allowing dissemination of the infection and consequent long-term illness.

Studies have revealed a long-term impact of Lyme borreliosis on a child's physical and intellectual functioning. Researchers at Columbia University found "deficits in visual and auditory attention, or in working memory and mental tracking" in children with cognitive problems associated with Lyme disease. They concluded that their study demonstrates that children whose diagnosis and treatment are delayed may suffer considerable impairment (Tager et al, 2001).

The education of children with persistent Lyme borreliosis becomes compromised, leading to inconsistent school attendance and performance. According to the NatCapLyme survey, 45 percent reported that their children with Lyme borreliosis missed school more than one day a week, and 42 percent reported that their children were tardy more than once a week. Studies on the long-term impact of Lyme borreliosis on children's physical and intellectual functioning have documented behavioral changes, forgetfulness, cognitive deficits, and partial complex seizure disorder (Bloom et al, 1998; Tager et al, 2001). Teachers notice changes in play behavior, declining school performance, excessive sleepiness and frequent trips to the school nurse. At home, parents notice that some children present with cognitive and behavioral issues, nightmares, trouble falling asleep, difficulty concentrating and learning difficulties.

Adolescents present special diagnostic and treatment challenges, since their new-found desire for privacy, normalcy and independence may prevent full-body tick checks by parents and compliance with keeping doctor appointments and taking prescribed medications. Lyme borreliosis can cause symptoms including fatigue, slurred speech, and confusion which can be misinterpreted as resulting from illegal drug or alcohol use. Although some school districts offer generous support through Individualized Educational Plans and home instruction, others resist. Sadly, some teenagers do turn to street drugs and alcohol to self-medicate unmanaged neurologic and rheumatologic pain.

Many teenagers, overwhelmed by the illness and socially isolated, find it increasingly difficult to cope with life. Parents of children 8 to 16 years old reported in the Columbia University study that 41 percent of their children had expressed suicidal thoughts and 11 percent had made a suicidal gesture (Tager et al, 2001). Among the most disturbing results of the NatCapLyme survey were that 54 percent of the respondents reported that their children with Lyme borreliosis suffered from depression and 13 percent reported that their children had attempted suicide. Such suicidal ideation arises from an understandable weariness from chronic illness. Most poignant is the simple statement from a Lyme-infected child, "I just don't want to live anymore."

*Patient Q, age 13 from Missouri, sick for 4 years:*

"The kids at school pick on me because I am now in a wheelchair. I have a pic line in my arm . . . I am very sad. I can't play sports and I am very tired all the time. Sometimes I wish I were not alive. I really have no friends. Who wants to be a friend of someone in a wheelchair or with an illness like mine?"

Relationships with friends and family become strained for some young people with Lyme borreliosis. Some children are confined at home by their illness. Their participation in normal activities, such as athletics or hobbies, becomes a vague memory. Persistent illness affects youths' ability to participate in normal rites of passage.

*Mother on behalf of Patient R from Florida, sick for more than 10 years:*

"Since R was not able to attend school for so many years, receiving home-bound tutoring through the school, she missed out on the normal social growth of a teenager. I think one of the most difficult moments for me was the night her only two friends brought their dates over to show off their prom finery, with the limo waiting outside. I thought my heart would break when my Cinderella ran upstairs after the kids left."

Parents understandably suffer along with their children. During periods when symptoms abate, hope of recovery rises, only to be dashed when symptoms return. Parents must make unimaginable decisions about putting their children on powerful painkillers or pursuing experimental treatments. They spend sleepless nights weighing the risks and benefits of committing their own child's life to one of the opposing treatment philosophies.

*Mother of Patient S from Virginia, sick for more than 8 years:*

"The treatment decisions often boil down to the lesser of two evils. I worry constantly about the potential long-term effects of all of these medications on her developing body, her reproductive capacity."

Parents wonder why there is a narrow focus of concern from physicians regarding the dangers of curative antibiotics while little concern is expressed regarding the dangers of all the other medications including painkillers and "black-box" medications for the treatment of symptoms. As the mother of an 8-year-old Maryland patient states, "There is also, as a parent, guilt . . . tremendous guilt if we make what later turns out to be the wrong choice."

Most parents share the goal of guiding their children to a happy, healthy, productive adulthood. To that end, many parents of children suffering from Lyme borreliosis stretch their resources of time, energy and money to the limit. When young adults expect to launch their independence via college and career, ongoing illness interferes with this natural process. As the years of illness accumulate, hopes of becoming a productive adult and having a family fade. Too many of these young people are forced to create new life plans, but how does one plan for life under these circumstances?

*Patient T, young adult from Virginia, sick for more than 10 years:*

"Lyme has taken what was supposed to be my decade of life, promise, and opportunities and turned it into a decade of intense struggle, betrayals, and constant disappointment. While I once celebrated the highest academic achievements, strove to draw that perfect sound from my instrument, and worried which boys' words rang true, I now celebrate making it to the bathroom, strive for ways to diminish my ever growing medical costs, and worry this time the insurance company will reject my claim because I'm too expensive and growing too weak to fight back. And when Lyme traps me in a twitching body that gasps for air, tries to vomit and feels crushed by an elephant all at the same time, I remember my past filled with promise, ponder my present filled with doctors who say if they can't figure out what's wrong it doesn't exist and family that says if you just try hard enough all problems will disappear, and then contemplate my future—wondering if there is still any hope left in it. They say that adversity builds character, but Lyme weaves darker paths in life that I hope my friends will never need to travel."

## Conclusion

Lyme borreliosis erodes every facet of an individual's life, decimates marriages, and causes children to leave the educational system. Life never returns to normal for many patients, as they must accommodate activity restrictions and ongoing health concerns. Recovery is further complicated by physicians who do not acknowledge the possibility of ongoing illness, and medical policymakers who do not consider additional avenues worthy of scientific exploration, in spite of mounting evidence of persistent infection.

Research remains inconclusive about optimal treatment. Yet state medical boards routinely penalize doctors for deviating from the Infectious Diseases Society of America's (IDSA) guidelines for treatment of Lyme disease (Wormser et al, 2006) by subjecting them to investigations and disciplinary procedures rarely visited on physicians treating other diseases. Consequently, a growing numbers of patients lose their doctors, who stop treating Lyme disease in fear of losing their licensing. Physicians are reluctant to treat Lyme and other tick-borne infections in a manner that contradicts the IDSA guidelines. This phenomenon appears to be unique to Lyme borreliosis. The government-sanctioned medical society favoring one treatment philosophy over another places an unnecessary burden on patients who are left to fend for themselves. In an ironic twist of the medical axiom "First do no harm," patients are left to wonder why the harm they endure from failure to receive treatment is not a rejection of that cherished standard.

The patient testimonies submitted illustrate that the conventional medical wisdom is seriously disserving Americans with tick-borne infections. They also support the frequent allegation that Lyme and associated tick-borne infections are major life-debilitating diseases that should be taken very seriously. Disease manifestations and treatment responses vary among patients. Some patients who are diagnosed and treated early respond well to IDSA-recommended treatment. Patients, whose diagnosis and treatment are delayed, often benefit from long-term or intermittent antibiotic therapy, which is why patients should have the right to pursue all treatment options.

Lyme patient support groups are encountering a growing number of people who were healthy prior to contracting Lyme borreliosis and have not returned to their former level of functioning after treatment. Patients across the United States report innumerable treatment failures. Worse yet, some people never receive treatment. It is unconscionable that so many people suffer for lack of an accurate diagnosis or effective treatment.

A recent study on the use of guidelines in medical negligence litigation in England and Wales concluded that, "there is a danger in applying the generalized prescription of guidelines in a rigid fashion to every patient" (Samanta et al, 2006). The authors noted that this interference with clinical freedom can result in "cookbook medicine." "In medical practice, many situations arise where the art of identifying patient problems and the application of clinical acumen to individual patient's needs remain removed from the science and technological advances of the discipline. Evidence-based medicine cannot fully capture the art of medical practice, and there remains a need for clinical judgment and discretion" (Samanta et al, 2006). Weak research data undermine the validity of treatment guidelines.

Clearly a serious gap between the conventional medical community's acknowledgment and patient reality is evident. Harvard Medical School professor Dr. Jonathan Edlow states in his book, *Bull's-Eye*, "We still have a lot to learn about Lyme disease, and more importantly, we still have a lot to learn about the scientific process" (Edlow, 2003). Patients hope that the Institute of Medicine's (IOM) Workshop will lay the foundation by bringing university and private-sector scientists and practicing physicians from different viewpoints together to collaborate on solving the problems of treatment failures and persistent illness. We must utilize the scarce resources available to reach out to new thinkers, to explore fresh approaches that will give us the answers to find a cure for all victims of *Borrelia burgdorferi*.

"The controversy in Lyme Disease research is a shameful affair. And I say that because the whole thing is politically tainted. Money goes to people who have, for the past 30 years produced the same thing. . . . Nothing."

Willy Burgdorfer, Entomologist who first identified the bacterial spirochete responsible for causing Lyme disease (Wilson, 2009).

### Recommendations

The National Capital Lyme and Tick-borne Disease Association recommends:

1. Improve surveillance by effective, thorough national oversight of tick-borne infections. Tick-borne infections are a serious health concern, and effective national surveillance of these diseases is needed in order to improve public awareness, prevention and diagnosis. Develop a more inclusive surveillance case definition that reflects the actual experiences of practicing physicians confronted with patients presenting with symptoms consistent with Lyme borreliosis. Suggestions to accomplish this are:

- Broaden the case definition for surveillance to include advanced late-manifestations of Lyme disease.
- Abandon the two-tier testing approach by eliminating the ELISA as a prescreening requirement before advancing to the Western Blot. The ELISA is too unreliable to be used as a preliminary screening test, given its extremely low sensitivity.
- Standardize national reporting forms by issuing brief, automated forms that will enable treating physicians to report cases easily. Reports should be held confidential and not disclosed to state medical boards or insurance companies and their service organizations in order to remove the physicians' fear of adverse consequences from treating patients with Lyme borreliosis.

2. Differentiate between the criteria for surveillance and clinical diagnosis. Once sufficient data have been gathered to form valid conclusions with respect to symptoms of Lyme borreliosis, develop a working clinical case definition for broad application within the medical community. Immediately, the CDC should inform all health service providers and health departments that the surveillance case definition is not intended to be used in clinical diagnosis.

3. Improve diagnostics by developing definitive, reproducible tests with a sensitivity of 95% or higher, that can detect active and latent infection of *Bb* and other tick-borne infections. The test should be reliable enough to be part of an annual physical examination.

4. Design a national survey. While both NatCapLyme and CALDA have conducted informal surveys which yielded useful information, their results point to the need for an unbiased national scientifically valid survey that collects reliable data on the experience of those suffering from Lyme and other tick-borne infections. Include the patient community in designing the survey.

5. Broaden clinical trials to include patients with persistent Lyme borreliosis. These patients are at the heart of the Lyme controversy. Broaden the entrance criteria for government-funded clinical trials to include entire classes of Lyme patients, whose disease expression and treatment response are poorly understood.

6. Base research grants for tick-borne infections on a non-biased approach. Given the recognized controversy over treatment of Lyme and other tick-borne infections, priority should be given to fund new researchers with innovative ideas and methods that would help to settle this controversy.
   - Many in the Lyme community believe that the Bayh-Dole Act of 1980 ultimately hindered advancement in Lyme disease research. Notably, the Alzheimer's Disease Neuroimaging Initiative (ADNI) researchers recently discovered significant new biomarkers. Under

the ADNI, researchers agree to share all data, make every finding public immediately, and renounce ownership and patent rights accruing to any individual researcher. According to Dr. John Trojanowski, a researcher at the University of Pennsylvania, ". . . we all realized that we would never get biomarkers unless all of us parked our egos and intellectual-property noses outside the door" (Kolata, 2010). NatCapLyme strongly advocates adoption of this model in the field of Lyme disease research.

- Conduct treatment trials that better mirror the variety of treatment regimens actually used by treating physicians.
- Research the unique attributes of *Bb* including multiple life forms and the incredible survivability of this organism in the host, genetic complexity, cell-wall deficient forms, its capacity for intercellular sequestration, antigenic variation, immune suppression, and the possible role of borrelial colonies and biofilms.
- Research the complex disease resulting from multiple tick-borne infections.

7. Create dialogue among the scientific research community, health agencies, medical societies, and the full spectrum of treating physicians, including those who view Lyme borreliosis and tick-borne diseases as a potential persistent and infectious process. NatCapLyme encourages all parties interested in Lyme and tick-borne diseases to work together to find solutions. NatCapLyme believes that true solutions to the dilemma of Lyme and tick-borne infections may be found only when all parties are willing to consider the views that each seeks to contribute.

8. Respect patients' right to choose treatment. Medical guidelines are designed to provide recommendations and not mandates. No monolithic treatment solution should be offered for such an unresolved area of medical research. While the overuse of antibiotics is a concern to all, some Lyme patients are reporting benefit from longer-term and combination antibiotic therapy.

9. Design a National Informed Consent Form to protect the patients' right to choose as well as protect the doctors' right to treat. The consent form should reflect fair and balanced treatment options and the benefits and risks of both short-term and long-term treatment choices. The committee that writes this should include medical and legal professionals who hold varied and conflicting points of view. This consent form must not favor any single treatment protocol. It should only include information necessary for fully informed patients to exercise their right to choose treatment.

10. Conduct Institute of Medicine Workshop on tick-borne infections, Part II. This workshop should address effective treatments for persistent and assimilated Lyme disease.

Our committee would be happy to discuss further these recommendations and the experiences of Lyme and tick-borne disease patients that led to our conclusions. We were asked to provide the IOM committee with insight into the patient experience. We concluded that a simple cathartic expression of the angst and suffering of patients and their families would be useless, unless it was combined with insights into the research and science that further illuminates that experience. There is an urgent need to broaden our understanding of tick-borne infections. It is our hope that the scientific community will address the chronic forms seriously and effectively, so that many more of Lyme victims will be able to return to useful, productive lives and the pursuit of happiness.

The National Capital Lyme and Tick-borne Disease Association thanks the Institute of Medicine committee members for allowing us to offer you the experience, thoughts, concerns, and needs of Lyme patients. Our hope is that the work of this committee will result in better care for patients and continued research to find a cure for this disease. We look forward to continuing to work with all governmental agencies and the medical community in hopes of finding successful treatment for all patients with tick-borne diseases.

**The NatCapLyme Working Group:** Monte Skall, Executive Director, NatCapLyme; Don Boileau, Professor; Barbara Cohen, Psychologist; Cindy Eisenhart, School Librarian; Susan Green, Attorney; Janis Ivicic, School Teacher; Helene Jorgensen, Economist; Linda Lobes, Advocate; Bill Merrigan, Legislative Attorney; Mimi Segal, Clinical Social Worker; Gregg Skall, Attorney; Lisa Torrey, Tick-Borne Disease Advocate; Joy Walker, Law Student; Judith Weeg, former CDC Health Educator; Sharon Whitehouse, Editor; Diane Wilcox, Professor.

**Acknowledgment:** We would like to thank the following organizations for their contributions to this paper: Lyme Disease United Coalition, Judith Weeg, President; Michigan Lyme Disease Association, Linda Lobes, President; National Tick-borne Disease Advocates, Lisa Torrey, President; and Parents of Children with Lyme.

**Correspondence:** Monte Skall, Executive Director, National Capital Lyme and Tick-borne Disease Association; phone: 703-821-8833; e-mail: Natcaplyme@natcaplyme.org.

## References

Aguero-Rosenfeld, M. E., G. Wang, I. Schwartz, and G. P. Wormser. 2005. Diagnosis of Lyme borreliosis. *Clinical Microbiology Reviews* 18(3):484-509.

Aucott, J., C. Morrison, B. Munoz, P. C. Rowe, A. K. Schwarzwalder, and S. West. 2009. Diagnostic challenges of early Lyme disease: Lessons from a community case series. *BMC Infectious Diseases* 9(79):1-8.

Barbour, A. 1996. *Lyme disease: The cause, the cure, the controversy.* Baltimore and London: The Johns Hopkins University Press. xiii.

Bloom, B. J., P. M. Wyckoff, H. C. Meissner, and A. C. Steere. 1998. Neurocognitive abnormalities in children after classic manifestations of Lyme disease. *Pediatric Infectious Disease Journal* 17(3):189-96.

CALDA (California Lyme Disease Association). 2009. *Lyme Policy Wonk: CALDA survey results are in!* (Attachment titled Surveysummary_09102009_blog_attach_872443128. pdf). http://www.lymedisease.org/news/lymepolicywonk/198.html (accessed July 15, 2010).

CDC (Centers for Disease Control and Prevention). 2004. Lyme disease-United States, 2001-2002. *Morbidity and Mortality Weekly Report* 53(17):365-9.

CDC, Division of Vector-Borne Infectious Diseases. 2006. *Average annual incidence of reported cases of Lyme disease by age group and sex, United States, 1999-2004.* http://www.cdc.gov/ncidod/dvbid/lyme/ld_MeanAnnualIncidence.htm (accessed July 2, 2010).

CDC, National Center for Public Health Informatics. 2010a. *Lyme disease (Borrelia burgdorferi). 2008 case definition.* http://www.casedef/lyme_disease_2008.htm (accessed July 17, 2010).

CDC, National Institute for Occupational Safety and Health. 2010b. *NIOSH Safety and Health Topics: Tick-borne diseases.* http://www.cdc.gov/niosh/topics/tick-borne/ (accessed July 28, 2010).

Depietropaolo, D. L., J. H. Powers, J. M. Gill, and A. Foy. 2005. Diagnosis of Lyme disease. *American Family Physician* 72(2):297-304.

DeVol, R., and A. Bedroussian. 2007. *An unhealthy America: The economic burden of chronic disease.* Santa Monica, CA: Milken Institute.

Donta, S. T. 1997. Tetracycline therapy for chronic Lyme disease. *Clinical Infectious Diseases* 25(Suppl 1):S52–6.

Duray, P. H. 1989. Clinical pathologic correlations of Lyme disease by stage. *Reviews of Infectious Diseases* 11(Suppl.6):S1487-93.

Edlow, J. A. 2003. *Bull's-eye: Unraveling the medical mystery of Lyme disease.* New Haven and London: Yale University Press. 197-8, 253.

Fallon, B. A., J. G. Keilp, K. M. Corbera, E. Petkova, C. B. Britton, E. Dwyer, I. Slavov, J. Cheng, J. Dobkin, D. R. Nelson, and H. A. Sackeim. 2008. A randomized, placebo-controlled trial of repeated IV antibiotic therapy for Lyme encephalopathy. *Neurology* 70(13):992-1003.

Green, C. 2009. Challenge to the clinical definition of late Lyme disease and post-Lyme disease syndrome. Unpublished paper. Los Altos, CA: Green Oaks Medical Center.

Jorgensen, H. 2010. *Sick and tired: How America's health care system fails its patients.* Sausalito, CA: Polipoint Press.

Kolata, G. 2010. Sharing of data leads to progress on Alzheimer's. *The New York Times,* August 13. http://www.nytimes.com/2010/08/13/health/research/13alzheimer.html (accessed August 13, 2010).

Klempner, M. S., L. T. Hu, J. Evans, C. H. Schmid, G. M. Johnson, R. P. Trevino, D. Norton, L. Levy, D. Wall, J. McCall, M. Kosinski, and A. Weinstein. 2001. Two controlled trials of antibiotic treatment in patients with persistent symptoms and a history of Lyme disease. *New England Journal of Medicine* 345(2):85-92.

Krause, P. J., S. R. Telford, A. Spielman, V. Sikand, R. Ryan, D. Christianson, G. Burke, P. Brassard, R. Pollack, J. Peck, and D. H. Persing. 1996. Concurrent Lyme disease and babesiosis. Evidence for increased severity and duration of illness. *JAMA* 275(2):1657-60.

Krupp, L. B., L. G. Hyman, R. Grimson, P. K. Coyle, P. Melville, S. Ahnn, R. Dattwyler, and B. Chandler. 2003. Study and treatment of post Lyme disease (STOP-LD): A randomized double masked clinical trial. *Neurology* 60(12):1923-30.

Landro, L. 2010, More tick infections begin at home. *The Wall Street Journal*, August 2. http://online.wsj.com/article/SB10001424052748703999304575399234058978228. html?KEYWORDS=Landro (accessed August 2, 2010).

Pachner, A. R. 1995. Early disseminated Lyme disease: Lyme meningitis. *American Journal of Medicine* 98(4A):30S-43S.

Pachner, A. R., K. Amemiya, M. Bartlett, H. Schaefer, K. Reddy, and W. F. Zhang. 2001. Lyme borreliosis in rhesus macaques: effects of corticosteroids on spirochetal load and isotype switching of anti-borrelia burgdorferi antibody. *Clinical and Diagnostic Laboratory Immunology* 8(2):225-32.

Samanta, A., M. M. Mello, C. Foster, J. Tingle, and J. Samanta. 2006. The role of clinical guidelines in medical negligence litigation: A shift from the Bolam standard? *Medical Law Review* 14(3):321-66.

Sapi, E., J. Bober, M. Montagna, M. Raman, M. Reddy, M. Hessberger, and A. Melillo. 2009. *Prevalence of tick-borne pathogens in Ixodes scapularis ticks from southern Connecticut.* Unpublished paper. New Haven, CT: New Haven University, CT.

Steere, A. C. 1989. Lyme disease. *New England Journal of Medicine* 321(9):586-96.

Tager, F. A., B. A. Fallon, J. Keilp, M. Rissenberg, C. R. Jones, and M. R. Liebowitz. 2001. A controlled study of cognitive deficits in children with chronic Lyme disease. *Journal Neuropsychiatry and Clinical Neurosciences* 13(4):500-7.

Tibbles, C. D., and J. A. Edlow. 2007. Does this patient have erythema migrans? *JAMA* 297(23):2617-27.

Wilcox, D. M., and C. Uram. 2009. *The impact of chronic Lyme disease on workplace performance: A survey of chronic Lyme patients.* (Addendum of tables and charts). Paper presented at the International Lyme and Associated Diseases Society Conference 2009, National Harbor, MD.

Wilson, A. A. 2009. *Under Our Skin.* Open Eye Pictures, Inc. http://underourskin.com/blog/?p=191 (Accessed August 5, 2010).

Wormser, G. P., R. J. Dattwyler, E. D. Shapiro, J. J. Halperin, A. C. Steere, M. S. Klempner, P. J. Krause, J. S. Bakken, F. Strle, G. Stanek, L. Bockenstedt, D. Fish, J. S. Dumler, and R. B. Nadelman. 2006. The clinical assessment, treatment, and prevention of Lyme disease, human granulocytic anaplasmosis, and babesiosis: Clinical practice guidelines by the Infectious Diseases Society of America. *Clinical Infectious Diseases* 43:1089-134.

Zhang, X., M. I. Meltzer, C. A. Pena, A. B. Hopkins, L. Wroth, and A.D. Fix. 2006. Economic impact of Lyme disease. *Emerging Infectious Diseases* 12(4):653-60.

## A4
## DIAGNOSIS OF TICK-BORNE DISEASES:
## *BORRELIA BURGDORFERI, BABESIA MICROTI,*
## AND *ANAPLASMA PHAGOCYTOPHILUM*

*David H. Persing, M.D., Ph.D.*
*Chief Medical and Technology Officer*
*Cepheid*
*Sunnyvale, CA*
*Consulting Professor of Pathology*
*Department of Pathology, Stanford University School of Medicine*

### Abstract

Lyme disease is the most common tick-borne zoonotic infection in the northern hemisphere. It is a complex multisystem disorder that may involve single or multiple organ systems. Infection with the causative agent, the spirochete *Borrelia burgdorferi*, may involve the skin, central and peripheral nervous systems, as well as targets within the cardiovascular and musculoskeletal systems. Patients at risk for Lyme disease are also at risk of acquiring infection or coinfection with other agents transmitted by the same tick vector, including *Babesia microti* and *Anaplasma phagocytophilum*. Since infection with all three agents can manifest initially as a nonspecific febrile illness with or without specific organ system involvement, the clinical diagnosis of a presenting patient can be challenging. Laboratory methods for detection of and discrimination among these infections are of significant value in the clinical evaluation of such patients. This review will describe the curious convergence of these tick-borne infections and the diagnostic challenges they pose, and will detail the laboratory procedures that can be used to decipher the complex array of diagnostic possibilities.

### Introduction

Although significant progress has been made over the past several decades in understanding the immunobiology of Lyme disease and in increasing awareness that this disease is an important public health problem, much about the disease still remains puzzling. Its pathogenesis is still poorly understood, and the interdependent problems of diagnosing the disease accurately and assessing therapeutic outcomes confound one another. One of the most curious aspects of Lyme disease in humans has been its inconsistent presentation, in terms of both disease severity and organ system involvement (Malawista and Steere, 1986; Rahn, 1991; Steere, 2001). By far, the most consistent finding is erythema migrans, often accompanied by a nonspecific febrile illness. However, even these findings may be absent or unrecognized in many cases, and subclinical or self-limiting infections may occur in a substantial proportion of exposed persons. Within a few weeks to months of infection, a wide array of signs may appear that affect certain subsets of infected patients. These signs (in roughly descending order) include arthritis, lymphadenopathy, meningitis, cranial neuritis (including Bell's palsy), myopericarditis, nonexudative sore throat, mild transient or recurrent hepatitis, and, less commonly, pancarditis, ocular involvement, and adult respiratory distress syndrome. Years after the onset of disease, occasional patients may develop migratory musculoskeletal disorders along with persistent malaise and fatigue or chronic encephalomyelitis (Logigian et al., 1990). These complications usually respond to therapies directed against *Borrelia burgdorferi*, but some patients have delayed responses and others do not respond at all.

In the United States, the apicomplexan blood parasite *Babesia microti* and the more recently recognized agent of human granulocytic anaplasmosis (HGA) are also transmitted by the deer tick (Pancholi et al., 1995; Spielman, 1976; Spielman et al., 1979; Telford et al., 1996). Both infections appear to be most intensely enzootic in established Lyme disease-endemic habitats, and Lyme disease coinfection with one or both of these organisms has been described in most of these areas in the upper Midwest and northeastern United States. In general, cardinal symptoms of babesiosis and anaplasmosis are often absent in co-infected patients, such that co-infected patients can be difficult to distinguish objectively from patients with uncomplicated Lyme disease. However, because the three infections may require different approaches to treatment, an understanding of the natural history of infection with *Babesia* and *Anaplasma* may become critical for understanding the biological variation of human Lyme disease and determining optimal medical management for affected patients. For these and other reasons, considerable effort in several laboratories has gone into further defining the transmission cycles of these agents, developing serological and molecular markers of infection for all three pathogens, propagating all three pathogens from human sources, and defining the extent of human exposure to these pathogens (Reviewed in Persing, 1997).

Several other tick-borne pathogens have been described in recent years, including the agent of human monocytic ehrlichiosis (reviewed in Bakken and Dumler, 2000) (Dumler et al., 2007; Thomas et al., 2009) and a novel babesia species *(B. duncani)* which is found primarily in the western U.S. (Persing et al., 1995; Quick et al., 1993). However, these organisms do not appear to be enzootic with Lyme disease and are not part of the Lyme disease transmission cycle. As a result, coinfection of these organisms with *B. burgdorferi*, though not impossible, is much less likely. The diagnosis of infection with these organisms should be considered on the basis of likelihood within their respective endemic areas, but the focus of this review will be on agents that are proven to be part of the Lyme disease ecology.

## B. microti Infection

B. microti infection has been diagnosed in residents of many areas in the northeastern and northern midwestern United States where Lyme disease is prevalent (Homer et al., 2000a; Krause et al., 2003; Pruthi et al., 1995; Vannier and Krause, 2009). It is interesting to note that B. microti was once considered to be a possible agent of Lyme disease, since many patients with babesiosis presented with an erythema migrans-like rash at the site of a deer tick bite. The initial symptoms of both illnesses somewhat overlap: like Lyme disease, babesiosis in humans often presents with non-specific symptoms including fever, fatigue, and other flu-like symptoms. Hemolytic anemia, which lasts from several days to a few months, may occur in patients with clinically severe cases, most commonly asplenic or elderly patients. However, most cases of human babesiosis in normosplenic, immunocompetent patients are probably subclinical and occur as a self-limiting illness (Krause et al., 1996d; Ruebush et al., 1977).

Seroepidemiological data suggest that ~10% of Lyme disease patients in Connecticut and perhaps even higher proportions of such patients in other areas have been exposed to B, microti (Filstein et al., 1980; Krause et al., 1991). However, these two studies did not provide proof of coinfection (vs. sequential infection) with both agents, because they were conducted retrospectively, and specimens for the direct demonstration of both pathogens were not collected. A prospective study by Krause et al. (Krause et al., 1996d) provided more convincing evidence of simultaneous infection with B. burgdorferi and B. microti in substantial numbers of patients with presumptive Lyme disease from coastal New England. Although not usually recognized as coinfected on clinical grounds, patients harboring both organisms often had more severe disease and a higher likelihood of persistent post-infectious fatigue.

Since antibiotic therapy for early Lyme disease is unlikely to be effective against coinfection with B. microti, it is easy to envision a scenario in which underlying babesiosis is responsible for the persistence of symptoms after therapy for early Lyme disease. However, since the clinical presentation is nonspecific, it will be difficult to know at the time of presentation whether a patient would benefit from therapy targeting babesial coinfection. The risks associated with antibabesial therapy such as atovaquone plus clindamycin are not insignificant, and given a low probability of coinfection, presumptive diagnosis and therapy would not appear to be warranted even in the most heavily endemic areas. It is important to note that the converse scenario does not appear to be true: among patients with case defined chronic fatigue syndrome and no history of antecedent Lyme disease, there is no evidence supporting a major role of coinfection with *B. burgdorferi* and/or *B. microti* (Macdonald et al., 1996). A more conservative approach would employ selective testing of patients, who based on clinical, epidemiological, and initial laboratory evaluations, may be at higher risk of coinfection (see below).

## Human Granulocytic Anaplasmosis

In 1994, Bakken et al. (Bakken et al., 1994) described a nonspecific febrile illness among patients in the Upper Midwest that was characterized by, thrombocytopenia, and neutrophilic inclusions (morulae). Genetic and serological analyses of patients' blood samples indicated that the agent of human granulocytic ehrlichiosis was closely related to *Ehrlichia equi* and *Ehrlichia phagocytophila*. Infections caused by a similar or identical agent were subsequently described in many states including New York, Connecticut, Massachusetts, Rhode Island, Minnesota, Wisconsin, and California (reviewed in Bakken and Dumler, 2000) (Dumler et al., 2007; Thomas et al., 2009). Since then, phylogenetic analyses have determined that the agent of human granulocytic ehrlichiosis is more closely related to the genus *Anaplasma* and the infection is now referred to as human granulocytic anaplasmosis (HGA) (Dumler et al., 2007).

The report of a case of HGA that occurred following a deer tick bite (Pancholi et al., 1995), together with recognition of the apparent overlap between areas where Lyme disease and HGA are endemic, prompted an investigation into whether the deer tick could also transmit HGA. *Ixodes* ticks collected from fields in several locations in Wisconsin where HGA cases have been described were analyzed retrospectively; the collection obtained from Wisconsin in 1993 and an earlier collection stored in alcohol since 1982 both contained *A. phagocytophilum*-infected PCR-positive specimens. Just as retrospective epidemiological studies of *B. burgdorferi* demonstrated the presence of pathogen DNA in suitable vectors (Persing et al., 1990b) or reservoirs (Marshall et al., 1994a) from historic specimens, the existence of the agent of HGA clearly preceded the first descriptions of the disease itself. Indeed, the increased incidence of HGA is likely to be due, in part, to the emergence of its recognition. In a subsequent study, Telford et al. (Telford et al., 1996) showed that the deer tick is competent to transmit an agent of HGA that was recovered from a patient on Nantucket Island. *Ixodes pacificus* may be the vector of HGA in the western United States; this tick is the primary vector of *E. equi,* which is the agent of HGA.

*Immunomodulatory Effects of* Babesia *and* Anaplasma: *Impact on Diagnostic Markers?*

The elucidation of the immunologic interplay of the microbial agents that exist with the transmission cycle of Lyme disease is likely to yield a better understanding of what can be expected in occasional human cases. In the case of multiple pathogens that coexist within a rodent reservoir involved in overlapping transmission cycles (as is the case for *B. burgdorferi, B. microti,* the HGA agent, and perhaps other organisms), it is reasonable to hypothesize that immune responses to one organism may have an impact on concurrent infections, especially if the underlying infection is associated with immune suppression. Infections by both *Babesia* and *Anaplasma* species are associated with substantial immunosuppressive or immunomodulatory effects (reviewed in Persing, 1997). Coinfection by the agent of HGA and *B. burgdorferi* or by *B. microti* and B. *burgdorferi* could have substantial theoretical effects on the immune response, but the practical questions are these: Are disease outcomes altered, and are immunologic effects severe enough to alter immune responses so that they can no longer be used as reliable indicators of infection?

Animal models are helpful in answering these questions. Consistent with the above predictions, experimental coinfection of *a* mouse model with *B. burgdorferi* and *A. phagocytophilum* increased the number of CD4+ cells and drove the cytokine responses toward a Th1 lymphocyte response (Zeidner et al., 2000). In another animal model, coinfection with *B. burgdorferi* and *A. phagocytophilum* led to increased pathogen burden in blood and tissue, and to more severe *Borrelia*-induced arthritis than single infection with *B. burgdorferi* alone (Thomas et al., 2001). However, during coinfection, levels of IL-12, gamma interferon, and tumor necrosis factor in serum were paradoxically decreased whereas levels of IL-6 were elevated. A similar study of coinfection in C3H/HeN mice evaluated the tissue distribution of tick-transmitted *B. burgdorferi* and *A. phagocytophilum* infection by quantitative PCR (Holden et al., 2005). Coinfected animals had increased spirochetal burdens in multiple tissues but *Anaplasma* numbers (found primarily in blood) remained constant. Although antibody responses were diminished somewhat for *A. phagocytophilum*, levels of antibody that developed against *B. burgdorferi* were not affected.

Although coinfection with *B. burgdorferi* and *B. microti* was found to be associated with increased disease severity and greater likelihood of spirochetemia in human subjects enrolled in a blinded clinical evaluation, experimental evidence of increased severity in animal models has been mixed. Initial studies showed immunologic effects of coinfection in some mouse strains but not others. C3H mice showed no evidence of increased severity, but normally Lyme disease-resistant Balb/c mice showed an increase in arthritis severity at day 30, along with reductions in levels of immunosuppressive cytokines IL-10 and IL-13 (Moro et al., 2006). Another mouse model showed that dual infection with *B. burgdorferi* and *B. microti* appeared to follow independent courses, with no apparent increase in Lyme disease severity (Coleman et al., 2005), although mouse strains used and inoculation times differed between the two studies. In both studies, serological responses to both agents appeared to be largely unaffected by coinfection.

Taken together, the data from animal models and human clinical studies suggest that coinfection with *A. phagocytophilum* and/or *B. microti* may have immunological effects during the course of *B. burgdorferi* infection, but these effects are not in themselves sufficient to completely abrogate cellular or humoral immune responses to the point of complicating the sero-diagnosis of Lyme disease. Likewise, the presence of concomitant infection with *B. burgdorferi* does not appear to suppress immune responses to either the HGA agent or *B. microti* to the point that infection cannot be detected in diagnostic assays. *A. phagocytophilum* infection may be associated with false positive serologic responses to *B. burgdorferi,* (Hofmeister et al., 1996; Wormser et al., 1996), but not false negative responses.

### Clinical and Initial Laboratory Evaluation of Tick-Borne Diseases

For patients exposed to ticks in areas where multiple tick-borne pathogens are endemic, it seems reasonable for clinicians to be aware of clinical signs that may be consistent with each infection alone or in combination, especially when patients with Lyme disease fail to respond promptly to antibiotic therapy. Patients with uncomplicated erythema migrans, without systemic symptoms, may require no further laboratory-based evaluation and can be treated presumptively for Lyme disease in many cases. More severe presentations may merit closer scrutiny. Symptoms including nausea and/or vomiting, fever, chills, sweats, severe malaise, and a delayed clinical response to antibiotic therapy for presumptive Lyme disease were characteristic of *Babesia*-co infected patients (Krause et al., 1996d). Fever, chills, myalgias, and severe headache are characteristic of granulocytic anaplasmosis (Thomas et al., 2009). Carditis has been described as a complication of Lyme disease, but has also been described in patients with HGA without evidence of *B. burgdorferi* infection (Jahangir et al., 1998).

Initial laboratory evaluations to be considered include examination of blood smears for the presence of intraerythrocytic inclusions (merozoites) typical of babesial infection and granulocytic morulae typical of HGA. However, the sensitivity of blood smear evaluations for immunocompetent, normosplenic patients has not been firmly established and may be relatively low for both diseases (see below). The presence of elevated liver enzymes or hematologic abnormalities may be especially useful in identifying coinfected patients, since both babesiosis and anaplasmosis have been associated with increases in the levels of alanine aminotransferase. Thromocytopenia may also be present in patients with either disease, but it is rarely a feature of uncomplicated Lyme disease. Thus, the presence of thromobocytopenia in patients presenting with early Lyme disease should trigger a suspicion of coinfection with one or the other agent.

*Laboratory Diagnosis of Tick-Borne Zoonoses*

In general terms, the available laboratory methods for the diagnosis of the tick-borne diseases described here fall into two categories: 1) Direct methods (microscopy, culture, or PCR, depending on the agent), and 2) indirect methods (detection of organism-specific immune responses). With some notable exceptions, direct methods are generally useful for characterization of acute or active infections, whereas detection of antibody responses is most useful for confirmation of clinical suspicion in post-acute and convalescent phases.

Irrespective of the diagnostic method used, an important consideration is the pre-test probability of infection. Since Lyme disease, HGA and human babesiosis are all characterized initially by seasonal occurrence of a non-specific febrile illness, the likelihood of tick-bite or tick exposure, guided by prevalence information for each of the infectious agents, should be a critical gating item for physician test ordering. Unfortunately, *I. scapularis* tick exposure is fairly common, and all three agents have been described in most of the areas endemic for Lyme disease, so laboratory testing plays an unusually prominent role in the diagnosis. However, since all of the laboratory methods currently in use have been shown to give rise to false-positive results, the positive predictive values of each of these methods may reach unacceptable levels, particularly when a multiplicity of tests is ordered. According to a recent treatment guideline from the American College of Physicians and the IDSA, patients with vague subjective complaints (headache, fatigue, and myalgia in the absence of respiratory symptoms) apart from other risk factors are at low risk for Lyme disease. They recommend against routine testing of such patients because the odds of a false positive result are greater than for obtaining a true positive result (Tugwell et al., 1997; Wormser et al., 2000b). Likewise, for patients with nonspecific persistent fatigue without a history of Lyme disease, even if living in or near endemic areas, seroprevalence rates for HGA and *B. microti* are low and these organisms are unlikely to be implicated (Macdonald et al., 1996).

*Hematologic Evaluation*

The complete blood count (CBC) with a manual differential (direct blood smear evaluation by a medical technologist) can be an extremely useful tool in the initial evaluation of patients with nonspecific presentations. blood counts and peripheral blood smears along with tests of liver function. Leukopenia, lymphopenia, granulocytopenia, and especially thrombocytopenia are found in HGA. Granulocytopenia is less commonly associated with uncomplicated Lyme disease but has been described in some cases. Anemia and hemolysis are more common in babesiosis, and especially thrombocytopenia is frequently evident in babesiosis and HGA infections.

Babesiosis and HGA can diagnosed directly by observing organisms on Giemsa-stained smears of peripheral blood. For patients with intact spleens, erythrocytes may show *B. microti* ring forms on thin blood smears; this proportion may be as high as 80% for asplenic patients (Homer et al., 2000a; Meldrum et al., 1992; Vannier and Krause, 2009). In one study (Krause et al., 1996b), most patients coinfected with *Borrelia* and *Babesia* species were smear negative for babesiosis at the time of presentation and at all time points thereafter.

Blood smear evaluation has been advocated for the diagnosis of HGA when the index of suspicion is high (Bakken and Dumler, 2006; Dumler et al., 2007; Thomas et al., 2009), but detection by this route is unlikely unless the examining technologist is alerted to the possibility of HGA. Moreover, visual inspection of blood smears for the length of time required to find a single morula may be impractical. In one study, a small subset of HGA patients with mild infection had intragranulocytic morulae detected on smears (Belongia et al., 2001), in contrast with symptomatic, untreated patients whose smear results were evaluated after several days of fever (Bakken et al., 1994). The blood smear evaluation for HGA should be carried out within a week of disease onset, as sensitivity is highest at this time (Bakken and Dumler, 2006). Blood samples should be collected prior to administering doxycycline therapy since morulae are eliminated from the blood within 24–72 h after the start of therapy (Thomas et al., 2009). However, the since the sensitivity for detecting *A. phagocytophilum* is only 25–75%, blood smear evaluation is useful if the results are positive but not particularly helpful if the results are negative.

False-positive results are possible; artifacts such as platelets superimposed on red cells or Howell-Jolly bodies can appear like *Babesia* (Matthews et al., 2003); and to an untrained eye, a well-separated nuclear segment within a neutrophil may give the appearance of a morula. Acridine orange stain, which intercalates into double stranded DNA, can help enhance detection of *B. microti* inclusions in red cells and avoid detection of platelet artifacts.

*Direct Detection Methods*

*Direct Detection of* B. burgdorferi

For direct detection of *B. burgdorferi*, a variety of approaches have been used in the clinical or research laboratories, including microscopic evaluation of tissues, detection of *B. burgdorferi*-specific proteins (by EIA or by immunohistochemistry) or nucleic acids (by PCR), and in vitro cultivation. Direct microscopic detection of *B. burgdorferi* has limited usefulness because of low throughput, low organism abundance in tissues (such as skin biopsies) that are confirmed positive by other methods, and the requirement for silver staining and a skilled operator. Antigen detection assays for detection of *B. burdorferi* have suffered similar limitations; although *B. burgdorferi* antigens can be detected by immunohistochemistry in tissues and by EIA within specimens from confined anatomical sites such as cerebrospinal fluid (CSF) and synovial fluid, where clearance of antigens is limited. Their presence in other samples such as urine has been more controversial (Dorward et al., 1991) (Hyde et al., 1989) (Klempner et al., 2001b) and has not stood up well to additional scrutiny. In contrast, culture and PCR techniques do appear to be diagnostically useful in certain circumstances, and we will limit the remainder of this section to these methods.

Culture-based methods for detection of *B. burgdorferi* were used for the initial establishment of the etiologic basis of Lyme disease, and have been used on and off for decades in the evaluation of various clinical samples for research protocols. However, their use for clinical diagnosis has been hampered by long incubation times, poor sensitivity (with the possible exception of skin biopsies from EM), and limited availability of the specialized growth medium for routine use.

The liquid media currently used for recovery of *B. burgdorferi* are modified versions of the original Kelly medium (Kelly, 1971) through various modifications made over time (Barbour, 1984) (Stoenner et al., 1982) (Barbour, 1986). The most commonly used medium (Barbour-Stoenner-Kelly II) is commercially available and is used for direct recovery of spirochetes from clinical specimens including plasma, CSF, whole blood and skin biopsies. Since serum supplementation is required for this medium, one source of variability in the efficiency of spirochete recovery has been the presence of anti-spirochetal antibodies in the serum (Pollack et al., 1993). Cultures are visually inspected by darkfield microscopy or after staining with specific antibodies or intercalating dyes. With newer modified media protocols, spirochetes can be detected within 5-7 days, but they may require incubation for up to three months at 30-34°C.

Recent studies of high-volume inoculation of whole blood or plasma have been surprisingly successful at recovering circulating spirochetes. For many years, rates of recovery of *B. burgdorferi* from blood samples collected from untreated patients with EM had been less than 5-10% (Wallach et al., 1993) (Steere et al., 1983). However, the inoculum volumes in these studies were generally small. Based on previous studies which showed that circulating bacteria in patients with sepsis are often rare, and that the volume of cultured blood is directly related to culture yield, a team of investigators at New York Medical College investigated the use of high volume inocula of blood or blood fractions. They showed the following: 1) recovery of *B. burgdorferi* was superior from serum or plasma compared to the same volume of whole blood (Wormser et al., 1998) and 2) the culture yields from plasma were significantly greater than that from serum (Wormser et al., 2000a). Recovery of *B. burgdorferi* from high-volume cultures (9 or more ml of plasma) inoculated into a modified BSK II medium was above 40%. However, increasing the volume of plasma from 9 ml to 18 ml for adult patients with EM met with diminishing returns; a mere 10% increase in culture yield was observed after doubling the inoculum volume (Wormser et al., 2000a).

PCR protocols for detection of *B. burgdorferi* have been in use since a few years after the description of PCR itself. PCR was initially promising as a study tool in studies of the retrospective epidemiology of *B. burgdorferi*, including detection of the organism in suitable tick vectors 30 years prior to the formal recognition of Lyme disease in the U.S. (Persing et al., 1990a) and in suitable animal reservoirs nearly a century earlier (Marshall et al., 1994b). However, its track record for dramatically improving the general lot of Lyme disease diagnostics has been more spotty, and in general disappointing (reviewed in Dumler, 2001), (Schmidt, 1997), (Aguero-Rosenfeld, 2003, 2008). A variety of chromosomal and/or plasmid targets have been used in the various PCR protocols with varying levels of sensitivity (Dumler, 2001), (Schmidt, 1997), (Aguero-Rosenfeld, 2003, 2008).

A number of studies have compared PCR to culture for detection of spirochetes in skin biopsies. Culture has proven to be roughly equivalent to PCR in several studies with a few exceptions (Moter et al., 1994) (Nowakowski et al., 2001) (Steere et al., 1998) as reviewed in (Aguero-Rosenfeld et al., 2005). Widely disparate results are likely to be attributable to differences in the various studies in the PCR protocols employed, including type of PCR and/or primer and target selection and/or method of tissue preservation, as well as differences in culture techniques, including size of the skin biopsy sample cultured and/or choice of culture medium. In one study of skin biopsy samples of 47 untreated patients with EM lesions, culture sensitivity was 51%, compared 81% by using a Taqman-based real-time PCR (Nowakowski et al., 2001).

In contrast to the experience with skin samples, the sensitivity of PCR for detection of *B. burgdorferi* in blood samples has been much lower in patients with EM (Goodman et al., 1995) (Oksi et al., 2001). In a prospective study of U.S. patients with EM, *B. burgdorferi* sensu stricto DNA was detected by PCR in only 14 of 76 (18.4%) plasma samples (Goodman et al., 1995). Detection of the spirochete in blood by PCR in blood samples for patients with disseminated disease has also been disappointing (Demaerschalck et al., 1995) (Liebling et al., 1993). This is likely due to the same issue that hampered early studies of culture in blood samples of Lyme disease patients, specifically the relative paucity of circulating spirochetes in the small volumes of blood that are typically extracted in a PCR procedure. Most PCR protocols test only 100 to 200 microliter samples, and these may simply be inadequate to capture enough circulating spirochetal DNA for detection, even by as sensitive a method as PCR. So it is no surprise that, given the relative lack of sensitivity of PCR in blood for detection of early, even disseminated disease, it would fare even more poorly in patients with later disease manifestations, despite positive serological findings in many of these patients (Klempner et al., 2001a).

Within anatomically confined compartments, PCR detection methods generally fare better. In a study of 60 U.S. patients with neuroborreliosis (16 with early and 44 with late neuroborreliosis), the sensitivity of PCR in CSF was 38% in early and 25% in late neuroborreliosis, and an inverse correlation was found between duration of antimicrobial treatment and PCR results (Nocton et al., 1996). In this study, four different PCR primer or probe sets were used, three targeting OspA genes and one targeting OspB genes, and concordance between the different assays was relatively poor which suggested low target number within the samples. Other studies from Europe have generated similar findings (Ornstein et al., 2002) (Lebech et al., 2000). Studies of synovial fluid, have provided the greatest clinical utility of PCR testing for the diagnosis of active Lyme arthritis and for monitoring the course of therapy (Aguero-Rosenfeld, 2008; Aguero-Rosenfeld et al., 2005; Bradley et al., 1994; Dumler, 2001; Eiffert et al., 1998; Jaulhac et al., 1996; Malawista et al., 1992; Nocton et al., 1994; Persing et al., 1994a). In a landmark study of 88 patients, *B. burgdorferi* DNA was detected in synovial fluid of 75 (85%) patients with Lyme arthritis (Nocton et al., 1994). Not surprisingly, the PCR detection rate was lower in patients who had received what should have been effective antibiotic therapy compared to untreated or undertreated patients. Of 73 patients who were untreated or treated with only short courses of oral antibiotics 70 (96%) had DNA detected by PCR in synovial fluid samples. In contrast, 7 of 19 (37%) patients who received either parenteral antibiotics or oral antibiotics for more than 1 month were still PCR positive (Nocton et al., 1994). The observation of higher sensitivity of PCR detection of plasmid-encoded OspA compared to multiple chromosomal loci (the 16S rRNA gene and flagellin) in synovial fluid specimens (Persing et al., 1994b; Nocton et al., 1994; Persing et al., 1994a) was referred to as "target imbalance." It has been speculated that

B. *burgdorferi* sensu stricto present in the synovium may selectively shed OspA DNA segments into the synovial fluid (Persing et al., 1994a). With the same or similar reagents, this phenomenon did not appear to occur in CSF specimens (Lebech et al., 1998).

A subsequent meta-analysis has largely confirmed the above assessment; it showed that PCR is a sensitive diagnostic tool for detection of B. *burgdorferi* DNA in skin biopsy and synovial fluid specimens whereas detection of the organism in blood or blood fractions and in CSF specimens is relatively low (Dumler, 2001). Given the paucity of supporting data for use of PCR as a diagnostic technique in samples other than skin and synovial fluid, extreme caution must be exercised in interpreting PCR test results from samples such as whole blood, urine, and cerebrospinal fluid. Even the best PCR laboratories have had problems with PCR amplicon contamination which, if sporadic, can give rise to undetected rates of false positive results which have been reported in a number of PCR assays, including those for B. *burgdorferi*. Because of the high credibility assigned to PCR by most clinicians, false positive PCR results can lead to inappropriate treatment and mismanagement, sometimes with fatal results (Molloy et al., 2001; Patel et al., 2000). Laboratories performing PCR should follow Good Laboratory Practices for controlling amplicon contamination, including strict separation of amplified material from areas where clinical samples are being prepared and inclusion of appropriate positive and negative controls in each run.

### Direct Detection of Babesia microti

*Babesia microti* has not been successfully grown in culture, despite multiple attempts, and animal inoculation of whole blood via the intraperitoneal route has been the mainstay of organism propagation for many years. This method is used primarily for organism isolation from patients with obvious parasitemia as demonstrated on Wright-Giemsa stained blood films, and it is limited for practical reasons to research laboratories. Hamster blood, which supports replication of B. *microti*, begins to show parasitemia at around day 7 after inoculation, and typically reaches peak levels at 2-3 weeks although samples with low numbers of parasites may take longer.

PCR has gained popularity as a diagnostic method, mainly for two reasons: 1) it provides good sensitivity levels and a broad dynamic range, making it suitable for parasitemic patients who are smear negative as well as smear positive, and 2) its turnaround time and general availability as a diagnostic procedure are far superior to comparable methods based on animal inoculation. Initial descriptions of PCR for detection of B. *microti* were based on conserved elements of the 18 S ribosomal gene, and showed that all strains of B. *microti* tested were reactive whereas DNA from *Plasmodium* and other related parasites were negative (Persing et al., 1992). The 3 hour method was much faster and easily 10- to 100-fold more sensitive than hamster inoculation when tested against a limiting dilution of parasites in whole blood (Persing et al., 1992). The same PCR assay was then used in several studies of babesial infection and co-infection with *B. burgdorferi* to demonstrate that it was more sensitive than blood smear evaluation for the diagnosis of babesial infection (Krause et al., 1996c) and that it could be used to detect *B. microti* infection in symptomatic and asymptomatic individuals including blood donors (Krause et al., 1998; Krause et al., 1996c; Krause et al., 1994; Krause et al., 1996b).

The utility of PCR for detection of *B. microti* was demonstrated in several prospective studies of exposed populations living in Block Island, RI, and Eastern Connecticut. Krause *et al* showed that patients with convincing evidence of simultaneous infection with *B. burgdorferi* and *B. microti* often had more severe disease and a higher likelihood of persistent post-infectious fatigue (Krause et al., 1996b). Coinfected patients also appeared to be more likely to be spirochetemic as determined by detection of *B. burgdorferi* DNA in their blood. In another landmark study (Krause et al., 1998), Krause *et al* showed 1) that patients with babesial infection often had prolonged and sometimes persistent parasitemia, as demonstrated by PCR, after primary infection, and 2) that many patients with primary infection with *B. microti* had infections that were subclinical and/or asymptomatic, and which, even if suspected, would not have been detected by blood smear evaluation (Krause et al., 1998). However, for practical purposes it has been found that virtually all patients who are symptomatic and PCR positive for *B. microti* are already also seropositive (Homer et al., 2000a; Krause et al., 1994), so the use of serologic methods, even in the initial diagnosis of babesial infection or coinfection with other tick borne organisms, is not unreasonable (see below).

These studies paved the way for a better understanding of the incidence of chronic, subclinical infection and the potential risk to the blood supply of blood donors who may unwittingly donate parasitemic blood to increasingly compromised populations including transplant patients, cancer patients, and other vulnerable recipients. Several studies have been done using serologic testing followed by PCR testing to identify asymptomatic carriers of *B. microti* in the blood donor population (Leiby et al., 2002; Leiby et al., 2005). In almost all cases, persons identified as asymptomatic carriers are blood smear negative and thus would have escaped detection upon routine examination, yet some of them are positive by hamster inoculation and all are considered potential persistent carriers of *B. microti*. In part due to the recent rise in the number of transfusion related deaths associated with *B. microti* infection, several new initiatives by the FDA and CDC are underway to institute screening measures by both serologic methods and PCR to detect asymptomatic donors in order to exclude infected units of blood from entering the U.S. blood supply (Leiby et al., 2002; Leiby et al., 2005). Because PCR may be able to detect parasitemia before serocoversion, it may play a pivotal role in such screening efforts.

### Direct Detection of Anaplasma phagocytophila

Direct cultivation of *Anaplasma phagocytophilum* was first accomplished by Goodman and colleagues (Goodman et al., 1996) in the few years after the first recognition the disease, by culture of whole blood in the promyelocytic leukemic cell line HL-60. Recovery of *A. phagocytophilum* from peripheral blood in cell culture can be used to definitively diagnose infection (Horowitz et al., 1998; Thomas et al., 2009). The bacteria develop within vacuoles to form morulae in the cytoplasm of infected cells, which can be detected using Wright or Giemsa staining. Intracellular organisms can be visualized as soon as 5 days postinoculation or can remain undetectable for more than 2 weeks. Culture of *A. phagocytophilum* in HL-60 cells is arguably the most sensitive method for the direct diagnosis of human anaplasmosis (HA), owing again to the relatively large volume of blood that can be analyzed compared to PCR methods (Aguero-Rosenfeld et al., 2000; Horowitz et al., 1998; Ravyn et al., 2001) However, as a routine diagnostic method, cell culture is rarely or ever used, and detection methods offered by most medical centers rely on demonstration of characteristic inclusion bodies on peripheral smears, immunoserologic methods, and PCR.

PCR is also a sensitive tool for detecting *A. phagocytophilum*. PCR was used early on to demonstrate the presence of the organism in blood samples and in initial studies that led to the identification of the deer tick as a vector (Pancholi et al., 1995). Several studies and reviews of the diagnostic performance of PCR for the diagnosis of HGA have been published (Aguero-Rosenfeld, 2003; Alberti and Sparagano, 2006; Comer et al., 1999; Krause et al., 2002; Walls et al., 2000). Sensitivity is approximately 67–90% for detecting *A. phagocytophilum* DNA (Horowitz et al., 1998), but just as for direct smear evaluation, the PCR sensitivity will likely be affected by the phase of infection and antibiotic therapy. After the first week, the bacteremic phase of infection rapidly wanes, thereby limiting the effectiveness of PCR as a diagnostic technique (Bakken and Dumler, 2006). In general, PCR positivity correlates with the concurrent presence of IgM antibodies and eventual IgG seroconversion.

### Immunodiagnostic Methods

For all of the tick-borne infections described here, the mainstay of the laboratory diagnosis is the detection of antibody responses in serum of affected individuals. Initial detection of organism-specific IgM antibodies during acute illness is accompanied by conversion to IgG during the convalescent phase, usually 10 to 14 days later. Serologic testing is more available than direct detection methods based on culture or PCR, and usually less expensive. Given the relative lack of sensitivity of direct detection methods, serologic testing is also usually more sensitive, especially for detection of *B. burgdorferi* infection. Multiple testing formats are available from commercial sources, including ELISA, IFA, and immunoblotting. This section will provide a summary of immunodiagnostic approaches for each of the three agents addressed by this review.

## B. burgdorferi

The regional antigenic variability and complexity of the antigenic components of *B. burgdorferi* have posed challenges for the serodiagnosis of LB. In Europe, Lyme borreliosis is caused primarily by the three species: *Borrelia burgdorferi* sensu stricto, *B. afzelii* and *B. garinii*. In the U.S., substantial genetic heterogeneity of *B. burgdorferi* sensu stricto exists, as assessed by pulsed-field gel electrophoresis (PFGE) typing, but the vast majority of human clinical isolates fall into a few closely related PFGE clusters of strains that have similar antigenic composition (Mathiesen et al., 1997). *B. burgdorferi* strains used in the U.S. for immunodiagnosis generally are drawn from these groups, so it is likely that sufficient serologic cross reactivity exists among these strains to allow for detection of antibody responses irrespective of the geographic location of the infection (Mathiesen et al., 1997). However, to complicate things, some immunodominant antigens or epitopes are expressed exclusively in vivo but not in cultures of organisms that are used to prepare antigens for diagnostic testing (Das et al., 1997) (Fikrig et al., 1997). This has led to the use of serological expression cloning to detect antigens that are expressed in vivo, which in some cases have led to the identification of diagnostically useful reagents.

Several initial studies of the immune response to *B. burgdorferi* recognized the flagellin protein as an immunodominant antigen that was recognized by IgG and IgM antibody subclasses within a few days of infection (Coleman and Benach, 1987; Craft et al., 1986). Unfortunately, the flagellin gene is conserved among multiple species of bacteria, so crossreactivity and nonspecific immune responses are quite common, especially on immunoblots where the protein is denatured (Fawcett et al., 1992) (Luft et al., 1993). Another immunodominant antigen recognized early during infection with *B. burgdorferi* sensu lato is the OspC protein which is encoded on a plasmid (Engstrom et al., 1995). OspC is upregulated by the spirochete while is still in the tick midgut and when it begins to migrate to the tick mouthparts prior to transmission. Some strains of *B. burgdorferi* cultured in vitro express little or no OspC; indeed, this antigen was unrecognized in early studies that used high-passage strains as the source of antigen. OspC is genetically and antigenically very heterogeneous (Theisen et al., 1993). Recently, conserved epitopes within the OspC protein have been identified comprising the C-terminal 10 amino acids of OspC (pepC10) (Mathiesen et al., 1998). Inclusion of this peptide in immunoassays may be an important step toward developing improved immunodiagnostic assays for Lyme disease (see below).

The so-called Vmp-like sequence expressed (VlsE) protein, a hypervariable immunodominant surface lipoprotein encoded by a linear plasmid, was described in conjunction with expression cloning experiments (Zhang et al., 1997a; Zhang and Norris, 1998a, 1998b). Although subject to extensive antigenic variation, presumably because of immunological pressure, within the variable regions a constant domain was identified called IR6 (or C6). Peptide mapping of this region showed that it is highly immunogenic (Lawrenz et al., 1999). Broad conservation of this region across multiple species of *B. burgdorferi* sensu lato have suggested that it would make a good immunodiagnostic reagent, and several studies have now been published that support its use alone or in combination with other immunodominant peptides. Several other antigens have been identified for potential immunodiagnostic use, including decorin binding protein (DBP1) (Heikkila et al., 2002) and a fibronectin binding protein (BBK32) (Fikrig et al., 2000).

## Testing Formats

Over the years, many commercial immunoassays to detect *B. burgdorferi* antibodies have been cleared for use in the United States by the Food and Drug Administration (FDA). Most of these assays use the B31 type strain of *B. burgdorferi* as the source of antigen, but several newer assays have employed recombinant antigens and/or peptides. In general, performance of these tests on blinded proficiency surveys of laboratories across the U.S. has been good, but a significant degree of performance variation still exists between test manufacturers and test methods (unpublished observation from 2009 CAP surveys). One potential source of variability is the method used for antigen preparation. For immunoassays using whole cell preparations, a surprising amount of antigenic variability will be encountered depending on growth conditions, medium used, incubation temperatures, growth phase of the organisms, and methods used to extract antigens, concentrate them and link them to specific substrates for test preparation. Lot-to-lot reproducibility and quality control are major concerns for methods based on whole cell lysates. In contrast, methods based on recombinant proteins or peptides are better defined and may lead to more lot consistency, but the presence of one or a few epitopes poses a different kind of limitation: the intrinsic variability of the human immune response. Thus, justification of the use of a variety of assay formats continues for a variety of reasons ranging from test performance to cost per test. In general, however, efforts to encourage better standardization should lead to better defined immunologic substrates, and challenging proficiency testing programs are one of the best ways to identify the strengths and weaknesses of individual tests and approaches, whether they are user-developed or commercial methods.

Indirect fluorescent antibody tests look for immunoadsorption of patient antibodies to cultured spirochetes attached to glass slides. A dilution series of patient serum is placed in adjacent wells, incubated on the substrate for a short time, and then detected by fluorescent microscopy after staining with fluorophore-congugated-human IgG or IgM antibody. Antibody titers of 1:64 or above are generally considered positive, though there may be considerable day-to-day and technologist-to-technologist variation in the determination of values because of the subjective nature of the procedure. Automated fluorescence readers have the potential to improve upon this, but variations in the procedural steps such as preparing the dilution series and washing stringency will continue to contribute to variability.

Enzyme immunoassay (EIA) is the most commonly used method for detection of immune responses to *B. burgdorferi*. Typically, antigen preparations comprising whole-cell sonicates of *B. burgdorferi* are bound to plastic EIA plates for detection of total Ig response or individual antibody subclasses. With EIAs using well prepared whole cell antigen preparations, about half of patients presenting within a week of the development of erythema migrans (EM) will register positive results. In untreated patients after one week, and in patients with multiple EM lesions or signs of systemic involvement, sensitivities of EIA approach 90% (Dressler et al., 1993). EIA is nearly uniformly positive in sera of patients with late manifestations of disease (Dressler et al., 1993).

False positive EIA reactions can and do occur in some patients with bacterial infections due to other organisms; this is thought to be due to cross reactivity with common bacterial antigens such as heat shock proteins, flagellin, and other conserved bacterial proteins (Fawcett et al., 1992) (Luft et al., 1993). Because all commercially available assays using whole cell sonicates contain the OspA protein, individuals who in the past have received the OspA vaccination will often generate false positive results (Aguero-Rosenfeld et al., 1999) (Molloy et al., 2000). EIAs based on strains that are negative for OspA (by virtue of losing the linear plasmid encoding the protein) or recombinant protein or peptide EIAs devoid of OspA epitopes will be non-reactive in these individuals (Zhang et al., 1997b). Because of the lack of specificity of EIA procedures, and because the pretest probability of having Lyme disease is often lower than the false positive rate (especially in non-endemic areas), EIA reactive sera should be confirmed by Western immunoblotting according to so-called two-tier testing guidelines.

Western immunoblotting is performed by carrying out electrophoretic separation of spirochetal antigens from whole cell sonicates, followed by transfer to nylon filters and detection of patient antibody reactivity to the denatured proteins on the blot by using labeled anti-IgG or IgM antibodies. Several commercial kits for WIB are available which employ a variety of *B. burgdorferi* strains. Choice of the strain and the growth conditions used will likely affect expression levels of many immundominant proteins, so significant variation has been seen in WIB performance between laboratories, as determined in proficiency testing surveys (Robertson et al., 2000). Rates of detection of IgM antibodies in patients with EM early in the course of disease have ranged from as low as 3% to as high as 84% (Engstrom et al., 1995; Dressler et al., 1993); some commercially available WIB kits failed to detect IgM responses even after several weeks of infection (Aguero-Rosenfeld et al., 1996; Aguero-Rosenfeld et al., 1993). For detection of IgG antibodies, performance has generally been better, especially for convalescent sera (Aguero-Rosenfeld, 2008; Dressler et al., 1993). Early IgG responses are dominated by antibody to OspC (assuming the strain used makes sufficient levels of OspC) and flagellin. As mentioned, flagellin responses are the least specific of all the IgG responses for reasons cited above. Later in the convalescent phase, additional reactivities are observed against a range of proteins including BmpA (39 kDa) and B31 proteins of 93-, 66-, 45-, 35-, 30-, and 18-kDa.

Interpretive criteria for IgG and IgM WIB have been established for U.S. patients (Recommendations for test performance and interpretation from the second national conference on serologic diagnosis of lyme disease, 1995). The IgM criteria of Engstrom et al. (1995) were adopted based on a study of early Lyme disease patients; they were established for use only within the first 4 weeks of illness. A positive IgM blot was defined by the presence of two of three reactive protein species in strain 297 (OspC, 41 or 39 kDa). The IgG criteria were based on work from Dr. Alan Steere's group (Dressler et al., 1993); these were intended for use at any time during the course of illness, although they were expected to be more informative and applicable to patients later in their disease course. IgG reactivity against at five of 10 protein species (93, 66, 58, 45, 41, 39, 30, 28, 21, or 18 kDa) in strain 39/40 was considered the minimum number to be considered positive. WIB may be more sensitive than EIA for detection of early Lyme disease, but the two methods are similar in sensitivity for convalescent and late-stage infection. In a study of 46 culture-confirmed patients with EM, IgM WIB was considered reactive in 43% of patients, compared with 33% by EIA (Aguero-Rosenfeld et al., 1996).

This is curiously the opposite of two-tier strategies used for viral serological testing, in which the first test is more sensitive, the second more specific. Operational aspects preclude the use of WIB as a screening test, however, and other factors may influence the performance of the WIB as a screening test. For example, many of the commercial WIB kits use strain B31, which was included in none of the studies that led to the standard interpretive criteria. Although each kit is supposed to have custom criteria that match the standard criteria, this is subject to interpretive error. Subtle differences in molecular weight of antigens, along with antigen degradation can lead to confusing results, even in experienced laboratories. In addition, as with EIA methods, false positives can occur from previous vaccination with the OspA-containing vaccine (Aguero-Rosenfeld et al., 1999; Molloy et al., 2000).

Despite this apparent role reversal of screening and confirmatory testing, the recommended use of two-tier testing has helped to resolve much diagnostic uncertainty in the diagnosis of Lyme disease in the U.S., largely because it improves overall specificity. In most studies of the two-tiered strategy, specificity levels have been 97 to 99%. The low false positive rate has been welcomed, especially in areas where the pre-test probability of infection is low, and among patients presenting with non-specific symptoms in endemic areas. The reduction of sensitivity for detection of early disease was an unfortunate compromise, since non-specific febrile illness can be presenting features of HGA, Lyme disease, and human babesiosis, where diagnostic differentiation is most critical. In 280 patients with various manifestations of Lyme disease, 38% of patients with EM during the acute phase were seroreactive; 67% were positive after antimicrobial treatment. (Bacon et al., 2003). The sensitivity increased in patients with evidence of more invasive disease; 87% of patients with early neuroborreliosis and to 97% of those with Lyme arthritis were seroreactive. Similar results were obtained in another study of 47 patients with clinically defined EM, for whom the sensitivities of the two-tier test were 40.4% in acute-phase sera and 66% during the convalescent phase after treatment (Nowakowski et al., 2001).

Newer antibody tests based on recombinant proteins or immunodominant peptides have the potential of maintaining current levels of specificity without sacrificing sensitivity, especially for detection of early disease. Many studies have been done on recombinant proteins, many of which have been mentioned above, with sensitivities ranging from 30% to nearly 100% depending on the antigen used and the stage of disease being tested reviewed recently in (Aguero-Rosenfeld, 2008). Specificity levels have been somewhat lower than expected (as low as 91%), perhaps because of the presence of small amounts of contaminating protein from the strains of bacteria or yeast used for protein expression. In general, however, no single recombinant protein has served as the universal solution for immunologic detection of both early and late disease (Aguero-Rosenfeld, 2008). Considerably more promise has been shown in combining immunodominant epitopes, especially those that derive from antigens that are recognized early in the course of disease.

In a different study of the same set of 839 serum samples (including those from 280 Lyme disease patients) cited above, antibody responses to recombinant VlsE1, the C6 peptide, and the conserved C terminal peptide from OspC (pepC10) were evaluated by kinetic enzyme-linked immunoassay (Bacon et al., 2003). At 99% specificity, the overall sensitivities for detecting IgG antibody to rVlsE1 or C6 in samples from patients with diverse manifestations of Lyme disease were equivalent to that of two-tiered testing. When data were considered in parallel, two combinations (IgG responses to either rVlsE1 or C6 in parallel with IgM responses to pepC10) maintained high specificity (98%) and were significantly more sensitive than two-tiered analysis in detecting antibodies to *B. burgdorferi* in patients with acute erythema migrans. In later stages of Lyme disease, the sensitivities of the in-parallel tests and two-tiered testing were high and statistically equivalent. In established cases of Lyme disease, the C6 ELISA may also be useful for tracking therapeutic responses (Marques et al., 2002; Philipp et al., 2003; Philipp et al., 2005; Wormser et al., 2008a; Wormser et al., 2008b). Although similar observations were made in other studies, some studies have not confirmed these findings (Peltomaa et al., 2003). Operational differences in the ways the assays were performed may account for this. Taken together, these data are supportive of the goal of potentially replacing two-tiered testing while improving the diagnosis for early Lyme disease patients.

### Serodiagnosis of Babesiosis

The serological testing methods for *B. microti* are not as developed as those for Lyme disease, mainly because the organism has not been propagated *in vitro*. The mainstay of the laboratory diagnosis is the IFA test, in which a standard 1:16 or 1:32 dilution of serum is dispensed onto wells of a microscope slide that has been previously coated with infected red blood cells, usually of hamster origin After a wash step, addition of fluorescent anti-human IgG or IgM, and an additional wash, the microscope wells are examined under a fluorescent microscope for staining of intraerythrocytic merozoite forms of the organism. If the screening serologic testing is positive, further 1:4 serial dilutions are performed to determine the serum titer. Determination of titer end point is somewhat subjective; it is usually associated with a significant, abrupt drop in the level of observed fluorescence. In most laboratories, a 1:64 cutoff titer has been established and is considered to be consistent with exposure to *B. microti*.

In animal models of infection, IgM antibodies precede IgG responses by 7 to 10 days, but in humans, by the time patients present (usually with nonspecific "flu-like" symptoms) they are already IgG positive (Benach et al., 1985; Homer et al., 2000a; Krause et al., 1996a; Krause et al., 1994). During the acute phase of infection in which patients are PCR positive, antibody titers typically reach 1: 512, 1:1024 or higher and then decline in the weeks and months after therapy. Even with therapy, however, antibody levels typically persist at 1:64 or above for years after the initial infection. Thus, the finding of an antibody titer at 1:64 during acute presentation should not be assumed to be due to active infection; it may simply reflect past exposure, especially if the patient is from an endemic area. PCR testing may be helpful in resolving this issue. On the other hand, titers of greater than 1:512 have been found to be consistently associated with acute infection and correlate with PCR positivity (Krause et al., 1996a; Krause et al., 1998; Krause et al., 1996e).

Enzyme immunoassays based on antigen preparations from infected hamster erythrocytes have been developed, but have been generally hampered by the presence of anti-rodent antibodies in serum of a few percent of patients. These confounding antibodies can to some extent be pre-adsorbed prior to testing to reduce this problem. Immunoblots made from partially purified antigens have also been developed (Houghton et al., 2002).

More recently, recombinant expression cloning efforts, using *B. microti* expression libraries screened with human serum, led to the discovery of several recombinant proteins that show promise as immunodiagnostic reagents (Homer et al., 2000b; Houghton et al., 2002). From two serocomplementary *B. microti*-specific antigens, peptide mapping was done to identify immunodominant epitopes that could be combined in a peptide EIA. The prototype peptide EIA was used to detect *B. microti*-specific antibodies in 15 sera taken before infection and 107 taken after infection from 59 individuals with known tick-borne infections previously confirmed by other methods. The combination peptide detected 98 out of 107 sera taken after infection that were immmunoblot positive; this included 12/12 samples that were PCR positive and six sera from smear-negative patients that were confirmed positive by PCR, immunoblot, or IFA.

In another interesting study, proteins of *B. microti* that are potentially secreted or surface exposed were identified by serologic expression cloning (Homer et al., 2003). This report described the identification and initial characterization of 27 clones representing seven genes or gene families that were isolated through serological expression cloning by using a technique that was specifically designed to screen for shed antigens. In this screen, sera from *B. microti*-infected SCID mice, putatively containing secreted or shed antigens from the parasites, were harvested and used to immunize syngeneic immunocompetent mice (BALB/c). After boosting, the sera from the BALB/c mice, containing antibodies against the immunodominant se-creted antigens, were used to screen a *B. microti* genomic expression library. Analyses of the putative peptides encoded by the novel DNA sequences revealed characteristics indicating that these peptides might be secreted. Initial serological data obtained with recombinant proteins and a patient serum panel demonstrated that several of the proteins could be useful in developing diagnostic tests for detection of *B. microti* antibodies and anti-gens in serum. Unfortunately, however, to date none of these recombinant peptides or proteins has been converted into an immunodiagnostic test that is widely available.

Unlike for Lyme disease serology, no proficiency testing programs yet exist for serodiagnosis of *B. microti* infection, mainly because of lack of demand for such a service. However, this leaves open the possibility that among laboratories performing serodiagnostic methods for this organism, significant inconsistencies may exist between laboratories and within labo-ratories from run-to-run.

*Serodiagnosis of HGA*

Like for *B. microti,* detection of antibody responses in patient serum by the indirect immunofluorescence (IFAT) assay is the most frequently used test for clinical purposes (Walls et al., 1999). However, unlike for *B. microti* infections, the onset of symptoms after tick bite is fairly abrupt, and symptomatic patients are frequently seronegative. IFA assays typically use HL-60 cells infected with *A. phagocytophilum* as a substrate, and screening and dilution series are typically performed as described above for *B. mi-croti.* Sensitivity is high 2–4 weeks following disease onset compared with a few days after onset for PCR, blood smear microscopy and cell culture. A diagnosis of *A. phagocytophilum* is confirmed by a fourfold increase in antibody titer between acute and convalescent sera or a seroconversion to a titer of 128 or higher (Walls et al., 1999) (Thomas et al., 2009). Like for *B. microti*, seropositivity for *A. phagocytophilum* often lasts for months and sometimes years after initial exposure (Aguero-Rosenfeld et al., 2000). Thus, like for *B. microti* and *B. burgdorferi*, an HGA antibody titer must be considered in light of other clinical evidence of infection and should not be used as the only criterion for diagnosis. False-positive or cross reactive serologic test results can be seen in cases of Rocky Mountain spotted fe-ver, typhus, Q fever, brucellosis, Lyme disease, Epstein–Barr infection and any variety of autoimmune disorders associated with production of auto antibodies (Dumler et al., 2007). Aguero-Rosenfeld *et al* evaluated the an-tibody responses by IFA in the sera of 24 patients with culture-confirmed HGA (Aguero-Rosenfeld et al., 2000). Patients were followed for up to 14 months. Seroconversion was observed in 21 of 23 patients (91.3%)

from whom convalescent-phase sera were obtained. Antibodies were first detected at an average of 11.5 days after onset of symptoms. Peak titers (>/=2,560 for 71.4% of patients and >/=640 for 95.2% of patients) were obtained an average of 14.7 days after onset of symptoms. Most patients were still considered seropositive after 6 months, and half of the patients were still seropositive after 11 months.

Some progress has been made toward development of recombinant serological reagents for the diagnosis of HGA, which might be more amenable to automated testing and or rapid immunodiagnostic assay formats (Lodes et al., 2001). Lodes et al described a panel of seven recombinant antigens, derived from the HGA agent, which were evaluated by class-specific ELISAs for utility in the diagnosis of the infection. Fourteen genomic fragments, obtained by serologic expression screening, contained open reading frames encoding 16 immunodominant antigens. Eleven of these antigens were members of the major surface protein (MSP) multigene family. In addition to two MSP recombinant antigens (rHGE-1 and -3) and a fusion protein of one of these antigens (rErf-1), five further recombinants were evaluated by ELISA. Two of these antigens (rHGE-14 and -15) were novel, while a third (rHGE-2), with no known function, had already been described. The final two recombinant antigens (rHGE-9 and -17) represented overlapping segments of the ankyrin gene. When serologic data for all recombinants were combined, 96.2% (26 of 27) of convalescent-phase patient serum samples and 85.2% (23 of 27) of acute-phase patient serum samples were detected, indicating the potential of these antigens for use in the development of a rapid serologic assay for the diagnoses of HGA.

*Conclusions*

The three identified infections transmissible by the bite of a deer tick in the United States—Lyme disease, HGA and human babesiosis—have distinct and overlapping clinical features that, in the case of infection by more than one organism, may confound each other. Each may require different treatment approaches, although one can argue that tetracycline derivatives, with activity against *B. burgdorferi* and HGA, should become the drug of choice for patients with confusing clinical pictures or features of more than one infection. Much of the management of patients with nonspecific presentations will depend on specific diagnostic test results. Fortunately, although babesiosis and HGA have immunosuppressive effects, these effects are not sufficient to confound the specific serologic responses to the cognate infectious agents. In the case of HGA and babesiosis, direct detection by blood smear, culture or PCR (HGA) or smear and PCR (babesiosis) are diagnostic options, but none of the direct detection approaches are very useful for the diagnosis of early Lyme disease. The diagnosis of all of these conditions may be improved by the use of next generation serologic testing and molecular diagnostic approaches, both of which are likely to make their way into increasing numbers of laboratories over the next decade.

## References

Aguero-Rosenfeld, M. E. 2003. Laboratory aspects of tick-borne diseases: Lyme, human granulocytic ehrlichiosis and babesiosis. *Mt Sinai J Med* 70(3):197-206.

———. 2008. Lyme disease: Laboratory issues. *Infect Dis Clin North Am* 22(2):301-313, vii.

Aguero-Rosenfeld, M. E., F. Kalantarpour, M. Baluch, H. W. Horowitz, D. F. McKenna, J. T. Raffalli, T. Hsieh, J. Wu, J. S. Dumler, and G. P. Wormser. 2000. Serology of culture-confirmed cases of human granulocytic ehrlichiosis. *J Clin Microbiol* 38(2):635-638.

Aguero-Rosenfeld, M. E., J. Nowakowski, S. Bittker, D. Cooper, R. B. Nadelman, and G. P. Wormser. 1996. Evolution of the serologic response to borrelia burgdorferi in treated patients with culture-confirmed erythema migrans. *Journal of Clinical Microbiology* 34(1):1-9.

Aguero-Rosenfeld, M. E., J. Nowakowski, D. F. McKenna, C. A. Carbonaro, and G. P. Wormser. 1993. Serodiagnosis in early lyme disease. *J Clin Microbiol* 31(12):3090-3095.

Aguero-Rosenfeld, M. E., J. Roberge, C. A. Carbonaro, J. Nowakowski, R. B. Nadelman, and G. P. Wormser. 1999. Effects of ospa vaccination on lyme disease serologic testing. *J Clin Microbiol* 37(11):3718-3721.

Aguero-Rosenfeld, M. E., G. Wang, I. Schwartz, and G. P. Wormser. 2005. Diagnosis of lyme borreliosis. *Clin Microbiol Rev* 18(3):484-509.

Alberti, A., and O. A. Sparagano. 2006. Molecular diagnosis of granulocytic anaplasmosis and infectious cyclic thrombocytopenia by pcr-rflp. *Ann N Y Acad Sci* 1081:371-378.

Bacon, R. M., B. J. Biggerstaff, M. E. Schriefer, R. D. Gilmore, Jr., M. T. Philipp, A. C. Steere, G. P. Wormser, A. R. Marques, and B. J. Johnson. 2003. Serodiagnosis of lyme disease by kinetic enzyme-linked immunosorbent assay using recombinant vlse1 or peptide antigens of borrelia burgdorferi compared with 2-tiered testing using whole-cell lysates. *J Infect Dis* 187(8):1187-1199.

Bakken, J. S., and J. S. Dumler. 2000. Human granulocytic ehrlichiosis. *Clin Infect Dis* 31(2):554-560.

———. 2006. Clinical diagnosis and treatment of human granulocytotropic anaplasmosis. *Ann N Y Acad Sci* 1078:236-247.

Bakken, J. S., J. S. Dumler, S. M. Chen, M. R. Eckman, L. L. Van Etta, and D. H. Walker. 1994. Human granulocytic ehrlichiosis in the upper midwest United States. A new species emerging? [see comments]. *Jama* 272(3):212-218.

Barbour, A. G. 1984. Isolation and cultivation of lyme disease spirochetes. *Yale Journal of Biology & Medicine* 57(4):521-525.

———. 1986. Cultivation of borrelia: A historical overview. *Zentralblatt Fur Bakteriologie, Mikrobiologie, Und Hygiene Series A, Medical Microbiology, Infectious Diseases, Virology, Parasitology* 263(1-2):11-14.

Belongia, E. A., K. D. Reed, P. D. Mitchell, N. Mueller-Rizner, M. Vandermause, M. F. Finkel, and J. J. Kazmierczak. 2001. Tickborne infections as a cause of nonspecific febrile illness in wisconsin. *Clin Infect Dis* 32(10):1434-1439.

Benach, J. L., J. L. Coleman, G. S. Habicht, A. MacDonald, E. Grunwaldt, and J. A. Giron. 1985. Serological evidence for simultaneous occurrences of lyme disease and babesiosis. *Journal of Infectious Diseases* 152(3):473-477.

Bradley, J. F., R. C. Johnson, and J. L. Goodman. 1994. The persistence of spirochetal nucleic acids in active lyme arthritis. *Ann Intern Med* 120(6):487-489.

Coleman, J. L., and J. L. Benach. 1987. Isolation of antigenic components from the lyme disease spirochete: Their role in early diagnosis. *J Infect Dis* 155(4):756-765.

Coleman, J. L., D. LeVine, C. Thill, C. Kuhlow, and J. L. Benach. 2005. Babesia microti and borrelia burgdorferi follow independent courses of infection in mice. *J Infect Dis* 192(9):1634-1641.

Comer, J. A., W. L. Nicholson, J. W. Sumner, J. G. Olson, and J. E. Childs. 1999. Diagnosis of human ehrlichiosis by pcr assay of acute-phase serum. *J Clin Microbiol* 37(1):31-34.

Craft, J. E., D. K. Fischer, G. T. Shimamoto, and A. C. Steere. 1986. Antigens of borrelia burgdorferi recognized during lyme disease. Appearance of a new immunoglobulin m response and expansion of the immunoglobulin g response late in the illness. *Journal of Clinical Investigation* 78(4):934-939.

Das, S., S. W. Barthold, S. S. Giles, R. R. Montgomery, S. R. Telford, 3rd, and E. Fikrig. 1997. Temporal pattern of borrelia burgdorferi p21 expression in ticks and the mammalian host. *J Clin Invest* 99(5):987-995.

Demaerschalck, I., A. Ben Messaoud, M. De Kesel, B. Hoyois, Y. Lobet, P. Hoet, G. Bigaignon, A. Bollen, and E. Godfroid. 1995. Simultaneous presence of different borrelia burgdorferi genospecies in biological fluids of lyme disease patients. *Journal of Clinical Microbiology* 33(3):602-608.

Dorward, D. W., T. G. Schwan, and C. F. Garon. 1991. Immune capture and detection of borrelia burgdorferi antigens in urine, blood, or tissues from infected ticks, mice, dogs, and humans. *Journal of Clinical Microbiology* 29(6):1162-1170.

Dressler, F., J. A. Whalen, B. N. Reinhardt, and A. C. Steere. 1993. Western blotting in the serodiagnosis of lyme disease. *J. Infect. Dis.* 167:392-400.

Dumler, J. S. 2001. Molecular diagnosis of lyme disease: Review and meta-analysis. *Mol Diagn* 6(1):1-11.

Dumler, J. S., J. E. Madigan, N. Pusterla, and J. S. Bakken. 2007. Ehrlichioses in humans: Epidemiology, clinical presentation, diagnosis, and treatment. *Clin Infect Dis* 45 Suppl 1:S45-51.

Eiffert, H., A. Karsten, R. Thomssen, and H. J. Christen. 1998. Characterization of borrelia burgdorferi strains in lyme arthritis. *Scand J Infect Dis* 30(3):265-268.

Engstrom, S. M., E. Shoop, and R. C. Johnson. 1995. Immunoblot interpretation criteria for serodiagnosis of early lyme disease. *J. Clin. Microbiol.* 33:419-427.

Fawcett, P. T., K. M. Gibney, C. D. Rose, S. B. Dubbs, and R. A. Doughty. 1992. Frequency and specificity of antibodies that crossreact with borrelia burgdorferi antigens. *J Rheumatol* 19(4):582-587.

Fikrig, E., S. W. Barthold, W. Sun, W. Feng, S. R. Telford, 3rd, and R. A. Flavell. 1997. Borrelia burgdorferi p35 and p37 proteins, expressed in vivo, elicit protective immunity. *Immunity* 6(5):531-539.

Fikrig, E., W. Feng, S. W. Barthold, S. R. Telford, 3rd, and R. A. Flavell. 2000. Arthropod- and host-specific borrelia burgdorferi bbk32 expression and the inhibition of spirochete transmission. *J Immunol* 164(10):5344-5351.

Filstein, M. R., J. L. Benach, D. J. White, B. A. Brody, W. D. Goldman, C. W. Bakal, and R. S. Schwartz. 1980. Serosurvey for human babesiosis in new york. *Journal of Infectious Diseases* 141(4):518-521.

Goodman, J. L., J. F. Bradley, A. E. Ross, P. Goellner, A. Lagus, B. Vitale, B. W. Berger, S. Luger, and R. C. Johnson. 1995. Bloodstream invasion in early lyme disease: Results from a prospective, controlled, blinded study using the polymerase chain reaction. *American Journal of Medicine* 99(1):6-12.

Goodman, J. L., C. Nelson, B. Vitale, J. E. Madigan, J. S. Dumler, T. J. Kurtti, and U. G. Munderloh. 1996. Direct cultivation of the causative agent of human granulocytic eh- rlichiosis. *New England Journal of Medicine* 334(4):209-215.

Heikkila, T., I. Seppala, H. Saxen, J. Panelius, H. Yrjanainen, and P. Lahdenne. 2002. Species-specific serodiagnosis of lyme arthritis and neuroborreliosis due to borrelia burgdorferi sensu stricto, B. Afzelii, and B. Garinii by using decorin binding protein A. *J Clin Microbiol* 40(2):453-460.

Hofmeister, E. K., J. Magera, L. Sloan, C. Kolbert, J. Hanson, and D. H. Persing. 1996. Borrelia burgdorferi proteins are recognized by antibodies from mice experimentally infected with the agent of human granulocytic ehrlichiosis. Paper read at Seventh International Congress on Lyme Borreliosis, San Francisco, CA.

Holden, K., E. Hodzic, S. Feng, K. J. Freet, R. B. Lefebvre, and S. W. Barthold. 2005. Coinfection with anaplasma phagocytophilum alters borrelia burgdorferi population distribution in c3h/hen mice. *Infect Immun* 73(6):3440-3444.

Homer, M. J., I. Aguilar-Delfin, S. R. Telford, 3rd, P. J. Krause, and D. H. Persing. 2000a. Babesiosis. *Clin Microbiol Rev* 13(3):451-469.

Homer, M. J., E. S. Bruinsma, M. J. Lodes, M. H. Moro, S. Telford, 3rd, P. J. Krause, L. D. Reynolds, R. Mohamath, D. R. Benson, R. L. Houghton, S. G. Reed, and D. H. Persing. 2000b. A polymorphic multigene family encoding an immunodominant protein from babesia microti. *J Clin Microbiol* 38(1):362-368.

Homer, M. J., M. J. Lodes, L. D. Reynolds, Y. Zhang, J. F. Douglass, P. D. McNeill, R. L. Houghton, and D. H. Persing. 2003. Identification and characterization of putative secreted antigens from babesia microti. *J Clin Microbiol* 41(2):723-729.

Horowitz, H. W., M. E. Aguero-Rosenfeld, D. F. McKenna, D. Holmgren, T. C. Hsieh, S. A. Varde, S. J. Dumler, J. M. Wu, I. Schwartz, Y. Rikihisa, and G. P. Wormser. 1998. Clinical and laboratory spectrum of culture-proven human granulocytic ehrlichiosis: Comparison with culture-negative cases. *Clin Infect Dis* 27(5):1314-1317.

Houghton, R. L., M. J. Homer, L. D. Reynolds, P. R. Sleath, M. J. Lodes, V. Berardi, D. A. Leiby, and D. H. Persing. 2002. Identification of babesia microti-specific immunodominant epitopes and development of a peptide eia for detection of antibodies in serum. *Transfusion* 42(11):1488-1496.

Hyde, F. W., R. C. Johnson, T. J. White, and C. E. Shelburne. 1989. Detection of antigens in urine of mice and humans infected with borrelia burgdorferi, etiologic agent of lyme disease. *J Clin Microbiol* 27(1):58-61.

Jahangir, A., C. Kolbert, W. Edwards, P. Mitchell, J. S. Dumler, and D. H. Persing. 1998. Fatal pancarditis associated with human granulocytic ehrlichiosis in a 44-year-old man. *Clin Infect Dis* 27(6):1424-1427.

Jaulhac, B., I. Chary-Valckenaere, J. Sibilia, R. M. Javier, Y. Piemont, J. L. Kuntz, H. Monteil, and J. Pourel. 1996. Detection of borrelia burgdorferi by DNA amplification in synovial tissue samples from patients with lyme arthritis. *Arthritis Rheum* 39(5):736-745.

Kelly, R. 1971. Cultivation of borrelia hermsi. *Science* 173(995):443-444.

Klempner, M. S., L. T. Hu, J. Evans, C. H. Schmid, G. M. Johnson, R. P. Trevino, D. Norton, L. Levy, D. Wall, J. McCall, M. Kosinski, and A. Weinstein. 2001a. Two controlled trials of antibiotic treatment in patients with persistent symptoms and a history of lyme disease. *N Engl J Med* 345(2):85-92.

Klempner, M. S., C. H. Schmid, L. Hu, A. C. Steere, G. Johnson, B. McCloud, R. Noring, and A. Weinstein. 2001b. Intralaboratory reliability of serologic and urine testing for lyme disease. *Am J Med* 110(3):217-219.

Krause, P. J., K. McKay, J. Gadbaw, D. Christianson, L. Closter, T. Lepore, S. R. Telford, 3rd, V. Sikand, R. Ryan, D. Persing, J. D. Radolf, and A. Spielman. 2003. Increasing health burden of human babesiosis in endemic sites. *Am J Trop Med Hyg* 68(4):431-436.

Krause, P. J., K. McKay, C. A. Thompson, V. K. Sikand, R. Lentz, T. Lepore, L. Closter, D. Christianson, S. R. Telford, D. Persing, J. D. Radolf, and A. Spielman. 2002. Disease-specific diagnosis of coinfecting tickborne zoonoses: Babesiosis, human granulocytic ehrlichiosis, and lyme disease. *Clin Infect Dis* 34(9):1184-1191.

Krause, P. J., R. Ryan, S. Telford, D. Persing, and A. Spielman. 1996a. Efficacy of immuno-globulin m serodiagnostic test for rapid diagnosis of acute babesiosis. *Journal of Clinical Microbiology* 34(8):2014-2016.

Krause, P. J., A. Spielman, S. R. Telford, 3rd, V. K. Sikand, K. McKay, D. Christianson, R. J. Pollack, P. Brassard, J. Magera, R. Ryan, and D. H. Persing. 1998. Persistent parasitemia after acute babesiosis. *N Engl J Med* 339(3):160-165.

Krause, P. J., S. R. Telford III, A. Spielman, V. J. Sikand, R. Ryan, D. Christianson, G. Burke, P. Brassard, R. Pollack, J. Peck, and D. H. Persing. 1996b. Concurrent lyme disease and babesiosis: Evidence for increased severity and duration of illness. *JAMA* 275:1657-1660.

Krause, P. J., S. Telford, 3rd, A. Spielman, R. Ryan, J. Magera, T. V. Rajan, D. Christianson, T. V. Alberghini, L. Bow, and D. Persing. 1996c. Comparison of pcr with blood smear and inoculation of small animals for diagnosis of babesia microti parasitemia. *J Clin Microbiol* 34(11):2791-2794.

Krause, P. J., S. D. Telford, R. Ryan, A. B. Hurta, I. Kwasnik, S. Luger, J. Niederman, M. Gerber, and A. Spielman. 1991. Geographical and temporal distribution of babesial infec-tion in connecticut. *Journal of Clinical Microbiology* 29(1):1-4.

Krause, P. J., S. R. Telford, R. Ryan, P. A. Conrad, M. Wilson, J. W. Thomford, and A. Spielman. 1994. Diagnosis of babesiosis: Evaluation of a serologic test for the detection of babesia microti antibody [see comments]. *Journal of Infectious Diseases* 169(4):923-926.

Krause, P. J., S. R. Telford, A. Spielman, R. Ryan, J. Magera, T. V. Rajan, D. Christianson, T. V. Alberghini, L. Bow, and D. Persing. 1996e. Comparison of pcr with blood smear and inoculation of small animals for diagnosis of babesia microti parasitemia. *Journal of Clinical Microbiology* 34(11):2791-2794.

Lawrenz, M. B., J. M. Hardham, R. T. Owens, J. Nowakowski, A. C. Steere, G. P. Wormser, and S. J. Norris. 1999. Human antibody responses to vlse antigenic variation protein of borrelia burgdorferi. *J Clin Microbiol* 37(12):3997-4004.

Lebech, A.-M., K. Hansen, F. Brandrup, O. Clemmensen, and L. Halkier-Sorensen. 2000. Di-agnostic value of pcr for detection of borrelia burgdorferi DNA in clinical specimens from patients with erythema migrans and lyme neuroborreliosis. *Mol Diagn* 5(2):139-150.

Lebech, A.-M., K. Hansen, P. Pancholi, L. Sloan, J. Magera, and D. H. Persing. 1998. Direct detection and genotyping of B. Burgdorferi in the cerebrospinal fluid of lyme neurobor-reliosis patients. *Molecular Diagnosis* 3(3):131-141.

Leiby, D. A., A. P. Chung, R. G. Cable, J. Trouern-Trend, J. McCullough, M. J. Homer, L. D. Reynolds, R. L. Houghton, M. J. Lodes, and D. H. Persing. 2002. Relationship between tick bites and the seroprevalence of babesia microti and anaplasma phagocytophila (pre-viously ehrlichia sp.) in blood donors. *Transfusion* 42(12):1585-1591.

Leiby, D. A., A. P. Chung, J. E. Gill, R. L. Houghton, D. H. Persing, S. Badon, and R. G. Cable. 2005. Demonstrable parasitemia among connecticut blood donors with antibodies to babesia microti. *Transfusion* 45(11):1804-1810.

Liebling, M. R., M. J. Nishio, A. Rodriguez, L. H. Sigal, T. Jin, and J. S. Louie. 1993. The polymerase chain reaction for the detection of borrelia burgdorferi in human body fluids. *Arthritis Rheum* 36(5):665-675.

Lodes, M. J., R. Mohamath, L. D. Reynolds, P. McNeill, C. P. Kolbert, E. S. Bruinsma, D. R. Benson, E. Hofmeister, S. G. Reed, R. L. Houghton, and D. H. Persing. 2001. Serodiag-nosis of human granulocytic ehrlichiosis by using novel combinations of immunoreactive recombinant proteins. *J Clin Microbiol* 39(7):2466-2476.

Logigian, E. L., R. F. Kaplan, and A. C. Steere. 1990. Chronic neurologic manifestations of lyme disease [see comments]. *New England Journal of Medicine* 323(21):1438-1444.

Luft, B. J., J. J. Dunn, R. J. Dattwyler, G. Gorgone, P. D. Gorevic, and W. H. Schubach. 1993. Cross-reactive antigenic domains of the flagellin protein of borrelia burgdorferi. *Res Microbiol* 144(4):251-257.

Macdonald, K. L., M. T. Osterholm, K. H. Ledell, K. E. White, C. H. Schenck, C. C. Chao, D. H. Persing, R. C. Johnson, J. M. Barker, and P. K. Peterson. 1996. A case-control study to assess possible triggers and cofactors in chronic fatigue syndrome. *American Journal of Medicine* 100(5):548-554.

Malawista, S. E., R. T. Schoen, T. L. Moore, D. E. Dodge, T. J. White, and D. H. Persing. 1992. Failure of multitarget detection of borrelia burgdorferi-associated DNA sequences in synovial fluids of patients with juvenile rheumatoid arthritis: A cautionary note. *Arthritis Rheum* 35(2):246-247.

Malawista, S. E., and A. C. Steere. 1986. Lyme disease: Infectious in origin, rheumatic in expression. [review]. *Advances in Internal Medicine* 31:147-166.

Marques, A. R., D. S. Martin, and M. T. Philipp. 2002. Evaluation of the c6 peptide enzyme-linked immunosorbent assay for individuals vaccinated with the recombinant ospa vaccine. *J Clin Microbiol* 40(7):2591-2593.

Marshall, W. F., 3rd, S. R. Telford, 3rd, P. N. Rys, B. J. Rutledge, D. Mathiesen, S. E. Malawista, A. Spielman, and D. H. Persing. 1994a. Detection of borrelia burgdorferi DNA in museum specimens of peromyscus leucopus. *J Infect Dis* 170(4):1027-1032.

Marshall, W. R., S. R. Telford, P. N. Rys, B. J. Rutledge, D. Mathiesen, S. E. Malawista, A. Spielman, and D. H. Persing. 1994b. Detection of borrelia burgdorferi DNA in museum specimens of peromyscus leucopus. *Journal of Infectious Diseases* 170(4):1027-1032.

Mathiesen, D. A., J. H. Oliver, C. P. Kolbert, E. D. Tullson, B. J. B. Johnson, G. L. Campbell, P. D. Mitchell, K. D. Reed, S. R. Telford, J. F. Anderson, R. S. Lane, and D. H. Persing. 1997. Genetic heterogeneity of borrelia burgdorferi in the United States. *Journal of Infectious Diseases* 175(1):98-107.

Mathiesen, M. J., A. Holm, M. Christiansen, J. Blom, K. Hansen, S. Ostergaard, and M. Theisen. 1998. The dominant epitope of borrelia garinii outer surface protein C recognized by sera from patients with neuroborreliosis has a surface-exposed conserved structural motif. *Infect Immun* 66(9):4073-4079.

Matthews, J., E. Rattigan, and H. Yee. 2003. Case 29-2003: A 60-year-old man with fever, rigors, and sweats. *N Engl J Med* 349(25):2467; author reply 2467.

Meldrum, S. C., G. S. Birkhead, D. J. White, J. L. Benach, and D. L. Morse. 1992. Human babesiosis in new york state: An epidemiological description of 136 cases. *Clinical Infectious Diseases* 15(6):1019-1023.

Molloy, P. J., V. P. Berardi, D. H. Persing, and L. H. Sigal. 2000. Detection of multiple reactive protein species by immunoblotting after recombinant outer surface protein A lyme disease vaccination [in process citation]. *Clin Infect Dis* 31(1):42-47.

Molloy, P. J., D. H. Persing, and V. P. Berardi. 2001. False-positive results of pcr testing for lyme disease. *Clin Infect Dis* 33(3):412-413.

Moro, M. H., O. L. Zegarra-Moro, and D. H. Persing. 2006. Babesia microti and borrelia burgdorferi coinfection associated with increased severity of arthritis. *J Infect Dis* 194(5):716.

Moter, S. E., H. Hofmann, R. Wallich, M. M. Simon, and M. D. Kramer. 1994. Detection of borrelia burgdorferi sensu lato in lesional skin of patients with erythema migrans and acrodermatitis chronica atrophicans by ospa-specific pcr. *J Clin Microbiol* 32(12):2980-2988.

Nocton, J. J., B. J. Bloom, B. J. Rutledge, D. H. Persing, E. L. Logigian, C. H. Schmid, and A. C. Steere. 1996. Detection of borrelia burgdorferi DNA by polymerase chain reaction in cerebrospinal fluid in lyme neuroborreliosis. *Journal of Infectious Diseases* 174(3):623-627.

Nocton, J. J., F. Dressler, B. J. Rutledge, P. N. Rys, D. H. Persing, and A. C. Steere. 1994. Detection of borrelia burgdorferi DNA by polymerase chain reaction in synovial fluid from patients with lyme arthritis. *N Engl J Med* 330(4):229-234.

Nowakowski, J., I. Schwartz, D. Liveris, G. Wang, M. E. Aguero-Rosenfeld, G. Girao, D. McKenna, R. B. Nadelman, L. F. Cavaliere, and G. P. Wormser. 2001. Laboratory diagnostic techniques for patients with early lyme disease associated with erythema migrans: A comparison of different techniques. *Clin Infect Dis* 33(12):2023-2027.

Oksi, J., H. Marttila, H. Soini, H. Aho, J. Uksila, and M. K. Viljanen. 2001. Early dissemination of borrelia burgdorferi without generalized symptoms in patients with erythema migrans. *APMIS* 109(9):581-588.

Ornstein, K., J. Berglund, S. Bergstrom, R. Norrby, and A. G. Barbour. 2002. Three major lyme borrelia genospecies (borrelia burgdorferi sensu stricto, B. Afzelii and B. Garinii) identified by pcr in cerebrospinal fluid from patients with neuroborreliosis in Sweden. *Scand J Infect Dis* 34(5):341-346.

Pancholi, P., C. P. Kolbert, P. D. Mitchell, K. D. Reed, J. S. Dumler, J. S. Bakken, S. R. Telford, and D. H. Persing. 1995. Ixodes dammini as a potential vector of human granulocytic ehrlichiosis. *Journal of Infectious Diseases* 172(4):1007-1012.

Patel, R., K. L. Grogg, W. D. Edwards, A. J. Wright, and N. M. Schwenk. 2000. Death from inappropriate therapy for lyme disease. *Clin Infect Dis* 31(4):1107-1109.

Peltomaa, M., G. McHugh, and A. C. Steere. 2003. Persistence of the antibody response to the vlse sixth invariant region (ir6) peptide of borrelia burgdorferi after successful antibiotic treatment of lyme disease. *J Infect Dis* 187(8):1178-1186.

Persing, D. H. 1997. The cold zone: A curious convergence of tick-transmitted diseases. *Clin Infect Dis* 25(Suppl 1):S35-42.

Persing, D. H., B. L. Herwaldt, C. Glaser, R. S. Lane, J. W. Thomford, D. Mathiesen, P. J. Krause, D. F. Phillip, and P. A. Conrad. 1995. Infection with a babesia-like organism in northern California. *New England Journal of Medicine* 332(5):298-303.

Persing, D. H., D. Mathiesen, W. F. Marshall, S. R. Telford, A. Spielman, J. W. Thomford, and P. A. Conrad. 1992. Detection of babesia microti by polymerase chain reaction. *Journal of Clinical Microbiology* 30(8):2097-2103.

Persing, D. H., B. J. Rutledge, P. N. Rys, D. S. Podzorski, P. D. Mitchell, K. D. Reed, B. Liu, E. Fikrig, and S. E. Malawista. 1994a. Target imbalance: Disparity of borrelia burgdorferi genetic material in synovial fluid from lyme arthritis patients. *Journal of Infectious Diseases* 169(3):668-672.

———. 1994b. Target imbalance: Disparity of borrelia burgdorferi genetic material in synovial fluid from lyme arthritis patients. *J Infect Dis* 169(3):668-672.

Persing, D. H., S. D. Telford, A. Spielman, and S. W. Barthold. 1990a. Detection of borrelia burgdorferi infection in ixodes dammini ticks with the polymerase chain reaction. *Journal of Clinical Microbiology* 28(3):566-572.

Persing, D. H., S. R. Telford, 3rd, P. N. Rys, D. E. Dodge, T. J. White, S. E. Malawista, and A. Spielman. 1990b. Detection of borrelia burgdorferi DNA in museum specimens of ixodes dammini ticks. *Science* 249(4975):1420-1423.

Philipp, M. T., A. R. Marques, P. T. Fawcett, L. G. Dally, and D. S. Martin. 2003. C6 test as an indicator of therapy outcome for patients with localized or disseminated lyme borreliosis. *J Clin Microbiol* 41(11):4955-4960.

Philipp, M. T., G. P. Wormser, A. R. Marques, S. Bittker, D. S. Martin, J. Nowakowski, and L. G. Dally. 2005. A decline in c6 antibody titer occurs in successfully treated patients with culture-confirmed early localized or early disseminated lyme borreliosis. *Clin Diagn Lab Immunol* 12(9):1069-1074.

Pollack, R. J., S. R. Telford, 3rd, and A. Spielman. 1993. Standardization of medium for culturing lyme disease spirochetes. *J Clin Microbiol* 31(5):1251-1255.

Pruthi, R. K., W. F. Marshall, J. C. Wiltsie, and D. H. Persing. 1995. Human babesiosis. *Mayo Clin Proc* 70(9):853-862.

Quick, R. E., B. L. Herwaldt, J. W. Thomford, M. E. Garnett, M. L. Eberhard, M. Wilson, D. H. Spach, J. W. Dickerson, S. R. Telford, K. R. Steingart, R. Pollock, D. H. Persing,

J. M. Kobayashi, D. D. Juranek, and P. A. Conrad. 1993. Babesiosis in washington state - a new species of babesia? *Annals of Internal Medicine* 119(4):284-290.

Rahn, D. W. 1991. Lyme disease: Clinical manifestations, diagnosis, and treatment. [review]. *Seminars in Arthritis & Rheumatism* 20(4):201-218.

Ravyn, M. D., C. B. Kodner, S. E. Carter, J. L. Jarnefeld, and R. C. Johnson. 2001. Isolation of the etiologic agent of human granulocytic ehrlichiosis from the white-footed mouse (peromyscus leucopus). *J Clin Microbiol* 39(1):335-338.

Recommendations for test performance and interpretation from the second national conference on serologic diagnosis of lyme disease. 1995. *MMWR Morb Mortal Wkly Rep* 44(31):590-591.

Robertson, J., E. Guy, N. Andrews, B. Wilske, P. Anda, M. Granstrom, U. Hauser, Y. Moosmann, V. Sambri, J. Schellekens, G. Stanek, and J. Gray. 2000. A european multicenter study of immunoblotting in serodiagnosis of lyme borreliosis. *J Clin Microbiol* 38(6):2097-2102.

Ruebush, T. D., D. D. Juranek, E. S. Chisholm, P. C. Snow, G. R. Healy, and A. J. Sulzer. 1977. Human babesiosis on nantucket island. Evidence for self-limited and subclinical infections. *New England Journal of Medicine* 297(15):825-827.

Schmidt, B. L. 1997. Pcr in laboratory diagnosis of human borrelia burgdorferi infections. *Clin Microbiol Rev* 10(1):185-201.

Spielman, A. 1976. Human babesiosis on nantucket island: Transmission by nymphal ixodes ticks. *Am. J. Trop. Med. Hyg.* 25:784-787.

Spielman, A., C. M. Clifford, J. Piesman, and M. D. Corwin. 1979. Human babesiosis on nantucket island, USA: Description of the vector, ixodes (ixodes) dammino, n. Sp. (acarina: Ixodidae). *J. Med. Entomol.* 15:218-234.

Steere, A. C. 2001. Lyme disease. *N Engl J Med* 345(2):115-125.

Steere, A. C., R. L. Grodzicki, A. N. Kornblatt, J. E. Craft, A. G. Barbour, W. Burgdorfer, G. P. Schmid, E. Johnson, and S. E. Malawista. 1983. The spirochetal etiology of lyme disease. *New England Journal of Medicine* 308(13):733-740.

Steere, A. C., V. K. Sikand, F. Meurice, D. L. Parenti, E. Fikrig, R. T. Schoen, J. Nowakowski, C. H. Schmid, S. Laukamp, C. Buscarino, and D. S. Krause. 1998. Vaccination against lyme disease with recombinant borrelia burgdorferi outer-surface lipoprotein A with adjuvant. Lyme disease vaccine study group [see comments]. *N Engl J Med* 339(4):209-215.

Stoenner, H. G., T. Dodd, and C. Larsen. 1982. Antigenic variation of borrelia hermsii. *J Exp Med* 156(5):1297-1311.

Telford, S. R., J. E. Dawson, P. Katavolos, C. K. Warner, C. P. Kolbert, and D. H. Persing. 1996. Perpetuation of the agent of human granulocytic ehrlichiosis in a deer tick-rodent cycle. *Proceedings of the National Academy of Sciences (USA)* 93:6209-6214.

Theisen, M., B. Frederiksen, A. M. Lebech, J. Vuust, and K. Hansen. 1993. Polymorphism in ospc gene of borrelia burgdorferi and immunoreactivity of ospc protein: Implications for taxonomy and for use of ospc protein as a diagnostic antigen. *J Clin Microbiol* 31(10):2570-2576.

Thomas, R. J., J. S. Dumler, and J. A. Carlyon. 2009. Current management of human granulocytic anaplasmosis, human monocytic ehrlichiosis and ehrlichia ewingii ehrlichiosis. *Expert Rev Anti Infect Ther* 7(6):709-722.

Thomas, V., J. Anguita, S. W. Barthold, and E. Fikrig. 2001. Coinfection with borrelia burgdorferi and the agent of human granulocytic ehrlichiosis alters murine immune responses, pathogen burden, and severity of lyme arthritis. *Infect Immun* 69(5):3359-3371.

Tugwell, P., D. T. Dennis, A. Weinstein, G. Wells, B. Shea, G. Nichol, R. Hayward, R. Lightfoot, P. Baker, and A. C. Steere. 1997. Laboratory evaluation in the diagnosis of lyme disease. *Ann Intern Med* 127(12):1109-1123.

Vannier, E., and P. J. Krause. 2009. Update on babesiosis. *Interdiscip Perspect Infect Dis* 2009:984568.

Wallach, F. R., A. L. Forni, J. Hariprashad, M. Y. Stoeckle, C. R. Steinberg, L. Fisher, S. E. Malawista, and H. W. Murray. 1993. Circulating borrelia burgdorferi in patients with acute lyme disease: Results of blood cultures and serum DNA analysis. *J Infect Dis* 168(6):1541-1543.

Walls, J. J., M. Aguero-Rosenfeld, J. S. Bakken, J. L. Goodman, D. Hossain, R. C. Johnson, and J. S. Dumler. 1999. Inter- and intralaboratory comparison of ehrlichia equi and human granulocytic ehrlichiosis (hge) agent strains for serodiagnosis of hge by the immunofluorescent-antibody test. *J Clin Microbiol* 37(9):2968-2973.

Walls, J. J., P. Caturegli, J. S. Bakken, K. M. Asanovich, and J. S. Dumler. 2000. Improved sensitivity of pcr for diagnosis of human granulocytic ehrlichiosis using epank1 genes of ehrlichia phagocytophila-group ehrlichiae. *J Clin Microbiol* 38(1):354-356.

Wormser, G. P., S. Bittker, D. Cooper, J. Nowakowski, R. B. Nadelman, and C. Pavia. 2000a. Comparison of the yields of blood cultures using serum or plasma from patients with early lyme disease. *J Clin Microbiol* 38(4):1648-1650.

Wormser, G. P., H. W. Horowitz, J. S. Dumler, I. Schwartz, and M. Aguero-Rosenfeld. 1996. False-positive lyme disease serology in human granulocytic ehrlichiosis [letter]. *Lancet* 347(9006):981-982.

Wormser, G. P., D. Liveris, K. Hanincova, D. Brisson, S. Ludin, V. J. Stracuzzi, M. E. Embers, M. T. Philipp, A. Levin, M. Aguero-Rosenfeld, and I. Schwartz. 2008a. Effect of borrelia burgdorferi genotype on the sensitivity of c6 and 2-tier testing in north American patients with culture-confirmed lyme disease. *Clin Infect Dis* 47(7):910-914.

Wormser, G. P., R. B. Nadelman, R. J. Dattwyler, D. T. Dennis, E. D. Shapiro, A. C. Steere, T. J. Rush, D. W. Rahn, P. K. Coyle, D. H. Persing, D. Fish, and B. J. Luft. 2000b. Practice guidelines for the treatment of lyme disease. The infectious diseases society of america. *Clin Infect Dis* 31(Suppl 1):1-14.

Wormser, G. P., J. Nowakowski, R. B. Nadelman, S. Bittker, D. Cooper, and C. Pavia. 1998. Improving the yield of blood cultures for patients with early lyme disease. *J Clin Microbiol* 36(1):296-298.

Wormser, G. P., J. Nowakowski, R. B. Nadelman, P. Visintainer, A. Levin, and M. E. Aguero-Rosenfeld. 2008b. Impact of clinical variables on borrelia burgdorferi-specific antibody seropositivity in acute-phase sera from patients in north america with culture-confirmed early lyme disease. *Clin Vaccine Immunol* 15(10):1519-1522.

Zeidner, N. S., M. C. Dolan, R. Massung, J. Piesman, and D. Fish. 2000. Coinfection with borrelia burgdorferi and the agent of human granulocytic ehrlichiosis suppresses IL-2 and ifn gamma production and promotes an IL-4 response in c3h/hej mice. *Parasite Immunol* 22(11):581-588.

Zhang, J.-R., J. M. Hardham, A. G. Barbour, and S. J. Norris. 1997a. Antigenic variation in lyme disease borreliae by promiscuous recombination of vmp-like sequence cassettes. *Cell Press* 89:275-285.

Zhang, J. R., and S. J. Norris. 1998a. Genetic variation of the borrelia burgdorferi gene vlse involves cassette-specific, segmental gene conversion. *Infection & Immunity* 66(8):3698-3704.

———. 1998b. Kinetics and in vivo induction of genetic variation of vlse in borrelia burgdorferi. *Infection & Immunity* 66(8):3689-3697.

Zhang, Y. Q., D. Mathiesen, C. P. Kolbert, J. Anderson, R. T. Schoen, E. Fikrig, and D. H. Persing. 1997b. Borrelia burgdorferi enzyme-linked immunosorbent assay for discrimination of ospa vaccination from spirochete infection. *Journal of Clinical Microbiology* 35(1):233-238.

## A5
## EHRLICHIOSES, RICKETTSIOSES, AND ANAPLASMOSIS IN THE UNITED STATES: CURRENT STATUS AND OPPORTUNITIES FOR NEW VACCINES

*Jere W. McBride,[5] Xue-jie Yu,[5] and Kelly Brayton[6]*

### Ehrlichioses

*Introduction*

*Ehrlichia* are obligately intracellular gram-negative bacteria that are associated with emerging, tick-transmitted, life-threatening zoonoses in humans. Human monocytotropic ehrlichiosis (HME) and human ehrlichosis ewingii (HEE) are now well established zoonoses in the United States caused by *E. chaffeensis* and *E. ewingii*, respectively. The first recognized case of human ehrlichiosis occurred in 1986 in a patient that acquired the infection in Arkansas (Maeda et al., 1987), and a previously unknown pathogen, *E. chaffeensis*, was later identified as the etiologic agent (Anderson et al., 1991). As epidemiologic and ecologic understanding of *E. chaffeensis* biology has developed, it is now considered a prototypical emerging pathogen (Paddock and Childs, 2003). Shortly after the emergence of *E. chaffeensis*, the canine pathogen, *E. ewingii*, associated with granulocytic ehrlichiosis in dogs, was molecularly identified in four patients from Missouri presenting with fever, headache and thrombocytopenia (Buller et al., 1999). The emergence of human ehrlichioses has been attributed to changes in biological, demographic and environmental factors, and these factors in addition to increased surveillance and diagnostic capability are likely to result in increasing recognized incidence of human ehrlichiosis in the future (Paddock and Childs, 2003). Thus, there is an immediate need for effective vaccines now for human ehrlichiosis and into the foreseeable future. In this review, we summarize the current status of vaccines and examine the status of new prospects for vaccine development for human ehrlichiosis.

---

[5] Department of Pathology, Center for Biodefense and Emerging Infectious Diseases, Institute for Human Infections and Immunity, University of Texas Medical Branch, Galveston, Texas.

[6] Department of Veterinary Microbiology and Pathology, College of Veterinary Medicine, School for Global Animal Health, Washington State University, Pullman, Washington.

Commissioned by the Institute of Medicine of the National Academies Committee on Lyme Disease and Other Tick-Borne Diseases: The State of the Science September 2010.

*Etiologic agents of the human ehrlichioses*

*Ehrlichia* species are in the subdivision of *Proteobacteria* and members of the family *Anaplasmataceae*, which also includes the genera *Anaplasma*, *Wolbachia*, and *Neorickettsia*. Organisms in the genus *Ehrlichia* include *E. chaffeensis*, *E. ewingii*, *E. canis*, *E. ruminantium*, and *E. muris*. *Ehrlichia* replicate in a membrane-bound cytoplasmic vacuole forming a microcolony called morula. Multiple morulae (1.0 to 6.0 µm) are often present in an infected cell, and by light microscopy they appear as dark blue-to-purple intracytoplasmic inclusions demonstrated by Romanovsky-type stains (Rikihisa, 1991). Morphologically individual ehrlichiae are coccoid and coccobacillary and exhibit two ultrastructural cell types, a larger reticulate cell (RC) (0.4 to 0.6 µm by 0.7 to 1.9 µm) and a smaller dense-cored cell (DC) (0.4 to 0.6 µm in diameter). Both forms have a gram-negative cell wall, characterized by a cytoplasmic membrane and rippled outer membrane separated by a periplasmic space. Reticulate cells are pleomorphic and have uniformly dispersed nucleoid filaments and ribosomes, and DC ehrlichiae are typically coccoid and have centrally condensed nucleoid filaments and ribosomes (Popov et al., 1995; Popov et al., 1998). Small and large morulae containing both RC and DC or exclusively containing DC or RC ehrlichiae usually in loosely packed clusters can be observed within a single infected cell (Popov et al., 1995; Popov et al., 1998). The intramorular space in some morulae contains a fibrillar matrix of ehrlichial origin (Popov et al., 1995). The DC ehrlichiae are infectious and attach to the host cell surface where they are rapidly internalized and transition into a replicating RC forms. RC replicate, doubling every 8 hrs, and then mature to DC within 72 hr after initial cell contact (Zhang et al., 2007).

The intracellular niche occupied by *Ehrlichia* has resulted in reductive evolutionary processes and corresponding severe loss of genes associated with metabolic processes provided by the host cell. Hence the genome sizes (~1-1.5 Mb) of *Ehrlichia* are relatively small compared to extracellular bacteria. The genomes of three *Ehrlichia* species have been sequenced (Collins et al., 2005; Dunning Hotopp et al., 2006; Mavromatis et al., 2006) and exhibit a high degree of genomic synteny, low G+C content (~30%) and one of the smallest genome coding ratios that is attributed to long non-coding regions and numerous long tandemly repeated sequences (TRs) (Frutos et al., 2006). These long non-coding regions and low G+C content in other related *Rickettsiales* members are speculated to represent degraded genes in the final stages of elimination and excess GC-to-AT mutations (Andersson and Andersson, 1999). Another feature of *Ehrlichia* genomes is the presence of a large number of long period TRs that appear to have evolved after divergence of the species (Frutos et al., 2007).

The identified agents of human ehrlichosis in the United States include

*E. chaffeensis* and *E. ewingii*. *E. chaffeensis* exhibits tropism for mononuclear phagocytes and causes mild to life-threatening disease in humans and mild to severe disease in dogs (Breitschwerdt et al., 1998b; Dawson and Ewing, 1992). *E. chaffeensis* is maintained in nature in a zoonotic cycle potentially involving many vertebrate species, and is transmitted primarily by the lone star tick, *Amblyomma americanum* (Paddock and Childs, 2003).

*E. ewingii* is an established canine pathogen first described in 1971 (Ewing et al., 1971). *E. ewingii* exhibits host cell tropism for granulocytes (neutrophils), and is also transmitted by the lone star tick, *A. americanum* (Anziani et al., 1990). Dogs are a reservoir for *E. ewingii*, and many individuals with documented infections reported contact with dogs before onset of symptoms (Buller et al., 1999). Most cases of HEE are manifested in immunocompromised patients, and thus, *E. ewingii* appears to be an opportunistic pathogen (Buller et al., 1999; Paddock et al., 2001).

*E. canis* is the type strain for the genus *Ehrlichia* and is the primary etiologic agent of canine monocytic ehrlichiosis (CME), a serious and sometimes fatal, globally distributed disease of dogs (Keefe et al., 1982). *E. canis* is transmitted by the brown dog tick, *Rhipicephalus sanguineus* (Groves et al., 1975), and infects monocytes/macrophages in dogs. *E. canis* was initially described in dogs in the United States in 1963 (Ewing, 1963), but received more attention after its identification as the agent responsible for outbreaks of a cryptogenic hemorrhagic disease called tropical canine pancytopenia in American and British military dog units on duty in southeast Asia (Huxsoll et al., 1969; Seamer and Snape, 1970; Wilkins et al., 1967). Human infections with *E. canis* have been reported in Venuzuela (Perez et al., 1996; Perez et al., 2006). The clinical manifestations of acute infection with *E. canis* are similar to those observed in humans infected with *E. chaffeensis*.

### Epidemiology and public health importance

Approximately 2,500 cases (passive surveillance) of HME have been formally reported to the Centers for Disease Control from 1999 to 2006, and HME and HEE are Nationally Notifiable Diseases on the public health information network. However, the incidence is likely underestimated since active surveillance studies performed in HME-endemic areas in Missouri, Tennessee and Georgia have revealed an incidence that is 10-100 times higher than reported by passive surveillance (Olano et al., 2003b). HME is a seasonal disease with most reported cases occurring in the spring and summer coinciding with higher tick activity, although cases can occur in the fall in more southern latitudes. The geographic distribution of HME follows the distribution of its vector *A. americanum* (lone star tick), that begins in west central Texas and extends east along the Gulf Coast, north through Oklahoma and Missouri, eastward to the Atlantic Coast and proceeds northeast through New Jersey, encompassing all the south central, southeastern and mid-Atlantic states. The main zoonotic reservoir is the white-tailed deer (*Odocoileus virginianus*), but other potentially important reservoirs are naturally infected with *E. chaffeensis* including goats, domestic dogs, and coyotes (Breitschwerdt et al., 1998b; Dugan et al., 2000; Kocan et al., 2000). The states with highest incidence include Arkansas, North Carolina, Missouri, Oklahoma, and New Jersey (McQuiston et al., 1999). Outside the USA, HME has been described in Cameroon where confirmation of the diagnosis was based on PCR detection of *E. chaffeensis* DNA from ill patients and dogs (Ndip et al., 2009a; Ndip et al., 2009b). *E. chaffeensis* has been found in 5 to 15% of *A. americanum* ticks collected from at least 15 states in endemic areas in the eastern US (Ijdo et al., 2000; Stromdahl et al., 2001;Whitlock et al., 2000). Human infections with *E. chaffeensis* or antigenically related ehrlichiae have been reported in Europe (Nuti et al., 1998), Asia (Heppner et al., 1997), South America (Ripoll et al., 1999), and Africa (Uhaa et al., 1992). Most reports of HME from other countries are based on serological studies, and therefore cannot be confirmed as *E. chaffeensis* infections.

The epidemiology of HEE remains poorly defined due to the lack of a specific serologic assay for this organism and absence of a dedicated reporting system for this disease. Laboratory diagnosis relies on nucleic acid amplification, but new serologic assays to detect *E. ewingii* antibodies have been recently developed (Zhang et al., 2008). Most cases of HEE have been reported in Tennessee, Missouri, and Oklahoma. However, *E. ewingii* infection in deer, dogs and ticks have been described throughout the range of the lone star tick, suggesting that human infection with this pathogen might be more widespread than is currently documented. All cases involving tick transmission have been described in immunocompromised patients (Buller et al., 1999; Paddock et al., 2001).

*Clinical spectrum and treatment*

HME and HEE manifest as undifferentiated febrile illnesses 1 to 3 weeks after the bite of an infected tick. For HME, the most frequent clinical findings reported anytime during the acute illness are fever, malaise, headache, dizziness, chills, and myalgias (Eng et al., 1990; Everett et al., 1994; Fishbein et al., 1989; Fishbein et al., 1994; Olano et al., 2003a; Olano et al., 2003b; Schutze and Jacobs, 1997). HME is more common in male (>2:1) patients >40 years of age; the majority (>80%) report a tick bite (Fishbein et al., 1994; Olano et al., 2003b). Many HME cases are associated with recreational or occupational activities that increase exposure of humans to tick infested environments (Petersen et al., 1989; Standaert et al., 1995). HME presents as a more severe disease in patients >60 years of age and in immunocompromised patients including persons with HIV/AIDS in whom severe complications can arise such as adult respiratory distress syndrome, acute renal failure, shock and CNS involvement (Paddock et al., 2001). Patients with HEE present with a milder disease with few complications suggesting that *E. ewingii* is less pathogenic (Buller et al., 1999). Hematologic and biochemical abnormalities usually include leukopenia, thrombocytopenia, anemia, mildly elevated serum hepatic transaminase activities, and hyponatremia (Fishbein et al., 1994; Olano et al., 2003b; Paddock et al., 2001). A high proportion of immunocompetent (41 to 62%) and immunocompromised patients (86%) require hospitalization (Fishbein et al., 1994; Olano et al., 2003b; Paddock et al., 2001) and delays in antibiotic treatment are associated with more pulmonary complications, increased transfer to intensive care, and longer duration of illness (Hamburg et al., 2008). Immunocompromised patients (human immunodeficiency virus-infected persons, transplant recipients, corticosteroid-treated patients) have a high risk of fatal infection associated with overwhelming infection not typically observed in immunocompetent patients (Paddock et al., 2001). No deaths have been reported as a result of infection with *E. ewingii* (Buller et al., 1999; Paddock et al., 2001).

*In vitro* susceptibility testing has shown that *E. chaffeensis* is resistant to representatives of most classes of antibiotics including aminoglycosides (gentamicin), fluoroquinolones (ciprofloxacin), -lactams (penicillin), macrolides and ketolides (erythromycin and telithromycin), and sulfa-containing drugs (co-trimoxazole) (Brouqui and Raoult, 1992). Patients with HME or HEE respond well to tetracyclines, which have bacteriostatic activities against *Ehrlichia* spp. and other rickettsial agents (Brouqui and Raoult, 1992; Horowitz et al., 2001). Doxycycline is preferred over tetracycline because of its pharmacokinetics and negligible staining of immature teeth. After the first trimester of pregnancy, doxycycline is contraindicated, and successful treatment with rifampin has been reported as an effective alternative (Buitrago et al., 1998).

Overview of Protective Immune Mechanisms

Numerous studies with multiple *Ehrlichia* spp. indicate that IFN-γ is an essential mediator of protection (Mahan et al., 1994b; Mahan et al., 1996; Mutunga et al., 1998; Totte et al., 1993; Totte et al., 1996). Moreover, CD4+ and CD8+ T cells both contribute to IFN- production (Bitsaktsis et al., 2004; Esteves et al., 2004a; Esteves et al., 2004b; Ismail et al., 2004). Notably, similar conclusions regarding the importance of MHC class I, CD4+ and CD8+ T cells, and the synergistic roles of IFN- and TNF- have been reported in mice infected with *E. muris* (Feng and Walker, 2004). An important role for CD4+ T cells in immunity to *E. ruminantium* and IOE has been suggested (Bitsaktsis et al., 2004; Byrom et al., 2000; Totte et al., 1997). Similarly, mice lacking functional MHC class II genes are unable to clear *E. chaffeensis* infection, suggesting that CD4+ T cells are essential for ehrlichial clearance (Ganta et al., 2002). The intradermal environment (natural route of inoculation) appears to promote the induction of protective type-1 responses characterized by increased CD4+ and CD8+ T cells and IFN- producing CD4+ T cells (Stevenson et al., 2006).

Antibody mediated immunity appears to play a significant role in protection against *E. chaffeensis* infection. Infection of SCID mice (B and T cell deficient) with *E. chaffeensis* results in an overwhelming infection (Li et al., 2001; Li et al., 2002; Winslow et al., 2000). Furthermore, mice lacking B cells or FcRI are unable to resolve an ordinarily sublethal infection by IOE, and passive transfer of antibodies in these mice results in significant reduction in bacterial load (Yager et al., 2005). Similarly, passive transfer of antibodies, but not Fab fragments, also protects mice against lethal infection (Feng and Walker, 2004). The specific anti-ehrlichial antibody-mediated mechanism is not fully understood, but appears to involve binding of antibody to the Fc receptor (Lee and Rikihisa, 1997; Yager et al., 2005) and subsequent generation of a proinflammatory cytokine response (Lee and Rikihisa, 1997) and generation of oxidative defenses (Yager et al., 2005).

### Vaccines: Current status and feasibility

Although *Ehrlichia* are responsible for serious diseases of livestock, companion animals and humans, there are no vaccines available for human ehrlichioses and only one infection-treatment immunization regimen is available for the veterinary ehrlichial disease heartwater, caused by *E. ruminantium*. *Ehrlichia* are maintained in nature through subclinical infections of vertebrate hosts (carriers) as well as ticks and have evolved mechanisms to persistently infect mammalian hosts by subverting the innate and adaptive immune responses (Harrus et al., 1998). Effective immune responses leading to the elimination of infections without treatment have been described in *E. canis*-infected dogs (Breitschwerdt et al., 1998a; Harrus et al., 1998), and infection and treatment strategies in Africa for *E. ruminantium* have been used for decades to provide protection against challenge (van der Merwe, 1987). Furthermore, experimental *E. ruminantium* vaccines (inactivated, live attenuated and recombinant) have demonstrated protection against homologous challenge, although less protection has been achieved against natural field challenge (Allsopp, 2009). Cell mediated immune responses and IFN- production correlate with protection against *Ehrlichia* spp. (Bitsaktsis et al., 2004; Totte et al., 1997), and antibodies also play an important role in immunity (Feng and Walker, 2004; Winslow et al., 2000; Yager et al., 2005). Thus, vaccines that stimulate humoral and cell mediated immune responses, prevent disease or minimize clinical signs, shorten duration of illness and/or prevent progression to a chronic infection appear to be feasible.

*Experimental vaccines*

The emergence of human ehrlichioses in the last decade and the risk to public health has elicited interest in the development of vaccines for HME. The use of vaccines to prevent HME may be especially useful for persons who are active outdoors and are at an increased risk level for acquiring the disease. Ehrlichioses, such as heartwater and CME, are important veterinary diseases. Thus, considerable effort has been made to develop vaccines for *E. ruminantium*, which causes large economic losses to the livestock industry in sub-Saharan Africa, and creates limitations on livestock production and export. Consequently, much of the knowledge base for ehrlichial disease vaccine development has involved *E. ruminantium*, where experimental vaccine compositions have been tested, including live, attenuated, nucleic acid and recombinant subunit candidates.

A small group of major immunoreactive proteins of *E. chaffeensis* and *E. canis* has been identified on the basis of immunoblot reactivity, and most of these proteins contain tandem repeats or ankyrin repeats, and most have been molecularly defined (Doyle et al., 2006; Luo et al., 2008; McBride et al., 2003; McBride et al., 2006; Yu et al., 1996). Moreover, many of these proteins are secreted effector proteins that have major species-specific antibody epitopes (Doyle et al., 2006; Luo et al., 2008; Luo et al., 2009; Luo et al., 2010; McBride et al., 2006; Nethery et al., 2007). However, there is relatively little information regarding the protective efficacy of specific immunoreactive proteins. Major immunoreactive *E. chaffeensis* proteins are 200-, 120-, 88-, 55-, 47-, 40-, 28- and 23-kDa (Chen et al., 1994; Rikihisa et al., 1994); *E. canis,* 200-, 140-, 95-, 75-, 47-, 36-, 28-, and 19-kDa (McBride et al., 2003); and *E. ruminantium,* 160-, 85-, 58-, 46-, 40-, 32- and 21-kDa (Mahan et al., 1994a). *E. chaffeensis* immunoreactive proteins (Ank200, TRP120, TRP47, TRP32 [VLPT], OMP-1 family [22 genes], and MAP2) have been molecularly characterized as well as the corresponding orthologs in *E. canis* (Ank200, TRP140, TRP36, TRP19 [VLPT], OMP-1 family [25 genes] and MAP2, respectively). Some of these immunoreactive orthologs have been molecularly identified and characterized in *E. ruminantium* including (MAP1 family [16 genes], MAP2, and mucin-like protein [clone hw26; TRP36/47 ortholog]) (Jongejan and Thielemans, 1989; Mahan et al., 1994a; Sulsona et al., 1999).

Major immunoreactive proteins identified in *Ehrlichia* spp. that have been the primary targets for experimental subunit vaccines include the major outer membrane proteins. Recombinant subunit and nucleic acid vaccines that contain a major surface protein ortholog of *Ehrlichia* spp. (designated MAP1 in *E. ruminantium*; p28 in *E. chaffeensis* and p28/p30 in *E. canis*), which is a member of a paralogous nonidentical multigene family of outer membrane protein genes (16 to 25 genes) in each respective *Ehrlichia* species. Partial protection using a recombinant version of the *E. chaffeensis* P28 protein has been demonstrated in mice after homologous challenge (Ohashi et al., 1998). Moreover, significant protection against homologous challenge using *E. ruminantium* MAP1 DNA vaccination and recombinant protein boost was demonstrated in a mouse model (Nyika et al., 2002). There is substantial divergence in *map1/p28* genes among different isolates of *E. ruminantium* and *E. chaffeensis,* and therefore this diversity may complicate development and implementation of vaccines utilizing this protein. Conversely, the *p28/p30* genes of *E. canis* appear to be highly conserved among geographically dispersed strains, and thus may facilitate more rapid development of effective vaccines utilizing this antigen. Most recently, several new vaccine candidates have been identified and molecularly characterized in *E. chaffeensis* that have major species specific epitopes within tandem repeat regions. These tandem repeat proteins (TRP120, TRP47 and TRP32) from *E. chaffeensis* are consistently recognized by antibodies in convalescent antisera. The ability of these proteins to protect against homologous challenge is currently under active investigation.

*Future prospects*

The emergence of human ehrlichioses in the late 20th century has focused new resources and efforts to improve diagnosis and treatment, and to understand pathogenic and protective immune mechanisms that will facilitate vaccine development. The completion of several *Ehrlichia* genome sequences has provided insight into their evolution, virulence mechanisms, clues to the unique strategies that they utilize to survive in both invertebrate and vertebrate hosts, and their interaction with and dependence on the host cell for survival. Molecular identification and characterization of the majority of the major immunoreactive proteins has been accomplished. These new vaccine prospects, coupled with a more complete understanding of ehrlichial pathobiology and interaction with the innate and adaptive host immune responses, and useful animal models, will undoubtedly stimulate the development of new and more effective nucleic acid or subunit vaccines for human and veterinary use in the future. New technologies including next-generation sequencing will provide researchers with the capability to rapidly and fully explore pathogen gene expression in order to define the dynamics of pathogen phenotype in invertebrate and vertebrate hosts, and new vaccine strategies will be identified through this exploration. New insights into immunoprotective mechanisms and molecular pathogen-host interactions have marked new areas of progress that have addressed key gaps in our knowledge that are required to make effective vaccines.

## Key Points

- Vaccination is the most cost-effective long-term means of controlling human ehrlichioses, and commercial interest and progress in vaccine development for heartwater and canine ehrlichiosis will enhance prospects for a human ehrlichiosis vaccine.
- Immunologically well characterized murine models are available for determining vaccine candidate efficacy and defining protective and pathologic immune mechanisms.
- Defining *Ehrlichia* proteins that elicit protective humoral and cell mediated immune responses is needed and is an area of active investigation.
- Understanding innate and adaptive immune evasion strategies of *Ehrlichia* will improve prospects of effective vaccine development.
- Effective vaccine development will depend on understanding ehrlichial biology and phenotype in mammalian and arthropod host environments.
- Major immunoreactive tandem and ankyrin repeat proteins of *Ehrlichia* have been recently molecularly characterized that contain major continuous species-specific antibody epitopes. Some of these proteins are known to be involved in complex molecular host interactions that may contribute to pathogen survival and may be blocked by the host immune response.

## References

Allsopp, B. A. (2009) Trends in the control of heartwater. Onderstepoort J Vet Res 76: 81-88.

Anderson, B. E., Dawson, J. E., Jones, D. C., and Wilson, K. H. (1991) Ehrlichia chaffeensis, a new species associated with human ehrlichiosis. J Clin Microbiol 29: 2838-2842.

Andersson, J. O. and Andersson, S. G. (1999) Genome degradation is an ongoing process in Rickettsia. Mol Biol Evol 16: 1178-1191.

Anziani, O. S., Ewing, S. A., and Barker, R. W. (1990) Experimental transmission of a granulocytic form of the tribe Ehrlichieae by Dermacentor variabilis and Amblyomma americanum to dogs. Am J Vet Res 51: 929-931.

Bitsaktsis, C., Huntington, J., and Winslow, G. (2004) Production of IFN-gamma by CD4 T cells is essential for resolving ehrlichia infection. J Immunol 172: 6894-6901.

Breitschwerdt, E. B., Hegarty, B. C., and Hancock, S. I. (1998a) Doxycycline hyclate treatment of experimental canine ehrlichiosis followed by challenge inoculation with two Ehrlichia canis strains. Antimicrob Agents Chemother 42: 362-368.

Breitschwerdt, E. B., Hegarty, B. C., and Hancock, S. I. (1998b) Sequential evaluation of dogs naturally infected with Ehrlichia canis, Ehrlichia chaffeensis, Ehrlichia equi, Ehrlichia ewingii, or Bartonella vinsonii. J Clin Microbiol 36: 2645-2651.

Brouqui, P. and Raoult, D. (1992) In vitro antibiotic susceptibility of the newly recognized agent of ehrlichiosis in humans, Ehrlichia chaffeensis. Antimicrob Agents Chemother 36: 2799-2803.

Buitrago, M. I., Ijdo, J. W., Rinaudo, P., Simon, H., Copel, J., Gadbaw, J. et al. (1998) Human granulocytic ehrlichiosis during pregnancy treated successfully with rifampin. Clin Infect Dis 27: 213-215.

Buller, R. S., Arens, M., Hmiel, S. P., Paddock, C. D., Sumner, J. W., Rikhisa, Y. et al. (1999) Ehrlichia ewingii, a newly recognized agent of human ehrlichiosis. N Eng J Med 341: 148-155.

Byrom, B., Barbet, A. F., Obwolo, M., and Mahan, S. M. (2000) CD8(+) T cell knockout mice are less susceptible to Cowdria ruminantium infection than athymic, CD4(+) T cell knockout, and normal C57BL/6 mice. Vet Parasitol 93: 159-172.

Chen, S. M., Dumler, J. S., Feng, H. M., and Walker, D. H. (1994) Identification of the antigenic constituents of Ehrlichia chaffeensis. Am J Trop Med Hyg 50: 52-58.

Collins, N. E., Liebenberg, J., de Villiers, E. P., Brayton, K. A., Louw, E., Pretorius, A. et al. (2005) The genome of the heartwater agent Ehrlichia ruminantium contains multiple tandem repeats of actively variable copy number. Proc Natl Acad Sci U S A 102: 838-843.

Dawson, J. E. and Ewing, S. A. (1992) Susceptibility of dogs to infection with Ehrlichia chaffeensis, causative agent of human ehrlichiosis. Am J Vet Res 53: 1322-1327.

Doyle, C. K., Nethery, K. A., Popov, V. L., and McBride, J. W. (2006) Differentially expressed and secreted major immunoreactive protein orthologs of Ehrlichia canis and E. chaffeensis elicit early antibody responses to epitopes on glycosylated tandem repeats. Infect Immun 74: 711-720.

Dugan, V. G., Little, S. E., Stallknecht, D. E., and Beall, A. D. (2000) Natural infection of domestic goats with Ehrlichia chaffeensis. J Clin Microbiol 38: 448-449.

Dunning Hotopp, J. C., Lin, M., Madupu, R., Crabtree, J., Angiuoli, S. V., Eisen, J. et al. (2006) Comparative genomics of emerging human ehrlichiosis agents. PLoS Genet 2: e21.

Eng, T. R., Harkess, J. R., Fishbein, D. B., Dawson, J. E., Greene, C. N., Redus, M. A. et al. (1990) Epidemiologic, clinical, and laboratory findings of human ehrlichiosis in the United States, 1988. J Am Med Assoc 264: 2251-2258.

Esteves, I., Vachiery, N., Martinez, D., and Totte, P. (2004a) Analysis of Ehrlichia ruminantium-specific T1/T2 responses during vaccination with a protective killed vaccine and challenge of goats. Parasite Immunol 26: 95-103.

Esteves, I., Walravens, K., Vachiery, N., Martinez, D., Letesson, J. J., and Totte, P. (2004b) Protective killed Ehrlichia ruminantium vaccine elicits IFN-gamma responses by CD4+ and CD8+ T lymphocytes in goats. Vet Immunol Immunopathol 98: 49-57.

Everett, E. D., Evans, K. A., Henry, R. B., and McDonald, G. (1994) Human ehrlichiosis in adults after tick exposure. Diagnosis using polymerase chain reaction. Annals of Internal Medicine 120: 730-735.

Ewing, S. A. (1963) Canine ehrlichiosis. J Am Med Assoc 143: 503-506.

Ewing, S. A., Roberson, W. R., Buckner, R. G., and Hayat, C. S. (1971) A new strain of Ehrlichia canis. J Am Vet Med Assoc 159: 1771-1774.

Feng, H. M. and Walker, D. H. (2004) Mechanisms of immunity to Ehrlichia muris: a model of monocytotropic ehrlichiosis. Infect Immun 72: 966-971.

Fishbein, D. B., Dawson, J. E., and Robinson, L. E. (1994) Human ehrlichiosis in the United States, 1985 to 1990. Ann Intern Med 120: 736-743.

Fishbein, D. B., Kemp, A., Dawson, J. E., Greene, N. R., Redus, M. A., and Fields, D. H. (1989) Human ehrlichiosis: prospective active surveillance in febrile hospitalized patients. J Infect Dis 160: 803-809.

Frutos, R., Viari, A., Ferraz, C., Morgat, A., Eychenie, S., Kandassamy, Y. et al. (2006) Comparative genomic analysis of three strains of Ehrlichia ruminantium reveals an active process of genome size plasticity. J Bacteriol 188: 2533-2542.

Frutos, R., Viari, A., Vachiery, N., Boyer, F., and Martinez, D. (2007) Ehrlichia ruminantium: genomic and evolutionary features. Trends Parasitol 23: 414-419.

Ganta, R. R., Wilkerson, M. J., Cheng, C., Rokey, A. M., and Chapes, S. K. (2002) Persistent Ehrlichia chaffeensis infection occurs in the absence of functional major histocompatibility complex class II genes. Infect Immun 70: 380-388.

Groves, M. G., Dennis, G. L., Amyx, H. L., and Huxsoll, D. L. (1975) Transmission of Ehrlichia canis to dogs by ticks (Rhipicephalus sanguineus). Am J Vet Res 36: 937-940.

Hamburg, B. J., Storch, G. A., Micek, S. T., and Kollef, M. H. (2008) The importance of early treatment with doxycycline in human ehrlichiosis. Medicine (Baltimore) 87: 53-60.

Harrus, S., Waner, T., Aizenberg, I., Foley, J. E., Poland, A. M., and Bark, H. (1998) Amplification of ehrlichial DNA from dogs 34 months after infection with Ehrlichia canis. J Clin Microbiol 36: 73-76.

Heppner, D. G., Wongsrichanalai, C., Walsh, D. S., McDaniel, P., Eamsila, C., Hanson, B. et al. (1997) Human ehrlichiosis in Thailand. Lancet 350: 785-786.

Horowitz, H. W., Hsieh, T. C., guero-Rosenfeld, M. E., Kalantarpour, F., Chowdhury, I., Wormser, G. P. et al. (2001) Antimicrobial susceptibility of Ehrlichia phagocytophila. Antimicrob Agents Chemother 45: 786-788.

Huxsoll, D. L., Hildebrandt, P. K., Nims, R. M., Ferguson, J. A., and Walker, J. S. (1969) Ehrlichia canis—the causative agent of a haemorrhagic disease of dogs? Vet Rec 85: 587.

Ijdo, J. W., Wu, C., Magnarelli, L. A., Stafford, K. C., III, Anderson, J. F., and Fikrig, E. (2000) Detection of Ehrlichia chaffeensis DNA in Amblyomma americanum ticks in Connecticut and Rhode Island. J Clin Microbiol 38: 4655-4656.

Ismail, N., Soong, L., McBride, J. W., Valbuena, G., Olano, J. P., Feng, H. M. et al. (2004) Overproduction of TNF-alpha by CD8+ type 1 cells and down-regulation of IFN-gamma production by CD4+ Th1 cells contribute to toxic shock-like syndrome in an animal model of fatal monocytotropic ehrlichiosis. J Immunol 172: 1786-1800.

Jongejan, F. and Thielemans, M. J. (1989) Identification of an immunodominant antigenically conserved 32-kilodalton protein from Cowdria ruminantium. Infect Immun 57: 3243-3246.

Keefe, T. J., Holland, C. J., Salyer, P. E., and Ristic, M. (1982) Distribution of Ehrlichia canis among military working dogs in the world and selected civilian dogs in the United States. J Am Vet Med Assoc 181: 236-238.

Kocan, A. A., Levesque, G. C., Whitworth, L. C., Murphy, G. L., Ewing, S. A., and Barker, R. W. (2000) Naturally occurring Ehrlichia chaffeensis infection in coyotes from Oklahoma. Emerg Infect Dis 6: 477-480.

Lee, E. H. and Rikihisa, Y. (1997) Anti-Ehrlichia chaffeensis antibody complexed with E. chaffeensis induces potent proinflammatory cytokine mRNA expression in human monocytes through sustained reduction of IkappaB-alpha and activation of NF-kappaB. Infect Immun 65: 2890-2897.

Li, J. S., Chu, F., Reilly, A., and Winslow, G. M. (2002) Antibodies highly effective in SCID mice during infection by the intracellular bacterium Ehrlichia chaffeensis are of picomolar affinity and exhibit preferential epitope and isotype utilization. J Immunol 169: 1419-1425.

Li, J. S., Yager, E., Reilly, M., Freeman, C., Reddy, G. R., Reilly, A. A. et al. (2001) Outer membrane protein-specific monoclonal antibodies protect SCID mice from fatal infection by the obligate intracellular bacterial pathogen Ehrlichia chaffeensis. J Immunol 166: 1855-1862.

Luo, T., Zhang, X., and McBride, J. W. (2009) Major species-specific antibody epitopes of the Ehrlichia chaffeensis p120 and E. canis p140 orthologs in surface-exposed tandem repeat regions. Clin Vaccine Immunol 16: 982-990.

Luo, T., Zhang, X., Nicholson, W. L., Zhu, B., and McBride, J. W. (2010) Molecular characterization of antibody epitopes of Ehrlichia chaffeensis ankyrin protein 200 and tandem repeat protein 47 and evaluation of synthetic immunodeterminants for serodiagnosis of human monocytotropic ehrlichiosis. Clin Vaccine Immunol 17: 87-97.

Luo, T., Zhang, X., Wakeel, A., Popov, V. L., and McBride, J. W. (2008) A variable-length PCR target protein of Ehrlichia chaffeensis contains major species-specific antibody epitopes in acidic serine-rich tandem repeats. Infect Immun 76: 1572-1580.

Maeda, K., Markowitz, N., Hawley, R. C., Ristic, M., Cox, D., and McDade, J. E. (1987) Human infection with Ehrlichia canis, a leukocytic rickettsia. N Engl J Med 316: 853-856.

Mahan, S. M., McGuire, T. C., Semu, S. M., Bowie, M. V., Jongejan, F., Rurangirwa, F. R. et al. (1994a) Molecular cloning of a gene encoding the immunogenic 21 kDa protein of Cowdria ruminantium. Microbiol 140 ( Pt 8): 2135-2142.

Mahan, S. M., Sileghem, M., Smith, G. E., and Byrom, B. (1996) Neutralization of bovine concanavalin-A T cell supernatant-mediated anti-Cowdria ruminantium activity with antibodies specific to interferon gamma but not to tumor necrosis factor. Parasite Immunol 18: 317-324.

Mahan, S. M., Smith, G. E., and Byrom, B. (1994b) Conconavalin A-stimulated bovine T-cell supernatants inhibit growth of Cowdria ruminantium in bovine endothelial cells in vitro. Infect Immun 62: 747-750.

Mavromatis, K., Doyle, C. K., Lykidis, A., Ivanova, N., Francino, M. P., Chain, P. et al. (2006) The genome of the obligately intracellular bacterium Ehrlichia canis reveals themes of complex membrane structure and immune evasion strategies. J Bacteriol 188: 4015-4023.

McBride, J. W., Comer, J. E., and Walker, D. H. (2003) Novel immunoreactive glycoprotein orthologs of Ehrlichia spp. Ann N Y Acad Sci 990: 678-684.

McBride, J. W., Corstvet, R. E., Gaunt, S. D., Boudreaux, C., Guedry, T., and Walker, D. H. (2003) Kinetics of antibody response to Ehrlichia canis immunoreactive proteins. Infect Immun 71: 2516-2524.

McBride, J. W., Doyle, C. K., Zhang, X., Cardenas, A. M., Popov, V. L., Nethery, K. A. et al. (2006) Identification of a glycosylated Ehrlichia canis 19-kDa major immunoreactive protein with a species-specific serine-rich glycopeptide epitope. Infect Immun 75: 74-82.

McQuiston, J. H., Paddock, C. D., Holman, R. C., and Childs, J. E. (1999) Human ehrlichioses in the United States. Emerg Infect Dis 5: 635-642.

Mutunga, M., Preston, P. M., and Sumption, K. J. (1998) Nitric oxide is produced by Cowdria ruminantium-infected bovine pulmonary endothelial cells in vitro and is stimulated by gamma interferon. Infect Immun 66: 2115-2121.

Ndip, L. M., Labruna, M. B., Ndip, R. N., Walker D.H., and McBride J.W. (2009a) Molecular and clinical evidence of Ehrlichia chaffeensis infection in Cameroonian patients with undifferentiated febrile illness. Ann Trop Med Parasit.

Ndip, L. M., Ndip, R. N., Esemu, S. N., Walker, D. H., and McBride, J. W. (2009b) Predominance of Ehrlichia chaffeensis in Rhipicephalus sanguineus ticks from kennel-confined dogs in Limbe, Cameroon. Exp Appl Acarol.

Nethery, K. A., Doyle, C. K., Zhang, X., and McBride, J. W. (2007) Ehrlichia canis gp200 contains dominant species-specific antibody epitopes in terminal acidic domains. Infect Immun 75: 4900-4908.

Nuti, M., Serafini, D. A., Bassetti, D., Ghionni, A., Russino, F., Rombola, P. et al. (1998) Ehrlichia infection in Italy. Emerg Infect Dis 4: 663-665.

Nyika, A., Barbet, A. F., Burridge, M. J., and Mahan, S. M. (2002) DNA vaccination with map1 gene followed by protein boost augments protection against challenge with Cowdria ruminantium, the agent of heartwater. Vaccine 20: 1215-1225.

Ohashi, N., Zhi, N., Zhang, Y., and Rikihisa, Y. (1998) Immunodominant major outer membrane proteins of Ehrlichia chaffeensis are encoded by a polymorphic multigene family. Infect Immun 66: 132-139.

Olano, J. P., Hogrefe, W., Seaton, B., and Walker, D. H. (2003a) Clinical manifestations, epidemiology, and laboratory diagnosis of human monocytotropic ehrlichiosis in a commercial laboratory setting. Clin Diagn Lab Immunol 10: 891-896.

Olano, J. P., Masters, E., Hogrefe, W., and Walker, D. H. (2003b) Human monocytotropic ehrlichiosis, Missouri. Emerg Infect Dis 9: 1579-1586.

Paddock, C. D. and Childs, J. E. (2003) Ehrlichia chaffeensis: a prototypical emerging pathogen. Clin Microbiol Rev 16: 37-64.

Paddock, C. D., Folk, S. M., Shore, G. M., Machado, L. J., Huycke, M. M., Slater, L. N. et al. (2001) Infections with Ehrlichia chaffeensis and Ehrlichia ewingii in persons coinfected with human immunodeficiency virus. Clin Infect Dis 33: 1586-1594.

Perez, M., Bodor, M., Zhang, C., Xiong, Q., and Rikihisa, Y. (2006) Human infection with Ehrlichia canis accompanied by clinical signs in Venezuela. Ann N Y Acad Sci 1078: 110-117.

Perez, M., Rikihisa, Y., and Wen, B. (1996) Ehrlichia canis-like agent isolated from a man in Venezuela: antigenic and genetic characterization. J Clin Microbiol 34: 2133-2139.

Petersen, L. R., Sawyer, L. A., Fishbein, D. B., Kelley, P. W., Thomas, R. J., Magnarelli, L. A. et al. (1989) An outbreak of ehrlichiosis in members of an Army Reserve unit exposed to ticks. J Infect Dis 159: 562-568.

Popov, V. L., Chen, S. M., Feng, H. M., and Walker, D. H. (1995) Ultrastructural variation of cultured Ehrlichia chaffeensis. J Med Microbiol 43: 411-421.

Popov, V. L., Han, V. C., Chen, S. M., Dumler, J. S., Feng, H. M., Andreadis, T. G. et al. (1998) Ultrastructural differentiation of the genogroups in the genus Ehrlichia. J Med Microbiol 47: 235-251.

Rikihisa, Y. (1991) The tribe Ehrlichieae and ehrlichial diseases. Clin Microbiol Rev 4: 286-308.

Rikihisa, Y., Ewing, S. A., and Fox, J. C. (1994) Western immunoblot analysis of Ehrlichia chaffeensis, E. canis, or E. ewingii infections in dogs and humans. J Clin Microbiol 32: 2107-2112.

Ripoll, C. M., Remondegui, C. E., Ordonez, G., Arazamendi, R., Fusaro, H., Hyman, M. J. et al. (1999) Evidence of rickettsial spotted fever and ehrlichial infections in a subtropical territory of Jujuy, Argentina. Am J Trop Med Hyg 61: 350-354.

Schutze, G. E. and Jacobs, R. F. (1997) Human monocytic ehrlichiosis in children. Pediatrics 100: E10.

Seamer, J. and Snape, T. (1970) Tropical canine pancytopaenia and Ehrlichia canis infection. Vet Rec 86: 375.

Standaert, S. M., Dawson, J. E., Schaffner, W., Childs, J. E., Biggie, K. L., Singleton, J. J. et al. (1995) Ehrlichiosis in a golf-oriented retirement community. N Eng J Med 333: 420-425.

Stevenson, H. L., Jordan, J. M., Peerwani, Z., Wang, H. Q., Walker, D. H., and Ismail, N. (2006) An intradermal environment promotes a protective type-1 response against lethal systemic monocytotropic ehrlichial infection. Infect Immun 74: 4856-4864.

Stromdahl, E. Y., Evans, S. R., O'Brien, J. J., and Gutierrez, A. G. (2001) Prevalence of infection in ticks submitted to the human tick test kit program of the U.S. Army Center for Health Promotion and Preventive Medicine. J Med Entomol 38: 67-74.

Sulsona, C. R., Mahan, S. M., and Barbet, A. F. (1999) The map1 gene of Cowdria ruminantium is a member of a multigene family containing both conserved and variable genes. Biochem Biophys Res Commun 257: 300-305.

Totte, P., Blankaert, D., Zilimwabagabo, P., and Werenne, J. (1993) Inhibition of Cowdria ruminantium infectious yield by interferons alpha and gamma in endothelial cells. Rev Elev Med Vet Pays Trop 46: 189-194.

Totte, P., McKeever, D., Martinez, D., and Bensaid, A. (1997) Analysis of T-cell responses in cattle immunized against heartwater by vaccination with killed elementary bodies of Cowdria ruminantium. Infect Immun 65: 236-241.

Totte, P., Vachiery, N., Martinez, D., Trap, I., Ballingall, K. T., MacHugh, N. D. et al. (1996) Recombinant bovine interferon gamma inhibits the growth of Cowdria ruminantium but fails to induce major histocompatibility complex class II following infection of endothelial cells. Vet Immunol Immunopathol 53: 61-71.

Uhaa, I. J., MacLean, J. D., Greene, C. R., and Fishbein, D. B. (1992) A case of human ehrlichiosis acquired in Mali: clinical and laboratory findings. Am J Trop Med Hyg 46: 161-164.

van der Merwe, L. (1987) The infection and treatment method of vaccination against heartwater. Onderstepoort J Vet Res 54: 489-491.

Whitlock, J. E., Fang, Q. Q., Durden, L. A., and Oliver, J. H., Jr. (2000) Prevalence of Ehrlichia chaffeensis (Rickettsiales: Rickettsiaceae) in Amblyomma americanum (Acari: Ixodidae) from the Georgia coast and barrier islands. J Med Entomol 37: 276-280.

Wilkins, J. H., Bowden, R. S., and Wilkinson, G. T. (1967) A new canine disease syndrome. Vet Rec 81: 57-58.

Winslow, G. M., Yager, E., Shilo, K., Volk, E., Reilly, A., and Chu, F. K. (2000) Antibody-mediated elimination of the obligate intracellular bacterial pathogen Ehrlichia chaffeensis during active infection. Infect Immun 68: 2187-2195.

Yager, E., Bitsaktsis, C., Nandi, B., McBride, J. W., and Winslow, G. (2005) Essential role for humoral immunity during Ehrlichia infection in immunocompetent mice. Infect Immun 73: 8009-8016.

Yu, X. J., Crocquet-Valdes, P., Cullman, L. C., and Walker, D. H. (1996) The recombinant 120-kilodalton protein of Ehrlichia chaffeensis, a potential diagnostic tool. J Clin Microbiol 34: 2853-2855.

Zhang, C., Xiong, Q., Kikuchi, T., and Rikihisa, Y. (2008) Identification of 19 polymorphic major outer membrane protein genes and their immunogenic peptides in Ehrlichia ewingii for use in a serodiagnostic assay. Clin Vaccine Immunol 15: 402-411.

Zhang, J. Z., Popov, V. L., Gao, S., Walker, D. H., and Yu, X. J. (2007) The developmental cycle of Ehrlichia chaffeensis in vertebrate cells. Cell Microbiol 9: 610-618.

# Rickettsiosis

## Introduction

*Rickettsia* are arthropod-borne, gram-negative, obligately intracellular bacteria that reside in the cytosol of host cells. Tick-borne *Rickettsia* include the most deadly bacterial organism, *R. rickettsii*, low pathogenic organisms such as *R. parkeri* and *R. sibirica*, and nonpathogenic organisms such as *R. peacockii*, *R. bellii*, and *R. montanensis*. Lethality of Rocky Mountain spotted fever (RMSF) caused by *R. rickettsii* in the pre-antibiotic era was as high as 80%. Even with the availability of effective rickettsiostatic antibiotic treatment, the mortality rate is around 3-5% for RMSF because of late diagnosis and delay in starting appropriate therapy (Paddock et al., 2002; Dumler et al., 2004). *R. rickettsii* not only causes severe disease naturally, is also a potential terrorism agent because it is highly infectious at a very low dose (Wike et al., 1972).

*Etiologic agents*

*Rickettsia* are small gram negative bacteria (0.3 – 0.5 × 0.8 – 1.0 µm). Rickettsial diseases are transmitted by arthropods including ticks, mites, lice, and fleas. Based on LPS antigens rickettsiae are classified into typhus group (TG) and spotted fever group (SFG). TG rickettsiae are transmitted by lice and fleas. SFG rickettsiae include more than 20 species and most of them are tick-borne except for mite-borne *R. akari* and flea-borne *R. felis*. The non-tick-borne *Rickettsia* will not be discussed further. All *Rickettsia* multiply in the cytoplasm of host cells, but SFG rickettsiae can also multiply in the nuclei of host cells. *Rickettsia* organisms have undergone genome reduction resulting in a smaller genome (approximately 1Mb), and have lost genes encoding enzymes for sugar metabolism, lipid biosynthesis, nucleotide synthesis and amino acid synthesis (Andersson et al., 1998). SFG rickettsiae spread from cell to cell via actin-based mobility (Teysseire et al., 1992).

*Epidemiology/Public health importance*

The distribution of tick-borne SFG rickettsioses is restricted to areas where their tick reservoirs are present such as Rocky Mountain spotted fever in the Americas, Mediterranean spotted fever in Europe, Africa and Asia, and Japanese spotted fever in Japan and Korea (Table A5-1).

Tick-borne rickettsiae are maintained in nature largely via transovarian transmission in ticks. Nonvirulent and low virulent tick-borne *Rickettsia* do not cause adverse effects on their tick vector, but virulent *Rickettsia* such as *R. rickettsii* and *R. conorii* are pathogenic for *Dermacentor* and *Rhipicephalus* ticks, respectively (Niebylski et al., 1999; Santos et al., 2002). Thus, virulent rickettsiae such as *R. rickettsii* need an animal host to amplify the organisms to establish new lines of transovarian rickettsial maintenance (e.g., *D. variabilis* ticks acquire *R. rickettsii* while feeding on rickettsemic cotton rats) (Niebylski et al., 1999). The vectors of Rocky Mountain spotted fever are *D. variabilis* (American dog tick) in the eastern two-thirds of the US and regions of the Pacific coast states, *D. andersoni* (wood tick) in the Rocky Mountain states, *Rhipicephalus sanguineus* (brown dog tick) in the southwestern US and northern Mexico, and *Amblyomma cajennense* and *A. aureolatum* in South America.

The seasonal and geographic distribution of each rickettsiosis reflects the months of activity of the vector and its contact with humans. Over 90% of cases of Rocky Mountain spotted fever occur during April through September. Approximately 250-1200 cases of Rocky Mountain spotted fever have been reported annually in the past (http://www.cdc.gov/ncidod/dvrd/rmsf/epidemiology.htm), and currently more than 2000 cases are reported each year.

**TABLE A5-1** Distribution of Tick-Borne Rickettsioses

| Disease | Rickettsia agent | Geographic Distribution |
|---|---|---|
| African tick-bite fever | *Rickettsia africae* | Sub-Saharan Africa, Caribbean islands |
| Far eastern spotted fever | *Rickettsia heilongjiangensis* | Far East of Russia and China |
| Flinders Island spotted fever | *Rickettsia honei* | Australia and southeastern Asia |
| Mediterranean spotted fever | *Rickettsia conorii* | Southern Europe, southern and western Asia, and Africa |
| North Asian tick typhus | *Rickettisa sibirica* | Asia, Europe, and Africa |
| Lymphangitis-associated Rickettsiosis | *Rickettsia sibirica mongolotimonae* | |
| Oriental spotted fever | *Rickettsia japonica* | Japan and Korea |
| Queensland tick typhus | *Rickettsia australis* | Australia |
| Rocky Mountain spotted fever | *Rickettsia rickettsii* | North, Central and South America |
| Tick-borne lymphadenopathy | *Rickettsia slovaca* | Europe |
| Unnamed | *Rickettsia parkeri* | North and South America |
| Unnamed | *Rickettsia massiliae* | Europe and North and South America |
| Unnamed | *Rickettsia aeschlimannii* | Europe and Africa |
| Unnamed | *Rickettsia monacensis* | Europe |
| Unknown | *Rickettsia helvetica* | Europe and Asia |

## Clinical spectrum and treatment

Rickettsial diseases are characterized at onset by fever, severe headache, and muscle aches. In Rocky Mountain spotted fever, the characteristic maculopapular rash typically appears 3 to 5 days later. In severe disease, petechiae may appear in the center of the maculopapules. However, up to 10% to 15% of people with RMSF never develop a rash, a condition often referred to as "Rocky Mountain *spotless* fever" (Sexton and Corey, 1992). Rashes are less frequent in less severe rickettsioses such as African tick bite fever and *R. parkeri* infection. Focal skin necrosis with a dark scab (an eschar) at the site of tick feeding is a common feature of boutonneuse fever, African tick bite fever, North Asian tick typhus, Queensland tick typhus, Japanese spotted fever, Flinders Island spotted fever, tick-borne lymphadenopathy, and the recently described infections in the US caused by *R. parkeri* and a novel strain 364 D, but is rare in Rocky Mountain spotted fever.

Tetracyclines are first-line treatment, and doxycycline may be used to avoid tooth staining in children. Tetracyclines are rickettsiostatic, not rickettsicidal. Ciprofloxacin and other fluoroquinolones are effective against certain rickettsiae. Because diagnostic tests can take time and may be insensitive, antibiotics are usually begun presumptively to prevent significant deterioration, death, and prolonged recovery.

## Overview of protective immune mechanisms

Most of our understanding of the immune response against *Rickettsia* is derived from *in vitro* studies as well as the murine models of rickettsioses. Proinflammatory cytokines such as IFN- and TNF- are essential for primary defense against rickettsial infection. These cytokines act in concert to activate endothelial cells, the major target cells of rickettsial infections, as well as other minor target cells to kill intracellular organisms via a nitric oxide synthesis-dependent mechanism. The sources of these protective cytokines are hypothesized to be the T lymphocytes and macrophages that infiltrate the perivascular space surrounding the vessels with infected endothelium.

Cell mediated immunity plays a critical role in host defenses against rickettsial infections(Walker et al., 2001). There are two important effector components of acquired immune response against *Rickettsia*, namely IFN-production by CD4+ and CD8+ type-1 cells, which activates intracellular bactericidal mechanisms of endothelial cells and macrophages, and the generation of *Rickettsia*-specific cytotoxic CD8+ T cells that lyse infected target cells via pathways involving perforin and/or granzymes. CD8+ T cells are more important in clearance of rickettsial infection against rickettsiae than CD4+ T cells (Walker et al., 2001). Although adoptive transfer of either CD4 or CD8 immune T lymphocytes control the infection and lead to survival, only depletion of CD8 T lymphocytes altered the outcome of infection, and depletion of CD4 cells had no observed effect on the course or outcome of infection (Walker et al., 2001).

Humoral response may play an important role in protection against infection and antibodies against surface protein antigens are very likely critical effectors of vaccines-induce protective immunity. In animal experiments, antibodies to *Rickettsia* or rickettsial outer membrane proteins can neutralize rickettsial infection (Anacker et al., 1987; Li et al., 1988). However, natural infection does not result in the production of protective antibodies prior to clearance of rickettsiae. Thus, humoral immunity may be more important in preventing reinfection as in vaccine-induced immunity than in clearance of primary infection.

## Vaccine feasibility and current status

Currently no commercial vaccine is available for any rickettsial disease. Infection with *R. rickettsii* and *R. conorii* is thought to provide long lasting immunity against re-infection. Thus, it is feasible to develop a vaccine against rickettsial diseases. In theory, a subunit vaccine targeting a conserved rickettsial protein such as OmpB may be developed to prevent all rickettsial diseases. The best rickettsial vaccine may be an attenuated organism that can multiply but does not cause disease in the host. Attenuated *Rickettsia* has been achieved with gene knockout technology, and more attenuated strains of *Rickettsia* will become available for vaccine evaluation.

## Experimental vaccines and other potential vaccine prospects

**Inactivated rickettsial vaccine.** The history of development of vaccines against Rocky Mountain spotted fever contains numerous failures and limited success in preventing or ameliorating disease. The first rickettsial vaccine was a killed *R. rickettsii* preparation from infected ticks (Spencer and Parker, 1925). The method of propagating *R. rickettsii* in yolk sac of embryonated chicken eggs was adapted soon after the development of this method in 1938 (Cox, 1939). A third killed Rocky Mountain spotted fever vaccine was prepared from cell culture-propagated *R. rickettsii* by the US Army in the 1970s (Kenyon et al., 1972).

A challenge trial in human volunteers was conducted in 1973. Neither the yolk sac vaccine nor the tick vaccine prevented the illness, which, of course, was treated promptly to prevent severe illness or death. The yolk sac vaccine was withdrawn from the market in 1978. Subsequent challenge trial of the killed-*R. rickettsii* vaccine prepared from cell culture yielded protection of 25% of the volunteers who received it. Evaluation of the recipients' immune responses revealed failure to stimulate sustained cellular immunity (Clements et al., 1983).

**Subunit vaccine for Rickettsia.** Two surface protein antigens of *R. rickettsii*, OmpA and OmpB, have been identified as major protective antigens and are candidates for use as subunit vaccines. The first evidence that OmpA and OmpB contain protective epitopes came from the studies of monoclonal antibodies to heat sensitive epitopes of OmpA and OmpB, which neutralized *R. rickettsii* toxicity in mice and infection in guinea pigs (Anacker et al., 1987; Li et al., 1988). Immunization with the *E. coli*-expressed OmpA N-terminal fragment partially protects guinea pigs against a lethal challenge dose of *R. rickettsii* (McDonald et al., 1988). A fragment from the N-terminus of *R. conorii* OmpA protects guinea pigs against experimental infection with *R. conorii* and partially protects guinea pigs from challenge with the heterologous *R. rickettsii* (Vishwanath et al., 1990). Fragments of the *ompA* and *ompB* genes have been tested as DNA vaccines. In a regime of DNA immunization followed by boosters of the corresponding peptide, mice immunized with one of several *R. rickettsii* *ompA* or *ompB* fragments are partially protected against a lethal challenge with heterologous *R. conorii* (Diaz-Montero et al., 2001). It is not known whether the incomplete protection of OmpA and OmpB to the heterologous *Rickettsia* species challenge in these experiments is caused by the antigenic differences between the rickettsial species, the immunization regime, or the antigen composition.

**Attenuation of Rickettsia by gene knockout.** Because of the difficulty of transforming *Rickettsia*, scientists have been unable to knock out rickettsial genes to test their function and to create an attenuated rickettsial vaccine until recently. The phopholipase D (*pld*) was the first rickettsial gene that was genetically knocked out. The *pld*- knockout Evir strain is avirulent for guinea pigs at the doses for which the Evir strain is virulent (Driskell et al., 2009). A Sca2 knockout strain of *R. rickettsii* has lost actin based mobility in cell culture, and in a guinea pig model of infection, the Sca2 mutant did not elicit fever, suggesting that Sca2 is a virulence factor of spotted fever group rickettsiae (Kleba et al., 2010).

## Future prospects

The protective immune response to rickettsial infection involves both innate and adaptive immune responses. A concerted action of CD8+ T cells, and CD4+ T cells producing IFN-, and antibodies is required to clear infection and to prevent reinfection. Live attenuated vaccine mimics the natural infection, thus *Rickettsia* that are genetically attenuated by gene knockout are the strongest future direction for developing a rickettsial vaccine.

## Key issues

*Rickettsia* are obligately intracellular bacteria and are transmitted by arthropods, including ticks.

*R. rickettsii* cause fatal disease that can be prevented by avoiding tick bites and removing attached ticks promptly.

There is no vaccine for rickettsial diseases despite the fact rickettsial infection stimulates long term immunity. Vaccines are needed for Rocky Mountain spotted fever.

Because diagnostic tests can take time and may be insensitive, antibiotic treatment should be initiated based on clinical and epidemiological information.

## References

Anacker,R.L., McDonald,G.A., List,R.H., and Mann,R.E. (1987) Neutralizing activity of monoclonal antibodies to heat-sensitive and heat-resistant epitopes of Rickettsia rickettsii surface proteins. Infect Immun 55: 825-827.

Andersson,S.G., Zomorodipour,A., Andersson,J.O., Sicheritz-Ponten,T., Alsmark,U.C., Podowski,R.M. et al. (1998) The genome sequence of Rickettsia prowazekii and the origin of mitochondria. Nature 396: 133-140.

Clements,M.L., Wisseman,C.L., Jr., Woodward,T.E., Fiset,P., Dumler,J.S., McNamee,W. et al. (1983) Reactogenicity, immunogenicity, and efficacy of a chick embryo cell-derived vaccine for Rocky Mountain spotted fever. J Infect Dis 148: 922-930.

Cox,H.R. (1939) Rocky Mountain spotted fever. Protective value for guinea pigs of vaccine prepared from rickettsiae cultivated in embryonic chick tissues. Public Health Rep 54: 1070-1077.

Diaz-Montero,C.M., Feng,H.-M., Crocquet-Valdes,P.A., and Walker,D.H. (2001) Identification of protective components of two major outer membrane proteins of spotted fever group rickettsiae. Am J Trop Med Hyg 65: 371-378.

Driskell,L.O., Yu,X.J., Zhang,L., Liu,Y., Popov,V.L., Walker,D.H. et al. (2009) Directed mutagenesis of the Rickettsia prowazekii pld gene encoding phospholipase D. Infect Immun 77: 3244-3248.

Kenyon,R.H., Acree,W.M., Wright,G.G., and Melchior,F.W., Jr. (1972) Preparation of vaccines for Rocky Mountain spotted fever from rickettsiae propagated in cell culture. J Infect Dis 125: 146-152.

Kleba,B., Clark,T.R., Lutter,E.I., Ellison,D.W., and Hackstadt,T. (2010) Disruption of the Rickettsia rickettsii Sca2 autotransporter inhibits actin-based motility. Infect Immun 78: 2240-2247.

Li,H., Lenz,B., and Walker,D.H. (1988) Protective monoclonal antibodies recognize heat-labile epitopes on surface proteins of spotted fever group rickettsiae. Infect Immun 56: 2587-2593.

McDonald,G.A., Anacker,R.L., Mann,R.E., and Milch,L.J. (1988) Protection of guinea pigs from experimental Rocky Mountain spotted fever with a cloned antigen of Rickettsia rickettsii. J Infect Dis 158: 228-231.

Niebylski,M.L., Peacock,M.G., and Schwan,T.G. (1999) Lethal effect of Rickettsia rickettsii on its tick vector (Dermacentor andersoni). Appl Environ Microbiol 65: 773-778.

Paddock,C.D., Holman,R.C., Krebs,J.W., and Childs,J.E. (2002) Assessing the magnitude of fatal Rocky Mountain spotted fever in the United States: comparison of two national data sources. Am J Trop Med Hyg 67: 349-354.

Raoult,D., Woodward,T., and Dumler,J.S. (2004) The history of epidemic typhus. Infect Dis Clin North Am 18: 127-140.

Santos,A.S., Bacellar,F., Santos-Silva,M., Formosinho,P., Gracio,A.J., and Franca,S. (2002) Ultrastructural study of the infection process of Rickettsia conorii in the salivary glands of the vector tick Rhipicephalus sanguineus. Vector Borne Zoonotic Dis 2: 165-177.

Sexton,D.J., and Corey,G.R. (1992) Rocky Mountain "spotless" and "almost spotless" fever: a wolf in sheep's clothing. Clin Infect Dis 15: 439-448.

Spencer,R.R., and Parker,R.R. (1925) Rocky Mountain spotted fever: vaccination of monkeys and man. Public Health Rep 40: 2159-2167.

Teysseire,N., Chiche-Portiche,C., and Raoult,D. (1992) Intracellular movements of Rickettsia conorii and R. typhi based on actin polymerization. Res Microbiol 143: 821-829.

Vishwanath,S., McDonald,G.A., and Watkins,N.G. (1990) A recombinant Rickettsia conorii vaccine protects guinea pigs from experimental boutonneuse fever and Rocky Mountain spotted fever. Infect Immun 58: 646-653.

Walker, D.H., Olano,J.P., and Feng,H.M. (2001) Critical role of cytotoxic T lymphocytes in immune clearance of rickettsial infection. Infect Immun 69: 1841-1846.

Wike, D.A., Tallent,G., Peacock,M.G., and Ormsbee,R.A. (1972) Studies of the rickettsial plaque assay technique. Infect Immun 5: 715-722.

## Anaplasmosis

*Introduction*

*Anaplasma* are gram-negative -Proteobacteria belonging to the order *Rickettsiales*, and family *Anaplasmataceae* (Figure A5-1) (Dumler et al., 2001). Like most *Rickettsiales*, organisms in the genus *Anaplasma* are small, ranging from 0.2-0.9 µm. Of the four genera in the family *Anaplasmataceae*, *Anaplasma* is most similar in lifestyle and evolutionary history to the closely related *Ehrlichia* spp. The genus *Anaplasma* contains five recognized species: *A. bovis*, *A. ovis*, *A. platys*, *A. marginale* and

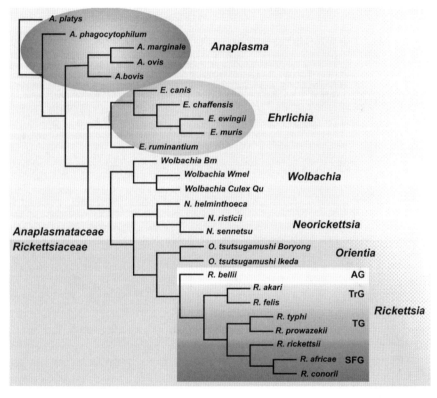

FIGURE A5-1 Phylogenetic tree of order *Rickettsiales*. [Genera in the families *Anaplasmataceae* (on yellow background) and *Rickettsiaceae* (on blue background) are shown. Species of interest are circled or boxed. The *Rickettsia* are subgrouped according to ancestral group (AG), transitional group (TrG), Typhus group (TG) and spotted fever group (SFG). The tree is based on a clustalW alignment of 16S ribosomal RNA gene sequences using POWER (http://power.nhri.org.tw/power/home.htm).]

A. *phagocytophilum*, with the first four species infecting animals, and the last being a zoonotic agent. The type species for the genus is A. *marginale*, a cattle pathogen that was recognized in the early 1900s (Theiler, 1910). Of these species, by far the most research has been done on the latter two species, A. *marginale* which causes anaplasmosis, and the human pathogen A. *phagocytophilum*, which causes human granulocytic anaplasmosis. All *Anaplasma* species are obligate intracellular organisms infecting mature or immature hematopoietic cells where they replicate within membrane bound vacuoles (Dumler et al., 2001). *Anaplasma* spp. are therefore blood-borne pathogens and are transmitted from host to host by Ixodid ticks. This manuscript will focus on the human pathogen, A. *phagocytophilum*.

*Etiologic agent*

A. *phagocytophilum* was previously classified as an *Ehrlichia* (the agent of human granulocytic ehrlichiosis). Accumulating genetic information on a number of pathogens originally named as *Ehrlichia* species drove the reorganization of the families Rickettsiaceae and Anaplasmataceae in 2001 wherein *Ehrlichia equi*, and *Ehrlichia phagocytophila* were unified as a single species with the agent of human granulocytic ehrlichiosis, to create the new species *Anaplasma phagocytophilum* (Dumler et al., 2001). Because anaplasmosis is recognized as a cattle disease, A. *phagocytophilum* is said to cause human granulocytic anaplasmosis (HGA).

A. *phagocytophilum* infects polymorphonuclear leucocytes (neutrophils), where it replicates within a membrane bound vacuole forming a morula or microcolony (Chen et al., 1994; Rikihisa, 1991). A. *phagocytophilum* has a biphasic developmental cycle with two morphologically distinct forms referred to as dense cored cells (DC) and reticulate cells (RC) (Popov et al., 1998). DCs are small electron dense bodies that predominate in early infection, are thought to be metabolically inert and play a role in attachment and invasion of the host cell (Munderloh et al., 1999). RCs are electron lucent larger pleomorphic cells that undergo binary fission and are thought to be the metabolically active form of the organism (Ismail et al., 2010; Troese and Carlyon, 2009).

The *Rickettsiales* are the closest extant relatives of the bacterial lineage that led to the mitochondria, and have undergone extensive genome reduction with individual species displaying small genome sizes between 0.8 and 1.5 Mb (Sallstrom and Andersson, 2005; Andersson et al., 1998; Viale and Arakaki, 1994). The A. *phagocytophilum* genome, completed in 2006, is 1,471,282 bp and is reported to contain 1264 protein coding genes as well as 37 tRNA and 3 rRNA genes (Dunning Hotopp et al., 2006). While this number of protein coding genes is greater than many of the closely related organisms (range = 805-1264), this difference is largely due to differences in annotation style (many small open reading frames were annotated) rather than a real difference in coding capacity (Brayton et al., 2008).

## Epidemiology/Public health importance

HGA was first identified as a human pathogen in 1990 when a patient in Wisconsin died after a short acute febrile illness (Dumler et al., 2005). HGA is increasingly recognized as a frequent cause of fever after tick bite in the Upper Midwest, New England, parts of the mid-Atlantic states, northern California (Figure A5-2), many parts of Europe and Asia (Dumler et al., 2005). In the United States, cases of HGA have increased since the CDC started tracking cases in 1999 (Figure A5-3) with 1009 cases reported in 2008 (Hall-Baker et al., 2010).

A. *phagocytophilum* infects many species including dogs, cats, horses, deer, cattle, sheep, mice, wood rats, bank voles, squirrels, opossums, skunks and raccoons (Foley et al., 2008; Hackett et al., 2006; Lester et al., 2005; Levin et al., 2002; Stuen and Bergstrom, 2001; Stuen et al., 2001a; Stuen et

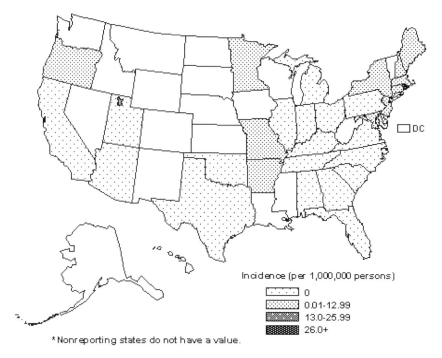

**FIGURE A5-2** Average annual incidence of HGA by state as reported in 2001-2002. Data from CDC National Electronic Telecommunications System for Surveillance.

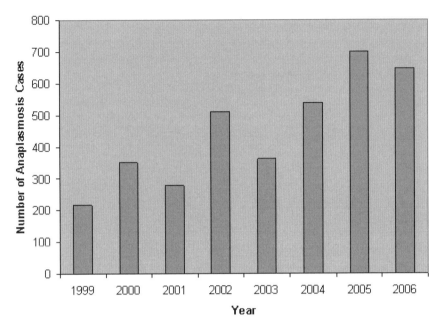

**FIGURE A5-3** Number of HGA cases reported by year from 1999-2002. Data from CDC National Electronic Telecommunications System for Surveillance.

al., 2001b; Stuen et al., 2001c; Pusterla et al., 1999). Humans are accidental, dead end hosts for *A. phagocytophilum*, typically becoming infected when humans encroach on small mammal-tick habitats (Dumler et al., 2005). The major mammalian reservoir is the white-footed mouse, which typically has a transient bacteremia (1-4 weeks). While white tailed deer can be persistently infected, they do not appear to harbor strains of *A. phagocytophilum* that cause HGA (Massung et al., 2005). Strain definition for *A. phagocytophilum* is not well defined; however, 1-2 nucleotide differences in the 16S ribosomal RNA gene and 1-3 bp differences in the GroESL gene have been used to identify strain variants (Stuen et al., 2003; Massung et al., 2002).

In the Midwestern and Eastern US *Ixodes scapularis* is the vector, while *I. pacificus* vectors *A. phagocytophilum* in the Western US. *I. ricinus* is the major vector in Europe, and *I. persulcatus* transmits disease in Asia. Tick infection is established after an infectious blood meal, and the bacterium is transstadially but not transovarially passed (Dumler et al., 2005). These ticks also transmit agents that cause Lyme disease, babesiosis and tick-borne meningoencephalitis, with about 10% of HGA patients showing serological evidence of co-infection with one of these agents (Ismail et al., 2010; Dumler et al., 2007; Dumler et al., 2005).

*Clinical spectrum/Treatment*

HGA presents with fever, headache, leukopenia, thrombocytopenia, absence of a skin rash and elevated liver enzymes. Symptoms typically begin a median of 9 days following tick bite, with the majority of patients seeking medical attention within the first 4 days of illness (Ismail et al., 2010; Dumler et al., 2005). Some individuals infected with *A. phagocytophilum* do not become ill or experience only very mild symptoms and do not seek medical treatment; however, at the other end of the spectrum, the disease can prove fatal, particularly in immunocompromised or elderly individuals (Thomas et al., 2009; Dumler et al., 2005).

Accurate diagnosis of HGA is often difficult due to the non-specific nature of the symptoms. An initial diagnosis is based on the patient's symptoms and a possible history of tick exposure. Diagnosis is confirmed by laboratory tests: 1) microscopic examination of Wright- or Giemsa-stained peripheral blood smears looking for dark staining morulae within neutrophils can be used early in infection, 2) a polymerase chain reaction (PCR) assay is the most sensitive test, provides rapid diagnostic evaluation and can discriminate between several tick-borne diseases that present with similar symptoms, 3) *A. phagocytophilum* can be cultivated within two weeks in the human promyelocytic leukemia cell line HL-60 by direct inoculation of cell cultures with peripheral blood from a potentially infected patient, and 4) serodiagnosis is most commonly used, but is not rapid, as it requires time for antibody to develop which typically takes longer than the onset of clinical symptoms; additionally, nonspecificity of this test may result from cross reactions with *Ehrlichia chaffeensis* (Ismail et al., 2010; Thomas et al., 2009).

The treatment of choice for both adults and children is a tetracycline antibiotic, usually doxycycline, which should be initiated promptly for improved outcomes and continued for 10-14 days (Hamburg et al., 2008; Chapman et al., 2006).

*Overview of protective immune mechanisms*

Relatively little is known about protective mechanisms of immunity to *A. phagocytophilum* infection except that protective immunity is mediated by cellular and humoral immune mechanisms. Development of high titer antibody responses is believed to be indicative of protective immunity (Ismail et al., 2010). Studies in sheep indicate that protection can last from a few months to > 1 year and that a measure of heterologous protection is afforded by some strains but not others (Stuen et al., 2003). Reinfection has been confirmed in some individuals which suggests that long-term immunity was not engendered; however, a lack of cross protection between different strains of *A. phagocytophilum* must also be considered (Levin et al., 2004; Horowitz et al., 1998).

Similar to *A. marginale*, *A. phagocytophilum* effects immune evasion through antigenic variation of the Msp2/p44 immunodominant surface protein (Granquist et al., 2010; Barbet et al., 2003). There is at least one expression site for *msp2*/P44 and ~100 functional pseudogenes which can recombine into the expression site to generate variation (Dunning Hotopp et al., 2006; Barbet et al., 2003). The Msp2/P44 protein is characterized by conserved amino- and carboxy-termini flanking a central hypervariable region (Murphy et al., 1998). Msp2/P44 functional pseudogenes are typically truncated at the 5' and 3' ends, and recombine into the expression site through a RecF dependent gene conversion mechanism (Lin et al., 2006).

*Current vaccine status, experimental vaccines, and potential vaccine prospects*

Vaccination against the cattle pathogen *A. marginale* is effected by infection with an avirulent strain, providing a measure of crossprotection without sterile immunity. This blood-based vaccine is not used in the U.S. due to the threat of transmitting emerging pathogens. There are no vaccines currently available for HGA. The search for vaccine candidates has focused on surface proteins as these are the interface for interactions with the host cell; however, these studies are in their infancy. Little is known about the surface proteins of *A. phagocytophilum*, aside from Msp2/P44, which due to rapid antigenic variation does not constitute a good vaccine candidate (Ge and Rikihisa, 2007). The genome sequence provides a useful tool to facilitate research to identify vaccine candidates and was recently used in combination with a proteomic approach to identify surface exposed proteins. Two proteins were identified, Asp55 and Asp62, that were also recognized by immune serum from a patient with HGA. Peptide anti-sera for these two proteins were able to partially neutralize *A. phagocytophilum* infection in the human promyelocytic leukemia cell line, HL-60 cells (Ge and Rikihisa, 2007).

Preliminary studies aimed at understanding the pathogen-tick interface have the long-term goal of developing transmission blocking vaccines, although this research has focused more on interrupting the transmission of the cattle pathogen *A. marginale* (de la Fuente et al., 2010; Ramabu et al., 2010; Noh et al., 2008). Novel approaches that could reduce the level of human contact with disease agents include the development anti-tick vaccines. An anti-tick vaccine based on the *Rhipicephalus microplus* gut protein Bm86 has been successful in field trials in Cuba; however, implementation of a similar vaccine was not successful in Australia (de la Fuente et al., 2007; Rodriguez Valle et al., 2004). A successful anti-tick vaccine would be introduced orally to the wildlife reservoirs in a similar fashion to rabies vaccine, and could eliminate the need for broad scale human vaccination (Slate et al., 2009). This strategy would reduce, but not eliminate risk of transmission. As yet, there are no candidates ready for testing for either of these strategies for ticks that transmit HGA.

*Theraupeutics and other biologics for prevention*

Preventative antibiotic therapy is contraindicated for individuals who have had recent tick bites but are not ill. Prevention is effected by avoidance of tick bites through the following strategies: 1) avoidance of tick dense areas, 2) wearing of light colored protective clothing (i.e., long pants, closed-toed shoes, etc.), 3) frequent checks for crawling and attached ticks, and 4) application of a repellant such as DEET (N,N-diethyl-m-toluamide). Should a person find an attached tick prompt removal reduces the threat of transmission, as studies have shown that a period of 4 to 24 hours may be necessary before successful transmission from tick to host takes place (Ismail et al., 2010; Bakken and Dumler, 2008; Katavolos et al., 1998).

*Key issues*

- Additional effort in identifying surface exposed targets that could illicit protective immune responses is needed. The genome is a key tool in this endeavor and the advent of affordable, widely available proteomic tools should facilitate these efforts. Understanding mechanisms of immune evasion will also help in assessment of vaccine candidates.
- Understanding the strain composition that makes up the *A. phagocytophilum* species will facilitate development of appropriate vaccine candidates; i.e., variation in leading vaccine candidate antigens may not be relevant if the variant strain does not infect humans. Representative *A. phagocytophilum* genome sequences from an array of hosts could assist in exploring the strain composition but this organism does not lend itself to high throughput, next generation sequencing strategies due to the highly repetitive nature of the genome sequence.
- Understanding of the transmission biology of *A. phagocytophilum* would facilitate the development of transmission blocking vaccines and potentially help elucidate targets for anti-tick vaccines as well.
- Understanding host differences in pathogenesis would aid in determining if vaccines tested in sheep, for example, would be relevant for humans.

## References

Andersson, S.G., Zomorodipour, A., Andersson, J.O., Sicheritz-Ponten, T., Alsmark, U.C., Podowski, R.M., et al (1998) The genome sequence of Rickettsia prowazekii and the origin of mitochondria. Nature. 396: 133-140.

Bakken, J.S. and Dumler, S. (2008) Human granulocytic anaplasmosis. Infect Dis Clin North Am. 22: 433-448, viii.

Barbet, A.F., Meeus, P.F., Belanger, M., Bowie, M.V., Yi, J., Lundgren, A.M., et al (2003) Expression of multiple outer membrane protein sequence variants from a single genomic locus of Anaplasma phagocytophilum. Infect Immun. 71: 1706-1718.

Brayton, K.A., Dark, M.J. and Palmer, G.H. (2008) Anplasma. In Genome Mapping and Genomics in Animal-Associated Microbes. Kole, C., and Nene, V.M. (eds.) Heidelberg, Germany: Springer Life Sciences,, pp. 85-116.

Chapman, A.S., Bakken, J.S., Folk, S.M., Paddock, C.D., Bloch, K.C., Krusell, A., et al (2006) Diagnosis and management of tickborne rickettsial diseases: Rocky Mountain spotted fever, ehrlichioses, and anaplasmosis—United States: a practical guide for physicians and other health-care and public health professionals. MMWR Recomm Rep. 55: 1-27.

Chen, S.M., Dumler, J.S., Bakken, J.S. and Walker, D.H. (1994) Identification of a granulo-cytotropic Ehrlichia species as the etiologic agent of human disease. J Clin Microbiol. 32: 589-595.

de la Fuente, J., Almazan, C., Canales, M., Perez de la Lastra, J.M., Kocan, K.M. and Willadsen, P. (2007) A ten-year review of commercial vaccine performance for control of tick infestations on cattle. Anim Health Res Rev. 8: 23-28.

de la Fuente, J., Kocan, K.M., Blouin, E.F., Zivkovic, Z., Naranjo, V., Almazan, C., et al (2010) Functional genomics and evolution of tick-Anaplasma interactions and vaccine development. Vet Parasitol. 167: 175-186.

Dumler, J.S., Barbet, A.F., Bekker, C.P., Dasch, G.A., Palmer, G.H., Ray, S.C., et al (2001) Reorganization of genera in the families Rickettsiaceae and Anaplasmataceae in the order Rickettsiales: unification of some species of Ehrlichia with Anaplasma, Cowdria with Ehrlichia and Ehrlichia with Neorickettsia, descriptions of six new species combinations and designation of Ehrlichia equi and 'HGE agent' as subjective synonyms of Ehrlichia phagocytophila. Int J Syst Evol Microbiol. 51: 2145-2165.

Dumler, J.S., Choi, K.S., Garcia-Garcia, J.C., Barat, N.S., Scorpio, D.G., Garyu, J.W., et al (2005) Human granulocytic anaplasmosis and Anaplasma phagocytophilum. Emerg Infect Dis. 11: 1828-1834.

Dumler, J.S., Madigan, J.E., Pusterla, N. and Bakken, J.S. (2007) Ehrlichioses in humans: epidemiology, clinical presentation, diagnosis, and treatment. Clin Infect Dis. 45 Suppl 1: S45-51.

Dunning Hotopp, J.C., Lin, M., Madupu, R., Crabtree, J., Angiuoli, S.V., Eisen, J., et al (2006) Comparative Genomics of Emerging Human Ehrlichiosis Agents. PLoS Genet. 2: e21.

Foley, J.E., Nieto, N.C., Adjemian, J., Dabritz, H. and Brown, R.N. (2008) Anaplasma phagocytophilum infection in small mammal hosts of Ixodes ticks, Western United States. Emerg Infect Dis. 14: 1147-1150.

Ge, Y. and Rikihisa, Y. (2007) Identification of novel surface proteins of Anaplasma phagocy-tophilum by affinity purification and proteomics. J Bacteriol. 189: 7819-7828.

Granquist, E.G., Stuen, S., Crosby, L., Lundgren, A.M., Alleman, A.R. and Barbet, A.F. (2010) Variant-specific and diminishing immune responses towards the highly variable MSP2(P44) outer membrane protein of Anaplasma phagocytophilum during persistent infection in lambs. Vet Immunol Immunopathol. 133: 117-124.

Hackett, T.B., Jensen, W.A., Lehman, T.L., Hohenhaus, A.E., Crawford, P.C., Giger, U. and Lappin, M.R. (2006) Prevalence of DNA of Mycoplasma haemofelis, 'Candidatus Mycoplasma haemominutum,' Anaplasma phagocytophilum, and species of Bartonella,

Neorickettsia, and Ehrlichia in cats used as blood donors in the United States. J Am Vet Med Assoc. 229: 700-705.

Hall-Baker, P.A., Nieves Jr, E., Jajosky, R.A., Adams, D.A., Sharp, P., Anderson, W.J., et al (2010) Summary of notifiable diseases—United States, 2008. MMWR Morb Mortal Wkly Rep. 57: 1-94.

Hamburg, B.J., Storch, G.A., Micek, S.T. and Kollef, M.H. (2008) The importance of early treatment with doxycycline in human ehrlichiosis. Medicine (Baltimore). 87: 53-60.

Horowitz, H.W., Aguero-Rosenfeld, M., Dumler, J.S., McKenna, D.F., Hsieh, T.C., Wu, J., et al (1998) Reinfection with the agent of human granulocytic ehrlichiosis. Ann Intern Med. 129: 461-463.

Ismail, N., Bloch, K.C. and McBride, J.W. (2010) Human ehrlichiosis and anaplasmosis. Clin Lab Med. 30: 261-292.

Katavolos, P., Armstrong, P.M., Dawson, J.E. and Telford, S.R., 3rd (1998) Duration of tick attachment required for transmission of granulocytic ehrlichiosis. J Infect Dis. 177: 1422-1425.

Lester, S.J., Breitschwerdt, E.B., Collis, C.D. and Hegarty, B.C. (2005) Anaplasma phagocytophilum infection (granulocytic anaplasmosis) in a dog from Vancouver Island. Can Vet J. 46: 825-827.

Levin, M.L., Coble, D.J. and Ross, D.E. (2004) Reinfection with Anaplasma phagocytophilum in BALB/c mice and cross-protection between two sympatric isolates. Infect Immun. 72: 4723-4730.

Levin, M.L., Nicholson, W.L., Massung, R.F., Sumner, J.W. and Fish, D. (2002) Comparison of the reservoir competence of medium-sized mammals and Peromyscus leucopus for Anaplasma phagocytophilum in Connecticut. Vector Borne Zoonotic Dis. 2: 125-136.

Lin, Q., Zhang, C. and Rikihisa, Y. (2006) Analysis of involvement of the RecF pathway in p44 recombination in Anaplasma phagocytophilum and in Escherichia coli by using a plasmid carrying the p44 expression and p44 donor loci. Infect Immun. 74: 2052-2062.

Massung, R.F., Courtney, J.W., Hiratzka, S.L., Pitzer, V.E., Smith, G. and Dryden, R.L. (2005) Anaplasma phagocytophilum in white-tailed deer. Emerg Infect Dis. 11: 1604-1606.

Massung, R.F., Mauel, M.J., Owens, J.H., Allan, N., Courtney, J.W., Stafford, K.C., 3rd and Mather, T.N. (2002) Genetic variants of Ehrlichia phagocytophila, Rhode Island and Connecticut. Emerg Infect Dis. 8: 467-472.

Munderloh, U.G., Jauron, S.D., Fingerle, V., Leitritz, L., Hayes, S.F., Hautman, J.M., et al (1999) Invasion and intracellular development of the human granulocytic ehrlichiosis agent in tick cell culture. J Clin Microbiol. 37: 2518-2524.

Murphy, C.I., Storey, J.R., Recchia, J., Doros-Richert, L.A., Gingrich-Baker, C., Munroe, K., et al (1998) Major antigenic proteins of the agent of human granulocytic ehrlichiosis are encoded by members of a multigene family. Infect Immun. 66: 3711-3718.

Noh, S.M., Brayton, K.A., Brown, W.C., Norimine, J., Munske, G.R., Davitt, C.M. and Palmer, G.H. (2008) Composition of the surface proteome of Anaplasma marginale and its role in protective immunity induced by outer membrane immunization. Infect Immun.

Popov, V.L., Han, V.C., Chen, S.M., Dumler, J.S., Feng, H.M., Andreadis, T.G., et al (1998) Ultrastructural differentiation of the genogroups in the genus Ehrlichia. J Med Microbiol. 47: 235-251.

Pusterla, N., Pusterla, J.B., Braun, U. and Lutz, H. (1999) Experimental cross-infections with Ehrlichia phagocytophila and human granulocytic ehrlichia-like agent in cows and horses. Vet Rec. 145: 311-314.

Ramabu, S.S., Ueti, M.W., Brayton, K.A., Baszler, T.V. and Palmer, G.H. (2010) Identification of Anaplasma marginale proteins specifically upregulated during colonization of the tick vector. Infect Immun. 78: 3047-3052.

Rikihisa, Y. (1991) The tribe Ehrlichieae and ehrlichial diseases. Clin Microbiol Rev. 4: 286-308.

Rodriguez Valle, M., Mendez, L., Valdez, M., Redondo, M., Espinosa, C.M., Vargas, M., et al (2004) Integrated control of Boophilus microplus ticks in Cuba based on vaccination with the anti-tick vaccine Gavac. Exp Appl Acarol. 34: 375-382.

Sallstrom, B. and Andersson, S.G. (2005) Genome reduction in the alpha-Proteobacteria. Curr Opin Microbiol. 8: 579-585.

Slate, D., Algeo, T.P., Nelson, K.M., Chipman, R.B., Donovan, D., Blanton, J.D., et al (2009) Oral rabies vaccination in north america: opportunities, complexities, and challenges. PLoS Negl Trop Dis. 3: e549.

Stuen, S. and Bergstrom, K. (2001) Persistence of Ehrlichia phagocytophila infection in two age groups of lambs. Acta Vet Scand. 42: 453-458.

Stuen, S., Bergstrom, K., Petrovec, M., Van de Pol, I. and Schouls, L.M. (2003) Differences in clinical manifestations and hematological and serological responses after experimental infection with genetic variants of Anaplasma phagocytophilum in sheep. Clin Diagn Lab Immunol. 10: 692-695.

Stuen, S., Djuve, R. and Bergstrom, K. (2001a) Persistence of granulocytic Ehrlichia infection during wintertime in two sheep flocks in Norway. Acta Vet Scand. 42: 347-353.

Stuen, S., Engvall, E.O., van de Poll, I. and Schouls, L.M. (2001b) Granulocytic ehrlichiosis in a roe deer calf in Norway. J Wildl Dis. 37: 614-616.

Stuen, S., Handeland, K., Frammarsvik, T. and Bergstrom, K. (2001c) Experimental Ehrlichia phagocytophila infection in red deer (Cervus elaphus). Vet Rec. 149: 390-392.

Theiler, A. (1910) Anaplasma marginale (gen. spec. nov.). The marginale points in the blood of cattle suffering from a specific disease. In Report of the government veterinary bacteriologist, 1908-1909. Theiler, A. (ed.) Transvaal, South Africa., pp. 7-64.

Thomas, R.J., Dumler, J.S. and Carlyon, J.A. (2009) Current management of human granulocytic anaplasmosis, human monocytic ehrlichiosis and Ehrlichia ewingii ehrlichiosis. Expert Rev Anti Infect Ther. 7: 709-722.

Troese, M.J. and Carlyon, J.A. (2009) Anaplasma phagocytophilum dense-cored organisms mediate cellular adherence through recognition of human P-selectin glycoprotein ligand-1. Infect Immun.

Viale, A.M. and Arakaki, A.K. (1994) The chaperone connection to the origins of the eukaryotic organelles. FEBS Lett. 341: 146-151.

# A6
# EMERGING AND RE-EMERGING TICK-BORNE DISEASES: NEW CHALLENGES AT THE INTERFACE OF HUMAN AND ANIMAL HEALTH

*Ulrike G. Munderloh and Timothy J. Kurtti*
*Department of Entomology, University of Minnesota*
*St. Paul, MN 55108*

## Introduction: Accelerated Increase and Uneven Distribution of Emerging Diseases

This manuscript is meant to be a synthesis of current knowledge about the forces that drive emergence of tick-borne diseases during this era of global change. This is an enormously complex field the components of which are in constant flux and change dynamically all the time. We therefore do not present here a comprehensive list of all tick-borne pathogens, but rather discuss those that have been researched in sufficient detail to allow assessment of their impact, how they have changed, and how they interact with their environment.

Globally, the great majority of emerging diseases are zoonoses that are predominantly vector-borne (Jones et al., 2008). In temperate climates, tick-borne pathogens are the leading cause of vector-borne diseases, whereas insects dominate the scene as vectors of pathogens in the tropics (Kalluri et al., 2007). The incidence of vector-borne diseases has increased disproportionately in relationship to other emerging diseases, and peaks at times of severe weather events and climate anomalies (Githeko et al., 2000; Gray et al., 2009), a reflection of the sensitivity to and reliance of arthropods on permissive conditions including rain. These effects may be seen relatively quickly, as for pathogens transmitted by mosquitoes, especially those maintained in the insect population transovarially, reducing the lag time before transmission can occur following acquisition. Development of mosquitoes from egg to adult can be completed in two weeks or less, during which larvae feed on microbes suspended in the water. Complete development takes months or years for ticks, but each life stage (except the males of certain species) may transmit pathogens during a blood meal. As for mosquitoes, dynamics of tick-borne disease activity are shaped by climate, though less by rapid weather changes. Availability of suitable larval habitat is of prime importance for maintenance and establishment of mosquito populations, whereas availability of hosts and host behavior are major determinants for ticks. Thus, human activities can shape expansion of different arthropod vectors in different ways, both by habitat modification as well as by altering host populations and their composition. In all, the relationships among factors governing the emergence and spread of vector-borne pathogens, including those that are tick-borne, are very complex. Seasonal and yearly variability determines how ecosystem components interact and contribute to provide habitat suitable for vector arthropods; arthropods, in turn, have evolved behaviors that allow them to take advantage of microclimate niches as needed to "weather" unpredictable conditions (Killilea et al., 2008). These complexities have not been sorted out to date at a global scale, and await a standardized approach to analysis before meaningful conclusions can be drawn.

Climate, weather and temperature directly influence poikilothermic arthropods by dictating periods when important activities, e.g., host seeking, mating, or egg development are possible. Thus climate restricts geographic range to regions with sufficient cumulative degree days to allow completion of these necessary activities and development to the next life stage. Unlike a hot, dry summer that affects ticks when they are normally active, cold winters are more readily tolerated by ticks that had time to prepare physiologically by seeking suitably protective habitat and accumulating protective anti-freeze compounds (Burks et al., 1996). A recent analysis of gene expression in black-legged ticks subjected to cold revealed that a glycoprotein with homology to a blood protein in cold water fish was more efficiently induced in ticks carrying the zoonotic bacterial pathogen *Anaplasma phagocytophilum* than in uninfected ones (Neelakanta et al., 2010), presumably providing a selective advantage to overwintering nymphs and adults. This would enhance northward dispersal of "anaplasma-winterized" ticks, and could introduce this pathogen to the mice, chipmunks, squirrels, raccoons and other reservoir hosts that live there (Levin et al., 2002). Davies et al., (2009) proposed that the range of mammals and their ability to expand into new habitats could be predicted by the variability of historic conditions in their range during the Quarternary period. Animals that have evolved to adapt to profound changes in the past are thought to more readily be able to exploit new opportunities. Although a comparable fossil record does not exist for arthropods, ectoparasites that remain on hosts for days at a time, as ticks do, are readily translocated during host movement (Bjöersdorff et al., 2001; McCoy et al., 2003; Ogden et al., 2008; Reed, 2003), thus historic tick host ranges could serve as a proxy for historic ranges of ticks, and their evolved potential to disperse could then be modeled similarly.

## Impact of Climate and Global Change Providing New Opportunities

The human population explosion has resulted in dramatic changes of the distribution and composition of natural habitat and land modified to sustain human needs in terms of living space and food production, and this is an ongoing, highly dynamic process. Changes in land use patterns favor establishment and expansion of ticks at the urban/agricultural interface and provide new habitat for highly adaptable wild hosts, as well as new domestic animal hosts for ticks. Even so, advancement of human settlements into virgin land has resulted in a reduction in species diversity and subsequent increase in the risk of tick-borne diseases. Much of the natural vegetation that would presumably cover the earth in the absence of humans ("potential vegetation"), and provide wildlife habitat, has been displaced by cropland and pastures (Foley et al., 2005). These managed agricultural systems lack the rich diversity of plant and animal species characteristic of undisturbed areas and are more prone to damage from diseases or either natural of human-made disasters such as floods, fires or pressure from invasive species. Rich assembly of plant and animal communities provides a buffer against such events, and enables affected regions to rebound in their wake. Moreover, reduced biodiversity has been linked to increased risk of vector-borne disease by depletion of natural hosts for vector and pathogen, as well as by provision of new hosts. Domesticated animals living close to farmers and herders, or sharing their dwellings, can act as new reservoirs and bridge hosts in the transfer of emerging diseases to humans (Keesing et al., 2006; LoGiudice et al., 2008; Vora, 2008). A recent example is the discovery of an active transmission focus of Rocky Mountain spotted fever (RMSF) rickettsiae, *Rickettsia rickettsii*, in Arizona, involving an introduced tick vector, the brown dog tick, *Rhipicephalus sanguineus*, and domestic dogs acting as reservoirs for the rickettsiae and hosts for the ticks (Demma et al., 2005). Since then, brown dog ticks infected with *R. rickettsii* have also been detected in California (Wikswo et al., 2007). This tick colonized the Americas along with humans and their dogs arriving from the Old World during the early colonial immigrations (Burlini et al., 2010). It is surprising that spotted fever group rickettsiae endemic to the Mediterranean region, *Rickettsia conorii* (Mumcuoglu et al., 1993), that are naturally transmitted by brown dog ticks, have thus far not been identified in the New World. The adaptation of *R. rickettsii* to a new tick vector is a good example of the host switching that can result when human-aided movement of animals and their parasites are introduced into new areas where they intermingle with resident hosts, parasites and disease agents (Hoberg et al., 2008). Such new combinations are more likely to turn up in the multiple host life cycle of tick-borne pathogens, especially when the vectors are non-specialized feeders as is the case with the black-legged tick *Ixodes scapularis*. In this situation, host switching without the need for subsequent adaptive evolution can occur in pathogens that inherently are equipped to take advantage of new opportunities provided by hosts undergoing range expansion in a process of ecological fitting (Brooks and Ferrao, 2005; Foley et al., 2008).

Human encroachment on wildlife habitat enhances contact with ticks as modern society embraces the concept of living with nature by building homes in natural settings and through engagement in outdoor sports such as hiking or camping. Regional and historical preferences for how and where homes are constructed, and how and where animals are housed or pastured have modified the zoonotic interface between humans and domestic and wild animals in ways that where not anticipated, but were predictable in retrospect. The desire to preserve natural vegetation such as mature stands of trees for aesthetic or practical reasons (e.g., to provide shade) has had the effect to attract wildlife to close proximity of human dwellings, enhancing contact with ticks and other arthropods that may carry disease agents. The increase in Lyme disease cases in residents of affluent housing developments in or near desirable natural wooded areas is a good example of this trend (Barbour and Fish, 1993; Linard et al., 2007). Although much research has been devoted to trying to describe the ecologic/sociologic interface that favors the presence of pathogens, vectors and reservoirs, and has resulted in large sets of data that do not easily coalesce into a single, well-fitting mosaic, few efforts have been made to systematically incorporate them into urban/suburban/agricultural planning (Ward and Brown, 2004). There is a clear need to apply what has been learned to new and existing urban and suburban as well as agricultural and recreational landscapes. Disease prevention through landscape management must, however, always be in balance with protection of natural habitat, and its meaningful incorporation into managed areas (Foley et al., 2005; Stafford III, 2007). Such decisions must be based on scientific knowledge, and biologists, medical scientists and public health researchers must be included in the planning processes alongside city planners and construction company employees.

Areas that are likely to experience increased or prolonged seasonal tick activity are most likely those located at the current extremes of the current range of distribution, areas where climate change will be felt most acutely. In the northern hemisphere, this will be at the northern edge, and in the southern hemisphere, tick distribution ranges will likely shift further south. A prerequisite is the presence of ecosystems with suitable land cover and hosts to receive the immigrants. Occupation of montane habitat by *Ixodes ricinus* in Europe has already shifted to greater altitudes (Materna et al., 2005), exposing alpine farming communities to new risk of infection. At these greater latitudes and altitudes, specialized plant communities are utilized by relatively few wild animals that can serve as tick hosts and impose constraints that may limit or curb further spread of the ticks. Domestic animals seasonally introduced into borderline habitat and the people tending them will experience a greater burden of tick bites.

### The Domestic Animal/Wildlife Interface

Driving flocks and herds out to pasture on a daily or weekly basis, or even turning live stock out onto range land for entire seasons, has been a tradition for centuries, and animal husbandry is thought to have been a source of human exposure to zoonoses since ancient times (Greger, 2007). A new and worrisome trend is the increasing practice of exotic animal farming and trade in exotic species. Exotic game farms have become popular with hunters seeking the thrill of a chance to shoot an African antelope without having to leave the USA, and offer farmers income from land that may be poorly suitable for traditional farming. Although animals imported from foreign countries must undergo rigorous testing for diseases and quarantine, any as yet unknown pathogens they may harbor may not be detected using existing diagnostics. In addition, tick-borne pathogens, e.g., the bovine anaplasmosis agent, *Anaplasma marginale*, which is widely present throughout the world, can chronically infect animals at undetectable levels (Eriks et al., 1989; Herrero et al., 1998), and other pathogens may do the same. There are numerous reports in recent history of accidental introduction of tick-borne animal pathogens or ticks into previously unaffected areas, with economically disastrous results. When imported ticks become established on wild animals, their eradication may be very difficult or impossible, as shown in New Caledonia (Barré et al., 2001) where cattle ticks and bovine babesiosis were accidentally imported. The cattle tick, *Rhipicephalus (Boophilus) microplus*, is the vector of bovine babesiosis, a disease with major consequences for cattle production wherever it is present. It has spread through most warm regions of the world from its origin in Asia by hitching a ride on imported cattle (Hoogstraal, 1956; Madder et al., 2010). This parasite has adapted well to wild ungulates in infested areas, providing alternate hosts when cattle are intensively treated with acaricides, unraveling control efforts (Cantu-C et al., 2009). After being nearly eradicated in the USA, this tick has recently expanded its range considerably in Texas, in part aided by development of acaricide resistance resulting from intense treatment regimes (George, 2008). There is no reason to believe that *R. microplus* would not adapt to exotic game on farms, as it has displaced other *Rhipicephalus* species in West Africa (Madder et al., 2010). Although the development of promising antigens raises the hope that a vaccine could protect cattle against this parasite (Canales et al., 2009), their effectiveness in essentially wild or feral exotic animal species remains unproven.

Much as exotic animals can be a source of exotic pathogens endangering resident fauna, pathogens endemic in areas into which non-endemic species are introduced may prove to be highly infectious for non-indigenous animals. Farming game, e.g., elk (or wapiti, *Cervus elaphus canadensis*), has been promoted as a sustainable alternative to raising cattle, because these animals are less demanding and are superior in their ability to utilize nutrients from natural pasture. They also produce lean meat that fetches premium prices on the market. In their natural range in the Rocky Mountains of the USA and Canada, elk do not encounter *I. scapularis* (black-legged ticks), but when raised in the Midwest or Northeast, they are exposed to a protozoan blood parasite, *Babesia odocoilei*, transmitted by ticks among white-tailed deer who do not show signs of infection (Waldrup et al., 1990). Elk and deer from outside the range of the vector tick may become severely ill, even suffer a fatal infection. Outbreaks of fatal illness have also been documented in a number of animals at zoos, e.g., reindeer (*Rangifer tarandus tarandus*) and caribou (*Rangifer tarandus caribou*), bovids such as musk oxen (*Ovibos moschatus*) and yak (*Bos grunniens*), as well as other ruminants, e.g., muntjac (*Muntiacus reevesi)* and markhor goat (*Capra falconeri*) (Schoelkopf et al., 2005; Bartlett et al., 2009). This list of susceptible species is not inclusive, but serves to demonstrate the enormous infection potential of tick-borne pathogens in animals that have not co-evolved with them. Importation of exotic species for uncontrolled release should be avoided for other reasons as well, because their impact on natural habitat is not easily predictable, and great environmental harm can result. One need only consider the devastation wrought by domestic goats released by sailors on many islands as a fresh food supply, or the disastrous release of European wild rabbits in Australia (Campbell and Donlan, 2005; Fenner, 2010).

### Changes in Climate Favor Establishment and Expansion of Ticks

The spread of human settlement is accompanied by changes in land use that have been linked with increasing risk of disease due to vector-borne pathogens (Hoogstraal, 1981; Harrus and Baneth, 2005). Global change is the sum of largely man-made ecologic disturbances resulting in rising temperatures and altered patterns of precipitation that promote the expansion of the geographic range where conditions are favorable for survival of vector arthropods. Changes in vector distribution and seasonal activity resulting in increased disease incidence arc likcly to be most pronounced at the geographic extremes of vector distribution (Ogden et al., 2005).

In temperate climates, pathogens transmitted by ticks are the causative agents of the most common vector-borne diseases, far outnumbering those carried by mosquitoes. The incidence of Lyme disease transmitted by *Ixodes* spp. in North America and Europe has been increasing steadily since the 1970s and 1980s (Gray et al., 2009). In the US Midwest, this steady pace accelerated at the beginning of the new century, with significant deviations from the average rate tied to unusually dry and hot weather, such as during the summer of 2003 that was followed by a rebound in 2004 (Minnesota Department of Health; http://www.health.state.mn.us/divs/idepc/diseases/anaplasmosis/casesyear.html). Human anaplasmosis caused by *A. phagocytophilum* is now the second most common tick-borne disease in the US, and is also transmitted by *I. scapularis*. Although still much less common than borreliosis, this disease has paralleled the upward trend of Lyme disease (http://www.cdc.gov/ticks/diseases/anaplasmosis/statistics.html), and may be subject to similar dynamics and constraints of climate and tick biology. Clearly, climate plays a prominent role in the shifting boundaries of tick populations, but it is certainly only one of multiple factors in the equation. Warmer winters with increased precipitation and thus deeper winter snow pack allow enhanced tick overwintering rates by providing critical protection from desiccation and chill injury (Burks et al., 1996), and result in expansion into formerly unsuitable regions—as seen in Canada with *I. scapularis* (Odgen et al., 2005, 2008). In currently endemic areas, greater humidity and higher temperatures earlier and later in the year extend periods of tick activity into a longer tick season while creating inviting conditions for human outdoor activity. This effectively prolongs risk of exposure and infection.

### Planning Ahead: Can Climate Models Predict Public Health Risk?

A number of research teams have attempted to model risk of infection with tick-borne pathogens. Intuitively, one should expect this to be possible in developed countries where there is a wealth of data on human disease cases, distribution of ticks and hosts, and climatologic data collected over decades. Areas that are currently considered to present high risk of encountering ticks can be identified at a regional level, and provide valuable guidance for the management of tick-borne disease risk through rational design of land use, and management of tick hosts and pathogen reservoirs (Ward and Brown, 2004; Stafford III, 2007). Risk assessments indicate that fragmented, patchy forest with a large proportion of edge habitat, support tick and mouse populations well (Allan et al., 2003; Brownstein et al., 2005; Foley et al., 2009; Eisen et al., 2010; Raizman et al., 2010). This agrees with the observation that disturbed ecosystems support larger numbers of ticks than intact ones, and reflects a variety of underlying reasons based in the biology of ecosystem participants. Deer, especially white-tailed deer, are important reproductive hosts for *Ixodes* ticks, and thrive in second growth forest that characterizes prime tick habitat (Foley et al., 2009). By contrast, intact old growth forests have much lower association with tick-bite risk, probably because they retain higher vertebrate species diversity that dilutes infection risk by interspecies competition and predation on reservoirs. This seeming discrepancy in the association of forests with tick bite risk is an example of the difficulties that analysts face when trying to make sense of the collective data set. The many abiotic and biotic factors that combine to shape the ecology of vector-borne diseases are highly complex, and published studies lack a standardized approach that would make them comparable (Kililea et al., 2008). Models that attempt to span expansive regions or to extend forecasts far ahead are often based on the assumption that current trends will remain continuous over long distances and into the future (Diuk-Wasser et al., 2006; Odgen et al., 2006). These assumptions remain to be validated, but nevertheless present plausible scenarios that have stimulated the debate about interventions and countermeasures. Long-term predictive models could be made more useful if they were continuously updated with new information to reflect the influence of changing populations and land use.

### Tick Species with the Greatest Potential for Expansion

Lessons learned from the two globally most widely distributed tick species, the cattle fever tick (pantropical blue tick), *Rhipicephalus (Boophilus) microplus* (Madder et al., 2010), and the brown dog tick, *Rhipicephalus sanguineus* (Burlini et al., 2010), indicate that human-facilitated dispersal of ectoparasites via movement on domestic hosts is by far the most effective mechanism. For ticks, this presents an ideal scenario that ensures a suitable or even preferred host is available at the new location. In the case of *R. (Bo.) microplus* this success was further enhanced by the fact that this is a one-host tick for which the eggs are the only off-host stage. Notwithstanding the great economic importance of *R. (Bo.) microplus* as a vector of livestock diseases agents, it does not parasitize humans, and therefore is of no relevance in tick-borne zoonoses.

The brown dog tick has likewise colonized the globe as a parasite of dogs accompanying humans (Burlini et al., 2010). It is found wherever dogs are kept in regions between the latitudes of 50° North and 30° South. It commonly infests kennels and even homes, seeking shelter in cracks, under window sills, and behind furniture. This tick preferentially parasitizes dogs, but may bite humans if dogs are not available, and does so apparently more readily in Europe where it has long been known to transmit *Rickettsia conorii*, the agent of boutonneuse fever, to people (Péter et al., 1984; Dantas-Torres, 2010). The recent identification of a North American focus of Rocky Mountain spotted fever with transmission of the agent among dogs and children (Demma et al., 2005) reinforces the zoonotic potential of this tick. Notably, brown dog ticks attack alternate hosts including humans more readily when ambient temperatures are high, can complete up to four generations a year, and may become more important vectors of human disease as climate warms in its current range (Dantas-Torres, 2010).

By contrast, tick dispersal on wild hosts is much less efficient, although it can account for increase of tick mobility to hundreds or thousands of miles on hosts such as deer or migratory birds (Klich et al., 1996; Björsdorff et al., 2001; Madhav et al., 2004; Odgen et al., 2008). Off host, *I. scapularis* ticks move at most a distance of a few meters (Carroll and Schmidtmann, 1996). Even though ticks can be carried great distances in these ways, there is no guarantee that their drop-off locations will present them with suitable habitat or hosts for subsequent life stages, but this will change as plant and animal communities respond to a warming climate.

## The Interface Between Ticks and Emerging Disease Agents

Tick-borne pathogens of humans causing emerging diseases are primarily reported in temperate climates, but this trend may be a distortion of the true picture, as public health systems and disease reporting are much less accurate and often inconsistent in less developed and tropical countries. As a result, emerging diseases in these countries are under-reported by comparison to those in the Western world (Jones et al., 2008). In Brazil, increasing numbers of suspected tick-borne spotted fever cases previously thought to be of viral origin are being identified (Labruna, 2009), and result in significant mortality. Brazilian spotted fever caused by a strain of *Rickettsia rickettsii* is now considered to cause the majority of such cases, but the true extent of its occurrence is not known (Rozental et al., 2006). *Amblyomma* spp. ticks have been implicated in transmitting the rickettsiae among rodents and opossums, although the presence of more abundant rickettsiae of undetermined pathogenicity has clouded the picture.

Ticks of greatest concern for human health are three-host generalist feeders, commonly utilizing small animals such as birds, rodents, squirrels and hedgehogs during the larval and nymphal stages, and feeding on larger hosts as nymphs and adults. They thus act as bridge vectors between animal reservoirs that are usually not affected by the pathogen, and humans who are dead-end hosts but suffer disease symptoms. A good example are ticks in the genus *Ixodes*, found around the globe in temperate and subtropical regions. In North America, the black-legged tick, *I. scapularis*, is probably the most notorious vector of zoonotic pathogens, capable of transmitting viruses (Powassan encephalitis virus; Pesko et al., 2010), bacteria (*Borrelia burgdorferi, A. phagocytophilum,* and possibly *Bartonella* spp. as well as a new *Ehrlichia muris*-like organism; Burgdorfer et al., 1982; Chen et al., 1994; Adelson et al., 2004; Pritt et al., 2009), and protozoa (*Babesia microti*; Piesman and Spielman, 1980). In Europe, the closely related tick species *Ixodes ricinus* is involved in a similarly broad spectrum of pathogen transmission, but has a much greater role in viral infections caused by tick-borne encephalitis viruses (Flaviviridae). Certainly, the many different types and species of vertebrates that are suitable hosts for *I. scapularis* and *I. ricinus* immature stages contribute significantly to their potential encounters with pathogens that are capable of colonizing and being transmitted by them. It is interesting to note that most zoonotic pathogens vectored by *Ixodes* species are maintained transstadially in ticks, even when infection rates in vertebrate reservoirs are low and of limited duration. This seems to be the case for *A. phagocytophilum* in white-footed mice that clear the infection within two weeks (Telford et al., 1996). *Anaplasma phagocytophilum* has been identified as an emerging human pathogen primarily in the US where it now is responsible for the second most common tick-borne illness (Chen et al., 1994). Serial re-infections of immune-intact laboratory mice (C57BL/6) by inoculation of culture-derived human-infectious *A. phagocytophilum* carrying different antibiotic and fluorescent marker genes suggests that mice do not develop a protective immune response to re-infection despite the fact that the bacteria are cleared after every inoculation (our unpublished results). If wild-type *A. phagocytophilum* behaves similarly in wild mice, sufficient levels of infected populations could thus be maintained, as per the susceptible-infected-susceptible model proposed by Kurtenbach et al. (2006).

Although transovarial transmission does occur in pathogens vectored by *Ixodes* ticks and contributes to viral maintenance in tick populations, this mechanism appears to be less important than horizontal transmission among co-feeding ticks, at least in European tick-borne encephalitis virus where it has been examined in greatest detail (Labuda et al., 1993; LaSala and Holbrook, 2010). Whether this preference also holds true for Powassan virus (Costero and Grayson, 1996) remains to be determined.

One of the notorious tick-borne diseases in North America has long been Rocky Mountain spotted fever, and as its name implies, it was first described in the Rocky Mountain region in the latter part of the 19th century. There, the agent, *R. rickettsii*, circulates among small to medium mammals and the Rocky Mountain wood tick, *Dermacentor andersoni*, in which it is maintained transovarially (Niebylski et al., 1999). Both ticks and mammals can serve the role of reservoir. Over the decades, the greatest disease incidence has shifted south and east, and North Carolina and Oklahoma now account for the highest number of cases (http://www.cdc.gov/ticks/diseases/rocky_mountain_spotted_fever/statistics.html). In these states, the main vector is the American dog tick, *Dermacentor variabilis*. In both tick vectors, infections are very low at less than 1%, making it hard to predict risk by sampling tick populations. Likewise, this makes it difficult to track how this geographic shift has occurred, if it has occurred, or whether the apparent redistribution of cases is a reflection of better diagnostics and surveillance. *Dermacentor* and *Amblyomma* spp. ticks, both of which are present in these states, carry a variety of more abundant related microbes of undetermined or low pathogenicity, e.g., *Rickettsia parkeri* and *Candidatus* Rickettsia amblyommii (Paddock, 2009) that are suspected of contributing to Rocky Mountain spotted fever. While *R. parkeri* is a proven though mild infectious agent, the status of *C. R. amblyommi* remains undetermined, and it could just as well exclude *R. rickettsii* from ticks in a manner as *Rickettsia peacockii* does (Burgdorfer et al., 1981).

### Pathogen Evolution Is a Dynamic, Ongoing Process

*Anaplasma phagocytophilum*, an obligate intracellular bacterium, has been known as a tick-borne pathogen of sheep, goats and cattle in Europe for decades where it was previously named *Cytoecetes phagocytophila* or *Ehrlichia phagocytophila* (Dumler et al., 2001; Woldehiwet, 2006). Ruminants remain persistently infected and experience cyclic bacteremia (Stuen, 2007). An organism named *Ehrlichia equi* was likewise known to infect Californian horses since the mid 1900s (Madigan and Gribble, 1987), but there, as in Europe, human cases are rare (Foley et al., 2009). Notably, *A. phagocytophilum* variants not found in human patients have been identified in deer in several locations of the US. One can imagine a scenario where European settlers unknowingly introduced infected livestock to North America, and American *Ixodes* ticks subsequently acquired and spread the agent which thrived in deer. Whether this strain later developed the ability to infect mice and humans (as well as dogs and horses), or whether the human-infectious strains were introduced separately, or even were already present in North America awaits further phylogenetic analysis.

In Minnesota, *I. scapularis* may be infected with different variants of *A. phagocytophilum* (Michalski et al., 2006; Baldridge et al., 2009), not all of which cause human anaplasmosis (HA). We are currently testing the hypothesis that a whole genome comparison of *A. phagocytophilum* (*Ap*) isolates that infect humans (*Ap*-ha) versus those that are pervasively found in ticks and wild animals (*Ap*-variants) will reveal genetic differences that underlie *Ap* pathogenicity. Research has focused on *Ap*-ha and we know little about the biology of the more recently described *Ap* variants (Massung et al., 2005, 2007; Baldridge et al., 2009). Besides their potential ability to regulate the epidemiology of HA (Massung et al., 2002), the genome sequence of *Ap*-variants would be a valuable resource to identify mechanisms of host specificity, virulence and tick transmission in *Ap*-ha. We found that 64% of *I. scapularis* and 45% of *Dermacentor albipictus* (the winter or moose tick) collected from whitetail deer (WTD) in the army base at Camp Ripley, MN, carried *Ap* variants, including two with 16S rRNA gene sequences identical to *Ap* variants from Wisconsin deer. The *D. albipictus* variants were transovarially transmitted to F1 larvae at efficiencies of up to 40%, the first evidence for vertical transmission of *Ap* to tick progeny. These represent the highest *Ap* prevalence rates reported for any location, notably in the absence of increased numbers of human HA cases, supporting the notion that Camp Ripley *Ap* variants are truly distinct from *Ap*-ha. Unlike human-infectious strains, they do not infect mice, and can only be cultured in a cell line from the vector tick, suggesting they are biologically very different (Massung et al., 2005, 2007). Using tick cell line ISE6, we obtained 8 isolates of *Ap* variants from ticks feeding on WTD hunted in Camp Ripley. One of these, MN-61-2, was infectious for a goat but not mice, similar to *Ap*-variant 1 from Rhode Island, suggesting that the Northeast and Midwest variants are related (Massung et al., 2007). All our variant *Ap* isolates have the same 16S rRNA sequences but different *ankA* gene sequences. Now that *Ap*-variant isolates are available, their genomes can be sequenced to address the salient differences between *Ap*-ha and *Ap* variants: what genes/operons determine infectivity for humans versus ruminants, and what do the genomes reveal about the evolution of this emerging pathogen?

Research with other agents reinforces the notion that genetic population structure of tick-borne pathogens affects the interaction of human-infectious and animal-infectious isolates in endemic areas. There is evidence that multiple genotypes of *B. burgdorferi* have arisen from multiple, distinct foci (Hoen et al., 2009), and that human infectious borreliae may displace non-human infectious genotypes in animal populations due to differential transmission by vector ticks (Girard et al., 2009). This suggests that factors affecting pathogen distribution are not limited to climate change, and include fitness determinants that regulate utilization of arthropods.

## The Interactive Bacterial Communities of Ticks

The mammalian host and vector tick are two quite divergent environments that tick-transmitted pathogens have adapted to in order to survive and invade new hosts. In addition to the well known pathogens that are acquired and transmitted during the blood meal, ticks are also colonized by symbionts and fortuitous microbes, the latter acquired from contact with animals during the blood meal or from the soil or plants while questing or surviving off the host. The life cycle of tick-borne bacteria is complex and controlled by the requirement for alternating between hosts with vastly different biological characteristics. Most ticks take weeks or months to complete each life stage, and take but a single blood meal each time. Human pathogens transmitted by ticks regulate gene expression to permit successful development in each host, as inappropriate timing of gene expression can abort transmission and infection.

Environmental changes are likely to introduce new environmental challenges and lead to altered tick-microbe and microbe-microbe associations, distributions and interactions. Arguably, the most important vector ticks with the greatest potential for expansion in North America are the *Ixodes, Amblyomma* and *Dermacentor* species. These ticks are three host ticks and generalist feeders (feed on different hosts in each of the life stages). Accordingly we focus herein on what is known about the microbial communities of *I. scapularis, Amblyomma americanum* (Lone Star tick), and *D. variabilis*. Though a variety of approaches have been used to delineate the bacterial communities of these ticks, we still need to address the question of how symbionts, fortuitous microbes and pathogens interact to affect pathogen acquisition or transmission and the emergence or re-emergence of tick borne disease agents.

Studies to determine the bacterial communities of ticks have generally focused on a given geographical region or tick developmental stage. The microbial community of *I. scapularis* is best described for ticks collected in areas endemic for Lyme disease, e.g., New York state (Moreno et al., 2006) or Massachusetts (Benson et al., 2004). Moreno et al. (2006) used temporal temperature gradient gel electrophoresis separation and sequencing of 16S DNA PCR-amplified products to detect specific bacteria in *I. scapularis* larvae, nymphs and adults, engorged and unfed. The most abundant were *Rickettsia, Pseudomonas* and *Borrelia,* whereas *Ralstonia, Anaplasma,* Enterobacteria, *Moraxella, Rhodococcus,* and "uncultured proteobacteria" were less common. There was considerable stage and fed/unfed variation, but in general, engorged nymphs and females harbored the most diverse bacteria, suggesting that the blood meal exerted major impact on the microbial diversity of the tick. The rickettsial endosymbiont of *I. scapularis* (REIS; Baldridge et al., 2010) was found in all ticks and stages, whether fed or not, and no correlations between REIS and presence or absence of *B. burgdorferi, A. phagocytophilum* or other microbes associated with *I. scapularis* have been found (Moreno et al., 2006; Steiner et al., 2008). REIS has also been referred to as "Rickettsia cooleyi" (Billings et al., 1998) or "Rickettsia midichlorii" (Parola et al., 2005). In contrast, four different genera of intracellular bacteria were detected in *I. scapularis* nymphs collected in Massachusetts: *Rickettsia, Anaplasma, Wolbachia* and *Cardinium* (Benson et al., 2004). The *Cardinium* species is closely related to a bacterium isolated from *I. scapularis* (Kurtti et al., 1996) that itself is closely related to *Cardinium hertigii* from mites and insects (Nakamura et al., 2009). Identification of *Wolbachia* and *Cardinium,* known to be involved in reproductive alterations in insects and mites, is intriguing, but no such effects have been reported for *I. scapularis*. Several of the nymphs were coinfected with two intracellular bacteria, but *Arsenophonus* spp. endosymbionts, found in a wide range of arthropods including *Amblyomma* and *Dermacentor* ticks (Novakova et al., 2009), were absent from *I. scapularis*.

The microbial communities of *A. americanum* and *D. variabilis* diverge from those reported for *I. scapularis* (Grindle et al., 2003; Clay et al., 2008; Dergouseff et al., 2010). *Rickettsia* spp. are associated with both ticks but unlike *I. scapularis*, they also harbor *Coxiella-* or *Francisella*-like endosymbionts that are members of the gammaproteobacteria. A *Coxiella* sp. is highly prevalent (100%) and *Rickettsia* sp. less so in *A. americanum*, but not *D. variabilis,* from several different states in the US (Jasinkas et al., 2007; Clay et al., 2008) (MD, OK, IN, MO, KY, GA, SC, and MS). Most of the *A. americanum* were infected with two to three microbes, and all ticks at all locations were infected with the *Coxiella* sp. endosymbiont that appears to have undergone genome reduction (Jasinskas et al., 2007). In contrast, a *Rickettsia* sp. with 99% similarity to *Candidatus* Rickettsia amblyommii was present in 45-61% of ticks, while prevalence of an *Arsenophonus* sp. was geographically spotty and varied from 0-90%. The *Coxiella* endosymbiont and *Pseudomonas* spp. were detected in larvae suggesting that both were transmitted transovarially. Coinfections involved the *Coxiella* endosymbiont and *Arsenophonus* or C. R. amblyommii and 26% of the ticks were infected with all three microbes. No sex ratio distortion was detected but a negative correlation between infection by *Arsenophonus* and *Rickettsia* sp. was noted, suggesting that one endosymbiont could potentially interfere with infection by another. In contrast to the wide presence of endosymbionts, pathogens, i.e., the monocytic ehrlichiosis agent, *Ehrlichia chaffeensis*, and *Borrelia lonestari*, were rare. The microbial community of *D. variabilis* ticks is less well characterized, though the most prevalent microbe in *Dermacentor* ticks is the symbiotic *Francisella* sp. (Scoles, 2004). Canadian *D. variabilis* also harbor *Arsenophonus* similar to that found in *D. variabilis* in eastern US (Dergouseff et al., 2010).

Most microbial surveys currently rely on the use of PCR technology to detect and identify microorganisms in ticks. Few culture isolates of tick-associated microorganisms are available which makes it difficult to characterize traits such as vertebrate infectivity and pathogenicity and hinders genome sequencing. An obligate intracellular gammaproteobacterium has recently been culture isolated in vertebrate cells from *I. ricinus* collected in Slovakia (Mediannikov et al., 2010). A polyphasic taxonomic approach showed it is most closely related to *Rickettsiella* spp, in the family Coxiellaceae. Bacteria belonging to this group are sometimes detected in ticks (Noda et al., 1997; Kurtti et al., 2002) but their influence on tick physiology or ability to cause human disease is unknown. Uncharacterized microbes isolated during an attempt to isolate pathogens in cell cultures may turn out to be potentially important regulators of tick biology and vectorial capacity. We isolated a bacterium from ticks collected in Connecticut that was later found to belong to the genus *Cardinium*, a group known to cause reproductive disorders in insects and mites (Nakamura et al., 2009). Our culture isolate from *I. scapularis* remains the only one for this important group of bacteria.

### The Dynamic Microbiomes of Vector Ticks

Studies outlined above suggest that tick-associate bacteria other than vertebrate pathogens modulate the vectorial capacity of ticks either by competition or possibly by exchange of genetic elements, and might provide tools to manipulate pathogen transmission. To exploit the microbial communities interacting with ticks, we propose that the microbiomes of major vector ticks be characterized. A microbiome is defined as "the totality of microbes, their genetic elements (genomes), and environmental interactions in a defined environment" (http://en.wikipedia.org/wiki/Microbiome). The microbiome of *I. scapularis* it is incomplete and weighted towards human pathogens transmitted by this tick (Table A6-1, completed and in progress). The only other microbial genome from *I. scapularis* is that of the REIS obtained during genome sequencing of the host tick (Van Zee et al., 2007). Pathogenic ehrlichiae and rickettsiae are so far the only characterized members of the microbiomes of *A. amblyommii* and *D. variabilis*, but other prominent microbes associated with these ticks should be considered for genome sequencing (Table A6-1, proposed). Because of its importance as a vector of Lyme disease and human

**TABLE A6-1** Prokaryotic Microbiomes of *Ixodes scapularis*, *Dermacentor variabilis*, and *Amblyomma americanum*

| | Microbe | Classification | Isolate | Reference |
|---|---|---|---|---|
| **Ixodes scapularis** | | | | |
| COMPLETED | | | | |
| | *Borrelia burgdorferi* | Spirochaetes | B31 | Fraser et al., 1997 |
| | *Anaplasma phagocyophilum* | *Alphaproteobacteria Anaplasmataceae* | HZ | Dunning Hotopp et al., 2006 |
| IN PROGRESS | | | | |
| | Borrelia burgdorferi | Spirochaetes | 297, CA8, DN127, JD1, N40 | unpublished (see NCBI Genome Project web page) |
| | REIS et al.[a] | *Alphaproteobacter Rickettsieai* | Wikel | Joardar et al., unpublished |
| | *Cardinium* sp. | *Bacteroidetes* | IsCLO | Noda et al., (unpublished, personal commun.) |
| PROPOSED | | | | |
| | REIS | *Alphaproteobacteria Rickettsieae* | ISO-7 | Kurtti, unpublished |
| | *Anaplasma phagocytophilum* | *Alphaproteobacteria Anaplasmataceae* | Ap-variant 1 | Massung et al., 2007 |
| | *Pseudomonas* spp (Symbiont) | *Gammaproteobacteria Pseudomonadaceae* | na[b] | Moreno et al., 2006 |
| **Dermacentor variabilis** | | | | |
| COMPLETED | | | | |
| | *Rickettsia rickettsii* | *Alphaproteobacteria Rickettsieae* | Iowa | Ellison et al., 2008 |
| PROPOSED | | | | |
| | *Francisella* sp endosymbiont | *Gammaproteobacteria Francisellaceae* | na | Niebylski et al., 1997a Scoles, 2004 |
| | *Arsenophonus* sp | *Gammaproteobacteria Enterobacteriales* | na | Grindle et al., 2003 |

*continued*

**TABLE A6-1** Continued

|  | Microbe | Classification | Isolate | Reference |
|---|---|---|---|---|
| *Amblyomma americanum* |  |  |  |  |
| COMPLETED |  |  |  |  |
|  | *Ehrlichia chaffeensis* | *Alphaproteobacteria Ehrlichieae* | Arkansas | Dunning Hotopp et al., 2006 |
| IN PROGRESS |  |  |  |  |
|  | *Ehrlichia chaffeensis* | Alphaproteobacteria Ehrlichieae | Sapulpa | Copeland et al. (unpublished) |
| PROPOSED |  |  |  |  |
|  | C. Rickettsia amblyommii | *Alphaproteobacteria Rickettsieae* | several available | Baldridge et al., 2010 |
|  | *Coxiella* sp. endosymbiont | *Gammaproteobacteria* Coxiellaceae | na | Jasinskas et al., 2007 Clay et al., 2008 |
|  | *Arsenophonus* sp endosymbiont | *Gammaproteobacteria* Enterobacteriales | na | Clay et al., 2008 |

[a] REIS = rickettsial endosymbiont of I. scapularis ("Rickettsia cooleyi" and "Rickettsia midichlorii").
[b] na = no available culture isolate.

anaplasmosis, comparing the microbiome of *I. scapularis* from different geographical regions should be a priority.

Tick-associated bacteria contain genes that encode molecular chaperones responsive to a wide range of stress conditions (Feder and Hofman, 1999), such as the small heat-shock protein genes (Hsps) found in *Rickettsia* and *Anaplasma* species. In most non-pathogenic rickettsiae *hsp2* is localized to plasmids and *hsp1* to the chromosome (Baldridge et al., 2008), suggesting expression may be controlled differently. Indeed, transcriptional regulation of host adaptive genes is facilitated by their location on plasmids as has been described in *B. burgdorferi* (Stewart et al., 2005). Hsps respond to a variety of stress effectors (pH, osmotic pressure, etc) and help to stabilize membrane proteins and nucleic acids. In the tick, intracellular bacteria face significant changes in temperature, pH, osmotic pressure, metabolite concentrations, and $CO_2$ and $O_2$ levels during the alternating periods of starvation and blood feeding (Munderloh et al., 2005), and the observed differential expression of Hsps in *A. phagocytophilum* growing in human versus tick cells implies a role in mitigating deleterious effects (Nelson et al., 2008). GenBank data derived from the *I. scapularis* genome project indicate that REIS carries at least three plasmids (pREIS1, 2 and 3) which is supported by pulsed field electrophoresis results of our REIS culture isolate (Baldridge et al., 2010). The presence of multiple plasmids in REIS is an enigma but may compensate for functional gene loss resulting in impaired ability to respond to environmental stressors such as elevated temperature and oxidation. The NCBI database for REIS indicates loss of a heat shock induced serine protease, HtrA, that degrades misfolded proteins. REIS also has a frame-shift in the poly-beta-hydroxybutyrate polymerase gene (*phbC*) that is upregulated in *R. conorii* in response to stress encountered in the skin of patients infected with Mediterranean spotted fever (Renesto et al., 2008). Diverse bacteria are associated with *I. scapularis*, and coinfections of a single tick with the *Cardinium* endosymbiont and REIS have been reported (Benson et al., 2004). This could facilitate horizontal gene transfer (hgt) between them, and is supported by the presence of closely related transposons in the *Dermacentor* tick symbiont *Rickettsia peacockii* and the *Cardinium* endosymbiont from *I. scapularis*. This transposon, likely acquired by hgt, is associated with extensive genomic reorganization and deletions in the *R. peacockii* genome (Felsheim et al., 2009). The potential for rickettsial plasmid mobility and hgt between intracellular bacteria cohabiting the same intracellular arena should be examined.

## Cohabitation and Horizontal Gene Transfer

Hgt has shaped the genomes of tick-transmitted pathogens and has played an important role in the acquisition of environmental adaptive traits and virulence determinants. There are two prominent hypotheses related to intracellular bacteria that can potentially infect the same host cell in a tick. The "intracellular arena hypothesis" posits that the coinhabitants can coexist, interact and exchange genetic material (Blanc et al., 2007). The "interference hypothesis" posits that interspecific competition between closely related species interferes with their ability to cohabit the same intracellular environment (Burgdorfer, 1981; Macaluso et al., 2002). There is considerable evidence for cohabitation of dissimilar intracellular microbes within the same host cell, especially among the symbionts that infect the ovarian cells of ticks. *Rickettsia peacockii* and a *Francisella*-like symbiont are present together in the interstitial ovarian cells of *D. andersoni* (Niebylski et al., 1997a). A *Coxiella*-like symbiont is found together with C. Rickettsia amblyommii in the ovarian cells of *A. americanum*. The evidence for interference between two closely related species derives mainly from research with *Rickettsia* and *Anaplasma*. On the other hand, the presence of mobile genetic elements (plasmids and transposons) suggests that *Rickettsia* spp. coinfecting the same host cell have the potential for the generation of genetic diversity, but it needs to be demonstrated that these genetic elements are indeed mobile. The ability to interact and acquire novel adaptive traits and virulence determinants is clearly germane to generation of new tick borne pathogens. The research tools to test these hypotheses have recently become available.

Discovered only recently (Ogata et al., 2005), plasmids appear to be surprisingly common in rickettsiae (Blanc et al., 2007; Baldridge et al., 2010), and several rickettsiae carry *tra* genes encoding type IV secretion system (T4SS) that may mediate rickettsial acquisition of foreign DNA, possibly via pili formation and conjugation (Ogata et al., 2005; Ogata et al., 2006; Blanc et al., 2007; Felsheim et al., 2009). Gillespie et al. (2010) proposed that the RvhB6 proteins (comparable to VirB6 in other bacterial species) in *Rickettsia* and *Anaplasma* play a role in DNA import and export in congener bacteria and create the potential for hgt. Tiling microarrays have detected host cell specific transcription patterns in the *rvhB6* genes of *A. phagocytophilum* during growth in human and *I. scapularis* cells in vitro (Nelson et al., 2008). Given the diversity of animals that *I. scapularis* feeds on and the temporal scale available for microbe-microbe interactions, hgt is most likely to take place in ticks. The experimental tools to examine genetic exchange between congeners of *Rickettsia* and *Anaplasma* have recently been developed (Felsheim et al., 2006; Baldridge et al., 2005).

*Mobile Genetic Elements: Future Directions in Laboratory Research on Tick-Borne Pathogens*

Research in rickettsiology has lagged far behind that on diseases caused by bacteria that can be propagated on axenic media, despite the pressing needs created by emergence and re-emergence of severe illnesses such as RMSF, anaplasmosis and ehlichiosis. Transformation of obligate intracellular bacteria has been a challenge that researchers have only recently been able to address, but this important tool is still in need of refinement (Baldridge et al., 2005; Felsheim et al., 2006; Liu et al., 2007). Original methods developed for rickettsial transformation, including homologous recombination (Rachek et al., 1998) and use of selectable markers with EZ:TN transposon vectors (Qin et al, 2004; Baldridge et al., 2005), had low efficiency, fueling our efforts to find better systems. The mariner class transposase, *Himar1*, which has shown broad activity in bacteria, proved useful in transforming *A. phagocytophilum* (Felsheim et al., 2006), enabling us to create mutants with defective phenotypes that can now be functionally characterized. This system is equally suited for rickettsial mutagenesis, but is still quite inefficient, yielding one or a few transformants at each electroporation. Nevertheless, an advantage of is the stability of resulting mutants when transposition occurs into the chromosome, making them well suited for in vivo tracking by live imaging applications such as time-lapse microscopy and tracking in vectors and vertebrate animals.

## Making the Most of Rickettsial Plasmids

With the discovery of plasmids in many *Rickettsi* spp. came the realization that they could be fashioned into an efficient transformation tool to facilitate studies on rickettsial functional genomics. Till now, analysis of rickettsial gene function has relied on cloning genes of interest into *E. coli* in the hope they would perform in this artificial system as they would "at home." To overcome this drawback, we set out to utilize rickettsial plasmids for direct analysis of rickettsial genes in rickettsiae themselves. To start we cloned the *Rickettsia monacensis* plasmid pRM (Baldridge et al, 2007) and *R. amblyommii* plasmids pRAM18 and pRAM23 (Baldridge et al., 2010) with the aim to design shuttle vectors that could be used as effective transformation systems. We modified pRAM18 to express a fluorescent (GFPuv) marker to successfully transform the nonpathogenic *R. bellii*. To create a more efficient plasmid we transferred the *parA* and *dnaA* genes of pRAM18 that regulate plasmid replication and partitioning into smaller (8.7 and 10.3 kbp) constructs that were efficiently transformed into three species, *R. montanensis*, *R. monacensis* and *R. bellii* (Burkhardt et al., 2010). While these initial results provide a good start towards eventual production of a shuttle vector system for efficient transformation of a wide range of rickettsiae, problems of incompatibility remain to be sorted out.

## Can the Paradigm of Paratransgenesis Be Realized in Rickettsiology?

The results of testing the "intracellular arena" and "interference" hypotheses have important implications for the potential application of paratransgenesis in the control of tick-borne diseases. The paratransgenesis paradigm involves the replacement or supplementation of an indigenous symbiont with a genetically altered (transformed) congener that interferes with the ability of the arthropod to transmit a pathogen without killing the arthropod. Manipulation of tick populations by subversion of their indigenous endosymbionts is an attractive concept because it targets a vehicle naturally restricted to the tick population. Systems for genetic modification of REIS could be applied to interfere with the transmission of *B. burgdorferi* or *A. phagocytophilum* by *I. scapulris*.

The relationship between ticks and their symbionts is not clear, and at this time, bacteria that could be regarded as "primary tick symbionts" analogous to those in insects (Dale and Moran, 2006) have not been identified. REIS and *R. peacockii* are regarded as the closest to being mutualistic endosymbionts among the known, non-pathogenic rickettsiae, because of their apparent inability to invade vertebrate cells. This is likely due to the disruption of rickettsial genes involved in mammalian cell invasion, such as *rompA* and *rickA* (Niebylski et al., 1997b; Simser et al., 2001, 2005).

The high prevalence of REIS in widely distributed *I. scapularis* popula-tions indicates that it is essential to *I. scapularis* survival. The sequenced genomes of *Rickettsiales*, including pathogens, have revealed a significant capacity to produce cofactors such as lipoate, protoheme, ubiquinone, and several amino acids, e.g., glutamine, glycine, diaminopimelate and aspar-tate (Dunning Hotopp et al., 2006). This suggests that even tick-borne pathogens may supply their tick hosts with some needed nutrients, acting like symbionts for their vector. In essence, there is much that remains to be learned about tick symbionts before they can be considered for paratrans-genic tick control. Clearly, there is a need to elucidate the relationships between ticks and the symbiotic and pathogenic microorganisms they carry and how the interactions are affected by environmental changes.

*Conclusions*

The reasons for the accelerated increase, expansion and uneven distri-bution of tick-borne emerging and re-emerging diseases are complex but several conclusions can be drawn. Human activities that modify habitats to support available hosts for maintaining tick populations while at the same time reducing species richness that could act to dilute risk. Weather and temperature regimes restricts the current range of tick populations, but global climate changes will provide new opportunities for the expansion of ticks into currently uncolonized regions. In addition, domestic animals can act as reservoirs for tick-borne pathogens and act as bridge hosts in the transfer of emerging and re-emerging pathogens to humans. Fragmenta-tion of wildlife habitats by human encroachment increases the contact with ticks and exposure to zoonotic disease agents (Allan et al., 2003). The areas likely to experience increased or prolonged seasonal tick activity are most likely located at the extremes of the current range of distribution. Long-term predictive models are complex and in need of refinement in order to predict public health risks associated with ticks and tick-borne pathogens. The expansion of three host ticks that feed on wild and domestic animals and humans show the greatest potential for expansion and acquisition and transmission of emerging pathogens. Introduction of ticks to new habi-tats or importation of exotic hosts are likely to increase the exposure of ticks to novel microbial communities. More information is needed about the potential for horizontal genetic exchange and interaction between the microorganisms within the tick's microbial community. Characterizing the microbiomes of major vector ticks from different geographical regions would assist in detecting and monitoring these interactions and determine their role in the generation of emerging and re-emerging tick-borne patho-gens. Characterizing the microbial communities would also assist in the identification of microbes that could complement the biological control of tick populations.

## References

Adelson, M. E., R. V. Rao, R. C. Tilton, K. Cabets, E. Eskow, L. Fein, J. L. Occi, and E. Mordechai. 2004. Prevalence of Borrelia burgdorferi, Bartonella spp., Babesia microti, and Anaplasma phagocytophila in Ixodes scapularis ticks collected in Northern New Jersey. Journal of Clinical Microbiology 42(6):2799-801.

Allan, B. F., F. Keesing, and R. S. Ostfeld. 2003. The effect of habitat fragmentation on Lyme disease risk. Conservation Biology 17:267-272.

Baldridge, G. D., N. Y. Burkhardt, M. J. Herron, T. J. Kurtti, and U. G. Munderloh. 2005. Analysis of fluorescent protein expression in transformants of Rickettsia monacensis, an obligate intracellular tick symbiont. Applied and Environmental Microbiology 71(4):2095-2105.

Baldridge, G. D., N. Y. Burkhardt, R. F. Felsheim, T. J. Kurtti, and U. G. Munderloh. 2008. Plasmids of the pRM/pRF family occur in diverse Rickettsia species. Applied and Environmental Microbiology 74(3):645-652.

Baldridge, G. D., G. A. Scoles, N. Burkhardt, B. Schloeder, T. J. Kurtti, and U. G. Munderloh. 2009. Transovarial transmission of Francisella-like endosymbionts and Anaplasma phagocytophilum variants in Dermacentor albipictus (Acari: Ixodidae). Journal of Medical Entomology 46:625-632.

Baldridge, G. D., N. Y. Burkhardt, M. B. Labruna, R. C. Pacheco, C. D. Paddock, P. C. Williamson, P. M. Billingsley, R. F. Felsheim, T. J. Kurtti, and U. G. Munderloh. 2010. Wide dispersal and possible multiple origins of low-copy-number plasmids in Rickettsia species associated with blood-feeding arthropods. Applied and Environmental Microbiology 76(6):1718-1731.

Barbour, A. G. and D. Fish. 1993. The biological and social phenomenon of Lyme disease. Science 260(5114):1610-1616.

Barré, N., M. Bianchi, and L. Chardonnet. 2001. Role of Rusa deer Cervus timorensis russa in the cycle of the cattle tick Boophilus microplus in New Caledonia. Experimental and Applied Acarology 25(1):79-96.

Bartlett, S. L., N. Abou-Madi, J. B. Messick, A. Birkenheuer, and G. V. Kollias. 2009. Diagnosis and treatment of Babesia odocoilei in captive reindeer (Rangifer tarandus tarandus) and recognition of three novel host species. Journal of Zoo and Wildlife Medicine 40(1):152-159.

Benson, M. J., J. D. Gawronski, D. E. Eveleigh, and D. R. Benson. 2004. Intracellular symbionts and other bacteria associated with deer ticks (Ixodes scapularis) from Nantucket and Wellfleet, Cape Cod, Massachusetts. Applied and Environmental Microbiology 70(1):616-620.

Billings, A. N., Tetlow, G. J., Weaver, S. C., and D. H. Walker. 1998. Molecular characterization of a novel Rickettsia species from Ixodes scapularis in Texas. Emerging Infectious Diseases 4(2):305-309.

Bjöersdorff, A., S. Bergström, R. F. Massung, P. D. Haemig, and B. Olsen. 2001. Ehrlichia-infected ticks on migrating birds. Emerging Infectious Diseases 7(5):877-879.

Blanc, G., H. Ogata, C. Robert, S. Audic, J.-M. Claverie, and D. Raoult. 2007. Lateral gene transfer between obligate intracellular bacteria: evidence from the Rickettsia massiliae genome. Genome Research 17:1657-1664.

Brooks, D., and A. Ferrao. 2005. The historical biogeography of co-evolution: emerging infectious diseases are evolutionary accidents waiting to happen. Journal of Biogeography 32:1291-1299.

Brownstein, J. S., D. K. Skelly, T. R. Holford, and D. Fish. 2005. Forest fragmentation predicts local scale heterogeneity of Lyme disease risk. Oecologia. 146(3):469-475.

Burgdorfer, W., S. F. Hayes, and A. J. Mavros. 1981. Non-pathogenic rickettsiae in Dermacentor andersoni: a limiting factor for the distribution of Rickettsia rickettsii. In Rickettsiae and Rickettsial Diseases, edited by W. Burdorfer and R. L. Anacker. Academic Press, New York, NY. Pp. 585-594, 650.

Burgdorfer, W., A. G. Barbour, S. F. Hayes, J. L. Benach, E. Grunwaldt, and J. P. Davis. 1982. Lyme disease-a tick-borne spirochetosis? Science. 216(4552):1317-1319.

Burkhardt, N. Y., G. D. Baldridge, P. C. Williamson, T. J. Kurtti, and U. G. Munderloh, 2010. Development of a shuttle vector for transformation of diverse Rickettsia species. Abstract of poster presented at the 24th meeting of the American Society for Rickettsiology. Stevenson, WA, July 31 to August 3rd.

Burks, C. S., R. L. Stewart Jr., G. R. Needham, and R. E. Lee Jr.. 1996. Cold hardiness in the ixodid ticks (Ixodidae). In Acarology IX, Proceedings, edited by R. Mitchell, D.J. Horn, G.R. Needham, and W.C. Wellbourn. Ohio Biological Survey, Columbus, Ohio. Vol. 1, Pp. 85-87.

Burlini, L., K. R. Teixeira, M. P. Szabó, and K. M. Famadas. 2010. Molecular dissimilarities of Rhipicephalus sanguineus (Acari: Ixodidae) in Brazil and its relation with samples throughout the world: is there a geographical pattern? Experimental and Applied Acarology. 50(4):361-374.

Campbell, K., and C. J. Donlan. 2005. Feral goat eradications on islands. Conservation Biology 19:1362-1374.

Canales, M., C. Almazán, V. Naranjo, F. Jongejan, and J. de la Fuente. 2009. Vaccination with recombinant Boophilus annulatus Bm86 ortholog protein, Ba86, protects cattle against B. annulatus and B. microplus infestations. BMC Biotechnology 9:29. http://www.biomedcentral.com/1472-6750/9/29

Cantu-C, A., J. A. Ortega-S, Z. García-Vázquez, J. Mosqueda, S. E. Henke, and J. E. George. 2009. Epizootiology of Babesia bovis and Babesia bigemina in free-ranging white-tailed deer in northeastern Mexico. Journal of Parasitology 95(3):536-542.

Carroll, J. F., and E. T. Schmidtmann. 1996. Dispersal of blacklegged tick (Acari:Ixodidae) nymphs and adults at the woods-pasture interface. Journal of Medical Entomology 33(4):554-558.

Chen, S. M., J. S. Dumler, J. S. Bakken, and D. H. Walker. 1994. Identification of a granulocytotropic Ehrlichia species as the etiologic agent of human disease. Journal of Clinical Microbiology 32(3):589-595.

Clay, K., O. Klyachko, N. Grindle, D. Civitello, D. Oleske, and C. Fuqua. 2008. Microbial communities and interactions in the lone star tick, Amblyomma americanum. Molecular Ecology 17:4371-4381.

Costero, A., and M. A. Grayson. 1996. Experimental transmission of Powassan virus (Flaviviridae) by Ixodes scapularis ticks (Acari:Ixodidae). American Journal of Tropical Medicine and Hygiene 55(5):536-546.

Dale, C., and N. A. Moran. 2006. Molecular interactions between bacterial symbionts and their hosts. Cell 126:453-464.

Dantas-Torres, F. 2010. Biology and ecology of the brown dog tick, Rhipicephalus sanguineus. Parasites and Vectors 3:26. http://www.parasitesandvectors.com/content/3/1/26

Davies, T. J., A. Purvis, amd J. L. Gittleman. 2009. Quaternary climate change and the geographic ranges of mammals. American Naturalist 174(3):297-307.

Demma, L. J., M. S. Traeger, W. L. Nicholson, C. D. Paddock, D. M. Blau, M. E. Eremeeva, G. A. Dasch, M. L. Levin, J. Singleton Jr, S. R. Zaki, J. E. Cheek, D. L. Swerdlow, and J. H. McQuiston. 2005. Rocky Mountain spotted fever from an unexpected tick vector in Arizona. New England Journal of Medicine 353(6):587-594.

Diuk-Wasser, M. A., A. G. Gatewood, M. R. Cortinas, S. Yaremych-Hamer, J. Tsao, U. Kitron, G. Hickling, J. S. Brownstein, E. Walker, J. Piesman, and D. Fish. 2006. Spatiotemporal patterns of host-seeking Ixodes scapularis nymphs (Acari: Ixodidae) in the United States. Journal of Medical Entomology 43(2):166-176.

Dumler, J. S., A. F. Barbet, C. P. Bekker, G. A. Dasch, G. H. Palmer, S. C. Ray, Y. Rikihisa, and F. R. Rurangirwa. 2001. Reorganization of genera in the families Rickettsiaceae and Anaplasmataceae in the order Rickettsiales: unification of some species of Ehrlichia with Anaplasma, Cowdria with Ehrlichia and Ehrlichia with Neorickettsia, descriptions of six new species combinations and designation of Ehrlichia equi and 'HGE agent' as subjective synonyms of Ehrlichia phagocytophila. International Journal of Systematic and Evolutionary Microbiology 51(6):2145-65.

Dunning Hotopp, J. C., M. Lin, R. Madupu, Crabtree, J., Angiuoli, and 35 others. 2006. Comparative genomics of emerging human ehrlichiosis agents. PLoS Genetics 2(2):e21.

Eisen, R. J., L. Eisen, Y. A. Girard, N. Fedorova, J. Mun, B. Slikas, S. Leonhard, U. Kitron, and R. S. Lane. 2010. A spatially-explicit model of acarological risk of exposure to Borrelia burgdorferi-infected Ixodes pacificus nymphs in northwestern California based on woodland type, temperature, and water vapor. Ticks and Tick Borne Diseases 1(1):35-43.

Ellison, D. W., T. R. Clark, D. E. Sturdevant, K. Virtaneva, S. F. Porcella, and T. Hackstadt. 2008. Genomic comparison of virulent Rickettsia rickettsii Sheila Smith and avirulent Rickettsia rickettsii Iowa. Infection and Immunity 76(2):542-550.

Eriks, I. S., G. H. Palmer, T. C. McGuire, D. R. Allred, and A. F. Barbet. 1989. Detection and quantitation of Anaplasma marginale in carrier cattle by using a nucleic acid probe. Journal of Clinical Microbiology 27(2):279-284.

Feder, M. E., and G. E. Hofman. 1999. Heat-shock proteins, molecular chaperones, and the stress response: evolutionary and ecological physiology. Annual Review of Physiology 61:243-282.

Felsheim, R. F., M. J. Herron, C. M. Nelson, N. Y. Burkhardt, A. F. Barbet, T. J. Kurtti, and U. G. Munderloh. 2006. Transformation of Anaplasma phagocytophilum. BMC Biotechnology 6:42. Doi:10.1186/1472-6750/6/42.

Felsheim, R. F., T. J. Kurtti, and U. G. Munderloh. 2009. Genome sequence of the endosymbiont Rickettsia peacockii and comparison with virulent Rickettsia rickettsii: identification of virulence factors. PLoS ONE 4(12): e8361. Doi:10.1371/journal.pone.0008361.

Fenner, F. 2010. Deliberate introduction of the European rabbit, Oryctolagus cuniculus, into Australia. Revue scientifique et technique 29(1):103-111.

Foley, J. A., R. Defries, G. P. Asner, C. Barford, G. Bonan, S. R. Carpenter, F. S. Chapin, M. T. Coe, G. C. Daily, H. K. Gibbs, J. H. Helkowski, T. Holloway, E. A. Howard, C. J. Kucharik, C. Monfreda, J. A. Patz, I. C. Prentice, N. Ramankutty, and P. K. Snyder. 2005. Global consequences of land use. Science 309(5734):570-4.

Foley, J., N. C. Nieto, P. Foley, and M. B. Teglas. 2008. Co-phylogenetic analysis of Anaplasma phagocytophilum and its vectors, Ixodes spp. ticks. Experimental and Applied Acarology 45(3-4):155-170.

Foley, J. E., N. C. Nieto, and P. Foley. 2009. Emergence of tick-borne granulocytic anaplasmosis associated with habitat type and forest change in northern California. American Journal of Tropical Medicine and Hygiene 81(6):1132-1140.

Fraser, C. M., S. Casjens, W. M. Huang, G. G. Sutton, R. Clayton, and 33 others. 1997. Genomic sequence of a Lyme disease spirochaete, Borrelia burgdorferi. Nature 390:580-586.

George, J. E. 2008. The effects of global change on the threat of exotic arthropods and arthropod-borne pathogens to livestock in the United States. Annals of the New York Academy of Sciences 1149:249-54.

Gillespie, J. J., K. A. Brayton, K. P. Williams, M. A. Quevedo Diaz, W. C. Brown, A. F. Azad, and B. W. Sobral. 2010. Phylogenomics reveals a diverse Rickettsiales type IV secretion system. Infection and Immunity 78(5):1809-1823.

Girard, Y. A., B. Travinsky, A. Schotthoefer, N. Fedorova, R. J. Eisen, L. Eisen L, A. G. Barbour AG, and R. S. Lane. 2009. Population structure of the Lyme disease spirochete Borrelia burgdorferi in the western black-legged tick (Ixodes pacificus) in Northern California. Applied and Environmental Microbiology 75(22): 7243-7252.

Githeko, A. K., Lindsay, S. W., Confalonieri, U.E., and J.A. Patz. 2000. Climate change and vector-borne diseases: a regional analysis. Bulletin of the World Health Organization 78(9):1136-1147

Gray, J. S., H. Dautel, A. Estrada-Peña, O. Kahl, and E. Lindgren. 2009. Effects of climate change on ticks and tick-borne diseases in Europe. Interdisciplinary Perspectives on Infectious Diseases. 2009:593232.

Greer, A., V. Ng, and D. Fisman. 2008. Climate change and infectious diseases in North America: the road ahead. Canadian Medial Association Journal 178(6):715-22.

Greger, M. 2007. The human/animal interface: emergence and resurgence of zoonotic infectious diseases. Critical Reviews in Microbiology 33(4):243-99.

Grindle, N., J. J. Tyner, K. Clay, and C. Fuqua. 2003. Identification of Arsenophonus-type bacteria from the dog tick Dermacentor variabilis. Journal of Invertebrate Pathology 83:264-266.

Harrus, S., and G. Baneth. 2005. Drivers for the emergence and re-emergence of vector-borne protozoal and bacterial diseases. International Journal of Parasitology 35(11-12): 1309-1318.

Herrero, M. V., E. Perez, W. L. Goff, S. Torioni de Echaide, D. P. Knowles, T. F. McElwain, V. Alvarez, A. Alvarez, and G. M. Buening. 1998. Prospective study for the detection of Anaplasma marginale Theiler, 1911 (Rickettsiales: Anaplasmataceae) in Costa Rica. Annals of the New York Academy of Sciences 849:226-233.

Hoberg, E. P., L. Polley, E. J. Jenkins, and S. J. Kutz. 2008. Pathogens of domestic and free-ranging ungulates: global climate change in temperate to boreal latitudes across North America. Revue scientifique et technique 27(2):511-28.

Hoen, A. G., G. Margos, S. J. Bent, M. A. Diuk-Wasser, A. Barbour, K. Kurtenbach, and D. Fish. 2009. Phylogeography of Borrelia burgdorferi in the eastern United States reflects multiple independent Lyme disease emergence events Proceedings of the National Academy of Sciences of the USA 106(35): 15013-8.

Hoogstraal, H. 1956. African ixodoidea. In. Ticks of the Sudan. (With special reference to Equatoria Province and with preliminary reviews of the genera Boophilus, Margaropus and Hyalomma). Research report NM 005 050. 29.07. Department of the Navy, Bureau of Medicine and Surgery, Washington. Vol. 1.

Hoogstraal, H. 1981. Changing patterns of tickborne diseases in modern society. Annual Review of Entomology 26:75-99.

Jasinskas, A., J. Zhong, and A. G. Barbour. 2007. Highly prevalent Coxiella sp. Bacterium in the tick vector Amblyomma americanum. Applied and Environmental Microbiology 73(1):334-336.

Jones, K. E., N. G. Patel, M. A. Levy, A. Storeygard, D. Balk, J. L. Gittleman, and P. Daszak. 2008. Global trends in emerging infectious diseases. Nature 451:990-994.

Kalluri, S., P. Gilruth, D. Rogers, and M. Szczur. 2007. Surveillance of arthropod vector-borne infectious diseases using remote sensing techniques: a review. PLoS Pathogens 3(10):1361-71.

Keesing, F., R. D. Holt, and R. S. Ostfeld. 2006. Effects of species diversity on disease risk. Ecology Letters 9(4):485-498.

Killilea, M. E., A. Swei, R. S. Lane, C. J. Briggs, and R. S. Ostfeld. 2008. Spatial dynamics of Lyme disease: a review. EcoHealth 5(2):167-95.

Klich, M., M. W. Lankester, and K. W. Wu. 1996. Spring migratory birds (Aves) extend the northern occurrence of blacklegged tick (Acari: Ixodidae). Journal of Medical Entomology 33:581-5.

Kurtenbach, K., K. Hanincová, J. I. Tsao, G. Margos, D. Fish D, and N. H. Ogden. 2006. Fundamental processes in the evolutionary ecology of Lyme borreliosis. Nature Reviews Microbiology 4(9):660-669.

Kurtti, T. J., U. G. Munderloh, T. G. Andreadis, L. A. Magnarelli, and T. N. Mather. 1996. Tick cell culture isolation of an intracellular prokaryote from the tick Ixodes scapularis. Journal of Invertebrate Pathology 67(3):318-321.

Kurtti, T. J., A. T. Palmer, and J. H. Oliver, Jr. 2002. Rickettsiella-like bacteria in Ixodes woodi (Acari: Ixodidae). Journal of Medical Entomology 39(3):534-540.

Labruna, M. B. 2009. Ecology of Rickettsia in South America. Annals of the New York Academy of Sciences 1166:156-166.

Labuda, M., V. Danielova, L. D. Jones, and P. A. Nuttall. 1993. Amplification of tick-borne encephalitis virus infection during co-feeding of ticks. Medical and Veterinary Entomology 7(4):339-342.

LaSala, P. R., and M. Holbrook. 2010. Tick-borne flaviviruses. Clinics in Laboratory Medicine 30(1):221-235.

Levin, M. L., W. L. Nicholson, R. F. Massung, J. W. Sumner, and D. Fish. 2002. Comparison of the reservoir competence of medium-sized mammals and Peromyscus leucopus for Anaplasma phagocytophilum in Connecticut. Vector-Borne and Zoonotic Diseases 2(3):125-136.

Linard, C., P. Lamarque, P. Heyman, G. Ducoffre, V. Luyasu, K. Tersago, S. O. Vanwambeke, and E. F. Lambin. 2007. Determinants of the geographic distribution of Puumala virus and Lyme borreliosis infections in Belgium. International Journal of Health Geographics 26:15.

Liu, Z.-M., A. M. Ticker, L. O. Driskell, and D. O. Wood. 2007. mariner-based transposon mutagenesis of Rickettsia prowazekii. Applied and Environmental Microbiology 73(20):6644-6649.

LoGiudice, K., S. T. Duerr, M. J. Newhouse, K. A. Schmidt, M. E. Killilea, and R. S. Ostfeld. 2008. Impact of host community composition on Lyme disease risk. Ecology 89(10):2841-9.

Macaluso, K. R., D. E. Sonenshine, S. M. Ceraul, and A. Azad. 2002. Rickettsial infection in Dermacentor variabilis (Acari: Ixodidae) inhbits transovarial transmission of a second Rickettsia. Journal of Medical Entomology 39(6):809-813.

Madder, M., E. Thys, L. Achi, A. Touré, and R. De Deken. 2010. Rhipicephalus (Boophilus) microplus: a most successful invasive tick species in West-Africa. Experimental and Applied Acarology Aug 15, 2010 [Epub ahead of print] http/www.springerlink.com/content/w812r4t206207135/fulltext.pdf.

Madhav, N. K., J. S. Brownstein, J. I. Tsao, and D. Fish. 2004. A dispersal model for the range expansion of blacklegged tick (Acari: Ixodidae). Journal of Medical Entomology 41(5):842-852.

Madigan, J. E., and D. Gribble. 1987. Equine ehrlichiosis in northern California: 49 cases (1968-1981). Journal of the American Veterinary Medical Association 190(4):445-448.

Massung, R. F., M. J. Mauel, J. H. Owens, N. Allan, J. W. Courtney, K. C. Stafford III, and T. N. Mather. 2002. Genetic variants of Ehrlichia phagocytophila, Rhode Island and Connecticut. Emerging Infectious Diseases 8:467-472.

Massung, R. F., J. W. Courtney, S. L. Hiratzka, V. E. Pitzer, G. Smith, and R. L. Dryden. 2005. Anaplasma phagocytophilum in white-tailed deer. Emerging Infectious Diseases 11(10):1604-1606.

Massung, R. F., M. L. Levin, U. G. Munderloh, D. J. Silverman, M. J. Lynch, J. K. Gaywee, and T. J. Kurtti. 2007. Isolation and propagation of the Ap-variant 1 strain of Anaplasma phagocytophilum in a tick cell line. Journal of Clinical Microbiology 45(7):2138-2143.

Materna, J., M. Daniel, and V. Danielová. 2005. Altitudinal distribution limit of the tick Ixodes ricinus shifted considerably towards higher altitudes in central Europe: results of three years monitoring in the Krkonose Mts. (Czech Republic). Central European Journal of Public Health 13(1):24-8.

McCoy, K. D., T. Boulinier, C. Tirard, and Y. Michalakis. 2003. Host-dependent genetic structure of parasite populations: differential dispersal of seabird tick host races. Evolution 57(2):288-96.

Mediannikov, O., S. Sekeyova, M.-L. Birg, and D. Raoult. 2010. A novel obligate intracellular gamma-proteobacterium associated with ixodid ticks, Diplorickettsia massiliensis, Gen. Nov., Sp. Nov. PLoS ONE 5(7): e11478. doi:10.1371/journal.pone.0011478.

Michalski, M. C., C. Rosenfeld, M. Erickson, R. Selle, K. Bates, D. Essar, and R. Massung. 2006. Anaplasma phagocytophilum in central and western Wisconsin: a molecular survey. Parasitology Research 99:694-699.

Moreno, C. X., F. Moy, T. J. Daniels, H. P. Godfrey, and F. C. Cabello. 2006. Molecular analysis of microbial communities identified in different developmental stages of Ixodes scapularis ticks from Westchester and Dutchess counties, New York. Environmental Microbiology 8(5):761-772.

Mumcuoglu, K. Y., K. Frish, B. Sarov, E. Manor, E. Gross, Z. Gat Z, and R. Galun. 1993. Ecological studies on the brown dog tick Rhipicephalus sanguineus (Acari: Ixodidae) in southern Israel and its relationship to spotted fever group rickettsiae. Journal of Medical Entomology 30(1):114-121.

Munderloh, U. G., S. D. Jauron, and T. J. Kurtti. 2005. The tick: a different kind of host for human pathogens. . In Tick-Borne Diseases of Humans, edited by J. L. Goodman, D. T. Dennis and D. E. Sonenshine. ASM Press, Washington, D.C. Pp 37-64.

Nakamura, Y., S. Kawai, F. Yukuhiro, S. Ito, T. Gotoh, R. Kisimoto, T. Yanase, Y. Matsumoto, D. Kageyama, and H. Noda. 2009. Prevalence of Cardinium bacteria in planthoppers and spider mites and taxonomic revision of "Candidatus Cardinium hertigii" based on detection of a new Cardinium group from biting midges. Applied and Environmental Microbiology 75(21):6757-6763.

Neelakanta, G., H. Sultana, D. Fish, J. F. Anderson, and E. Fikrig. 2010. Anaplasma phagocytophilum induces Ixodes scapularis ticks to express an antifreeze glycoprotein gene that enhances their survival in the cold. Journal of Clinical Investigation 120(9):3179-3190.

Nelson, C. M., M. J. Herron, R. F. Felsheim, B. R. Schloeder, S. M. Grindle, A. O. Chavez, T. J. Kurtti, and U. G. Munderloh. 2008. Whole genome transcription profiling of Anaplasma phagocytophilum in human and tick host cells by tiling array analysis. BMC Genomics 2008, 9:364 doi:10.1186/1471-2164-9-364.

Niebylski, M. L., M. G. Peacock, E. R. Fischer, S. F. Porcella, and T. G. Schwan. 1997a. Characterization of an endosymbiont infecting wood ticks, Dermacentor andersoni, as a member of the genus Francisella. Applied and Environmental Microbiology 63(10):3933-3940.

Niebylski, M. L., M. E. Schrumpf, W. Burgdorfer, E. R. Fischer, E. R. Gage, and T. G. Schwan. 1997b. Rickettsia peacockii sp. nov., a new species infecfting wood ticks, Dermacentor andersoni, in western Montana. International Journal Systematic Bacteriology 47:446-452.

Niebylski, M. L., M. G. Peacock, and T. G. Schwan. 1999. Lethal effect of Rickettsia rickettsii on its tick vector (Dermacentor andersoniI). Applied and Environmental Microbiology 65(2):773-778.

Noda, H., U. G. Munderloh, and T. J. Kurtti. 1997. Endosymbionts of ticks and their relationship to Wolbachia spp. and tick-borne pathogens of humans and animals. Applied and Environmental Microbiology 63(10):3926-3932.

Novakova, E., V. Hypsa, and N. A. Moran. 2009. Arsenophonus, an emerging clade of intracellular symbionts with a broad host distribution. BMC Microbiology 2009, 9:143doi:10.1186/1471-2180-9-143.

Ogata, H., P. Renesto, S. Audic, C. Robert, G. Blanc, P.E. Fournier, H Parinello, J.-M. Claverie, and D. Raoult. 2005. The genome sequence of Rickettsia felis identifies the first putative conjugative plasmid in an obligate intracellular parasite. PLoS Biology 3(8):e248.

Ogata, H., B. La Scola, S. Audic, P. Renesto, G. Blanc, C. Robert, , P.-E. Fournier, J.-M. Claverie, and D. Raoult. 2006. Genome sequence of Rickettsia bellii illuminates the role of amoebae in gene exchanges between intracellular pathogens. PLoS Genetics 2(5): e76. DOI: 10:1371/journal.pgen.0020076.

Ogden, N. H., A. Maarouf, I. K. Barker, M. Bigras-Poulin, L. R. Lindsay, M. G. Morshed, C. J. O'Callaghan, F. Ramay, D. Waltner-Toews, and D. F. Charron. 2005. Climate change and the potential for range expansion of the Lyme disease vector Ixodes scapularis in Canada. International Journal for Parasitology 36:63-70.

Ogden, N. H., L. R. Lindsay, K. Hanincová, I. K. Barker, M. Bigras-Poulin, D. F. Charron, A. Heagy, C. M. Francis, C. J. O'Callaghan, I. Schwartz, and R. A. Thompson. 2008. Role of migratory birds in introduction and range expansion of Ixodes scapularis ticks and of Borrelia burgdorferi and Anaplasma phagocytophilum in Canada. Applied and Environmental Microbiology 74(6):1780-1790.

Paddock, C. D. 2009. The science and fiction of emerging rickettsioses. Annals of the New York Acadmies of Science 1166:133-143.

Parola, P., C. D. Paddock, and D. Raoult. 2005. Tick-borne rickettsioses around the world: emerging diseases challenging old concepts. Clinical Microbiology Reviews 18:710-756.

Pesko, K., F. Torres-Perez, B. Hjelle, and G. D. Ebel. 2010. Molecular epidemiology of Powassan virus in North America. Journal of General Virology Jul 14. [Epub ahead of print] http://vir.sgmjournals.org/cgi/rapidpdf/vir.0.024232-0v1.pdf

Péter, O., W. Burgdorfer, A. Aeschlimann, and P. Chatelanat. 1984. Rickettsia conorii isolated from Rhipicephalus sanguineus introduced into Switzerland on a pet dog. Zeitschrift für Parasitenkunde 70(2):265-70.

Piesman, J., and A. Spielman. 1980. Human babesiosis on Nantucket Island: prevalence of Babesia microti in ticks. American Journal of Tropical Medicine and Hygiene 29(5):742-6.

Pritt, B. S., L. M. Sloan, S. A. Cunningham, J. J. Franson, R. Patel, M. P. Wilhelm, D. F. Neitzel, U. G. Munderloh, C. M. Nelson, D. K. Hoang Johnson, J. McQuiston, K. M. McElroy, J. D. McFadden, C. R. Steward, K. Bogumill, M. E. Bjorgaard, J. P. Davis, D. M. Warshauer, and M. E. Eremeeva. 2009. Emergence of novel human ehrlichiosis in the Mid West United States, 2009. Late-breaker abstract; poster presented at the ASTMH Annual Meeting, Washington D.C., Nov. 18-22, 2009.

Qin, A., A. M. Tucker, A. Hines, and D. O. Wood. 2004. Transposon mutagenesis of the obligate intracellular pathogen Rickettsia prowazekii. Applied and Environmental Microbiology 70(5):2816-2822.

Rachek, L. I., A. M. Tucker, H. H. Winkler, and D. O. Wood. 1998. Transformation of Rickettsia prowazekii to rifampin resistance. Journal of Bacteriology 180(8):2118-2124.

Raizman, E. A., J. D. Holland, L. M. Keefe, and M. H. Moro. 2010. Forest and surface water as predictors of Borrelia burgdorferi and its vector Ixodes scapularis (Acari: Ixodidae) in Indiana. Journal of Medical Entomology 47(3):458-65.

Reed, K. D. 2003. Birds, Migration and Emerging Zoonoses: West Nile Virus, Lyme Disease, Influenza A and Enteropathogens. Clinical Medicine & Research 1:5-12.

Renesto, P., C. Rovery, J. Schrenzel, Q. Leroy, A. Huyghe, W. Li, H. Lepidi, P. Francois, and D. Raoult. 2008. Rickettsia conorii transcriptional response within inoculation eschar. PLoS ONE 3(11): e3681. doi:10.1371/journal.pone.0003681.

Rozental, T., M. E. Eremeeva, C. D. Paddock, S. R. Zaki, G. A. Dasch, and E. R. Lemos. 2006. Fatal case of Brazilian spotted fever confirmed by immunohistochemical staining and sequencing methods on fixed tissues. Annals of the New York Academy of Sciences 1078:257-259.

Schoelkopf, L., C. E. Hutchinson, K. G. Bendele, W. L. Goff, M. Willette, J. M. Rasmussen, and P. J. Holman. 2005. New ruminant hosts and wider geographic range identified for Babesia odocoilei (Emerson and Wright 1970). Journal of Wildlife Diseases 41(4):683-90.

Scoles, G. A. 2004. Phylogenetic analysis of the Francisella-like endosymbionts of Dermacentor ticks Journal of Medical Entomology 41(3):277-286.

Simser, J. A., A. T. Palmer, U. G. Munderloh, and T. J. Kurtti. 2001. Isolation of a spotted fever group rickettsia, Rickettsia peacockii, in a Rocky Mountain wood tick, Dermacentor andersoni, cell line. Applied and Environmental Microbiology 67(2)546-552.

Simser, J. A., M. S. Rahman, S. M. Dreher-Lesnick, and A. Azad. 2005. A novel and naturally occurring transposon, ISRpe1 in Rickettsia peacockii genome disrupting the rickA gene involved in actin-based motility. Molecular Microbiology 58(1):71-79.

Stafford, K. C. III. 2007. Tick Control Handbook. Bulletin 1010; The Connecticut Agricultural Experiment Station. http://www.cdc.gov/ncidod/dvbid/lyme/resources/handbook. pdf

Steiner, F. E., R. R. Pinger, C. N. Vann, N. Grindle, D. Civitello, K. Clay, and C. Fuqua. 2008. Infection and co-infection rates of Anaplasma phagocytophilum variants, Babesia spp., Borrelia burgdorferi, and the rickettsial endosymbiont in Ixodes scapularis (Acari: Ixodidae) from sites in Indiana, Maine, Pennsylvania, and Wisconsin. 2008. Journal of Medical Entomology 45(2):289-297.

Stuen, S. 2007. Anaplasma phagocytophilum - the most widespread tick-borne infection in animals in Europe. Veterinary Research Communications. 31:79-84, Supplement 1.

Telford, S. R. 3rd, J. E. Dawson, P. Katavolos, C. K. Warner, C. P. Kolbert, and D. H. Persing. 1996. Perpetuation of the agent of human granulocytic ehrlichiosis in a deer tick-rodent cycle. Proceedings of the National Academy of Sciences of the USA. 93(12):6209-6214.

Uspensky, I., and I. Ioffe-Uspensky. 2002. The dog factor in brown dog tick Rhipicephalus sanguineus (Acari: Ixodidae) infestations in and near human dwellings. International Journal of Medical Microbiology 291:156-63, Suppl 33.

Van Zee, J. P., N. S. Geraci, F. D. Guerrero, S. K. Wikel, J. J. Stuart, V. M. Nene, and C. A. Hill. 2007. Tick genomics: the Ixodes genome project and beyond. International Journal for Parasitology 37:1297-1305.

Vora, N. 2008. Impact of anthropogenic environmental alterations on vector-borne diseases. Medscape Journal of Medicine 10(10):238.

Waldrup, K. A., A. A. Kocan, R. W. Barker, and G. G. Wagner. 1990. Transmission of Babesia odocoilei in white-tailed deer (Odocoileus virginianus) by Ixodes scapularis (Acari: Ixodidae). Journal of Wildlife Diseases 26(3):390-391

Ward, S. E., and R. D. Brown. 2004. A framework for incorporating the prevention of Lyme disease transmission into the landscape planning and design process. Landscape and Urban Planning 66:91-106.

Wikswo, M. E., R. Hu, M. E. Metzger, and M. E. Eremeeva. 2007. Detection of Rickettsia rickettsii and Bartonella henselae in Rhipicephalus sanguineus ticks from California. Journal of Medical Entomology 44(1):158-62.

Woldehiwet, Z. 2006. Anaplasma phagocytophilum in ruminants in Europe. Annals of the New York Academy of Sciences 1078:446-60.

A7

# LYME BORRELIOSIS AND OTHER IXODID TICK-BORNE DISEASES—A EUROPEAN PERSPECTIVE

*Susan O'Connell, M.D.*
*Consultant Medical Microbiologist*
*Head, Lyme Borreliosis Unit*
*Health Protection Agency*
*Southampton, UK*

## Ixodid Ticks in Europe, Their Geographic Distribution and Ecological Requirements

Ticks of the *Ixodes ricinus* complex are vectors of *Borrelia burgdorferi* and several other bacterial and viral infectious agents. In Europe the main tick vector for these organisms is *Ixodes ricinus*, commonly called the sheep tick or castor bean tick, and in Asia it is *Ixodes persulcatus*, the taiga tick. There is an area of overlap in the range of these species in parts of eastern Europe including the Baltic republics and western regions of Russia (See Figure A7-1). *Ixodes ricinus* is widely distributed, from countries on the western seaboard eastwards to Russia and it overlaps with *I persulcatus* in western Russia, the Baltic republics and eastern Europe.

*Ixodes ricinus* ticks have three active stages in their life-cycle, usually over two to three years, and at each stage they take a single blood meal lasting from about three to seven days (See Figure A7-2; European Union Concerted Action on Lyme Borreliosis [EUCALB], 2010). There is a high mortality throughout the process, with few ticks surviving to complete the life-cycle from an initial egg batch of about 2,000. The essential habitat requirements for tick survival are high humidity to maintain water balance and presence of suitable animal species as feeding hosts. Ticks survive only in areas where there is good vegetation cover, with a mat of decaying vegetation (leaf litter etc) that will maintain a relative humidity of 80-85% during the driest periods, providing protection against desiccation during the long interstadial development periods. Immature ticks can feed on a wide variety of mammalian and ground-feeding avian hosts which may be reservoir-competent for *Borrelia burgdorferi* and other potential human pathogens. Adult female ticks usually feed successfully only on large mammals such as deer, sheep, cattle and horses, underlining the importance of those hosts to the reproductive stage of the tick life-cycle.

These essential requirements are optimally provided in mixed deciduous woodland. They can also occur in coniferous forests provided that there is enough vegetation litter and a moist microclimate. Some heathland,

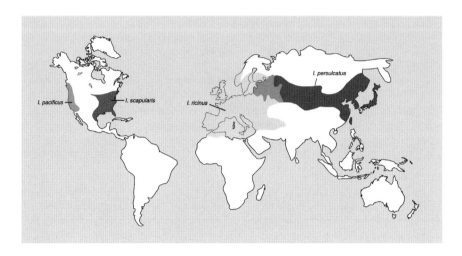

**FIGURE A7-1** Distribution of *Ixodes ricinus* complex ticks *Courtesy of Professor J Gray and Mr B Kaye and taken with permission from the European Union Concerted Action on Lyme Borreliosis (EUCALB) website.*

moorland and pastureland habitats of regions with mild, damp climates, such as the British Isles, also provide suitable conditions. In these environments large animals are likely to be feeding hosts for all three stages of the tick life-cycle (Gray, 1991, 1998). Many areas in southern Europe are too hot and dry for survival of *Ixodes ricinus*. Areas experiencing repeated droughts or episodes of severe flooding are also less favourable for tick survival.

There is evidence for changing distribution of ixodid tick populations in some parts of Europe, which may be related to changing climate. This is demonstrated most significantly at the geographic distribution limits of *Ixodes ricinus*. Few ticks are found in altitudes greater than about 1100 metres, but this altitude limit has risen significantly over 30 years from an earlier maximal altitude of 700 metres, as shown by well-documented studies in the Czech Republic and Switzerland (Lindgren and Jaenson, 2006). An extension in the northerly distribution of ixodid ticks into higher latitudes has occurred in Scandinavia in the past 20 years, associated with less severe winter temperatures and a greater number of days with temperature >10°C.

More generally in Europe, changing climate has led to milder and shorter winters in many regions with earlier onset of spring (on average two weeks earlier than seen before the 1980s) and longer autumns, leading to earlier start of tick feeding activity and potentially greater tick survival. Conversely, conditions will become less favourable for ixodid ticks if areas

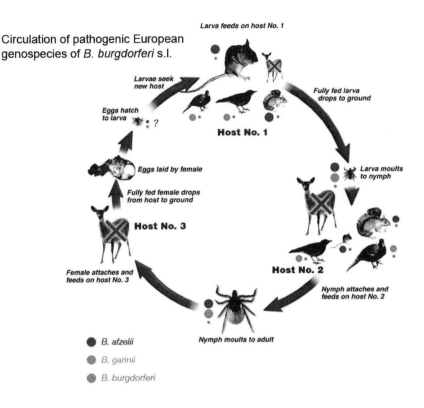

Circulation of pathogenic European genospecies of *B. burgdorferi* s.l.

Larva feeds on host No. 1

Larvae seek new host

Eggs hatch to larva

Fully fed larva drops to ground

**Host No. 1**

Eggs laid by female

Fully fed female drops from host to ground

Larva moults to nymph

**Host No. 3**

Female attaches and feeds on host No. 3

**Host No. 2**

Nymph attaches and feeds on host No. 2

*B. afzelii*

*B. garinii*

*B. burgdorferi*

Nymph moults to adult

**FIGURE A7-2** Ixodes ricinus lifecycle *Courtesy of Professor J Gray and Mr B Kaye and taken with permission from the EUCALB website.* http://meduni09 .edis.at/eucalb/cms/index.php?option=com_content&task=view&id=53&Ite mid=84. The relative size of the animals approximates their significance as hosts for the different tick life-cycle stages in a typical woodland habitat.

of hotter, more arid conditions expand in southern Europe. Tick survival and activity is also affected by more localized and short-term weather conditions. Other ecological aspects include changes in biodiversity. The possible effects of these and other factors on *Ixodes ricinus* and Lyme borreliosis in Europe were addressed in a World Health Organisation (WHO) publication in 2006, and this continues to be an important area of research (Lindgren and Jaenson, 2006). The summary of findings and recommendations of a 2007 workshop on environmental change and infectious diseases disease burden in Europe, organised by the European Centre for Disease Control (ECDC) is another valuable data source, as is a review published in 2009 (ECDC, 2007; Gray et al., 2009).

Other factors contributing to increased tick populations include changes in land use, particularly agriculture and forestry practice, with reforestation projects and pine monoculture being replaced by mixed forestry in many parts of Europe (see Figure A7-3 and A7-3a). Increased deer population densities are reported from many areas, which can also promote

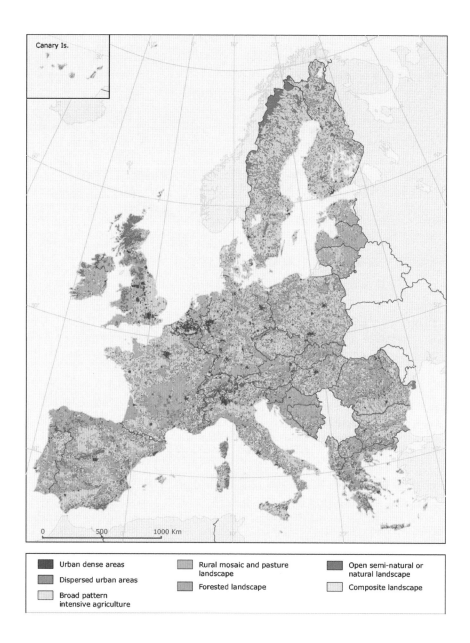

tick reproductive success, as deer are the most important feeding hosts for ticks' reproductive life-cycle stage. Wider geographic range of deer caused by deer population pressure has also resulted in expansion of tick populations into new areas in many parts of Europe. A report from the WHO Regional Office for Europe published in 2004 provided a comprehensive survey of vector-borne diseases, including tick-transmitted infections, and ecological, environmental and human behavioural factors influencing their incidence (WHO, 2004).

Human factors must be considered when assessing risks of tick-transmitted infections. These include residential, occupational and recreational factors. People living and working in tick habitats are at obvious risk

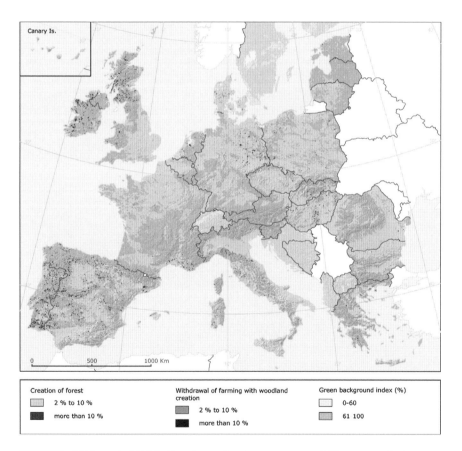

FIGURE A7-3 and A7-3A Dominant landscape types of Europe and changes. (European Environment Agency). http://www.eea.europa.eu/data-and-maps/figures/dominant-landscape-types-of-europe-based-on-corine-land-cover-2000-1.

of acquiring tick-transmitted infections. Housing developments in previously semi-rural and rural environments can expose new populations to these risks, as has been seen in many parts of Europe. Occupational risks include forestry and game management, and there have been significant changes in these industries in the past fifty years. Recreational aspects are important, with the high and increasing popularity of outdoor activities in tick-permissive environments, which can expose participants with little previous awareness of ticks to risk of tick-transmitted infections. Epidemiological studies from various European countries suggest that recreational activities, including those undertaken on vacation in other countries, are major factors for acquisition of Lyme borreliosis. This can have important economic implications for tourism in endemic areas.

Human beings can be incidental hosts for all three stages of the *Ixodes ricinus* life-cycle, although in practice the nymphal stage feed is the most likely to result in transmission of *Borrelia burgdorferi*, which is the most common tick-transmitted infection, as the organism rarely infects larval ticks transovarially. Few ticks survive to adulthood and in general only female adults take significant feeds. Because of their larger size adults are more likely to be noticed and removed earlier in the feeding period than earlier-stage ticks. The immature stages of *Ixodes persulcatus* appear not to feed readily on human beings and most transmission of infectious agents from this *Ixodes* species results from adult feeds (Korenberg et al., 2001). Human behavioural factors related to tick-transmitted diseases are addressed in more detail in a later section.

Ixodid feeding activity is affected by several factors, including diapause (dormancy) mechanisms, day-length, temperature and availability of hosts (see Figures A7-4, A7-5, and A7-6; EUCALB, 2010). These latter features produce some variations throughout Europe. In general *Ixodes ricinus* ticks feed between March and October, peaking in May to July, with a smaller secondary peak in the early autumn, but in countries with mild winters there can be a low level of feeding activity and potential risk of infection on warmer winter days. *Ixodes persulcatus* appears to have a similar level of activity in spring and early summer but is rarely active in autumn. Tick feeding seasonality affects the epidemiology of tick-transmitted infections, with peak incidence of tick-borne encephalitis in the late spring and early summer months. Lyme borreliosis presentations peak slightly later, reflecting the longer incubation period.

### Ixodid Ticks and Micro-Organism Carriage

A variety of micro-organisms have been identified in *Ixodes ricinus* and *I persulcatus* ticks but organism carriage or DNA positivity must be distinguished from vector-competence. To establish vector-competence a

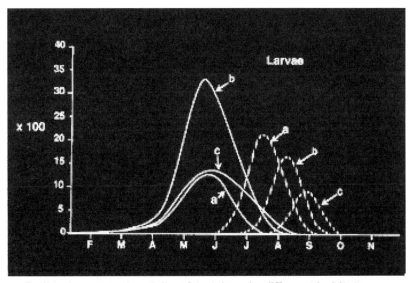

Stylised seasonal activity of *I. ricinus* in different habitats

solid line = spring population
broken line = autumn population

a = exposed meadow;
b = dense hill vegetation or scondary deciduous woodland;
c = highly sheltered woodland;
d = spring-derived but autumn-feeding.

**FIGURE A7-4** Stylized seasonal activity of *I. ricinus* in different habitats: Larvae. *Courtesy of Professor Jeremy Gray and Mr Bernard Kaye and taken, with permission, from the EUCALB website.* http://meduni09.edis.at/eucalb/cms/index.php?option=com_content&task=view&id=54&Itemid=89.

tick must be capable of maintaining organisms obtained at an earlier feed or transovarially and able to transmit them during a subsequent feed.

*Ixodes ricinus* and *I persulcatus* are known to be vector-competent for the flavivirus agents of tick-borne encephalitis virus and louping-ill. The latter is a well-recognised pathogen of sheep, cattle, goats and grouse, and also causes rare cases of human disease in the UK and Ireland. Several other viruses have been identified in *Ixodes ricinus*, including Tribec, Tettnang and Eyach viruses, but the public health importance of these agents seems to be very limited (WHO, 2004).

Tick-borne encephalitis is focally endemic in many parts of western, central and eastern Europe and in southern Scandinavia. It is mandatorily

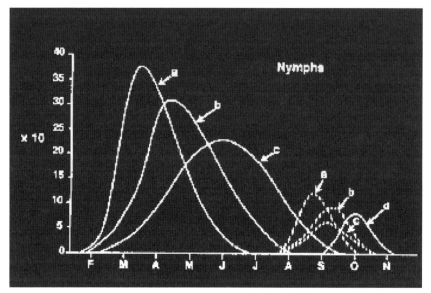

Stylised seasonal activity of *I. ricinus* in different habitats

solid line = spring population
broken line = autumn population

a = exposed meadow;
b = dense hill vegetation or scondary deciduous woodland;
c = highly sheltered woodland;
d = spring-derived but autumn-feeding.

**FIGURE A7-5** Stylized seasonal activity of *I. ricinus* in different habitats: Nymphs. *Courtesy of Professor Jeremy Gray and Mr Bernard Kaye and taken, with permission, from the EUCALB website.* http://meduni09.edis.at/eucalb/cms/index .php?option=com_content&task=view&id=54&Itemid=89.

notifiable in most states in which it occurs and between 2,000 and 3,000 cases are reported annually from European countries, including the Baltic states. It has an estimated mortality of between 0.5% and 2%, and significant long-term morbidity following meningoencephalitis, especially in older people. There is evidence of increased range and incidence into higher latitudes and altitudes in some regions, which may in part be due to changing climate, but other biological and human behavioural factors also play significant roles. Studies suggest that in the long-term the incidence may decrease in the more southerly regions as climate change alters tick seasonal dynamics, disrupting synchrony of larval and nymph co-feeding on rodent reservoirs. Co-feeding

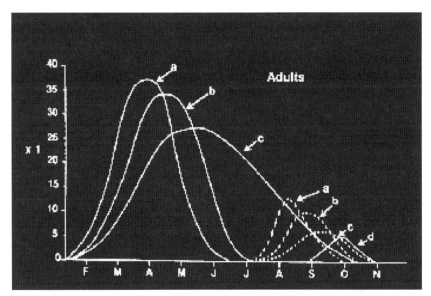

Stylised seasonal activity of *I. ricinus* in different habitats

solid line = spring population
broken line = autumn population

a = exposed meadow;
b = dense hill vegetation or scondary deciduous woodland;
c = highly sheltered woodland;
d = spring-derived but autumn-feeding.

FIGURE A7-6 Stylized seasonal activity of *I. ricinus* in different habitats: Adults. *Courtesy of Professor Jeremy Gray and Mr Bernard Kaye and taken, with permission, from the EUCALB website.* http://meduni09.edis.at/eucalb/cms/index .php?option=com_content&task=view&id=54&Itemid=89.

appears to be an important factor in maintaining enzootic cycles of TBE (ECDC, 2007; Randolph, 2001). An effective TBE vaccine is available.

*Ixodes ricinus* is vector-competent for *Borrelia burgdorferi* sensu lato, the causes of Lyme borreliosis, which is by far the most common tick-transmitted disease in Europe. European Lyme borreliosis will be described in more detail later. It is also a vector for *Borrelia miyamotoi*, a member of the relapsing fever group of borreliae, which was first identified in Japan in 1995 and has been found in tick populations in many parts of Russia and Europe. At present it is unclear if this organism has human pathogenic potential (Karan et al., 2007).

*Anaplasma phagocytophilum* and rickettsioses, including *Rickettsia helvetica* are also tick-transmitted. *Anaplasma phagocytophilum* is widely distributed in Europe and livestock infections are common, causing a significant financial burden (Bown et al., 2009). Fewer than 100 human cases have been reported since the first European case was identified in Slovenia in 1997. Seroprevalence studies have found antibodies in 1.5-21% of forestry workers and other people exposed to ticks in northern and central Europe but significant systemic disease appears to be very uncommon (Parola, Davoust, et al., 2005).

*Rickettsia helvetica* was first isolated from *Ixodes ricinus* ticks in Switzerland in 1979 and subsequently identified in many European countries. Few human cases of clinical disease have been serologically confirmed, mainly presenting with relatively mild, self-limited illnesses with headache and myalgias and less frequently with a rash and/or an eschar. A condition characterised by eschar, usually on the scalp and accompanied by regional lymphadenopathy following bites from *Dermacenter spp* ticks have been documented from France and Hungary, where the condition has been termed tick-borne lymphdenopathy (TIBOLA). It is caused by *R slovaca*, which is widely distributed in *Dermacenter spp* ticks in Europe, and was first isolated in 1968. With molecular methods allowing more sensitive detection and refinement of speciation the range of rickettsial agents associated with *Ixodes spp* and other tick species is likely to increase, as extensively reviewed in 2005 (Parola, Paddock, et al., 2005).

*Ixodes ricinus* can also transmit *Babesia spp*, which are intraerythrocytic protozoa. *Babesia divergens* is the cause of redwater fever in cattle and also causes occasional cases of human disease, which can be overwhelming in asplenic or otherwise immunocompromised patients. About 40 cases have been reported in Europe in the past ten years, and numbers are likely to rise with increased awareness of tick-transmitted infections and rising numbers of potentially susceptible individuals. A few cases of *Babesia venatorum* (previously termed *Babesia*-EU1) infection have been reported in splenectomised patients, causing less severe clinical presentations than those seen with *B divergens*. This organism and several *Babesia divergens*-like strains have been identified in European deer. A human case of European-acquired *Babesia microti* infection was reported in 2007 and the species has been identified in ticks and animal reservoirs in several regions of Europe. Data on babesial infection has recently been reviewed and it is likely that other babesial species and reservoir hosts will be identified (Gray et al., 2010).

*Francisella tularensis*, the agent of tularaemia, and *Coxiella burnetii*, which causes Q fever, can also be transmitted to human beings through tick bites, but other transmission routes are more important for these organisms. The authors of the 2004 WHO report on vector-borne diseases in Europe concluded that a large outbreak of tularaemia in Kosovo that occurred in 1999-2000 was associated with food or water contamination from a rodent source, related to post-war disruption and poor living conditions. Another outbreak in north-central Sweden in 1981 was thought to be related mainly to transmission by mosquitoes. Sporadic cases of tick-transmitted tularaemia are well-documented, particularly in eastern Europe and Scandinavia, highlighting the importance of raising public and healthcare worker awareness of this risk to enable early recognition and treatment. Tick transmission may be significant in maintaining enzootic infection cycles of both tularaemia and Q fever.

There is debate about the vector-competence of ixodid ticks for *Bartonella spp* including *Bartonella henselae*, the agent of catscratch disease. Bartonellae are common mammalian haemoparasites and there is increasing appreciation of the range of clinical presentations found in human infections. *Bartonella* DNA has been identified in many tick species, including *I ricinus*. This is not surprising, given the significant prevalence of *Bartonella* spp infection in rodent tick-feeding hosts, but transmission to human beings from *I ricinus* or *I scapularis* has not been proven. Only one study, published in 1996, showed successful culture of a *Bartonella* species from an *I ricinus* tick, suggesting that the organisms may not easily remain viable in ticks. The issue was recently reviewed in some detail and on currently available evidence it appears that *Ixodes spp* ticks are unlikely to be significant vectors of bartonellosis (Angelakis et al., 2010).

## Borrelia Burgdorferi *Sensu Lato in Europe*

At least fifteen genospecies of *Borrelia burgdorferi* sensu lato have been identified and three cause the bulk of Lyme borreliosis in Europe: *Borrelia afzelii*, *Borrelia garinii* and *Borrelia burgdorferi* sensu stricto (EUCALB website). *Borrelia garinii* OspA serotype 4 has recently been designated *B bavariensis*. Another genospecies, *B spielmanii*, has been isolated occasionally from erythema migrans lesions but seems to cause little systemic ill-effects. *Borrelia valaisiana* appears to be non-pathogenic and is found in many parts of Europe, including the UK and Ireland, where it has been identified as the major infecting borrelia in some tick populations. This may account in part for the lower incidence of Lyme borreliosis in these countries by comparison to other European regions, where most infected ticks carry more pathogenic genospecies. *Borrelia lusitaniae* is rare, with foci mainly on the Iberian peninsula, and there have been only a few reports of associated human disease.

Many mammalian species are reservoir-competent for *Borrelia burgdorferi* sensu lato. The most important are rodents, particularly *Apodemus spp* mice, voles and squirrels. *Borrelia afzelii* is strongly associated with these species, and *B bavariensis* (previously *B garinii* OspA serotype 4) with *Apodemus spp.* Birds, particularly ground-feeding species such as thrushes, blackbirds and pheasants are potential reservoirs of *B valaisiana* and *B garinii*. Some lizard species appear to be reservoir-competent for *B lusitaniae* (EUCALB, 2010). Ungulates (deer, sheep, goats, cattle and pigs) are crucially involved in the eco-epidemiology of Lyme borreliosis as maintenance hosts for ticks, but they are not significant as reservoir hosts.

The mammalian and avian reservoir host differences for *B afzelii* and *B garinii* are thought to be linked to differences in sensitivity of these genospecies to the host serum complement. Borrelial complement regulator-acquiring surface proteins (CRASPs) bind host immune regulators that protect spirochaetes from complement lysis. The CRASP repertoire of *B garinii* protects the spirochaete from avian complement lysis, whereas the CRASPs of *B afzelii* and *B bavariensis* protect these organisms from lysis by rodent sera (Piesman and Schwan, 2010).

Geographic distribution of different European genospecies has some effect on incidence and distribution of various clinical presentations of Lyme borreliosis in different parts of the continent. A useful meta-analysis based on publications between 1986 and 2003 summarised tick infection rates and genospecies identified in studies from 24 European countries (Rauter and Hartung, 2005). All pathogenic genospecies can cause erythema migrans. *B burgdorferi* sensu stricto is arthritogenic and causes disease presentations similar to those found in the USA, but is the least common of the major pathogenic genospecies in Europe. Lyme arthritis is a less frequent European complication than neuroborreliosis, predominantly caused by *B garinii*, the most neurotropic genospecies, which is widespread particularly in western Europe. The most common genospecies in central and eastern European countries and Scandinavia is *B afzelii*, which causes erythema migrans lesions that are less rapidly progressive and have less evidence of inflammatory response than those caused by *B burgdorferi* sensu stricto or *B garinii*. (Strle et al., 1999) They are also less likely to have extracutaneous manifestations, but can cause acrodermatitis chronica atrophicans, an indolent gradually progressive skin condition which may persist for years if left untreated, and occasional cases of neuroborreliosis.

*Epidemiology of Lyme Borreliosis in Europe*

There is no centralised reporting or surveillance system for Lyme borreliosis or tick-borne encephalitis in Europe. A ECDC-funded initiative is underway to collate all currently available data on Lyme borreliosis and will report during 2011. It aims to provide a pan-European assessment of the epidemiological patterns, laboratory diagnostic and reporting criteria and the overall impact of Lyme borreliosis on human populations throughout the EU and EFTA countries. Data is also being sought from the current EU Candidate countries and from a number of European Neighbourhood Policy countries. A similar programme is underway for tick-borne encephalitis.

Epidemiological evidence for Lyme borreliosis is available piecemeal from numerous sources, including national or regional mandatory notification schemes in a few countries, surveillance schemes in some endemic regions, primary care surveys, seroprevalence studies and reporting systems based on laboratory-confirmed cases. About 85,000 cases are reported annually in Europe but this is a considerable underestimate, both because of inconsistent case reporting mechanisms and under-recognition of disease manifestations, particularly erythema migrans (Lindgren and Jaenson, 2006). In 2002 it was estimated that at least 60,000 cases are likely to occur annually in Germany alone, giving an approximate incidence rate of 75/100,000 in that country (Mehnert and Krause, 2005). A more recent study estimated the incidence in Germany as about 32/100,000 in 2009 (Poggensee and Adlhoch, 2010). Reviewing data from various sources it is likely that there are over 200,000 cases annually in Europe, with a bimodal age incidence, peaking in the 5-15 and 45-65 age groups.

Overall national figures have only limited value, especially in the larger, more industrialised countries where most of the population is urban-dwelling, as they do not indicate regional and sub-regional variations in risk, which can be very marked. Regional and local data analysis is important for the appropriate targeting of public health and clinical interventions.

*Mandatory Notification Schemes*

Few countries have mandatory notification schemes for Lyme borreliosis. Erythema migrans and other manifestations of the disease are mandatorily notifiable in Slovenia, with a reported incidence rate in 2005 of 206/100,000 (Smith and Takkinen, 2006) and 312/100,000 in 2009. Notifications are incomplete, especially for erythema migrans, but data related to disseminated and late complications are more accurate because most Slovenian patients with these presentations are managed within a few research-orientated institutions. Neuroborreliosis has been notifiable in Denmark since 1994; with an annual average of 83 cases (1.5/100,000), ranging from 41 in 3002 to 104 in 2006 (Christiansen and Mølbak, 2005) and 61 cases (1.1/100,000) in 2009 (EpiNorthData, 2011). Cases of disseminated and late borreliosis have been notifiable in Norway since 1995. Annual incidence of neuroborreliosis varied from 75 to 200 cases in the ten years 1995-2004 (average 3/100,000), with a marked increase of nearly 100 cases between 2003 and 2004 (Nygard et al., 2005). There were 273 notifications in 2009, a rate of 5.6 /100,000 (EpiNorthData, 2011). As neurological complications are the most significant manifestations of disseminated and late Lyme borreliosis in Europe data on neuroborreliosis obtained from the Slovenian, Danish and Norwegian notification schemes can give useful information on epidemiological trends in widely geographically separated areas of Europe. Pan-European monitoring methods for neuroborreliosis would be a welcome epidemiological initiative.

*Regional Clinical Surveillance and Prospective Studies*

In some countries case surveillance is regionally focussed on areas of known high endemicity, e.g. Alsace and Limousin in France and in six eastern states of Germany (*La maladie de Lyme. Données du réseau de surveillance de la maladie en Alsace*, Institut Veille Sanitaire, 2008; Fülöp and Poggensee, 2008; Mehnert and Krause, 2005). A French national primary care-based prospective study estimated an overall national incidence rate of 9.4/100,000, (Letrilliart et al., 2005), whereas data from the Alsace study suggested a regional rate of 180-232/100,000, which varied from 30 to 511/100,000 between individual cantons in the region. Erythema migrans was the only manifestation of disease in 90% of the cases; a further 5% had evidence of neuroborreliosis. Similar detailed and useful study reports are available for several other regions of France from L'Institut Veille Sanitaire. A prospective study performed in the Wurzburg region of Germany in 1996 followed an extensive awareness campaign and reported an incidence rate of 111/100,000 (313 cases). Erythema migrans was the only manifestation in 89% of cases. (Huppertz et al., 1999) It is notable that in these and other recent prospective studies erythema migrans was the presenting feature in around 90% of cases. In an earlier primary care-based prospective study performed in endemic counties of southern Sweden in 1992-1993 the overall annual incidence was 69/100,000 (1471 cases) and ranged focally from 26 to 160/100,000 (Berglund et al., 1995). Erythema migrans was the presenting feature in 77% of patients; 16% had neuroborreliosis and 7% had arthritis. Prospective community-based studies can provide longer-term benefits in addition to their epidemiological value, through raising awareness of the condition, its clinical features, management and prevention within primary and secondary care health care providers and the general community.

*Laboratory-Based Surveillance*

Some countries use laboratory-based surveillance, and erythema migrans cases are certainly under-reported in these schemes. Variability in test requesting patterns and diagnostic methods limit the validity of direct comparisons of laboratory-based surveillance findings between countries.

Nevertheless, some useful demographic, geographic and seasonality data can be obtained and year-on-year data compared in stable data collection systems, especially in schemes that approach referring clinicians and patients for additional clinical and tick exposure risk information such as the enhanced surveillance system in England and Wales, where the great majority of specialised laboratory tests for Lyme borreliosis are performed in a single reference facility. Annual incidence of laboratory-confirmed cases rose from 268 (0.5/100,000) in 2001 to 973 (1.79/100,000) in 2009, with a rate of 15/100,000 in one focal area. At least 18% of reported cases in 2009 had been acquired in other countries. Neuroborreliosis accounts for between 10% and 20% of laboratory-confirmed cases each year and appears to be a useful sentinel for year-on-year comparison. It has been estimated that there may be 2,000-3,000 cases of Lyme borreliosis annually in the UK (Health Protection Agency, 2011).

Seroprevalence studies have been performed in many parts of Europe. Population groups studied include healthy blood donors and people whose residence, occupation or recreational interests place them at higher risk of acquiring *Borrelia burgdorferi* infection. The overall picture shows a trend of increasing seroprevalence from west to east in Europe, which is consistent with findings from prospective studies and other surveillance methods. The findings from some of these studies and the prospective studies also suggest significant incidence of asymptomatic infections.

## Clinical Presentations of Lyme Borreliosis in Europe

Clinical case definitions for use in Europe were published in 1996 by the European Union Concerted Action on Lyme Borreliosis (EUCALB, 2010; Stanek et al., 1996). A recent review by the EUCALB group has affirmed the robust nature of the 1996 definitions, as more recently published evidence has necessitated only minor additions to the definitions, which were updated in 2010 (Stanek et al., 2011). The 1996 case definitions have been cited in various diagnosis and treatment guidelines and recommendations from European specialist societies and national groups, which were summarised in a presentation at the 2010 European Conference on Clinical Microbiology and Infectious Diseases (ECCMID) (O'Connell, 2010).

The EUCALB case definitions acknowledge similarities between the major manifestations of Lyme borreliosis and North America, including erythema migrans, early neuroborreliosis and Lyme arthritis. They also recognise the broader spectrum of clinical presentations seen in Europe, eg borrelial lymphocytoma, acrodermatitis chronica atrophicans and late encephalomyelitis, all of which are rarely reported in association with American-acquired infections. The 2011 case definitions also describe rare ocular manifestations, including conjunctivitis, uveitis and papillitis and discuss objective and subjective long-term sequelae of *Borrelia burgdorferi* infection. They describe the requirement for laboratory supporting evidence for the diagnosis of all manifestations other than erythema migrans. A brief resume of the principal features is given here.

### Erythema Migrans in Europe

The variety of pathogenic borrelial genospecies in Europe can cause some variation in presentations of erythema migrans. For example, a rash caused by *B afzelii* usually expands more slowly and is more likely to have central clearing than one caused by *B burgdorferi* sensu stricto, and less likely to be accompanied by significant systemic symptoms (Strle et al., 1999). Erythema migrans caused by *B garinii* is usually more homogeneous than that caused by *B afzelii*, and it is more frequently accompanied by systemic symptoms. Overall the clinical picture of *B garinii* infection suggests greater acute pathogenicity than caused by *B afzelii*.

### Other Skin Manifestations of European Lyme Borreliosis

Borrelial lymphocytoma is an uncommon early manifestation, presenting as a bluish-red nodule or plaque, usually on the earlobe, ear helix, nipple or scrotum, occurring more frequently in children than adults. It has a distinctive histological appearance, with an intense B-lymphocytic infiltrate and has occasionally been misdiagnosed as cutaneous B-cell lymphoma.

Acrodermatitis chronica atrophicans (ACA) is an uncommon later manifestation of active infection, which is usually seen in older adults, predominantly women. It presents with bluish-red discolouration, usually on the extensor surfaces of one or more limbs. There can be doughy swelling and atrophic changes developing later. Local involvement of peripheral nerves can cause an axonal polyneuropathy, usually presenting with predominantly mild sensory symptoms. *B afzelii* causes the great majority of ACA presentations, which occur more frequently in Scandinavia and central Europe than in the west of the continent.

### Neuroborreliosis in Europe

Neuroborreliosis is the most common complication of European Lyme borreliosis and most cases appear to be caused by *B garinii*, which is the most neurotropic of the pathogenic genospecies. The European Federation of Neurological Societies (EFNS) recently published guidelines for diagnosis and treatment, giving detailed descriptions of presentations in adults and children (Mygland et al., 2010). About 95% of European neuroborreliosis cases present acutely, usually within twelve weeks of infection, and early neuroborreliosis is often self-limiting. The most common manifestation in adults is a painful meningoradiculitis (Garin-Bujadoux-Bannwarth syndrome). Pain may be very severe and paresis can affect muscles innervated by the facial (unilateral or bilateral) or other cranial nerves and those of the trunk and limbs. In children the most common presentations of acute neuroborreliosis are facial palsy, which may be an isolated clinical feature, other cranial nerve palsies and lymphocytic meningitis, and headache can be a prominent feature. Painful radiculopathy is very uncommon in children.

Although the differences between presentations of European and American Lyme neuroborreliosis have been stressed over the years, they may have been overemphasised in the case of early neuroborreliosis (Halperin, 2008). This is also supported by clinical experience in the UK, where between 10 and 20% of patients with serologically confirmed Lyme borreliosis acquired infections abroad, in mainland Europe or USA (HPA, 2011). Clinicians in the UK have noted marked similarities in acute neurological presentations of patients with USA-acquired infection and those acquired in the UK and other parts of Europe (Dillon et al., 2010).

Less than 5% of European neuroborreliosis patients present with late neuroborreliosis, with duration of symptoms from six months to several years (Mygland et al., 2010). This condition is likely to have a chronic course if left untreated and can affect the central and peripheral nervous systems.

Central nervous system manifestations of late neuroborreliosis include encephalitis or encephalomyelitis with tetraspastic syndrome, spastic-ataxic gait disorder and disturbed micturition, which may lead to misdiagnosis with other conditions such as multiple sclerosis if the possibility of neuroborreliosis is overlooked. Clinical awareness of this possibility is crucial, as antibiotic treatment will arrest progression. The degree of clinical recovery following microbiological cure depends on the severity of tissue damage. Recovery may be slow, especially in older patients, and can be incomplete, particularly in those who had been severely affected prior to treatment.

Peripheral nervous system manifestations include radiculopathy and mononeuropathy. Occasional patients, mainly in the older age groups, present with radiculopathy of gradual onset, progressing over many months and resulting in severe debilitating pain. This most commonly affects a lower limb and can be misdiagnosed as nerve entrapment conditions such as sciatica. The patient may not be aware of, or may have forgotten an earlier tick bite or erythema migrans. It is important that clinicians are aware of this condition, as antibiotic treatment usually brings rapid reduction in pain. It has been suggested that this more slowly evolving manifestation of radiculopathy may be related to direct spread of borreliae from the inoculation site along nerves to the nerve roots (Rupprecht et al.,

2008). A polyneuropathy can also occur in association with acrodermatitis chronica atrophicans, which is an uncommon late manifestation of cutaneous *B afzelii* infection.

## Lyme Arthritis in Europe

Lyme arthritis is less prominent a feature of Lyme borreliosis in Europe than in the USA although myalgias and arthralgias frequently occur in early disease. *Borrelia burgdorferi* sensu stricto, which is less prevalent in Europe than *B afzelii* or *B garinii*, appears to be the predominant cause of Lyme arthritis, which occurs most frequently in areas of Europe where this genospecies is most prevalent. The clinical and laboratory findings and outcomes are similar to those seen in North American-acquired infection, where it is caused exclusively by the same genospecies.

## Diagnostic Tests for Lyme Borreliosis in Europe

The EUCALB case definitions, EFNS guidelines for neuroborreliosis and other European guidelines and consensus documents recommend that laboratory support should be sought for the clinical diagnosis of all manifestations of Lyme borreliosis other than erythema migrans, as clinical features of later stage presentations are not unique to *Borrelia burgdorferi* infection. (Stanek et al., 2011; Mygland et al., 2010; O'Connell, 2010). In all cases the clinical presentation and tick exposure risk should be carefully evaluated and tests performed only on patients in whom there is a significant likelihood of Lyme borreliosis, i.e., the pre-test likelihood of infection should be evaluated. In recent years there has been a tendency for "tests for Lyme disease" to be included as part of a broad serological investigation panel for patients with a wide range of clinical presentations, without adequate consideration of its appropriateness in the individual patient's case. Indiscriminate testing without significant clinical indications can lead to misleading results, as the positive predictive value in such circumstances is low.

The European Society of Clinical Microbiology and Infectious Diseases (ESCMID) published guidelines for the laboratory diagnosis of bacterial tick borne diseases in Europe, including Lyme borreliosis, in 2004 (Brouqui et al., 2004). The German Society of Hygiene published recommendations for test use and performance in 2000 (Wilske et al., 2000). These have been widely used in Europe. Testing for Lyme borreliosis in Europe as recommended by these authorities has many similarities to standard practices recommended in North America and a recent publication gives an excellent overview of the issues in European and American infections (Wang et al., 2010).

Antibody detection is the most widely available and useful method and there have been significant improvements in both sensitivity and specificity of tests in recent years, particularly with developments in recombinant antigens derived from the major pathogenic genospecies. Direct testing methods using culture or DNA detection have more limited practical value, similar to the situation in North America (Aguero-Rosenfeld et al., 2005; Wilske et al., 2007).

The greater heterogeneity of pathogenic genospecies in Europe must be considered when evaluating test methods. In the case of DNA detection, borrelial DNA targets should be capable of detecting all pathogenic genospecies. A variety of target sequences are currently used in Europe, including those based on OspA, flagellin, 16s RNA and 5S-23S rRNA intergenic spacer region. Sensitivity of the method is similar to that of culture on tissues (about 70% overall for erythema migrans and as high as 90% for ACA). In neuroborreliosis only about 10-30% of DNA detection tests on CSF are positive, and highest rates are obtained on samples taken within the first two weeks of a clinical presentation. It is considerably more sensitive than culture for synovial tissue and fluid, for which culture has rarely been successful (Wilske et al., 2007). Borrelial DNA detection in blood culture samples from European erythema migrans patients has a lower yield than those taken in American-acquired infections, most likely because *B afzelii*, the most common infecting organism, has a lower frequency of haematogenous dissemination than *B burgdorferi* sensu stricto and because smaller sample volumes have been used in European studies.

Several factors are significant in relation to antibody testing for European Lyme borreliosis. These include genospecies variation and also variations within genospecies; heterogeneity of immunodominant epitopes, speed of immune response development to individual infecting genospecies and duration of infection prior to testing. Generally, *Borrelia burgdorferi* sensu stricto seems to cause the most acute infection presentations of the three major infecting genospecies, and immune response development is brisker than that seen in most *B afzelii* infections, which have slower development of rash, and lower incidence of significant systemic symptoms. The immune response to early *B garinii* infection also seems to be detectable earlier than that of *B afzelii* in many cases.

Patients with prolonged infection prior to antibody testing usually exhibit a broad expansion of immune response. Patients with ACA and late neuroborreliosis are usually strongly seropositive, with reactions on IgG immunoblot to many borrelial antigens, similar to findings in European and American patients with well-established Lyme arthritis. In response to concerns regarding seronegativity in patients with late stage infection the EUCALB case definition revision group reviewed published case reports of suspected seronegative late Lyme borreliosis. They concluded: *"The diagnosis of so called 'seronegative chronic Lyme disease' in supposed long-standing infections is highly unsatisfactory, requiring further clinical and laboratory investigations Seronegative late LB, if it occurs at all, is extremely rare and there have been only two reported cases of apparently seronegative ACA and one of seronegative Lyme arthritis in immunocompetent patients. There are no reliable reports of seronegative late-stage Lyme neuroborreliosis"* (Stanek et al., 2011).

Most European countries follow a two-tier antibody testing approach, similar to the American system, with a first-stage test using a sensitive screening immunoassay and second-tier test to assess specificity, usually immunoblot. There is increasing interest in using more highly specific immunoassays such as those based on C6 synthetic peptide or recombinant VlsE antigens rather than immunoblots as second tests (Nyman et al., 2006). Assessments of this simpler approach are underway in several European centres. It would be a significant gain if this approach were found to be equivalent or superior to the traditional second-tier immunoblot system, as it involves less complex laboratory procedures and interpretation is objective, although immunoblots would still be necessary in some situations. Development of a highly sensitive and specific single tier system remains the ultimate aim.

Developments in antibody test formats, incorporating recombinant antigens (including homologous proteins from different genospecies) in immunoassays and immunoblots have increased the sensitivity of new-generation tests. These are now widely used in European laboratories and some are available on automated test platforms. Some specificity problems remain, particularly with IgM tests, including immunoblots, and false-positive IgM results frequently lead to misdiagnosis if the results are not critically evaluated in the light of the patient's clinical presentation. Generally, IgM test use should be restricted to patients with short duration of illness and later follow-up samples tested if there is diagnostic uncertainty as to the specificity of an IgM result.

European criteria for IgG immunoblot positivity require fewer reactions to be present than the CDC criteria (i.e., two or three out of eight to ten candidate bands compared to five of ten in the CDC criteria) but European candidate bands exclude some less specific antigens such as p41 and p60 that are included in the CDC candidates. The European criteria also reflect the slightly slower evolution of antibody response generally seen in European infections. Experts emphasise the need for strict attention to performance and interpretation of reaction (cut-off) controls, to avoid inappropriate scoring of very weak non-specific reactions, which is a frequent cause of false-positive immunoblots and potential misdiagnosis. High background seropositivity (between 5% and 20% in many European endemic regions) can also cause confusion and potential misdiagnosis if the clinical significance of a result is not carefully assessed in the circumstances of the patient's history and clinical findings (Stanek et al., 2011; Wilske et al., 2007).

The formal diagnosis of neuroborreliosis in Europe requires CSF evaluation, including white cell count and assessment of intrathecal antibody synthesis, including CSF/serum antibody index, although in practice many clinicians do not perform CSF sampling routinely in patients whose history and clinical examination are strongly indicative of neuroborreliosis and have positive serum antibody tests. In very acute presentations of neuroborreliosis some patients may have antibodies in CSF before seroconversion in peripheral blood (Mygland et al., 2010; Stanek et al., 2011). Lymphocytic pleiocytosis is almost always present in both early and late neuroborreliosis and many patients have raised protein and oligoclonal IgG bands. Patients with ACA-associated neuropathy often have normal CSF as this is essentially a localised peripheral manifestation.

## Tests That Are Not Recommended for Diagnosis of Lyme Borreliosis in Europe

The EUCALB case definitions, the EFNS guidelines and numerous other European guidelines and consensus documents do not recommend certain tests that have been marketed as Lyme-diagnostic tests. These include live microscopy of blood, urinary borrelial antigen or PCR tests, unvalidated antibody test methods, immunoblots interpreted using poorly specific criteria, lymphocyte transformation (LTT) tests and CD57 lymphocyte subpopulation typing, as they lack specificity (Duerden, 2006; Duerden et al., 2010; Mygland et al., 2010; Stanek et al., 2011; Wilske et al., 2007).

## Outcome Data of Treated Infections

Several recent publications have reviewed outcome data in adults and children treated for various manifestations of Lyme borreliosis. A Norwegian population-based study prospectively enrolled all children in with suspected neuroborreliosis between 1996 and 2006 (Oymar and Tveitnes, 2009). All 143 children received antibiotic treatment (mainly two weeks of ceftriaxone). Following treatment four children had minor residual facial palsy; the remainder had recovered completely. This valuable paper gives an excellent illustration of clinical presentations of paediatric neuroborreliosis and the associated laboratory findings, with high rates of seropositivity and CSF pleiocytosis at presentation.

A recent Swedish prospective paediatric neuroborreliosis study of 177 children also enrolled a healthy control group (Skogman et al., 2008). Outcomes were evaluated at six months after treatment and were good, with no evidence of progressive or recurrent abnormalities. About 10%

of the children had some residual facial weakness, but no other objective findings were present. Non-specific symptoms such as headache and fatigue were reported less frequently by patients than controls. Antibiotic choice (doxycycline or ceftriaxone) did not affect outcomes.

A Slovenian prospective study comparing outcomes of treatment with doxycycline or cefuroxime axetil for erythema migrans in 285 adults also enrolled a healthy control group. Outcomes were good, with no significant differences between the treatment groups, and the incidence of non-specific symptoms at six and twelve months follow-up did not exceed those of the control group. Both of these studies illustrate a significant rate of non-specific symptoms such as headache and fatigue in non-infected healthy control populations.

A Norwegian prospective double-blind study compared outcomes of oral doxycycline or parenteral ceftriaxone treatment in adults with neuroborreliosis (Ljøstad and Mygland, 2010). Patients with early neuroborreliosis, defined as pre-treatment duration of less than six months, were followed up for one year. Out of 85 patients 41 had remaining complaints (14 with objective findings, 27 with subjective symptoms). Remaining complaints were associated with longer (>6 weeks) pre-treatment duration, higher CSF cell count and female gender. Objective findings, but not subjective symptoms, were associated with pre-treatment duration of >6 weeks, underlying the importance of early diagnosis and treatment. There were no differences in outcomes between the antibiotic treatment groups.

### Persisting Symptoms Following Treated Lyme Borreliosis

Further work is required to understand the incidence, causes and best management of persisting symptoms following appropriately treated infection. The two European trials described above that incorporated healthy non-infected controls showed significant incidence of non-specific symptoms in the control groups, and it would be helpful if further studies on patients with a broader range of Lyme borreliosis presentations incorporated healthy control subjects, in order to provide a better assessment of the true incidence of post-treatment non-specific symptoms that are attributable to Lyme borreliosis.

Persisting symptoms are well-documented following other systemic infections, and risk seems to correlate with severity of symptoms during the acute events (Hickie et al., 2006). Studies in patients with continuing symptoms following Lyme borreliosis have not shown evidence of persisting infection nor of sustained benefit from extended antibiotic treatment. Further research is required to review possible causes including immunological mechanisms. A recent publication of a study on samples from patients with persisting symptoms provided some intriguing data on heightened reactivity of anti-neural antibodies in patients with persisting symptoms compared to healthy post-Lyme borreliosis healthy and normal healthy controls, suggesting the possibility of a differential immune system response in post-Lyme-syndrome patients (Chandra et al., 2010).

### Nonstandard Medical Practices in Europe Associated with Lyme Borreliosis

Some European patients have been diagnosed with Lyme borreliosis or chronic Lyme disease on the basis of poorly specific clinical criteria and non-standard laboratory tests, including live blood microscopy, lymphocyte transformation tests or inadequately validated antibody tests including unorthodox immunoblot criteria (Duerden, 2006; Duerden et al., 2010; Stanek et al., 2011). False-positive IgM tests (including immunoblots) appear to be a particularly significant problem leading to misdiagnosis. Unorthodox treatment modalities include multiple or very prolonged courses of oral or parenteral antibiotics and parasitic agents. Some patients have received other agents including arsenicals. Misdiagnosis and inappropriate treatment can cause significant harm to patients, both from potential adverse effects and loss of opportunity for correct diagnosis and appropriate management.

### Prevention of Lyme Borreliosis and Other Tick-Transmitted Infections

No vaccine for Lyme borreliosis is currently available in Europe and none is likely to be available in the near future. Antibiotic prophylaxis following tick bites is not routinely recommended, although some European guidelines and consensus documents suggest post-exposure antibiotics could be used under certain very restricted circumstances, for example, in immunodeficient individuals (SPILF, 2007).

An effective vaccine is available for tick-borne encephalitis. A very active immunisation and tick awareness programme in Austria resulted in a marked decline in TBE incidence from a peak of 677 cases in 1979, just prior to the vaccine's introduction, to 41 in 1999 (WHO, 2004). The vaccine is recommended for residents of TBE-endemic regions throughout Europe and for visitors whose outdoor activities expose them to risk of tick bite. It is now widely promoted in travellers' health clinics and through outdoor-recreation interest groups and media outlets. The vaccine's efficacy should not be allowed to distract users from the continuing need for tick bite avoidance strategies, particularly to prevent Lyme borreliosis, which is far more prevalent and widespread in distribution than TBE in Europe.

Primary prevention of tick-borne infections entails awareness of ticks and their potential for transmitting a variety of infections, most commonly

Lyme borreliosis, so public education is an important measure. Many countries' public health authorities and special interest groups such as sporting associations and voluntary groups have annual publicity campaigns, often timed to coincide with the start of the tick-feeding season. Raising health professionals' awareness of tickborne infections, their prevention, recognition and management is essential to minimise risk of missed diagnosis or inadequate treatment. ECDC recently issued an educational toolkit on tickborne diseases, with modules for adults, children and healthcare professionals. The toolkit is designed to be modifiable by national public health authorities as appropriate for local circumstances (ECDC, 2010).

People should avoid tick infested areas if possible, but if this is not practicable they should take personal measures to reduce tick bite risk. These include minimising the amount of exposed skin, using DEET-containing insect repellents and frequently checking for attached ticks. People such as forestry workers who have frequent and potentially heavy contact with ticks should consider wearing permethrin-treated clothing.

Lyme borreliosis is unlikely to be transmitted within the first hours of a blood meal, so early removal of attached ticks is a valuable protection measure. There is some experimental evidence in animals to suggest that *Borrelia afzelii* can be transmitted at a relatively early stage of an *I ricinus* feed, with a steadily rising risk from about 24 hours of attachment (Crippa et al., 2002; Kahl et al., 1998). Although this differs from the North American situation, where there is a longer lag phase before *Ixodes scapularis* transmits *Borrelia burgdorferi* sensu stricto, a thorough search for attached ticks at the end of each day in a tick-infested area remains a very valuable protective measure against Lyme borreliosis in Europe.

Environmental aspects of tickborne disease prevention have been considered by a number of European authorities, including the European Centre for Disease Control and the World Health Organization Regional Office for Europe (ECDC, 2007; Lindgren and Jaenson, 2006). Possible measures included widespread use of acaricides, removal of deer populations and controlled burning of tick-permissive vegetation. None are regarded as feasible or acceptable for large-scale use. Modification of local vegetation by landscaping and removal of leaf litter and undergrowth in gardens and parks may be helpful in reducing tick and host animal abundance in residential settings. Personal protection against tick bites remains the most important measure.

*Health Promotion in Relation to Tick-Borne Infections; Presentation*
*of Evidence-Based Medicine and Science to Patients, Support Groups,*
*and the Wider Public*

The ECDC educational toolkit is a welcome initiative, particularly if it is taken up by national and regional public health authorities or stimulates more locally based activities, especially in populations with low awareness of ticks. A UK Rural Economy and Land Use (RELU) multidisciplinary research project included a study of educational needs of residents, workers and visitors for prevention of tick-borne infection in Lyme-endemic areas that are heavily used for recreational purposes. It also surveyed Lyme borreliosis awareness and knowledge amongst Lyme borreliosis patients and health professionals in urban and rural practice. The project is due to report in 2011. Preliminary feedback has been useful in assessing the differing educational needs of diverse groups and was presented at the Health Protection Agency Conference 2010 (Marcu et al., 2010).

Much information on tickborne infections available from media sources, including the Internet is of variable quality, ranging from highly accurate, valuable content for raising awareness and disease prevention, to poor quality and misleading, a recent example being the promotion of Lyme borreliosis as an inducer of autism. There is a need to develop methods of presenting the best scientific evidence on conditions such as Lyme borreliosis to the general public, reaching out in ways that are accessible but not condescending to readers and viewers who do not have a scientific background. An important example causing misunderstanding is a frequently-quoted statement that "tests for Lyme are highly inaccurate," alluding to statistics for antibody positivity in early infection, but implying that these figures are correct for all stages of disease. The work of organisations such as Sense About Science, building understanding and trust between scientists, clinicians and the media and public may be useful in helping to model new approaches to this important aspect of tickborne diseases (Sense About Science, 2008 *I've Got Nothing to Lose by Trying It*).

A proactive approach has already been taken by the ALSUntangled group of clinician/scientists, an international scientific effort to help people with amyotrophic lateral sclerosis investigate alternative and off-label therapies. They reviewed claims of a causal link between ALS and Lyme borreliosis and published a report on Lyme disease testing and treatment in 2009, concluding that there was no convincing evidence to support such a link (ALSUntangled Update 1: Investigating a bug (Lyme Disease) and a drug (Iplex) on behalf of people with ALS, 2009).

*Possible Directions for Future Research Related to Lyme Borreliosis and Other Tick-Transmitted Infections*

Many further developments are required in the broad range of basic sciences associated with tickborne diseases, including biology of ticks, feeding hosts, infecting agents and ecosystems, in addition to greater understanding of human disease processes. Many areas of basic research are beyond the scope of this paper and are addressed by others, but some important issues already discussed here can be summarised.

*Ecology and Epidemiology in Europe*

- Multidisciplinary work on ecological changes affecting tick populations and their distribution, reservoir hosts and human interaction with the environment is ongoing and greater co-ordination of effort should be encouraged.
- More systematic epidemiological data collection on tickborne diseases is necessary and preliminary work funded by ECDC, due to report in 2011, should lay a firm base for future improvements.

*Diagnostic Tests for Lyme Borreliosis*

- Diagnostic tests have improved significantly, particularly through developments in recombinant and synthetic peptide based antigens, but testing algorithms and the two-tier testing approach have not been reviewed to take account of these changes. There is an urgent need to for a Europe-wide (and inter-continental) assessment, with a view to minimising the need for immunoblot tests. The experience of Scandinavian workers would be particularly helpful, as immunoblots are less widely used in that region, without apparent harm. The value of currently available IgM tests should be carefully scrutinised, as experience of many laboratory workers and clinicians suggests that their potential for misleading results may outweigh their benefit.
- Further developments in antibody tests, aiming for increased sensitivity without loss of specificity would be most welcome, although this may be difficult to achieve because of the relatively slow development of antibody response to *B burgdorferi* by comparison to many other infectious agents.
- A reference repository of large volumes of sera with well-defined clinical provenance should be created, for use in development and evaluation of new diagnostic tests and to allow comparison with currently available laboratory assays.
- Research into development of laboratory markers of response to treatment would be valuable.

- There is an urgent need for educational efforts to encourage clinicians in the appropriate use of laboratory tests, particularly in the assessment of pre-test probability of disease likelihood and predictive values of test results.
- Diagnostic tests for other tickborne infections should be developed further.

*Persisting Symptoms Following Treatment of Lyme Borreliosis*

- Further research is urgently required into the incidence and possible mechanisms of persistent post-infection symptoms, which can occur following many systemic infections, including Lyme borreliosis. Lyme borreliosis could be a useful model for studying mechanisms of post-infection syndromes, from a host immune response perspective and other host factors as well as pathogen aspects. This could be a focus for international research collaboration.
- Development of optimal management strategies for patients affected by persisting symptoms following infections should be a priority.

*Prevention*

- Vaccine development against Lyme borreliosis in Europe is an active area of research.
- A broader approach to education about ticks, infection risks and tick bite prevention should be encouraged.

*Communication Issues*

- Further multidisciplinary work is urgently required in this area, as outlined above. This should include patients, support groups and members of the general public in addition to the wide range of professionals working in the field of Lyme borreliosis and other tickborne infections. The diverse needs of different communities should be taken into consideration in assessing needs.

*Acknowledgements*

I am most grateful to Mr Derek V Nudd, Dr Robert MM Smith, Mrs Anne Southwell, Dr Peter R Hawtin and Dr Adriana Basarab for their valuable and constructive comments and support; to Professor Jeremy Gray for his advice on aspects of tick ecology and biology and to Professor Gray and Mr Bernard Kaye of University College Dublin for their generosity in allowing me to include their illustrations.

## References

Aguero-Rosenfeld, Maria E., Guiqing Wang, Ira Schwartz, and Gary P. Wormser. 2005. Diagnosis of Lyme Borreliosis. *Clin. Microbiol. Rev.* 18 (3):484-509.

ALSUntangled Update 1: Investigating a bug (Lyme Disease) and a drug (Iplex) on behalf of people with ALS. 2009. *Amyotrophic Lateral Sclerosis* 10 (4):248-250.

Angelakis, E., S. A. Billeter, E. B. Breitschwerdt, B. B. Chomel, and D. Raoult. Potential for Tick-borne Bartonelloses. Emerg Infect Dis 16 (3):385-91.

Berglund, Johan, Rickard Eitrem, Katharina Ornstein, Anders Lindberg, Åke Ringnér, Henrik Elmrud, Mikael Carlsson, Arne Runehagen, Catarina Svanborg, and Ragnar Norrby. 1995. An epidemiologic study of Lyme disease in southern Sweden. *New England Journal of Medicine* 333 (20):1319-1324.

Bown, K. J., X. Lambin, N. H. Ogden, M. Begon, G. Telford, Z. Woldehiwet, and R. J. Birtles. 2009. Delineating Anaplasma phagocytophilum ecotypes in coexisting, discrete enzootic cycles. *Emerg Infect Dis* 15 (12):1948-54.

Brouqui, P., F. Bacellar, G. Baranton, R. J. Birtles, A. Bjoersdorff, J. R. Blanco, G. Caruso, M. Cinco, P. E. Fournier, E. Francavilla, M. Jensenius, J. Kazar, H. Laferl, A. Lakos, S. Lotric Furlan, M. Maurin, J. A. Oteo, P. Parola, C. Perez-Eid, O. Peter, D. Postic, D. Raoult, A. Tellez, Y. Tselentis, and B. Wilske. 2004. Guidelines for the diagnosis of tick-borne bacterial diseases in Europe. *Clin Microbiol Infect* 10 (12):1108-32.

Chandra, A., G. P. Wormser, M. S. Klempner, R. P. Trevino, M. K. Crow, N. Latov, and A. Alaedini. 2010. Anti-neural antibody reactivity in patients with a history of Lyme borreliosis and persistent symptoms. *Brain Behav Immun* 24 (6):1018-24.

Christiansen, A. H., and K. Mølbak. 2005. Neuroborreliosis 1994-2004. *Statens Serum Institut Report* (33):1.

Crippa, M., O. Rais, and L. Gern. 2002. Investigations on the mode and dynamics of transmission and infectivity of Borrelia burgdorferi sensu stricto and Borrelia afzelii in Ixodes ricinus ticks. *Vector Borne Zoonotic Dis* 2 (1):3-9.

Dillon, R., O'Connell S, and Wright S. 2010. Lyme disease in the UK: clinical and laboratory features and response to treatment. Clin Med 10 (5):454-457.

Duerden, B. I. 2006. *Unorthodox and unvalidated laboratory tests in the diagnosis of Lyme Borreliosis and in relation to medically unexplained symptoms*. Department of Health, 2006 [cited Oct 8 2010]. Available from http://www.dh.gov.uk/prod_consum_dh/groups/dh_digitalassets/@dh/@en/documents/digitalasset/dh_4138917.pdf.

Duerden, B. I. (Chair) on behalf of the Independent Review Panel. 2010. Independent appraisal and review of the ILADS 2004 "Evidence-based guidelines for the management of Lyme disease". Health Protection Agency. Available from http://www.hpa.org.uk/web/HPAwebFile/HPAweb_C/1294739293177 (accessed 16th March 2011)

ECDC. 2007. *Meeting Report, Workshop: Environmental Change and Infectious Disease* 2007 [accessed Oct 8 2010]. Available from http://www.ecdc.europa.eu/en/publications/Publications/0703_MER_Environmental_Change_and_Infectious_Disease.pdf.

———. 2010. *Spotlight: Tick-borne diseases* 2010 [accessed Oct 8 2010]. Available from http://www.ecdc.europa.eu/en/healthtopics/spotlight/spotlight_tickborne/Pages/home.aspx.

EpiNorthData. 2011. http://www.epinorth.org/eway/default.aspx?pid=230&trg=Area_5279 &MainArea_5260=5279:0:15,2937:1:0:0:::0:0&Area_5279=5291:44530::1:5290:1:::0: 0&diseaseid=20 Accessed March 16 2011

EUCALB. 2010. *European Union Concerted Action on Lyme Borreliosis - Spirochaete, reservoir hosts* 2010 [cited Oct 8 2010]. Available from http://meduni09.edis.at/eucalb/cms/index.php?option=com_content&task=view&id=59&Itemid=93.

Fülöp, Balazs, and Gabriele Poggensee. 2008. Epidemiological situation of Lyme borreliosis in Germany: Surveillance data from six Eastern German States, 2002 to 2006. *Parasitology Research* 103 (0):117-120.

Gray, J. S. 1991. The development and seasonal activity of the tick Ixodes ricinus: a vector of Lyme borreliosis. *Review of Medical and Veterinary Entomology* 79 (6):323-333.

———. 1998. Review The ecology of ticks transmitting Lyme borreliosis. *Experimental and Applied Acarology* 22 (5):249-258.

Gray, J. S., H. Dautel, A. Estrada-Pena, O. Kahl, and E. Lindgren. 2009. Effects of climate change on ticks and tick-borne diseases in Europe. *Interdiscip Perspect Infect Dis* 2009.

Gray, Jeremy, Annetta Zintl, Anke Hildebrandt, Klaus-Peter Hunfeld, and Louis Weiss. 2010. Zoonotic babesiosis: Overview of the disease and novel aspects of pathogen identity. *Ticks and Tick-borne Diseases* 1 (1):3-10.

Halperin, John J. 2008. Nervous System Lyme Disease. *Infectious disease clinics of North America* 22 (2):261-274.

Health Protection Agency. 2011. Lyme borreliosis: epidemiological data. Accessed March 16 2011 at: http://www.hpa.org.uk/Topics/InfectiousDiseases/InfectionsAZ/LymeDisease/EpidemiologicalData/

Hickie, I., T. Davenport, D. Wakefield, U. Vollmer-Conna, B. Cameron, S. D. Vernon, W. C. Reeves, and A. Lloyd. 2006. Post-infective and chronic fatigue syndromes precipitated by viral and non-viral pathogens: prospective cohort study. *BMJ* 333 (7568):575.

Huppertz, H. I., M. Bohme, S. M. Standaert, H. Karch, and S. A. Plotkin. 1999. Incidence of Lyme borreliosis in the Wurzburg region of Germany. *Eur J Clin Microbiol Infect Dis* 18 (10):697-703.

*I've Got Nothing to Lose by Trying It.* 2010. Sense about Science 2008 [Accessed March 16 2011]. Available from http://www.senseaboutscience.org.uk/pdf/I%27ve%20got%20nothing%20to%20lose%20by%20trying%20it%20FINAL.pdf.

Kahl, O., C. Janetzki-Mittmann, J. S. Gray, R. Jonas, J. Stein, and R. de Boer. 1998. Risk of infection with Borrelia burgdorferi sensu lato for a host in relation to the duration of nymphal Ixodes ricinus feeding and the method of tick removal. *Zentralbl Bakteriol* 287 (1-2):41-52.

Karan, L. S., N.A. Rudnikova, A.E. Platonov, and et al. 2007. Ixodes tick-borne borrelioses in Russia. In *Abstract book of 5th International Conference on Emerging Zoonoses*. Limassol, Cyprus.

Korenberg, E. I., L. Y. Gorban, Y. V. Kovalevskii, V. I. Frizen, and A. S. Karavanov. 2001. Risk for human tick-borne encephalitis, borrelioses, and double infection in the pre-Ural region of Russia. *Emerg Infect Dis* 7 (3):459-62.

*La maladie de Lyme. Données du réseau de surveillance de la maladie en Alsace.* 2010. Institut Veille Sanitaire 2008 [accessed September 11 2010]. Available from http://www.invs.sante.fr/publications/2005/lyme_alsace/index.html.

Letrilliart, L., B. Ragon, T. Hanslik, and A. Flahault. 2005. Lyme disease in France: a primary care-based prospective study. *Epidemiol Infect* 133 (5):935-42.

Lindgren, Elisabet, and Thomas G. T. Jaenson. 2006. Lyme borreliosis in Europe: influences of climate and climate change, epidemiology, ecology and adaptation measures. Copenhagen, Denmark: WHO Regional Office for Europe. http://www.euro.who.int/document/E89522.pdf.

Ljøstad, U., and Å Mygland. 2010. Remaining complaints 1 year after treatment for acute Lyme neuroborreliosis; frequency, pattern and risk factors. *European Journal of Neurology* 17 (1):118-123.

Marcu, Afrodita, Julie Barnett, David Uzzell, and Sue O'Connell. 2010. Lyme disease patients' information needs and their preferences for future precautionary measures. In *Health Protection Agency Conference*. University of Warwick, Coventry, UK.

Mehnert, W. H., and G. Krause. 2005. Surveillance of Lyme borreliosis in Germany, 2002 and 2003. *Euro Surveill* 10 (4):83-5.

Mygland, A., U. Ljostad, V. Fingerle, T. Rupprecht, E. Schmutzhard, and I. Steiner. 2010. EFNS guidelines on the diagnosis and management of European Lyme neuroborreliosis. *Eur J Neurol* 17 (1):8-16, e1-4.

Nygard, K., A. B. Brantsaeter, and R. Mehl. 2005. Disseminated and chronic Lyme borreliosis in Norway, 1995 - 2004. *Euro Surveill* 10 (10):235-8.

Nyman, D., L. Willen, C. Jansson, S. A. Carlsson, H. Granlund, and P. Wahlberg. 2006. VlsE C6 peptide and IgG ELISA antibody analysis for clinical diagnosis of Lyme borreliosis in an endemic area. *Clin Microbiol Infect* 12 (5):496-7.

O'Connell, S. 2010. Recommendations for the diagnosis and treatment of Lyme borreliosis: guidelines and consensus papers from specialist societies and expert groups in Europe and North America http://www.hpa.org.uk/web/HPAwebFile/HPAweb_C/1287144781602 (Accessed 16th March 2011)

Oymar, K., and D. Tveitnes. 2009. Clinical characteristics of childhood Lyme neuroborreliosis in an endemic area of northern Europe. *Scand J Infect Dis* 41 (2):88-94.

Parola, P., B. Davoust, and D. Raoult. 2005. Tick- and flea-borne rickettsial emerging zoonoses. *Vet Res* 36 (3):469-92.

Parola, P., C. D. Paddock, and D. Raoult. 2005. Tick-borne rickettsioses around the world: emerging diseases challenging old concepts. *Clin Microbiol Rev* 18 (4):719-56.

Piesman, J., and T. G. Schwan. 2010. Ecology of borreliae and their vectors. In *Borrelia, Molecular Biology, Host Interactions and Pathogenesis*, edited by D. S. Samuels and J. D. Radolf. Norfolk, UK: Caister Academic Press.

Poggensee, G., and C. Adlhoch. 2010. Lyme-Borreliosis: ein Situationsbericht aus den sechs ostlichen Bundeslanden 2007-2009. UMID 2, 5-8.

Randolph, S. E. 2001. The shifting landscape of tick-borne zoonoses: tick-borne encephalitis and Lyme borreliosis in Europe. *Philos Trans R Soc Lond B Biol Sci* 356 (1411):1045-56.

Rauter, Carolin, and Thomas Hartung. 2005. Prevalence of Borrelia burgdorferi Sensu Lato Genospecies in Ixodes ricinus Ticks in Europe: a Metaanalysis. *Appl. Environ. Microbiol.* 71 (11):7203-7216.

Rupprecht, T. A., U. Koedel, V. Fingerle, and H. W. Pfister. 2008. The pathogenesis of lyme neuroborreliosis: from infection to inflammation. *Mol Med* 14 (3-4):205-12.

Sense About Science (UK Registered Charity 11101114) http://www.senseaboutscience.org.uk/index.php (Accessed 16th March 2011).

Skogman, Barbro Hedin, Stefan Croner, Maria Nordwall, Mattias Eknefelt, Jan Ernerudh, and Pia Forsberg. 2008. Lyme Neuroborreliosis in Children: A prospective study of clinical features, prognosis, and outcome. *The Pediatric Infectious Disease Journal* 27 (12):1089-1094 10.1097/INF.0b013e31817fd423.

Smith, R., and J. Takkinen. 2006. Lyme borreliosis: Europe-wide coordinated surveillance and action needed? *Euro Surveill* 11 (6):E060622 1.

SPILF. 2007. Borréliose de Lyme : démarches diagnostiques, thérapeutiques et préventives. Texte court. *Médecine et Maladies Infectieuses* 37 (4):187-193.

Stanek, G., V. Fingerle, K. P. Hunfeld, B. Jaulhac, R. Kaiser, A. Krause, W. Kristoferitsch, S. O'Connell, K. Ornstein, F. Strle, and J. Gray. 2011. Lyme borreliosis: Clinical case definitions for diagnosis and management in Europe. *Clin Microbiol Infect*. 17(1):69-79.

Stanek, G., S. O'Connell, M. Cimmino, E. Aberer, W. Kristoferitsch, M. Granstrom, E. Guy, and J. Gray. 1996. European Union Concerted Action on Risk Assessment in Lyme Borreliosis: clinical case definitions for Lyme borreliosis. *Wien Klin Wochenschr* 108 (23):741-7.

Strle, F., R. B. Nadelman, J. Cimperman, J. Nowakowski, R. N. Picken, I. Schwartz, V. Maraspin, M. E. Aguero-Rosenfeld, S. Varde, S. Lotric-Furlan, and G. P. Wormser. 1999. Comparison of culture-confirmed erythema migrans caused by Borrelia burgdorferi sensu stricto in New York State and by Borrelia afzelii in Slovenia. *Ann Intern Med* 130 (1):32-6.

Wang, G., M. E. Aguero-Rosenfeld, G.P. Wormser, and I. Schwarz. 2010. Detection of Borrelia burgdorferi. In *Borrelia, Molecular Biology, Host Interactions and Pathogenesis*, edited by D. S. Samuels and J. D. Radolf. Norfolk, UK: Caister Academic Press.

WHO. 2004. *The vector-borne human infections of Europe: their distribution and burden on public health*. WHO Regional Office for Europe 2004 [accessed October, 8 2010]. Available from http://www.euro.who.int/__data/assets/pdf_file/0008/98765/e82481.pdf.

Wilske, B., V. Fingerle, and U. Schulte-Spechtel. 2007. Microbiological and serological diagnosis of Lyme borreliosis. *FEMS Immunol Med Microbiol* 49 (1):13-21.

Wilske, B., L Zöller, V. Brade, H. Eiffert, U.B. Gobel, G. Stanek, and H.W. Pfister. 2000. Lyme-Borreliosis. In *MiQ: mikrobiologisch-infektiologische Qualitätstandards(MiQ); Qualitätsstandards in der mikrobiologisch-infektiologischen Diagnostik*, edited by H. Mauch and R. Lutticken. Munich: Urban und Fischer.

# A8

# THE TICK MICROBIOME: DIVERSITY, DISTRIBUTION, AND INFLUENCE OF THE INTERNAL MICROBIAL COMMUNITY FOR A BLOOD-FEEDING DISEASE VECTOR

Authors: *Keith Clay and Clay Fuqua*
*Department of Biology*
*Indiana University*

## Abstract

Ticks are well established as important vectors for human disease, accounting for a growing number of zoonotic infections. Certain primary pathogens such as the Lyme disease agent, have received great attention. Less well understood is the overall microbial community that is harbored within ticks, in addition to human pathogens. A variety of powerful molecular detection approaches have revealed a constrained but significant microbial community associated with ticks, including vertically-transmitted symbionts, opportunistic pathogens, and more transient guest commensals, which include viruses, bacteria, protozoans, and fungi. Ticks join a growing number of arthropod and filarial systems in which microbial symbionts can have profound and extensive effects on the activity of their host and in certain cases, a direct impact on human disease. The recognized human pathogens are in fact vastly outnumbered by these other microorganisms, and pathogens represent a relatively small fraction of the total microbial community in ticks. The tick-borne microbial community affords the opportunity for functional interactions between microorganisms, which can have significant influence on the relative population sizes of the different resident microbial taxa. In ticks, limited evidence suggests that specific microbes or the overall microbial community can influence the acquisition, transmission and virulence of known pathogens such as *Borrelia burgdorferi, Anaplasma phagocytophilum*, or *Babesia microti*, as well as newly emerging pathogens. This area remains understudied at this point and represents a current gap in our knowledge. Future research efforts are required in light of recent results from other arthropod systems such as aphids and *Drosophila*, and will greatly benefit from new technologies for in-depth profiling of the tick microbiome, allowing high sampling depth for ecological investigations and for experimental laboratory approaches.

### Introduction

Ticks (Class Arachnida, Order Acari) are blood-feeding arthropods that feed on terrestrial vertebrates and vector a diverse group of human and wildlife pathogens, including viral, bacterial, and protozoan disease agents (Sonenshine and Mather 1994; Goodman, Dennis, and Sonenshine 2005). Ticks vector more human pathogens than any other arthropod, and are the primary source of vector-borne infectious disease in many temperate areas (Asia, Europe, North America). Unlike other blood-feeding arthropods such as mosquitos, fleas and lice, ticks exhibit extended time periods between blood meals of up to a year or more. Ticks can acquire pathogens during blood meals but transmission of pathogens to susceptible vertebrate hosts depends on ticks maintaining their infections during transstadial molts (from larvae to nymphs and from nymphs to adults) (Sonenshine 1991). Most hard ticks (Ixodidae) have a three-stage life cycle (larvae, nymph, adult) and each blood meal may be from a different host species. As a result, pathogens are potentially spread widely among vertebrate species, making ticks important sources of zoonotic disease.

Ticks have been well-studied because of their human health impacts but new microbial associations continue to be described (Jasinskas, Zhong, and Barbour 2007; Grindle et al. 2003; Morimoto, Kurtti, and Noda 2006) and new emerging diseases are being recognized (e.g. Paddock and Yabsley 2007, STARI, Loftis et al. 2008, Panola Mountain *Ehrlichia*, LaSala and Holbrook 2010, viral haemorrhagic fevers). In addition to pathogens, ticks serve as hosts for a variety of endosymbiotic, vertically-transmitted bacteria, including *Coxiella-, Francisella-* and *Rickettsia*-like organisms (Perotti et al. 2006; Noda, Munderloh, and Kurtti 1997; Sun et al. 2000; Morimoto, Kurtti, and Noda 2006), and

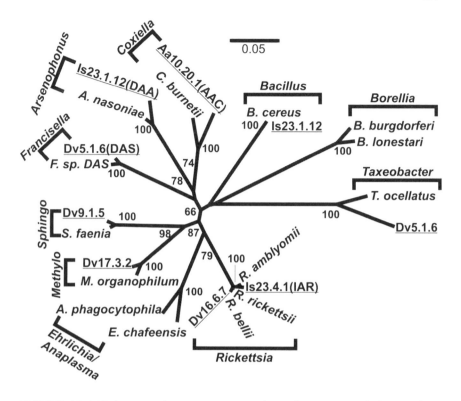

FIGURE A8-1 Phylogram of representative a subset of 16s-rDNA phylotypes from ticks. Brackets indicate genera. Underlined entries from recent tick isolates. Dv, *D. variabilis*; Aa, *A. americanum*; Is, *I. scapularis*. Numbers at nodes are boot strap support.
SOURCE: Clay and Fuqua, unpublished.

newly described symbionts of tick mitochondria (Sassera et al. 2006; Epis et al. 2008). Tick endosymbionts are often closely related to virulent human pathogens (Figure A8-1). It is likely that ticks are host to a larger diversity of, as yet undiscovered, microbes.

Changing environmental conditions, including climate change, land-use patterns, wildlife populations and agricultural practices, are acting to alter host and tick ecology and their geographical distributions, leading to new regions of tick activity, overlapping distributions and emerging disease (Childs and Paddock 2003; McDiarmid et al. 2000; Masuzawa et al. 2008; Sun et al. 2008; van Overbeek et al. 2008; Randolph 2010). These dynamic changes are providing new opportunities for pathogen host shifts and mixed infections, including new microbial community associations (Eisen, Meyer, and Eisen 2007; Eisen 2008; Randolph and Rogers 2010).

## Methodologies for Identifying and Enumerating Microbes in Ticks

The field of microbiology has relied for over a century on the ability to cultivate microorganisms derived from natural environments. Although this approach remains one of the most commonly employed and useful means of identifying microbes, it excludes the detection of a potentially vast range of microorganisms. Estimates from soil environments suggest that greater than 99% of active microorganisms are not detectable by conventional cultivation methods (Rondon et al. 2000; Hugenholz, Goebel, and Pace 1998). It is particularly clear that ticks and other arthropods frequently harbor microbes that have obligate intracellular life histories, either as commensals or pathogens, or are very difficult to cultivate (Dale and Moran 2006). Although traditional microscopy and histological staining can provide presumptive identifications of tick-associated microbes, the information is often ambiguous and of limited utility.

Powerful molecular approaches now enable the detection of microorganisms independent of the limitations of cultivation. Microbes can be identified and phylogenetically characterized, often to the level of genus and species, using nucleic acid or antibody probes directed towards highly conserved macromolecules (Clements and Bullivant 1991). Although a range of conserved proteins, fatty acids and nucleic acids have been used as targets for this purpose, small subunit ribosomal RNAs (SSUs) such as bacterial 16S rRNA, are the most generally applied, and often the most informative (Stahl 1995). No area of investigation has benefited more from these approaches than arthropod-microbe interactions. Molecular analyses have revealed diverse arthropod-associated microbes for a variety of systems (Dale and Moran 2006). Many of these microbes have not yet been cultured and their identification would be virtually impossible without cultivation-independent methods. Likewise, the study of tick-borne pathogens increasingly relies on molecular detection approaches to identify, distinguish and compare pathogens among different tick species and populations (Sun et al. 2000; Schabereiter-Gurtner, Lubitz, and Rölleke 2003; Burkot et al. 2001).

A number of studies have utilized Polymerase Chain Reaction (PCR) to amplify conserved microbial sequences, such as 16S rRNA gene sequences from total DNA extracts isolated from ticks, either as individuals or in small pools (Heise, Elshahed, and Little 2010; Clay et al. 2008; Benson et al. 2004). In the gene library sequence approach, these amplicons are ligated *en masse* into standard PCR cloning vectors, transformed into a cloning host such as *Escherichia coli*, and the plasmids are isolated from the initial transformants. The 16S rRNA amplicons carried on these plasmids are then sequenced and the source microorganism is deduced by comparison with rRNA gene sequence databases, such as the Ribosomal Database Project (http://rdp.cme.msu.edu/). This cultivation-independent approach has been tremendously informative, and has revealed a number of tick-associated microbes that would have never been identified otherwise (Adar, Simaan, and Ulitzur 1992; Grindle et al. 2003; Heise, Elshahed, and Little 2010; Jasinskas, Zhong, and Barbour 2007; Schabereiter-Gurtner, Lubitz, and Rölleke 2003). A major limitation is however numerical—each clone must be sequenced individually. Hundreds of plasmids may be generated from a single tick, and sequencing to significant depth per tick is extremely expensive and time consuming. In depth analysis of large numbers of individual ticks becomes prohibitive. This problem is exacerbated by the trend for there to be a single, highly abundant type of microbe that colonizes each tick to high density, and therefore a large fraction the 16 S rRNA gene sequences determined are from this one taxon.

Molecular community fingerprinting techniques such as denaturing gradient gel electrophoresis (DGGE) and terminal restriction fragment length polymorphisms (T-RFLP) analysis, ostensibly provide efficient snapshots of microbial community composition (Muyzer and Smalla 1998; Osborn, Moore, and Timmis 2000). These approaches also utilize PCR to amplify diagnostic sequences from samples, again most typically 16S rRNA genes. The underlying microbial diversity in any given community is revealed by electrophoretic separation of amplicons with different sequences, providing a microbial fingerprint. Specific microbial identification is also possible with both DGGE and T-RFLP approaches, but in practice this is considerably less reliable than the library sequencing approach for microbial identification. These techniques have proven useful in analyzing certain microbial communities, but have only been employed sparingly to analyze tick microbiota (Schabereiter-Gurtner, Lubitz, and Rölleke 2003). They provide somewhat course resolution on microbial diversity, revealing the major trends in composition, and therefore the numerical dominance of a single symbiont taxon cited above also creates problems for this approach.

The molecular approaches described above provide a way to gauge diversity in a microbial community, but are not an efficient way to determine the presence or absence of specific microbes in a sample. Nor do they provide robust information on relative abundances of a given microbe. Once specific microbial taxa of interest have been identified, these microbes can be targeted directly. Direct and nested PCR based assays with primer sets specific to diagnostic sequences (often, but not always 16S rRNA genes) for targeted microbial groups allows highly sensitive detection (Clay et al. 2008). Fluorescent in situ hybridization (FISH) analysis of sectioned ticks with specific oligonucleotide probes allows visualization of the site(s) of colonization for specific microbial taxa (Figure A8-2; Klyachko et al.

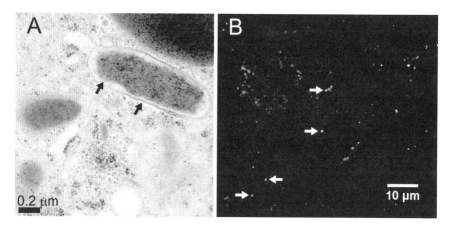

**FIGURE A8-2** Visualization of *Coxiella*-type symbiont from *A. americanum*. (A) Transmission electron microscopy of thin sectioned ovarian tissue from a engorged female. Arrows demarcate presumptive outer and inner membrane structures (B) FISH microscopy of tissue section from a dissected ovary *A. americanum* show oocytes stained with a *Coxiella*-specific probe labeled with Cy5. Arrows highlight fluorescent punta resulting from probing and indicate of the *Coxiella*-type symbiont. SOURCE: Klyachko et al. 2007.

2007; Hammer et al. 2001). These taxon-specific assays are able to detect microbes at very low relative abundance that often escape the more general community approaches. Furthermore, quantitative PCR allows the relative abundance of specific microbes to be determined (Jasinskas, Zhong, and Barbour 2007). The directed approaches, however, also suffer from several limitations and complexities. Investigators must know precisely which microbe they aim to detect, and they must have high confidence that the specific PCR primer set they employ is not confounded by cross-amplification of other microbes. Even minor divergence in the targeted sequences can lead to loss of detection, and it is difficult to trust PCR failures of a single target sequence as evidence for the absence of specific pathogens or other symbionts. Multilocus sequence typing (MLST) approaches target multiple conserved genes (usually 5-10) in a targeted microbe, again using PCR, but following this by sequencing of the amplicons (Maiden et al. 1998). Specific microbial lineages, or sequence types, are defined by the complete set of sequences obtained. This technique generally relies on the physical isolation of the targeted microbe from the sample, however, most typically by cultivation, and has been used only to analyze closely related tick microbiota (Margos et al. 2008).

The advent of high-throughput, next generation sequencing techniques promises to surmount many of the limitations in current molecular approaches to microbial diversity studies described above. The ability to obtain hundreds of thousands of individual sequences in a single run provides tremendous power to probe the depth and breadth of a wide range of microbial communities. In the analysis of microbial communities, short segments of the 16S rRNA gene are PCR amplified using specific primer sets to generate 16S "tags" (Sogin et al. 2006). These amplified tags are then subjected to high-throughput sequencing such as pyrosequencing using a 454 sequence analyzer (http://www.454.com/). Current 454 technology provides from 400-600 bp sequence reads per fragment, allowing complete coverage of each amplicon. Upwards of 100,000 individual sequences can be obtained from a single 454 experiment. The primers used to perform the initial tag amplification contain specific identifier sequencers or "bar codes" outside of the region of the primer that anneals to the target sequence. These bar codes allow correlation of the sequences, obtained *en masse*, back to an original sample. For example, bar coding allows the simultaneous sequencing of greater than 100 individual ticks in a single experiment, generating hundreds of individual 16S rRNA tag sequences that can be correlated back to each specific source tick. Each sequence is then analyzed using the sequence databases (such as the RDP described above) to provide phylogenetic information about each microbe. Because of the depth of sequencing afforded, the number of sequences matching a specific taxon also provides information on the relative abundance of the microbe within the original sample. In our own studies we have found good agreement between abundances determined by tag sequencing and those determined by more direct assays such as targeted Q-PCR (Silvanose et al. in preparation).

All of these molecular approaches depend on PCR to amplify targeted genes and thus are all subject to any biases introduced by the PCR reaction itself. It is clear that there are no truly universal primer sets, and that in any given experiment it is possible to miss an important community member simply because of poor amplification. Conversely, some microbes may be overrepresented due to aberrantly efficient PCR. High-throughput sequencing may offer the answer here as well. New sequencing technologies, such as that provided by Solexa sequencing on Illumina instruments (http://www.illumina.com/technology/sequencing_technology.ilmn), can generate staggeringly high numbers of sequences, now up to $2 \times 10^{11}$ bp in a single experiment. At a read length of roughly 100 bp this represents greater than $10^9$ individual sequences (generally much shorter in length than those obtained by 454). With Illumina sequencing and other emerging technologies the ability to acquire sequence information from samples will no longer be the rate-limiting issue (Morozova and Marra 2008). With this sequencing power it may be possible to analyze total DNA from ticks directly, obtaining the tick genome and its microbial colonist's genomes, without the need for PCR, and avoiding the bias described above. As with many of these sequence-based technologies, the true challenge will be analyzing the bio-informatic data to obtain reliable information on the microbiome.

Molecular approaches have also begun to show great utility in studying tick host-microbiome interactions. Several groups have generated expressed sequence tag (EST) cDNA libraries from ticks that provide information not only on gene content, but also gene activity at the time of sampling (Wang et al. 2007; Hill and Gutierrez 2000). These libraries can also provide infor-mation about the microbiome. Our own analysis of several *A. americanum* EST libraries revealed a strikingly large percentage of cDNAs derived from a bacterial symbiont, indicating active expression of symbiont genes (Smith et al., in preparation). The sequence information gained from such libraries also facilitates construction of DNA microarrays to analyze gene expres-sion (Colbourne et al. 2007). Whole genomic sequence projects for *Ixodes scapularis* and *Boophilus microplus* are well underway (Pagel Van Zee et al. 2007; Guerrero et al. 2006), and this information should provide even more comprehensive information for construction of DNA microarrays. With these microarrays, the expression patterns induced in ticks under a va-riety of conditions, including variable composition of the microbiome, may be monitored readily (Rodriguez-Valle et al. 2010). Even more powerful for these purposes may be massively parallel sequencing of transcripts, or RNASeq, using next generation sequencing technology to generate informa-tion on the genes being expressed and their level of expression (Ronning et al. 2010). This is as yet a new approach and we are not aware of its appli-cation to ticks or tick-borne disease, but the technique has great potential.

## Microbial Communities of Ticks

Over the past two decades, research has revealed unsuspected microbial diversity in arthropods. For example, it is estimated that *Wolbachia* occurs in over 65% of all insect species (Hilgenboecker et al. 2008) and other prokaryotes (e.g., *Cardinium*, *Arsenophonus*, *Rickettsia*) are also highly represented (Perlman, Hunter, and Zchori-Fein 2006; Duron, Wilkes, and Hurst 2010; Duron et al. 2008; Weinert et al. 2009; Novakova, Hypsa, and Moran 2009). These microbes are often associated with reproductive altera-tions in hosts such as feminization, induced parthenogenesis or reproductive incompatibilities (Werren, Baldo, and Clark 2008). More specific arthropod families or genera are often associated with other bacterial endosymbionts such as *Buchnera* in aphids that play a role in nutrition of their hosts by provisioning critical amino acids (Douglas 1998; Oliver et al. 2010). Other insect groups (e.g., beetles, cockroaches, termites) are also associated with specific groups of microbes with enzymatic capabilities for the digestion of cellulose-rich food materials (Dillon and Dillon 2004; Vasanthakumar et al. 2008; Sabree, Kambhampati, and Moran 2009). A growing literature suggests that bacterial symbionts can also play an important role in host defense against biotic enemies (Oliver, Moran, and Hunter 2005; Oliver et al. 2009; Jaenike et al. 2010), and also against abiotic stresses such as heat and cold (Montllor, Maxmen, and Purcell 2002; Neelakanta et al. 2010). Except for pathogens of humans and domestic animals, the functional role and impact of most microbial associations in ticks is unknown. It is likely that some endosymbionts play a nutritional role during blood feeding.

Most attention has been given to pathogenic bacteria vectored by ticks but they are also capable of transmitting pathogenic piroplasms (e.g., *Babesia* and *Theileria*) (Florin-Christensen and Schnittger 2009; Bishop et al. 2004) and a variety of viral pathogens. For example, tick-borne encephalitis is major human health threat worldwide (LaSala and Holbrook 2010; Charrel et al. 2004) and there is growing concern over deer tick or Powassan virus (Flavivirus) in *Ixodes*-endemic areas (Tokarz et al. 2010; Ebel 2010). In addition to tick-borne Flaviviruses, Colorado tick fever is caused by a Coltivirus transmitted by *Dermacentor andersoni* in the western United States and Canada (Brackney et al. 2010). Other pathogenic viruses could potentially be transmitted by ticks but standard methodologies for detecting bacteria would not detect them. The panviral Virochip approach would represent one possible method for quickly screening tick samples for viruses. Their blood-feeding lifestyle makes ticks potential vectors for a wide range of blood-borne pathogens.

Ticks may be co-infected by multiple pathogens (Schouls et al. 1999; Mixson et al. 2006; Moreno et al. 2006; Tokarz et al. 2010). Moreover, because of the high prevalence of vertically-transmitted endosymbionts in ticks, including multiple endosymbionts within the same tick (Scoles 2004; Goethert and Telford 2005; Carmichael and Fuerst 2006; Clay et al. 2008), pathogen infections almost always co-occur with resident endosymbionts (Yabsley et al. 2009; Jasinskas, Zhong, and Barbour 2007; Sun et al. 2000; Niebylski et al. 1997; Noda, Munderloh, and Kurtti 1997). Prior studies of the relationships among ticks, vertebrate hosts and pathogens have generally given little consideration to how microbial interactions and the entire microbial community within ticks, including endosymbionts and other microbes of unknown function, impact tick-borne disease (Table A8-1). These associations might affect the colonization, transmission and virulence of human or animal pathogens.

Ticks could become co-infected by pathogens while consuming a single blood meal containing multiple pathogens, or by transfer of pathogens between co-feeding ticks (Piesman and Happ 2001). It is less likely that ticks become infected by a diversity of pathogens from sequential feeding on multiple animals given that the hard tick life cycle includes only three blood meals that are well-separated in time. In contrast, co-infections of vertebrates by tick-borne pathogens could easily result from sequential

**TABLE A8-1** Tick-Borne Bacteria and Human Diseases

| Tick Genus | Species | Bacteria | Human Disease | Reference |
|---|---|---|---|---|
| Ixodes[a] | Is, Ir | *Borrelia burgdorferi* | Lyme Disease | Burgdorfer et al. 1982 |
| | Is | *Anaplasma phagocytophila* | Anaplasmosis | Belongia et al. 1997 |
| | Is, Ir | *Rickettsia* symbiont | None recognized | Noda, Munderloh, and Kurtti 1997 |
| | Is, Ip | *Arsenophonus* symbiont | None recognized | Grindle et al. (Unpublished) |
| | Ir | *Cytophaga* symbiont | None recognized | Morimoto, Kurtti, and Noda 2006 |
| | Ir | *Midichloria mitochondrii* | None recognized | Beninati et al. 2004 |
| | Ir | *Diplorickettsia massiliensis* | None recognized | Mediannikov et al. 2010 |
| Dermacentor[b] | Dv | *Rickettsia rickettsii* | Rocky Mountain Spotted Fever | Shepard and Goldwasser 1960 |
| | Dv, Da | *Rickettsia montana* | None recognized | Steiner et al. (Unpublished) |
| | Dv, Da | *Francisella* symbiont[c] | None recognized | Sun et al. 2000 |
| | Dv, Da | *Arsenophonus* symbiont | None recognized | Grindle et al. 2003 |
| Amblyomma[d] | Aa | *Borrelia lonestari* | Southern Tick-Associated Rash Illness (STARI) | Varela et al. 2004 |
| | Aa | *Ehrlichia chafeensis* | Ehrlichiosis | Anderson et al. 1991 |
| | Aa | *Rickettsia amblyommii* | None recognized | Clay et al. 2008 |
| | Aa | *Arsenophonus* symbiont | None recognized | Clay et al. 2008 |
| | Aa | *Coxiella* symbiont[c] | None recognized | Jasinskas, Zhong, and Barbour 2007; Klyachko et al. 2007 |

[a] Is, I. scapularis; Ir, I. ricinus; Ip, I. Pacificus.
[b] Dv, D. variabilis; Da, D. andersoni.
[c] The mammalian pathogens Coxiella burnettii (Q-Fever) and Francisella tularensis (Tularemia) can be occasionally harbored and transmitted by multiple tick species.
[d] Aa, A. americanum.

and independent tick bites given that a large animal host could have a tick burden in the hundreds or thousands (Ginsberg 2008). Moreover, hosts may be bitten by ticks co-infected with multiple pathogens as described above. Human co-infections are most likely to arise from the bite of a single co-infected tick. Simultaneous infections by multiple tick-borne pathogens occur frequently in mammalian hosts, including humans. For example, of 96 patients in Wisconsin and Minnesota infected with *Borrelia burgdorferi*, five were co-infected with *Anaplasma phagocytophilum*, two with *Babesia microti* and two with all three pathogens (Mitchell, Reed, and Hofkes 1996). In New York, 60-90% of patients diagnosed with Human Granulo-cytic Anaplasmosis (*A. phagocytophilum*) tested positive for *B. burgdorferi*, a higher than expected rate based on pathogen prevalence (Wormser et al. 1997, see also Mitchell, Reed, and Hofkes 1996). Tick-borne co-infections may result in increased severity and duration of illness (Alekseev et al. 2001; Nyarko, Grab, and Dumler 2006) and misdiagnosis resulting from symptom overlap (Belongia et al. 1997). Co-infections with tick-borne pathogens have also been reported from domestic and wild animals including dogs (Kordick et al. 1999), deer (Little et al. 1998), rodents (Zeidner et al. 2000), cattle (Marufu et al. 2010) and horses (Parola, Davoust, and Raoult 2005).

Co-infections within ticks and competitive or facilitative interactions among microbes can affect the colonization and transmission of other tick-borne pathogens (Lively et al. 2005; Burgdorfer, Hayes, and Mavros 1981; Macaluso et al. 2002; de la Fuente, Blouin, and Kocan 2003; Ginsberg 2008) and the severity of ensuing disease (Korenberg 2004). For example, *Ixodes* ticks may be simultaneously infected by *B. burgdorferi* and other *Borrelia* species, *B. microti*, *A. phagocytophilum*, *Bartonella henselae* and Powassan virus (Tokarz et al. 2010; Goodman, Dennis, and Sionenshine 2005). Similarly, *Amblyomma* ticks may simultaneously harbor *Borrelia lonestari*, *Ehrlichia spp.*, and *Rickettsia amblyommii* (Heise, Elshahed, and Little 2010; Clay et al. 2008; Castellaw et al. 2010). If colonization of ticks by a particular microbe leads to the exclusion or facilitation of other microbes, this would be manifested as a significant statistical deviation from random co-occurrence. For example, Mather et al. (Mather, Riberiro, and Spielman 1987) suggested that the agents of Lyme Disease and Babesiosis occurred together in ticks more frequently than expected. In contrast, Schauber et al. (Schauber et al. 1998) found that infection of *I. scapularis* by *B. burgdorferi* and *A. phagocytophilum* were independent of each other. Likewise, *A. phagocytophilum* and *B. burgdorferi* were acquired by mice regardless of their prior infection status by the opposite agent and were transmitted independently (Levin and Fish 2000).

Analysis of microbial exclusion or facilitation requires explicit re-porting of co-infection rates. In a recent meta-analysis, 44% of the *Ixo-des* tick populations (8 of 18) meeting criteria for inclusion significantly deviated from expected co-infection frequencies under the assumption of independent infection of *A. phagocytophilum* and *B. burgdorferi* (Civitello, Rynkiewicz, and Clay 2010; Ginsberg 2008). In contrast, there was no evidence of deviation from expected rates of co-occurrence of five microbial taxa in *Amblyomma americanum* (Clay et al. 2008). However, the *Coxiella* endosymbiont occurred at 100% prevalence and two recognized human pathogens (*E. chaffeensis* and *B. lonestari*) occurred at very low frequencies, leading to limited statistical power to detect deviations from independent association.

Competition and crossover of vertebrate host immune response may be greatest between closely related strains (Barthold 1999; Pal et al. 2001). For example, infection by some Spotted Fever Group *Rickettsia* in *Dermacentor variabilis* prevents establishment and vertical transmission of related *Rickettsia* (Macaluso et al. 2002) see also (Burgdorfer, Hayes, and Mavros 1981). Price (Price 1953) described a different form of interaction between virulent and non virulent rickettsiae where guinea pigs injected with both forms were protected from the effects of the virulent rickettsiae, possibly as a result of immunological cross-protection. We expect that vertically-transmitted tick endosymbionts should inhibit or exclude pathogens if those pathogens cause some harm to tick hosts (e.g., Niebylski, Peacock, and Schwan 1999). It is to the evolutionary benefit of vertically-transmitted endosymbionts to exclude pathogens from the tick microbial community because infection by a virulent pathogen condemns that endosymbiont community to extinction (Lively et al. 2005). It is clear that complex communities of microorganisms can coordinate activities within hosts or interfere with other microbes via cell-cell communication, and such mechanisms may be relevant to the interactions between tick-borne endosymbionts and pathogens (Fuqua and Greenberg 2002).

Overall, these studies demonstrate that ticks harbor a diversity of pathogens and symbionts, potentially allowing for ecological interactions among microbes within ticks. Microbial interactions could affect pathogen prevalence and transmission within tick populations. The role of microbial interactions in the organization of microbial communities within vectors and hosts needs further critical evaluation. An important first step is the evaluation and enumeration of microbial diversity within ticks.

## Diverse Microbiome of Ticks

In preliminary studies of eastern North American ticks, we have examined the prokaryotic diversity of ticks by 16S rRNA tag sequencing using a 454 approach for amplicons from DNA extracts of *A. americanum*, *D. variabilis* and *I. scapularis* collected from the wild. All individuals were adult, questing ticks that were rigorously surface sterilized before DNA extraction and sample preparation. The proportion of annotated sequences corresponding to the 10 most frequent taxa are presented in Figure A8-3 for each species. The number of sequences from a given taxon is presumed to reflect the density of that microbe within the tick. For *A. americanum*, the most abundant sequences were from the *Coxiella* endosymbiont (approx. 40% of all sequences) with *Rickettsia* being the second most common (approx. 5% of total), in good agreement with our direct probing data (Clay et al. 2008). We did not distinguish species of *Rickettsia* (and other groups) with accuracy so only present generic classifications. More than 40% of the identified sequences were from a large variety of other microbes. For *D. variabilis*, an *Arsenophonus* endosymbiont was the most frequently identified prokaryote followed by *Methylobacterium* and *Francisella*. Nearly 40% of the identified sequences were from a large number of rare taxa. Finally, for *I. scapularis*, *Rickettsia* represented nearly 75% of the total sequences with *Bacillus* making up approximately 10% of the total. The "other" category was relatively small in *Ixodes*.

The prevalence of prokaryotes across individual ticks provides another measure of the tick microbiome (Figure A8-4). 100% of the sampled *A. americanum* ticks were host to *Coxiella* with over 90% host also to *Methylobacterium* and *Sphingomonas*. 75% were infected by *Rickettsia*. Notably, *Rhizobium*, usually associated with nitrogen fixation, was also detected in 75% of the sampled ticks. For *D. variabilis*, the three most prevalent microbes were *Methylobacterium*, *Francisella* and *Sphingomonas*, each found from 19 of 22 (86%) sampled ticks. Three-quarters of *I. scapularis* hosted *Rickettsia* with no other microbe found in greater than 53% of the samples. *Bradyrhizobium*, another known N-fixing group, was found in 37% of the sampled *Ixodes* ticks. Although these findings are preliminary and subject to modification based on additional experiments, they do clearly indicate the potentially significant microbial diversity in ticks.

Known human pathogens were occasionally detected (data not shown because of their low density and prevalence) including *Ehrlichia* from *Amblyomma* and *Borrelia* from *Ixodes*. In *Amblyomma* we also occasionally detected sequences from *Cardinium*, another commonly-reported arthropod endosymbiont (Duron et al. 2008) that has never before been reported from ticks. *Arsenophonus* is another widespread insect endosymbiont (Novakova, Hypsa, and Moran 2009) that has recently been reported from several tick species (Dergousoff and Chilton 2010; Grindle et al. 2003; Clay et al. 2008). While our results are preliminary and need to be repeated with a larger sample of tick species and individuals, they clearly point to the fact that the dominant members of the tick microbiome are endosymbionts and/or microbes of unknown specificity and function. A similar result was recently obtained by Andreotti et al. (2011), who used 16S pyrosequencing to enumerate bacterial diversity in

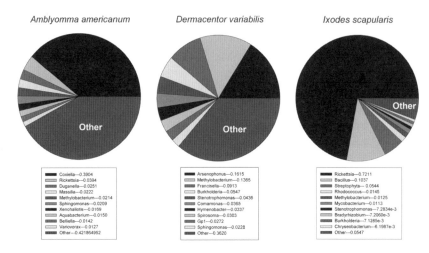

**FIGURE A8-3** Density of annotated bacterial sequences in *Amblyomma americanum* (N=32), *Dermacentor variabilis* (N=22) and *Ixodes scapularis* (N=19) based on 454 sequencing. All ticks were collected from various sites in Indiana. The top 10 most abundant sequences are given for each species; other indicates all remaining sequences.
SOURCE: Clay and Fuqua, unpublished.

the cattle tick, Rhipicephalus (Boophilus) microplus. They found from 53–61 bacterial genera in adult males, eggs and females, respectively, with the very large majority not typically recognized as tick-borne pathogens. It is likely that some of these microbes play a nutritional role by helping to provision critical amino acids, vitamins, or otherwise help ticks survive on a limited diet of blood. Parallel microbiome studies of sap-sucking insects point to a critical role for nutritional endosymbionts, and a recurrent theme of convergent evolution for these symbionts (Sabree, Kambhampati, and Moran 2009; Oliver et al. 2010).

*Future Directions*

Ticks represent a compelling yet challenging system for the study of microbiomes and microbial interactions. They require blood meals prior to molting, their symbionts are difficult to cure and to deliberately inoculate, and their genomes are highly complex. The microbes that colonize ticks also can be very difficult to work with since many have not yet been cultivated or are obligate intracellular symbionts. Little is currently known about the

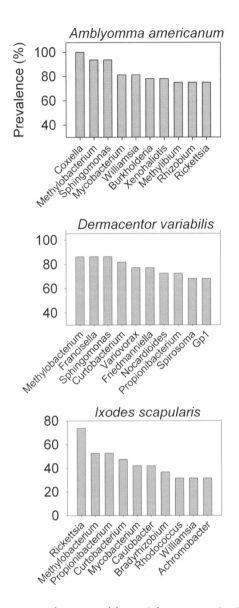

**FIGURE A8-4** Density of annotated bacterial sequences in *Amblyomma americanum* (N=32), *Dermacentor variabilis* (N=22) and *Ixodes scapularis* (N=19) based on 454 sequencing. All ticks were collected from various sites in Indiana. The top 10 most abundant sequences are given for each species; other indicates all remaining sequences.
SOURCE: Clay and Fuqua, unpublished.

roles and activities of many of these microorganisms. Additionally, they can have plastic genetic content, and the features which separate a benign commensal from a significant pathogen are not always clear or well understood. Now that it is clear that there can be multiple microorganisms colonizing the same tick and even the same tissues, the prospects for genetic exchange between these microbes are quite distinct, and it is conceivable that an otherwise benign commensal microbe might acquire virulence functions through this route. Likewise, synergistic or antagonistic interactions between microbes may be manifested by the emergence of new polymicrobial diseases or, alternatively, the decline of a current disease agent.

Although more efficient arthropod systems exist for fundamental investigations into microbial-host interactions, few have the human health impact of ticks and the microbes they vector. Ultimately, it is the importance of ticks to human health that drives active research in this area rather than their utility as a model system. The increasing availability of genomic information for ticks and tick-associated microbes creates significant opportunities to broaden the range of analyses that can be performed. Several tick-vectored pathogens have had their genomes sequenced (Seshadri et al. 2003) and several whole tick genome sequences should be forthcoming (Guerrero et al. 2006; Pagel Van Zee et al. 2007). Genomic sequencing of non-pathogenic symbionts is thus far less common, but would add to the understanding of the tick-borne community, affording opportunities for comparative genomics between related pathogens and non-pathogens, and yielding insights into acquisition and transmission processes. In addition, the ability to simultaneously evaluate tick gene expression as well as those of their resident microbiota, through DNA microarrays and RNA-Seq, should begin to unravel these tight and stable arthropod-microbe interactions.

As with other efforts rooted in genomic science a major hurdle lies within the bioinformatics. Acquisition of sequence or expression data is no longer rate limiting, but rather the ability to distill the potentially massive amount of data down to manageable segments or significant patterns is very challenging, and efficient progress will require interdisciplinary teams of microbiologists, epidemiologists and bioinformaticians.

While technological advances and deep sequencing has revealed unsuspected microbial diversity, many basic questions remain unanswered. What are the evolutionary origins and means of spread of these microbes? What is their functional role or are they simply highly abundant guest commensals? For example, *Methylobacterium* was highly represented in all tick sequences and occurred at very high prevalence in all tick species examined (Figures A8-3 and A8-4). What is the functional role of the highly abundant endosymbionts such as *Arsenophonus*, *Coxiella*, *Francisella* and *Rickettsia*? What distinguishes hereditary endosymbionts from virulent human pathogens (e.g.. *Coxiella* endosymbiont of *A. americanum* vs. *C. burnetti* (Jasinskas, Zhong, and Barbour 2007; Klyachko et al. 2007; Seshadri et al. 2003)? Could horizontal gene exchange between related pathogens and endosymbionts give rise to new virulent pathogens? More generally, are there characteristic microbial communities associated with different tick species and what regulates the structure of these tick-associated microbial communities? Addressing these questions will require more genomic data from non-pathogens combined with efficient inoculation and disinfection strategies. Greater understanding of the dynamics and organization of tick-associated microbial communities may also contribute to the development of more accurate epidemiological and disease risk models.

The increasing homogenization of Earth's biota and human domination of terrestrial ecosystems may be increasing, rather than decreasing human health risks. Ticks and their pathogens are highly dispersible and thrive in many human-dominated habitats. Increasing wildlife populations, such as deer and turkey, may also contribute increasing risk of tick encounters (Childs and Paddock 2003). For example, annual incidence of Lyme disease is increasing despite greater awareness and prompt medical responses. Climate change may further alter geographical ranges of ticks, pathogens and vertebrate hosts (Randolph 2010), potentially leading to host and vector shifts of tick-associated microbes and the composition of their microbial communities. Tick-borne pathogens are just one component of larger, diverse microbial communities. Genetic exchange between pathogens and symbionts, exchange of virulence factors, new mechanisms for contagious transmission and new host associations all need to considered in light of larger scale ecological and environmental changes.

## References

Adar, Y. Y., M. Simaan, and S. Ulitzur. 1992. Formation of the LuxR protein in the *Vibrio fischeri lux* system is controlled by HtpR through the GroESL proteins. *Journal of Bacteriology* 174 (22):7138-7143.

Alekseev, A. N., H. V. Dubinina, I. Van De Pol, and L. M. Schouls. 2001. Identification of *Ehrlichia* spp, and *Borrelia burgdorferi* in *Ixodes* ticks in the Baltic regions of Russia. *Journal of Clinical Microbiology* 39 (6):2237-2242.

Anderson, B. E., J. E. Dawson, D. C. Jones, and K. H. Wilson. 1991. *Ehrlichia chaffeensis*, a new species associated with Human Ehrlichiosis. *Journal of Clinical Microbiology* 29 (12):2838-2842.

Andreotti, R., A. A. P. de Leon, S. E. Dowd, F. D. Guerrero, K. G. Bendele, and G. A. Scoles. 2011. Assessment of bacterial diversity in the cattle tick Rhipicephalus (Boophilus) microplus through tag-encoded pyrosequencing. BMC Microbiology 11:6.

Barthold, S. W. 1999. Specificity of infection-induced immunity among *Borrelia burgdorferi* sensu late species. *Infection and Immunity* 67 (1):36-42.

Belongia, E. A., K. D. Reed, P. D. Mitchell, C. P. Kolbert, D. H. Persing, J. S. Gill, and J. J. Kazmierczak. 1997. Prevalence of granulocytic *Ehrlichia* infection among white-tailed deer in Wisconsin. *Journal of Clinical Microbiology* 35:1465-1468.

Beninati, T., N. Lo, L. Sacchi, C. Genchi, H. Noda, and C. Bandi. 2004. A novel alpha-proteobacterium resides in the mitochondria of ovarian cells of the tick *Ixodes ricinus*. *Applied and Environmental Microbiology* 70 (5):2596-2602.

Benson, M. J., J. D. Gawronski, D. E. Eveleigh, and D. R. Benson. 2004. Intracellular symbionts and other bacteria associated with deer ticks (*Ixodes scapularis*) from Nantucket and Wellfleet, Cape Cod, Massachusetts. *Applied and Environmental Microbiology* 70 (1):616-20.

Bishop, R., A. Musoke, S. Morzaria, M. Gardner, and V. Nene. 2004. *Theileria*: intracellular protozoan parasites of wild and domestic ruminants transmitted by ixodid ticks. *Parasitology* 129:S271-S283.

Brackney, M. M., A. A. Marfin, J. E. Staples, L. Stallones, T. Keefe, W. C. Black, and G. L. Campbell. 2010. Epidemiology of Colorado Tick Fever in Montana, Utah, and Wyoming, 1995-2003. *Vector-Borne and Zoonotic Diseases* 10 (4):381-385.

Burgdorfer, W., A. G. Barbour, S. F. Hayes, J. L. Benach, E. Grunwaldt, and J. P. Davis. 1982. Lyme Disease - A tick-borne spirochetosis. *Science* 216 (4552):1317-1319.

Burgdorfer, W., S. F. Hayes, and A. J. Mavros. 1981. Nonpathogenic rickettsiae in *Dermacentor andersoni*: a limiting factor for the distribution of *Rickettsia rickettsii*. In *Rickettsiae and Rickettsial Diseases*, edited by W. Burgdorfer and R. L. Anacker. New York: Academic Press.

Burkot, T. R., G. R. Mullen, R. Anderson, B. S. Schneider, C. M. Happ, and N. S. Zeidner. 2001. *Borrelia lonestari* DNA in adult *Amblyomma americanum* ticks, Alabama. *Emerging Infectious Disease* 7:471-473.

Carmichael, J. R., and P. A. Fuerst. 2006. A rickettsial mixed infection in a *Dermacentor variabilis* tick from Ohio. In *Century of Rickettsiology: Emerging, Reemerging Rickettsioses, Molecular Diagnostics, and Emerging Veterinary Rickettsioses*, edited by K. E. Hechemy, J. A. Oteo, D. Raoult, D. Silverman and J. R. Blanco.

Castellaw, A. H., J. Showers, J. Goddard, E. F. Chenney, and A. S. Varela-Stokes. 2010. Detection of Vector-Borne Agents in Lone Star Ticks, *Amblyomma americanum* (Acari: Ixodidae), From Mississippi. *Journal of Medical Entomology* 47 (3):473-476.

Charrel, R. N., H. Attoui, A. M. Butenko, J. C. Clegg, V. Deubel, T. V. Frolova, E. A. Gould, T. S. Gritsun, F. X. Heinz, M. Labuda, V. A. Lashkevich, V. Loktev, A. Lundkvist, D. V. Lvov, C. W. Mandl, M. Niedrig, A. Papa, V. S. Petrov, A. Plyusnin, S. Randolph, J. Suss, V. I. Zlobin, and X. de Lamballerie. 2004. Tick-borne virus diseases of human interest in Europe. *Clinical Microbiology and Infection* 10 (12):1040-1055.

Childs, J. E., and C. D. Paddock. 2003. The ascendancy of *Amblyomma americanum* as a vector of pathogens affecting humans in the United States. *Annual Review of Entomology* 48:307-37.

Civitello, D. J., E. Rynkiewicz, and K. Clay. 2010. Meta-analysis of co-infections in ticks. *Israel Journal of Ecology and Evolution* (in press).

Clay, K., O. Klyachko, N. Grindle, D. Civitello, D. Oleske, and C. Fuqua. 2008. Microbial communities and interactions in the lone star tick, *Amblyomma americanum*. *Molecular Ecology* 17:4371-4381.

Clements, K. D., and S. Bullivant. 1991. An unusual symbiont from the gut of surgeonfishes may be the largest known prokaryote. *Journal of Bacteriology* 173:5359-5362.

Colbourne, J. K., B. D. Eads, J. Shaw, E. Bohuski, D. J. Bauer, and J. Andrews. 2007. Sampling *Daphnia*'s expressed genes: preservation, expansion and invention of crustacean genes with reference to insect genomes. *BMC Genomics* 8:217.

Dale, C., and N. A. Moran. 2006. Molecular interactions between bacterial symbionts and their hosts. *Cell* 126 (3):453-65.

de la Fuente, J., E. F. Blouin, and K. M. Kocan. 2003. Infection exclusion of the rickettsial pathogen anaplasma marginale in the tick vector *Dermacentor variabilis*. *Clinical and Diagnostic Laboratory Immunology* 10 (1):182-4.

Dergousoff, S. J., and N. B. Chilton. 2010. Detection of a new *Arsenophonus*-type bacterium in Canadian populations of the Rocky Mountain wood tick, Dermacentor andersoni. *Experimental and Applied Acarology* 52 (1):85-91.

Dillon, R. J., and V. M. Dillon. 2004. The gut bacteria of insects: Nonpathogenic interactions. *Annual Review of Entomology* 49:71-92.

Douglas, A. E. 1998. Nutritional interactions in insect-microbial symbioses: Aphids and their symbiotic bacteria Buchnera. *Annual Review of Entomology* 43:17-37.

Duron, O., D. Bouchon, S. Boutin, L. Bellamy, L. Q. Zhou, J. Engelstadter, and G. D. Hurst. 2008. The diversity of reproductive parasites among arthropods: *Wolbachia* do not walk alone. *Bmc Biology* 6.

Duron, O., T. E. Wilkes, and G. D. D. Hurst. 2010. Interspecific transmission of a male-killing bacterium on an ecological timescale. *Ecology Letters* 13 (9):1139-1148.

Ebel, G. D. 2010. Update on Powassan Virus: Emergence of a North American Tick-Borne Flavivirus. *Annual Review of Entomology* 55:95-110.

Eisen, L. 2008. Climate change and tick-borne diseases: A research field in need of long-term empirical field studies. *International Journal of Medical Microbiology* 298:12-18.

Eisen, L., A. M. Meyer, and R. J. Eisen. 2007. Climate-based model predicting acarological risk of encountering the human-biting adult life stage of *Dermacentor andersoni* (Acari : Ixodidae) in a key habitat type in Colorado. *Journal of Medical Entomology* 44 (4):694-704.

Epis, S., D. Sassera, T. Beninati, N. Lo, L. Beati, J. Piesman, L. Rinaldi, K. D. McCoy, A. Torina, L. Sacchi, E. Clementi, M. Genchi, S. Magnino, and C. Bandi. 2008. Midichloria mitochondrii is widespread in hard ticks (Ixodidae) and resides in the mitochondria of phylogenetically diverse species. *Parasitology* 135 (4):485-494.

Florin-Christensen, M., and L. Schnittger. 2009. Piroplasmids and ticks: a long-lasting intimate relationship. *Frontiers in Bioscience* 14:3064-3073.

Fuqua, C., and E. P. Greenberg. 2002. Listening in on bacteria: Acyl-homoserine lactone signalling. *Nature Reviews Molecular Cell Biology* 3 (9):685-695.

Ginsberg, H. S. 2008. Potential effects of mixed infections in ticks on transmission dynamics of pathogens: comparative analysis of published records. *Experimental and Applied Acarology* 46 (1-4):29-41.

Goethert, H. K., and S. R. Telford. 2005. A new *Francisella* (Beggiatiales : Francisellaceae) inquiline within *Dermacentor variabilis* say (Acari : Ixodidae). *Journal of Medical Entomology* 42 (3):502-505.

Goodman, J. L., D. T. Dennis, and D. E. Sionenshine, eds. 2005. *Tick-borne disease of humans*. Washington, D.C.: ASM Press.

Grindle, N., J.J. Tyner, K. Clay, and C. Fuqua. 2003. Identification of *Arsenophonus*-type bacteria from the dog tick *Dermacentor variabilis*. *Journal of Invertebrate Pathology* 83:264-266.

Guerrero, F. D., V. M. Nene, J. E. George, S. C. Barker, and P. Willadsen. 2006. Sequencing a new target genome: the *Boophilus microplus* (Acari: Ixodidae) genome project. *Journal of Medical Entomology* 43 (1):9-16.

Hammer, B., A. Moter, O. Kahl, G. Alberti, and U. B. Gobel. 2001. Visualization of *Borrelia burgdorferi sensu lato* by fluorescence in situ hybridization (FISH) on whole-body sections of *Ixodes ricinus* ticks and gerbil skin biopsies. *Microbiology* 147 (Pt 6):1425-36.

Heise, S. R., M. S. Elshahed, and S. E. Little. 2010. Bacterial diversity in *Amblyomma americanum* (Acari: Ixodidae) with a focus on members of the genus *Rickettsia*. *Journal of Medical Entomology* 47 (2):258-268.

Hilgenboecker, K., P. Hammerstein, P. Schlattmann, A. Telschow, and J. H. Werren. 2008. How many species are infected with *Wolbachia*? - a statistical analysis of current data. *FEMS Microbiology Letters* 281 (2):215-220.

Hill, C. A., and J. A. Gutierrez. 2000. Analysis of the expressed genome of the Lone Star Tick, *Amblyomma americanum* (Acari: Ixodidae) using an expressed sequence tag approach. *Micro. Comp. Genomics* 5:89-101.

Hugenholz, P., B. M. Goebel, and N. R. Pace. 1998. Impact of culture-independent studies on the emerging phylogenetic view of bacterial diversity. *Journal of Bacteriology* 180:4765-4774.

Jaenike, J., R. Unckless, S. N. Cockburn, L. M. Boelio, and S. J. Perlman. 2010. Adaptation via symbiosis: Recent spread of a *Drosophila* defensive symbiont. *Science* 329 (5988):212-215.

Jasinskas, A., J. Zhong, and A. G. Barbour. 2007. Highly prevalent *Coxiella* sp. bacterium in the tick vector *Amblyomma americanum*. *Applied and Environmental Microbiology* 73 (1):334-6.

Klyachko, O., B. D. Stein, N. Grindle, K. Clay, and C. Fuqua. 2007. Localization and visualization of a coxiella-type symbiont within the lone star tick, Amblyomma americanum. *Applied and Environmental Microbiology* 73 (20):6584-94.

Kordick, S. K., E. B. Breitschwerdt, B. C. Hegarty, K. L. Southwick, C. M. Colitz, S. I. Hancock, J. M. Bradley, R. Rumbough, J. T. McPherson, and J. N. MacCormack. 1999. Coinfection with multiple tick-borne pathogens in a Walker Hound kennel in North Carolina. *Journal of Clinical Microbiology* 37:2631-2638.

Korenberg, E. I. 2004. Problems in the study and prophylaxis of mixed infections transmitted by ixodid ticks. *International Journal of Medical Microbiology* 293:80-85.

LaSala, P. R., and M. Holbrook. 2010. Tick-Borne Flaviviruses. *Clinics in Laboratory Medicine* 30 (1):221-+.

Levin, M. L., and D. Fish. 2000. Acquisition of coinfection and simultaneous transmission of *Borrelia burgdorferi* and *Ehrlichia phagocytophila* by I*xodes scapularis* ticks. *Infection and Immunity* 68:2183-2186.

Little, S. E., D. E. Stallknecht, J. M. Lockhart, J. E. Dawson, and W. R. Davidson. 1998. Natural coinfection of a white-tailed deer (*Odocoileus virginianus*) population with three *Ehrlichia* spp. *Journal of Parasitology* 84:897-901.

Lively, C. M., K. Clay, W. J. Wade, and C. Fuqua. 2005. Competitive coexistence of vertically and horizontally transmitted parasites. *Evolutionary Ecology Research* 7:1183-1190.

Loftis, A. D., T. R. Mixson, E. Y. Stromdahl, M. J. Yabsley, L. E. Garrison, P. C. Williamson, R. R. Fitak, P. A. Fuerst, D. J. Kelly, and K. W. Blount. 2008. Geographic distribution and genetic diversity of the Ehrlichia sp from Panola Mountain in Amblyomma americanum. *Bmc Infectious Diseases* 8.

Macaluso, K. R., D. E. Sonenshine, S. M. Ceraul, and A. F. Azad. 2002. Rickettsial infection in *Dermocentor variabilis* (Acari:Ixodidae) inhibits transovarial transmission of a second *Rickettsia*. *Journal of Medical Entomology* 39:809-813.

Maiden, M. C., J. A. Bygraves, E. Feil, G. Morelli, J. E. Russell, R. Urwin, Q. Zhang, J. Zhou, K. Zurth, D. A. Caugant, I. M. Feavers, M. Achtman, and B. G. Spratt. 1998. Multilocus sequence typing: a portable approach to the identification of clones within populations of pathogenic microorganisms. *Proceedings of the National Academy of Sciences, USA* 95 (6):3140-5.

Margos, G., A. G. Gatewood, D. M. Aanensen, K. Hanincova, D. Terekhova, S. A. Vollmer, M. Cornet, J. Piesman, M. Donaghy, A. Bormane, M. A. Hurn, E. J. Feil, D. Fish, S. Casjens, G. P. Wormser, I. Schwartz, and K. Kurtenbach. 2008. MLST of housekeeping genes captures geographic population structure and suggests a European origin of *Borrelia burgdorferi*. *Proceedings of the National Academy of Sciences, USA* 105 (25):8730-5.

Marufu, M. C., M. Chimonyo, K. Dzama, and C. Mapiye. 2010. Seroprevalence of tick-borne diseases in communal cattle reared on sweet and sour rangelands in a semi-arid area of South Africa. *Veterinary Journal* 184 (1):71-76.

Masuzawa, T., I. G. Kharitonenkov, Y. Okamoto, T. Fukui, and N. Ohashi. 2008. Prevalence of *Anaplasma phagocytophilum* and its coinfection with *Borrellia afzefii* in *Ixodes ricinus* and *Ixodes persulcatus* ticks inhabiting Tver Province (Russia) - a sympatric region for both tick species. *Journal of Medical Microbiology* 57 (8):986-991.

Mather, T. N., J. M. C. Riberiro, and A. Spielman. 1987. Lyme disease and babesiosis: acaricide focused on potentially infected ticks. *American Journal of Tropical Medicine Hygene* 36:609-614.

McDiarmid, L., T. Petney, B. Dixon, and R. Andrews. 2000. Range expansion of the tick *Amblyomma triguttatum*, an Australian vector for Q fever. *International Journal of Parasitology* 30:791-793.

Mediannikov, O., Z. Sekeyova, M. L. Birg, and D. Raoult. 2010. A Novel Obligate Intracellular Gamma-Proteobacterium Associated with Ixodid Ticks, *Diplorickettsia massiliensis*, Gen. Nov., Sp Nov. *Plos One* 5 (7).

Mitchell, P. D., K. D. Reed, and J. M. Hofkes. 1996. Immunoserologic evidence of coinfection with *Borrelia burgdorferi*, *Babesia microti* and human granulocytic *Ehrlichia* species in residents of Wisconsin and Minnesota. *Journal of Clinical Microbiology* 34:724-727.

Mixson, T. R., S. R. Campbell, J. S. Gill, H. S. Ginsberg, M. V. Reichard, T. L. Schulze, and G. A. Dasch. 2006. Prevalence of *Ehrlichia*, *Borrelia*, and Rickettsial agents in *Amblyomma americanum* (*Acari*: *Ixodidae*) collected from nine states. *Journal of Medical Entomology* 43 (6):1261-8.

Montllor, C. B., A. Maxmen, and A. H. Purcell. 2002. Facultative bacterial endosymbionts benefit pea aphids *Acyrthosiphon pisum* under heat stress. *Ecological Entomology* 27 (2):189-195.

Moreno, C. X., F. Moy, T. J. Daniels, H. P. Godfrey, and F. C. Cabello. 2006. Molecular analysis of microbial communities identified in different developmental stages of *Ixodes scapularis* ticks from Westchester and Dutchess Counties, New York. *Environmental Microbiology* 8 (5):761-772.

Morimoto, S., T. J. Kurtti, and H. Noda. 2006. In vitro cultivation and antibiotic susceptibility of a *Cytophaga*-like intracellular symbiote isolated from the tick *Ixodes scapularis*. *Current Microbiology* 52 (4):324-329.

Morozova, O., and M. A. Marra. 2008. Applications of next-generation sequencing technologies in functional genomics. *Genomics* 92 (5):255-64.

Muyzer, G., and K. Smalla. 1998. Application of denaturing gradient gel electrophoresis (DGGE) and temperature gradient gel electrophoresis (TGGE) in microbial ecology. *Antonie van Leeuwenhoek* 73:127-141.

Neelakanta, G., H. Sultana, D. Fish, J. F. Anderson, and E. Fikrig. 2010. *Anaplasma phagocytophilum* induces *Ixodes scapularis* ticks to express an antifreeze glycoprotein gene that enhances their survival in the cold. *Journal of Clinical Investigation* 120 (9):3179-3190.

Niebylski, M. L., M. G. Peacock, and T. G. Schwan. 1999. Lethal effect of *Rickettsia rickettsii* on its tick vector *Dermacentor andersoni*. *Applied and Environmental Microbiology* 65:773-778.

Niebylski, M. L., M. G. Peacock, E. R. Fischer, S. F. Porcella, and T. G. Schwan. 1997. Characterization of an endosymbiont infecting wood ticks, *Dermacentor andersoni*, as a member of the genus *Francisella*. *Applied and Environmental Microbiology* 63:3933-3940.

Noda, H., U. G. Munderloh, and T. J. Kurtti. 1997. Endosymbionts of ticks and their relationship to *Wolbachia* spp. and tick-borne pathogens of humans and animals. *Applied and Environmental Microbiology* 63:3926-3932.

Novakova, E., V. Hypsa, and N. A. Moran. 2009. *Arsenophonus*, an emerging clade of intra-cellular symbionts with a broad host distribution. *Bmc Microbiology* 9.

Nyarko, E., D. J. Grab, and J. S. Dumler. 2006. Anaplasma phagocytophilum - infected neu-trophils enhance transmigration of Borrelia burgdorferi across the human blood brain barrier in vitro. *International Journal for Parasitology* 36 (5):601-605.

Oliver, K. M., P. H. Degnan, G. R. Burke, and N. A. Moran. 2010. Facultative symbionts in aphids and the horizontal transfer of ecologically important traits. *Annual Review of Entomology* 55:247-266.

Oliver, K. M., P. H. Degnan, M. S. Hunter, and N. A. Moran. 2009. Bacteriophages Encode Factors Required for Protection in a Symbiotic Mutualism. *Science* 325 (5943):992-994.

Oliver, K. M., N. A. Moran, and M. S. Hunter. 2005. Variation in resistance to parasitism in aphids is due to symbionts not host genotype. *Proceedings of the National Academy of Sciences U. S. A.*102 (36):12795-12800.

Osborn, A. M., E. R. B. Moore, and K. N. Timmis. 2000. An evaluation of terminal-restriction fragment length polymorphism (T-RFLP) analysis for the study of microbial community structure and dynamics. *Environmental Microbiology* 2:39-50.

Paddock, C. D., and M. J. Yabsley. 2007. Ecological havoc, the rise of white-tailed deer, and the emergence of Amblyomma americanum - Associated zoonoses in the United States. In *Wildlife and Emerging Zoonotic Diseases: The Biology, Circumstances and Conse-quences of Cross-Species Transmission.*

Pagel Van Zee, J., N. S. Geraci, F. D. Guerrero, S. K. Wikel, J. J. Stuart, V. M. Nene, and C. A. Hill. 2007. Tick genomics: the *Ixodes* genome project and beyond. *International Journal of Parasitology* 37 (12):1297-305.

Pal, U., R. R. Montgomery, D. Lusitani, P. Voet, V. Weynants, S. E. Malawista, Y. Lobet, and E. Fikrig. 2001. Inhibition of *Borrelia burgdorferi*-tick interactions in vivo by outer surface protein A antibody. *Journal of Immunology* 166 (12):7398-7403.

Parola, P., B. Davoust, and D. Raoult. 2005. Tick- and flea-borne rickettsial emerging zoono-ses. *Veterinary Research* 36 (3):469-492.

Perlman, S. J., M. S. Hunter, and E. Zchori-Fein. 2006. The emerging diversity of Rickettsia. *Proceedings of the Royal Society B-Biological Sciences* 273 (1598):2097-2106.

Perotti, M. A., H. K. Clarke, B. D. Turner, and H. R. Braig. 2006. Rickettsia as obligate and mycetomic bacteria. *Faseb Journal* 20 (13):2372-+.

Piesman, J., and C. M. Happ. 2001. The efficacy of co-feeding as a means of maintaining *Borrelia burgdorferi*: a North American model system. *Journal of Vector Ecology* 26 (2):216-220.

Price, W. H. 1953. Interference phenomenon in animal infections with rickettsiae of Rocky Mountain spotted fever. *Proceedings of the Society for Experimental Biology and Medi-cine* 82:180-184.

Randolph, S. E. 2010. To what extent has climate change contributed to the recent epidemiol-ogy of tick-borne diseases? *Veterinary Parasitology* 167 (2-4):92-94.

Randolph, S. E., and D. J. Rogers. 2010. The arrival, establishment and spread of exotic dis-eases: patterns and predictions. *Nature Reviews Microbiology* 8 (5):361-371.

Rodriguez-Valle, M., A. Lew-Tabor, C. Gondro, P. Moolhuijzen, M. Vance, F. D. Guerrero, M. Bellgard, and W. Jorgensen. 2010. Comparative microarray analysis of *Rhipicephalus* (*Boophilus*) *microplus* expression profiles of larvae pre-attachment and feeding adult female stages on *Bos indicus* and *Bos taurus* cattle. 11:437.

Rondon, M. R., P. R. August, A. D. Bettermann, S. F. Brady, T. H. Grossman, M. R. Liles, K. A. Loiacono, B. A. Lynch, I. A. MacNeil, C. Minor, C. L. Tiong, M. Gilman, M. S. Osburne, J. Clardy, J. Handelsman, and R. M. Goodman. 2000. Cloning the soil metage-nome: a strategy for accessing the genetic and functional diversity of uncultured micro-organisms. *Applied and Environmental Microbiology* 66:2541-2547.

Ronning, C. M., L. Losada, L. Brinkac, J. Inman, R. L. Ulrich, M. Schell, W. C. Nierman, and D. Deshazer. 2010. Genetic and phenotypic diversity in *Burkholderia*: contributions by prophage and phage-like elements. *BMC Microbiology* 10:202.

Sabree, Z. L., S. Kambhampati, and N. A. Moran. 2009. Nitrogen recycling and nutritional provisioning by *Blattabacterium*, the cockroach endosymbiont. *Proceedings of the National Academy of Sciences U. S. A.*106 (46):19521-19526.

Sassera, D., T. Beninati, C. Bandi, E. A. P. Bouman, L. Sacchi, M. Fabbi, and N. Lo. 2006. 'Candidatus *Midichloria mitochondrii*', an endosymbiont of the tick *Ixodes ricinus* with a unique intramitochondrial lifestyle. *International Journal of Systematic and Evolutionary Microbiology* 56:2535-2540.

Schabereiter-Gurtner, C., W. Lubitz, and S. Rölleke. 2003. Application of broad-range 16S rRNA PCR amplification and DGGE fingerprinting for detection of tick-infecting bacteria. *Journal of Microbiological Methods* 52:251-260.

Schauber, E. M., S. J. Gertz, W. T. Maple, and R. S. Ostfeld. 1998. Coinfection of blacklegged ticks (Acari : Ixodidae) in Dutchess County, New York, with the agents of Lyme disease and human granulocytic ehrlichiosis. *Journal of Medical Entomology* 35 (5):901-903.

Schouls, L.M., I. van De Pol, G.T. Rijpkema, and C.S. Schot. 1999. Detection and identification of *Ehrlichia*, *Borrelia burgdorferi* sensu lato, and *Bartonella* species in Dutch *Ixodes ricinus* ticks. *Journal of Clinical Microbiology* 37:2215-2222.

Scoles, G. A. 2004. Phylogenetic analysis of the Francisella-like endosymbionts of Dermacentor ticks. *Journal of Medical Entomology* 41 (3):277-286.

Seshadri, R., I. T. Paulsen, J. A. Eisen, T. D. Read, K. E. Nelson, W. C. Nelson, N. L. Ward, H. Tettelin, T. M. Davidsen, M. J. Beanan, R. T. Deboy, S. C. Daugherty, L. M. Brinkac, R. Madupu, R. J. Dodson, H. M. Khouri, K. H. Lee, H. A. Carty, D. Scanlan, R. A. Heinzen, H. A. Thompson, J. E. Samuel, C. M. Fraser, and J. F. Heidelberg. 2003. Complete genome sequence of the Q-fever pathogen *Coxiella burnetii*. *Proceedings of the National Academy of Sciences U.S.A.* 100 (9):5455-5460.

Sogin, M. L., H. G. Morrison, J. A. Huber, D. Mark Welch, S. M. Huse, P. R. Neal, J. M. Arrieta, and G. J. Herndl. 2006. Microbial diversity in the deep sea and the underexplored "rare biosphere". *Proceedings of the National Academy of Sciences U. S. A.*103 (32):12115-20.

Sonenshine, D. E. 1991. *Biology of Ticks*. Vol. 1. New York: Oxford University Press.

Sonenshine, D. E., and T. N. Mather. 1994. *Ecological Dynamics of Tick-Borne Zoonoses*. New York: Oxford University Press.

Stahl, D. A. 1995. Application of phylogentically base hybridization probes to microbial ecology. *Molecular Ecology* 4:535-542.

Sun, J. M., Q. Y. Liu, L. Lu, G. Q. Ding, J. Q. Guo, G. M. Fu, J. B. Zhang, F. X. Meng, H. X. Wu, X. P. Song, D. S. Ren, D. M. Li, Y. H. Guo, J. Wang, G. C. Li, J. L. Liu, and H. L. Lin. 2008. Coinfection with four genera of bacteria (*Borrelia, Bartonella, Anaplasma*, and *Ehrlichia)* in *Haemaphysalis longicornis* and I*xodes sinensis* Ticks from China. *Vector-Borne and Zoonotic Diseases* 8 (6):791-795.

Sun, L. V., G. A. Scoles, D. Fish, and S. L. O'Neill. 2000. Francisella-like endosymbionts of ticks. *Journal of Invertebrate Pathology* 76:301-303.

Tokarz, R., K. Jain, A. Bennett, T. Briese, and W. I. Lipkin. 2010. Assessment of polymicrobial infections in ticks in New York State. *Vector-Borne and Zoonotic Diseases* 10 (3):217-221.

van Overbeek, L., F. Gassner, C. L. van der Plas, P. Kastelein, U. N. D. Rocha, and W. Takken. 2008. Diversity of *Ixodes ricinus* tick-associated bacterial communities from different forests. *Fems Microbiology Ecology* 66 (1):72-84.

Varela, A. S., M. P. Luttrell, E. W. Howerth, V. A. Moore, W. R. Davidson, D. E. Stallknecht, and S. E. Little. 2004. First culture isolation of *Borrelia lonestari*, putative agent of southern tick-associated rash illness. *Journal of Clinical Microbiology* 42 (3):1163-1169.

Vasanthakumar, A., J. Handelsman, P. D. Schloss, L. S. Bauer, and K. F. Raffa. 2008. Gut microbiota of an invasive subcortical beetle, Agrilus planipennis Fairmarine, across various life stages. *Environmental Entomology* 37 (5):1344-1353.

Wang, M., F. D. Guerrero, G. Pertea, and V. M. Nene. 2007. Global comparative analysis of ESTs from the southern cattle tick, *Rhipicephalus (Boophilus) microplus. BMC Genomics* 8:368.

Weinert, L. A., J. H. Werren, A. Aebi, G. N. Stone, and F. M. Jiggins. 2009. Evolution and diversity of *Rickettsia* bacteria. *Bmc Biology* 7.

Werren, J. H., L. Baldo, and M. E. Clark. 2008. *Wolbachia*: master manipulators of invertebrate biology. *Nature Reviews Microbiology* 6 (10):741-751.

Wormser, G. P., H. W. Horowitz, J. Nowakowski, D. McKenna, J. S. Dumler, S. Varde, I. Schwartz, C. Carbano, and M. AgueroRosenfeld. 1997. Positive Lyme disease serology in patients with clinical and laboratory evidence of human granulocytic ehrlichiosis. *American Journal of Clinical Pathology* 107:142-147.

Yabsley, M. J., T. N. Nims, M. Y. Savage, and L. A. Durden. 2009. Ticks and tick-borne pathogens and putative symbionts of black bears (*Ursus americanus floridanus*) from Georgia and Florida. *Journal of Parasitology* 95 (5):1125-1128.

Zeidner, N. S., T. R. Burkot, R. Massung, W. L. Nicholson, M. C. Dolan, J. S. Rutherford, B. J. Biggerstaff, and G. O. Maupin. 2000. Transmission of the agent of human granulocytic ehrlichiosis by *Ixodes spinipalpis* ticks: Evidence of an enzootic cycle of dual infection with *Borrelia burgdorferi* in northern Colorado. *Journal of Infectious Diseases* 182:616-619.

## A9
## MANAGING SUSPECTED, ATYPICAL LYME DISEASE IN NON-REFERRAL PRACTICES

*Matthew H. Liang, M.D., M.P.H., F.A.C.P., F.A.C.R.*
*Massachusetts Veterans Epidemiology and Research Center,*
*Section of Rheumatology*
*Boston VA Healthcare System, Boston, MA*
*Division of Rheumatology, Immunology and Allergy,*
*Brigham & Women's Hospital, Boston, MA*

### Summary

Lyme disease is the most common vector borne disease in Europe and North America. In the U.S. alone, over 50,000 cases have been reported to the U.S. Centers for Disease Control since 1988 from the Northeast, upper Mideast and far West with some reported incidence rates as high as 1192 cases/100,000 (Nantucket Island, Massachusetts).

Based on actual cost data from the Maryland Eastern Shore from 1997 to 2000, the mean per patient direct medical costs of early-stage LD decreased from \$1,609 to \$464, and the mean per patient direct medical cost of late-stage LD decreased from \$4,240 to \$1,380 (Zhang et al., 2006). The estimated median of all costs (direct medical cost, indirect medical cost, nonmedical cost, and productivity loss) aggregated across all patients, was ~\$281 per patient; as with many cost of illness studies, a small number of LD patients accounted for the majority of the costs.

To approximate the annual economic impact of LD nationwide, these results can be extrapolated to the total number of LD cases reported nationwide, 23,763 LD cases in 2002 corresponds to ~\$203 million (in 2002 dollars). LD cases reported using the CDC surveillance case definition underreport the true incidence; therefore, the estimate is likely to be low. The decline in average cost per LD case is observed in all cost categories, drug costs, hospital days, diagnostic testing, and may be related to successful adoption of personal protection measures and/or prompt consultation and treatment after exposure or tick bite. It may also be reporting bias.

The description of Lyme disease in the U.S. in 1976 and subsequent characterization of its mode of transmission, causative organism and treatment is an important saga in the history of medicine. In theory, Lyme disease could be prevented and eradicated but in practice it continues to grow as a public health problem and many biological and clinical questions remain unanswered. Typical acute Lyme Disease, by definition, is fairly straightforward to diagnose and treat. However, acute Lyme may not present typically and acute Lyme with persistent symptoms respond to recommended antibiotic regimens. Both forms in practice are major challenges in non-referral practices.

## My frame of reference

I live and work in Massachusetts where Lyme Disease can be endemic. Nevertheless, I missed diagnosing chronic Lyme in a physician's wife from Vermont. Her husband and I did internship and residency together, and it has haunted me since. This was an object lesson again that Lyme Disease is always in the differential.

I am a salaried general internist and primary care physician and board-eligible rheumatologist seeing patients since 1969. I am a general internist for patients at the Brigham and Women's Hospital, an academic health center, and in the Veterans Administration. As a clinician-scientist, I study health services, the epidemiology of systemic rheumatic disease, health disparities, determinants of health outcomes, and have done more than 25 investigator-initiated clinical trials.

I also bring the view of a patient with chronic illness having had a six-vessel coronary by-pass operation in 2000 and a strept millerei lung abscess and empyema in 2003 from a dental procedure. I am doing very well, thank you. I am inevitably drawn in as a coach for my extended family when they have a health problem, doing telephone consultations for my three 30+ year old children who work harder than I but are underinsured, internet inhabitants, and use alternative and over the counter therapies whenever they can, as does my bride. I am happy coaching.

## Atypical acute Lyme Disease

A major challenge of ministering to patients in non-referral practices is not missing treatable illnesses that might present atypically. A study of consecutive patients with possible early Lyme disease either self- or physician-referred to a general internist with infectious disease training in a region with endemic Lyme disease (Aucott et al., 2009) suggests that about 39% of such patients do not meet CDC criteria nor alternative diagnostic criteria.

Of these nearly 40% had negative Lyme serology and an acute, viral-like illness without objective findings. Many of these patients had already been treated with antibiotics. In a quarter, another diagnosis could be made, including parvovirus, Ramsay Hunt syndrome or varicella zoster virus. About a third had a rash which did not meet criteria for EM and were thought to be local hypersensitivity reactions to tick bites or nonspecific or non-diagnosable lesions.

EM was the most common presentation of early Lyme disease in this case-series. However, prior misdiagnosis were common, similar to experiences reported from other endemic areas. While 80% of EM in the United States are uniformly red, only 19% have the stereotypical bull's-eye appearance. Typically circular or oval, it can also be triangular, rectangular or distorted in other ways when occurring in areas such as the neck. Atypical EM may appear erythematous with central induration, urticarial-like, confluent red-blue lesions, vesicles, and with central necrosis.

If erythema migrans goes unnoticed, the disease may present months after the initial tick bite when the spirochete has disseminated. Disseminated Lyme disease often has symptoms of malaise, fatigue, or generalized or regional lymphadenopathy. Patients may have multiple, slow-growing erythema migrans lesions. Joint inflammation occurs in up to 70% of untreated patients with dessiminated disease and is typically mono- or oligo-articular, migratory, and involves the large joints and often recurring over several years.

Neurological Lyme involvement manifests as meningitis, cranial neuritis or radiculoneuritis. The most pronounced symptom is painful radiculoneuritis involving the chest or abdomen and like most neuropathies, prominent at night. The facial nerve is the cranial nerve most commonly involved and can be bilateral.

*Diagnosis* (Corapi et al., 2008)

Early Lyme disease is best diagnosed by recognizing an erythema migrans lesion, which is present in 70-90% of cases. Laboratory testing should be used to confirm a clinician's suspicion of Lyme disease rather than to be the sole basis of diagnosis. Serology is often negative early in the disease and may take three to four weeks for IgM antibodies to borrelia to appear and four to six weeks for IgG to be present. The American College of Physicians guidelines indicates that a patient with a high index of suspicion for Lyme disease in an endemic area for the disease may require no testing and that a diagnosis can be made solely on the clinical picture.

Serological testing is used to confirm Lyme disease in patients with disseminated disease with arthritis, carditis, or neurological involvement. Unfortunately the options for testing are not ideal and the results can be unreliable. One study demonstrated that 14-21% of laboratories failed to correctly identify positive samples (Bakken et al., 1997).

A two-test algorithm for active disease and for previous infection using a sensitive enzyme immunoassay (EIA) or immunofluorescent assay (IFA) followed by a Western immunoblot is recommended by the CDC (CDC, 1995). Specimens positive or equivocal by the EIA or IFA should be tested by a standardized Western immunoblot. Specimens negative by a sensitive EIA or IFA need not be tested further. When Western immunoblot is used during the first 4 weeks of disease (early LD), both IgM and IgG procedures should be used. A positive IgM test result alone is not recommended for determining active disease in persons with illness greater than 1 month's duration because the likelihood of a false-positive test result for a current infection is high for these persons. If a patient with suspected early LD has a negative serology, serologic evidence of infection is best sought by obtaining acute and convalescent serum samples. Serum samples from persons with disseminated or late-stage LD almost always have a strong IgG response to Borrelia burgdorferi antigens.

It was recommended that IgM immunoblots be considered positive if two of the following three bands are present: 24 kDa (OspC), 39 kDa (BmpA), and 41 kDa (Fla) (1). It was further recommended that an that IgG immunoblot be considered positive if five of the following 10 bands are present: 18 kDa, 21 kDa (OspC), 28 kDa, 30 kDa, 39 kDa (BmpA), 41 kDa (Fla), 45 kDa, 58 kDa (not GroEL), 66 kDa, and 93 kDa. This serial testing has a specificity of 99-100%, but low sensitivity due to variable interpretation of results across laboratories.

Culture is labor-intensive, expensive, and time-consuming. Polymerase chain reaction (PCR) detects the genetic material of the spirochete; positive results do not neccesarily indicate active infections. PCR may be helpful in suspected cases of co-infection or to confirm a clinical suspicion of Lyme disease. While PCR is useful for identifying the spirochete in skin, the technique is of marginal usefulness, as these cases can be diagnosed clinically.

Therefore, clinicians have to work with the limitations of the technology available. In most situations, as with most diagnostic testing, if the test result will not change how one treats or follows a patient or what they tell them, it should not be done. Serodiagnostics indicate exposures and whether the exposure has been recent or remote. Re-exposure and/or treatment can alter the results. The diagnostic test performance characteristics (i.e., its sensitivity, specificity, predictive value positive, and predictive value negative) of any test or testing algorithm is determined by the prior probability of the disease given a particular combination of symptoms and signs.

*Treatment of early Lyme Disease*

The aims in treating Lyme disease are to relieve symptoms and prevent the late stage complications. Delay in treatment increases a patient's risk for treatment failure. In patients who present with or shortly after a tick bite, the question of antibiotic prophylaxis arises. A randomized, double-blind, placebo-controlled trial in a hyper-endemic area showed that Doxycycline as a single 200 mg dose was associated with fewer cases of subsequent erythema migrans; the primary endpoint of the study (Nadelman et al., 2001). While these results are significant, it is important to note that only a small number of subjects in the control group developed Lyme disease, resulting in a wide confidence interval. Also important is that 30% of patients treated with doxycyline experienced a drug adverse event such as nausea, vomiting, and diarrhea.

The 2006 IDSA guidelines suggest antibiotic prophylaxis only if all of the following four conditions are met: the attached tick is positively identified as an adult or nymphal Ixodes scapularis tick which has been attached for more than 36 hours, prophylaxis can be started within 72 hours of tick removal, local ecologic information demonstrates that local ticks have a borrelia burgdorferi infection rate of greater than 20%, and there are no contraindications to doxycycline use (Wormser et al., 2006). For pregnant or lactating women and children less than 8, in whom doxycycline should not be used, the guidelines do not recommend the use of substitute prophylaxis. Whether or not patients meet the criteria for antibiotic prophylaxis, the guidelines recommend that all patients who remove a tick should be observed for thirty days and treated promptly Lyme disease, human granulocytic anaplasmosis, or babesia.

When a patient presents with signs and symptoms suggestive of early

Lyme disease, whether localized or disseminated, doxycycline, amoxicillin, and cefuroxime axetil are effective. The IDSA recommends 10-21 days of oral doxycycline (100mg twice daily), 14-21 days of amoxicillin (500mg three times daily), or 14-21 days of cefuroxime (500mg twice per day) for the treatment of early, localized or disseminated disease. While 10 days may be a sufficient course of doxycycline, at least two weeks is needed for beta-lactam antibiotics because of their shorter half-lives (Wormser et al., 2003).

Doxycycline is the drug of choice as it is also effective against human granulocytic anaplasmosis, which may occur as a co-infection with Lyme disease. Amoxicillin is used when there is a contra-indication to using doxycycline. When a patient is unable to take both doxycycline and amoxicillin, cefuroxime or erythromycin may be used. Cefuroxime is as efficacious as doxycycline but is more expensive.

A randomized, double-blind, placebo-controlled study of one hundred and eighty patients with erythema migrans compared the efficacy of 10 days of oral doxycycline versus 20 days of oral treatment and combination oral doxycycline and intravenous ceftriaxone. The study concluded that treating patients for 10 days with oral doxycycline was as efficacious as the two other regimens studied (Wormser et al., 2003). More than 83% of patients in each treatment group described complete resolution of symptoms at the 30 month evaluation.

While antibiotics for the treatment of early Lyme disease are effective, 10-17% of patients continue to have problems (Wormser et al., 2003) and it is not clear as to why some patients with early Lyme disease improve and others do not.

Some patients with early Lyme disease have central nervous system involvement, such as radiculopathy, neuropathy, meningitis, or facial nerve palsy. Such patients require treatment with intravenous ceftriaxone (2g once daily) for 10-28 days. Alternatives to ceftriaxone include intravenous penicillin G or intravenous cefotaxime. Ceftriaxone has the advantage of once-daily dosing, making it the preferred agent. Intravenous administration is preferred to ensure adequate penetration of the blood-brain barrier. Data from Europe show that oral regimens, particularly doxycycline are also efficacious in neuroborreliosis. There is no definitive data to establish the superiority of either oral or parenteral therapy in the treatment patients with CNS involvement. Patients with evidence of increased intracranial pressure (papilledema, sixth cranial nerve palsy), may benefit from the addition of steroids, serial lumbar punctures, or CSF shunting. Although antibiotic treatment may not hasten the resolution of facial nerve palsy, treatment is recommended to prevent further sequelae such as Lyme arthritis.

Patients with cardiac involvement, namely first or second-degree atrioventricular block, should be treated with either oral or parenteral antibiotics for 14 days. Patients presenting with syncope, chest pain, or other cardiac symptoms, require hospitalization to allow for continuous monitoring. The degree of heart block associated with Lyme disease is known to fluctuate and therefore careful monitoring is required. Intravenous ceftriaxone is felt to be useful in the management of hospitalized patients with cardiac involvement, but there are no studies addressing this. The placement of a cardiac pacemaker may be indicated in cases of severe heart block. Patients may switched to the standard oral antibiotic treatment for early Lyme disease once they are stable enough to be followed as outpatients.

Lyme arthritis can be treated with either oral or intravenous antibiotics. The majority of patients improve with one month of oral antibiotics, either doxycycline or amoxicillin. If arthritis persists after the initial course of treatment, then a second course should be tried. The improvement may be slow. A minority of patients continue to have arthritic symptoms, and non-steroidal anti-inflammatory drugs (NSAIDs), intra-articular corticosteroid injections, and hydroxychloroquine, methotrexate, or infliximab have been used successfully.

The optimal length of intravenous antibiotics in late Lyme disease has not been determined. A prospective, open-label, randomized, multi-center study with one hundred and forty-three participants compared a 14- to 28-day regimen. All participants had a history of erythema migrans at least 3 months, dermatological, rheumatological, and neurological manifestations of disease, and no prior treatment for Lyme disease. The 14 days of ceftriaxone relieved the symptoms of late Lyme disease in 70% of patients; the same improvement rate was observed in the 28 day treatment group. Patients in both groups had higher cure rates at 12 months than when evaluated at 3 months; demonstrating that patients continue to improve even after completion of treatment (Wormser et al., 2003). Of note, 30% of patients remained symptomatic at the end of this study.

Approximately 15% of patients experience a Jarisch Herxheimer-like reaction in the first 24 hours of starting treatment. This involves worsening of systemic symptoms and an increase in the size and intensity of skin lesions. The majority of patients notice improvement by the end of the course of treatment. Erythema migrans lesions usually respond first and typically resolve within one to two weeks. Systemic symptoms, however, take longer to resolve. Three months after treatment, one in four patients may still have systemic complaints. Patients should be forewarned that they may still experience symptoms at the end of treatment and be reassured that in most cases they will improve steadily with time.

*Treatment of persons with persistent symptoms after*
*treatment for Lyme Disease*

Some patients experience symptoms following treatment with appropriate antibiotic therapy for Lyme disease, a phenomenon known as post-Lyme syndrome (PLS). While the IDSA guidelines used the term PLS (Wormser et al., 2006), the International Lyme and Associated Diseases Society (ILADS) uses the term "chronic Lyme disease" (Cameron et al., 2004). The IDSA proposes a definition of the post-Lyme syndrome as persons who develop subjective symptoms within 6 months of their Lyme disease diagnosis, which last at least a further 6 months. Symptoms include cognitive dysfunction, fatigue, or persistent musculoskeletal complaints. The ILADS lists similar symptoms under their discussion of chronic Lyme disease.

The IDSA definition points out the importance of excluding pre-existing or concomitant disease that may account for the symptoms. Some of these may occur in "healthy" persons. For example, chronic fatigue occurs in up to 20-30% of the population. When a patient fails to respond to accepted antibiotic therapy it is important to consider the possibility of co-infection with another tick borne illness. Controversy exists as to whether PLS reflects persistent infection or not, and this has implications in the debate over how to manage such patients.

Two randomized controlled trials examined whether antibiotics are efficacious in PLS. One study examined fatigue and cognitive impairment as endpoints; the other improvement in quality of life. The first compared 28 days of placebo or intravenous ceftriaxone in 55 patients with PLS. While ceftriaxone improved fatigue, there was no improvement in either group in cognitive function. The authors concluded that antibiotics had no role in the treatment of PLS and pointed out that 7% of patients receiving ceftriaxone experienced serious side effects requiring hospitalization (Krupp et al., 2003).

The second study, of one hundred and twenty-nine patients, received either one month intravenous ceftriaxone followed by 60 days of oral doxycycline or placebo. Of note, none of the participants had evidence of persistent infection with borrelia burgdorferi by culture and PCR. The study was stopped after a planned interim analysis revealed no difference between the two groups in terms of quality of life (Klempner et al., 2001). While the authors conclude that antibiotics do not improve health related quality of life in patients with PLS, the findings could be interpreted more specifically that the antibiotic regimen of intravenous ceftriaxone and oral doxycycline does not benefit PLS patients.

The IDSA guidelines present the case against persistent infection in PLS while the ILADS guidelines support the idea. One expert guideline states that patients with chronic symptoms of Lyme disease do not benefit from antibiotics, while the other expert group advocates their use. That two expert panels differ underscores the need to elucidate the pathogenesis of PLS and to develop improved treatment. Crucial to this effort will to develop a universally accepted definition of PLS to provide a framework in which to work.

*Chronic previously unexplained symptoms attributed to Lyme Disease*

As problematic as post-Lyme syndrome is the association of chronic previously unexplained symptoms (often cognitive difficulties and fatigue) with Lyme Disease. These persons have usually had exhaustive unproductive evaluations eventually having serologic testing for Lyme Disease which may be "positive." One school of thought maintains that this is a subset of Lyme; the other believe that chronic Lyme disease is only the latest syndrome postulated to attribute previously unexplained symptoms to particular infections—other examples that have lost credibility being "chronic candida syndrome" and "chronic Epstein–Barr virus infection." A review stated in no uncertain terms:

> "The assumption that chronic, subjective symptoms are caused by persistent infection with B. burgdorferi is not supported by carefully conducted laboratory studies or by controlled treatment trials. Chronic Lyme disease, which is equated with chronic B. burgdorferi infection, is a misnomer, and the use of prolonged, dangerous, and expensive antibiotic treatments for it is not warranted." (Feder et al., 2007)

*When there is no answer*

For some individuals, this declaration, although technically correct and the dominant opinion, provides no comfort nor acknowledgment of their suffering. Furthermore it may be heard or felt as being dismissive or disbelief in their symptoms.

I schedule an open-ended appointment, try to review all previous records before the visit or shortly after the encounter, and write my summary of what has been done. I take a careful review of systems and "park" anything that needs more detail to complete or check later., Some patients have found me by word of mouth or Googling and these patients don't walk into my practice but I have screened them . . . so they come prepared. I ask them to keep a 24 diary of their routine and symptoms noting what has been tried, helped a little or not at all, and any side effects in case some treatments might be recycled or gradually increased to tolerance. It's important as one marches through trials of therapy that options are not abandoned if they have not had a chance to work.

I use my network of senior doctors for help. Nowadays I might even ask the question of Google. If there is any inkling, I have no reticence to refer the patient. When I don't know or I don't have any ideas, I think I am secure enough to tell the patient. I follow the adage, primum non nocere, and deconstruct what I am looking for and why and ask them to help me help them. Reassurance is not about saying something is ruled out but saying

Unexplained fatigue, cognitive dysfunction, lancinating pain without focal abnormalities occur but when they persist are a source of consternation for both the person and the physician asked to sort it out and treat. The exhaustive differential diagnosis is in theory long but after a year or 2 in diagnostic pursuit of a label, and the symptoms unchanged is unlikely to be related to life-threatening disease but it is a major source of suffering.

The longer the symptoms and the higher the number of previous unsuccessful therapy, the less probable is it that I will come up with a new possibility (although I have) or that all symptoms will vanish with treatment. It's important to be honest in establishing expectations that they be attainable.

I try never start a treatment with potential side effects if I cannot state à priori what the criteria of success will be. It's essential that the criteria for success be discussed with the person affected and that they agree and believe it (Daltroy, 1993). I give my rationale as to why the medication might be helpful, its mode of action, and guess how likely it is to work, all conceivable side effects. I might increase the dose to what is a therapeutic dose by increasing the medication to tolerance and/or effect. Cost is almost never a consideration unless the patient is paying for it. Interestingly, some patients elect the most expensive option because they believe it to be better ("you pay for what you get"). The decision should never be made on one visit.

When I can find no objective evidence of Lyme exposure nor make an alternative diagnosis to explain the symptoms, there is no book on what to do next. Being older, acknowledging my inability to make a specific diagnosis doesn't make me feel anxious or less competent. I am also comfortable asking, "Could this be due to depression or stress?" It may help validate and legitimize their feelings and give them permission to discuss difficulties instead of a medical problem.

I explain that we are not always able to find a reason for many symptoms but this does not prevent us from trying things that might help balancing harms and benefits for the most troubling symptoms while providing support (Aronowitz, 2001). Every person and patient is slightly different but the trials of therapy have a patient chart and rate their symptoms and moves from realistic assessment of what we can do, revising expectations often, to life style modification ("working and living within their ability") before trials of medications directed at sleep disturbance, pain management.

## Prevention of Lyme Disease

Not emphasized enough and unfortunately not covered in the reimbursement of health care is the teachable moment or opportunity that is afforded when a person comes in with suspected Lyme Disease in an endemic area. Prevention strategies directed at the environment, ticks and/ or the vector, reviewed elsewhere, theoretically could put a stop to Lyme disease (Corapi et al., 2007; Hayes and Piesman, 2003). Protective behaviors, tick-avoidance or tick checking and removal, can be highly effective, voluntary, economical, and suitable for residents and visitors to endemic areas. Avoidance involves recognition and reduction of time spent in high-risk areas (woods, brush, and tall grass). Protective clothing, such as long-sleeved shirts and long pants, should be light colored so that ticks can be easily detected. Tick repellents can be applied to skin or clothing. The repellant DEET (N,N-diethyl-meta-toluamide, Morflex® Inc. Greensboro, NC) may be used on the skin; however, it is harmful to children in large doses, is neurotoxic, and must be reapplied every few hours for maximal effect. Permethrin, a repellant applied to clothing, kills ticks upon exposure, but should not come into contact with skin.

Effective tick check and removal behaviors are truly "green" approaches and take advantage of the fact that an infected tick has to be attached and feed for anywhere from 24 to 72 hours to transmit infection. The messages must be combined with an appreciation of the barriers to their practice (Shadick et al., 1997). A daily visual and manual search of exposed skin after visiting tick-infested areas provides an opportunity to identify and remove feeding ticks. A novel effective theory-based public education intervention demonstrating tick avoidance and removal health behaviors directed towards travelers to an epidemic area reduced the incidence of disease and is a model that could be implemented elsewhere (Daltroy et al., 2007).

In 1998 a recombinant vaccine against Lyme disease was approved by the FDA but was withdrawn after 4 years due to poor sales. This probably occurred due to lingering concerns about its long-term safety and because its immunization schedule was inconvenient requiring 3 injections before transmission season started to ensure optimum antibody levels and boosters because protective antibody titers declined rapidly.

Vaccination is cost effective where the incidence of Lyme disease is greater than 1% (Hsia et al., 2002; Shadick et al., 2001; Sigal, 2002) and would only be recommended for persons who reside, work, or do recreational activities in high-risk areas. A vaccine is unlikely to be 100%

effective, and would not protect against other tick-borne illnesses; therefore, efforts to avoid contact with ticks would still be required.

## Conclusion

Lyme disease continues to be a problem and even grow as hosts, vectors and man live closer together with the reduction of the forest habitat. While effective antibiotics have been identified for the early localized and disseminated stages of Lyme disease considerable uncertainty surrounds the management of patients with post-Lyme syndrome. More research needs to be done to understand the pathophysiology of persistent symptoms.

Educating patients on prevention strategies is essential in decreasing the annual incidence. Health educational programs in endemic areas beginning in the school and others focused on vacationers in these areas should be a priority. Another vaccine may be developed but is likely to face the same problems in gaining acceptance and reinforce complacency with tick avoidance and tick removal behaviors.

## Acknowledgments

I am indebted to Dr. Lynn Gerber who made suggestions on an earlier draft.

## References

Aronowitz, R. A. 2001. When do symptoms become a disease? *Ann Intern Med* 134 (9 Pt 2):803-8.

Aucott, J., C. Morrison, B. Munoz, P. C. Rowe, A. Schwarzwalder, and S. K. West. 2009. Diagnostic challenges of early Lyme disease: lessons from a community case series. *BMC Infect Dis* 9:79.

Bakken, L. L., S. M. Callister, P. J. Wand, and R. F. Schell. 1997. Interlaboratory comparison of test results for detection of Lyme disease by 516 participants in the Wisconsin State Laboratory of Hygiene/College of American Pathologists Proficiency Testing Program. *J Clin Microbiol* 35 (3):537-43.

Cameron, D., A. Gaito, N. Harris, G. Bach, S. Bellovin, K. Bock, S. Bock, J. Burrascano, C. Dickey, R. Horowitz, S. Phillips, L. Meer-Scherrer, B. Raxlen, V. Sherr, H. Smith, P. Smith, and R. Stricker. 2004. Evidence-based guidelines for the management of Lyme disease. *Expert Rev Anti Infect Ther* 2 (1 Suppl):S1-13.

CDC. 1995. Recommendations for test performance and interpretation from the Second National Conference of. *MMWR: Morbidity & Mortality Weekly Report* 44 (31):590.

Corapi, K. M., M. I. White, C. B. Phillips, L. H. Daltroy, N. A. Shadick, and M. H. Liang. 2007. Strategies for primary and secondary prevention of Lyme disease. *Nat Clin Pract Rheumatol* 3 (1):20-5.

Corapi, Kristin M, Samardeep Gupta, and Matthew H Liang. 2008. Management of Lyme disease. *Expert Review of Anti-infective Therapy* 6 (2):241-250.

Daltroy, L. H. 1993. Doctor-patient communication in rheumatological disorders. *Baillieres Clin Rheumatol* 7 (2):221-39.

Daltroy, L. H., C. Phillips, R. Lew, E. Wright, N. A. Shadick, and M. H. Liang. 2007. A controlled trial of a novel primary prevention program for Lyme disease and other tick-borne illnesses. *Health Educ Behav* 34 (3):531-42.

Feder, H. M., Jr., B. J. Johnson, S. O'Connell, E. D. Shapiro, A. C. Steere, G. P. Wormser, W. A. Agger, H. Artsob, P. Auwaerter, J. S. Dumler, J. S. Bakken, L. K. Bockenstedt, J. Green, R. J. Dattwyler, J. Munoz, R. B. Nadelman, I. Schwartz, T. Draper, E. McSweegan, J. J. Halperin, M. S. Klempner, P. J. Krause, P. Mead, M. Morshed, R. Porwancher, J. D. Radolf, R. P. Smith, Jr., S. Sood, A. Weinstein, S. J. Wong, and L. Zemel. 2007. A critical appraisal of "chronic Lyme disease". *N Engl J Med* 357 (14):1422-30.

Hayes, Edward B., and Joseph Piesman. 2003. How Can We Prevent Lyme Disease? *New England Journal of Medicine* 348 (24):2424-2430.

Hsia, E. C., J. B. Chung, J. S. Schwartz, and D. A. Albert. 2002. Cost-effectiveness analysis of the Lyme disease vaccine. *Arthritis Rheum* 46 (6):1651-60.

Klempner, M. S., L. T. Hu, J. Evans, C. H. Schmid, G. M. Johnson, R. P. Trevino, D. Norton, L. Levy, D. Wall, J. McCall, M. Kosinski, and A. Weinstein. 2001. Two controlled trials of antibiotic treatment in patients with persistent symptoms and a history of Lyme disease. *N Engl J Med* 345 (2):85-92.

Krupp, L. B., L. G. Hyman, R. Grimson, P. K. Coyle, P. Melville, S. Ahnn, R. Dattwyler, and B. Chandler. 2003. Study and treatment of post Lyme disease (STOP-LD): a randomized double masked clinical trial. *Neurology* 60 (12):1923-30.

Nadelman, R. B., J. Nowakowski, D. Fish, R. C. Falco, K. Freeman, D. McKenna, P. Welch, R. Marcus, M. E. Aguero-Rosenfeld, D. T. Dennis, and G. P. Wormser. 2001. Prophylaxis with single-dose doxycycline for the prevention of Lyme disease after an Ixodes scapularis tick bite. *N Engl J Med* 345 (2):79-84.

Shadick, N. A., L. H. Daltroy, C. B. Phillips, U. S. Liang, and M. H. Liang. 1997. Predictors of tick avoidance behaviors in an endemic area for Lyme Disease. *American Journal of Preventive Medicine* 13:265-270.

Shadick, N. A., M. H. Liang, C. B. Phillips, K. Fossel, and K. M. Kuntz. 2001. The cost-effectiveness of vaccination against Lyme disease. *Arch Intern Med* 161 (4):554-61.

Sigal, L. H. 2002. Vaccination for lyme disease: Cost-effectiveness versus cost and value. *Arthritis & Rheumatism* 46 (6):1439-1442.

Wormser, G. P., R. J. Dattwyler, E. D. Shapiro, J. J. Halperin, A. C. Steere, M. S. Klempner, P. J. Krause, J. S. Bakken, F. Strle, G. Stanek, L. Bockenstedt, D. Fish, J. S. Dumler, and R. B. Nadelman. 2006. The clinical assessment, treatment, and prevention of lyme disease, human granulocytic anaplasmosis, and babesiosis: clinical practice guidelines by the Infectious Diseases Society of America. *Clin Infect Dis* 43 (9):1089-134.

Wormser, G. P., R. Ramanathan, J. Nowakowski, D. McKenna, D. Holmgren, P. Visintainer, R. Dornbush, B. Singh, and R. B. Nadelman. 2003. Duration of antibiotic therapy for early Lyme disease. A randomized, double-blind, placebo-controlled trial. *Ann Intern Med* 138 (9):697-704.

Zhang, X., M. I. Meltzer, C. A. Pena, A. B. Hopkins, L. Wroth, and A. D. Fix. 2006. Economic impact of Lyme disease. *Emerg Infect Dis* 12 (4):653-60.

# A10
# DISEASE SURVEILLANCE AND CASE DEFINITIONS
# IN TICK-BORNE DISEASES

*Prepared for the IOM Committee on Lyme Disease*
*and Other Tick-Borne Diseases: The State of the Science*
*James L. Hadler, M.D., M.P.H.*
*September 20, 2010*

This briefing on case definitions and surveillance for tick-borne disease is presented in three main sections: Background on surveillance and methods, particularly as they relate to tickborne diseases and nationally notifiable diseases; Lyme disease surveillance and case-definitions; and Public Health Surveillance for other tick-borne diseases in the United States.

## Background

Public health surveillance is the ongoing, systematic collection, analysis, interpretation, and dissemination of data regarding a health-related event for use in public health action to reduce morbidity and mortality and to improve health (CDC, 2001). For any given public health surveillance activity, it is critical to define the purpose of surveillance, use surveillance methods that are efficient and appropriate to achieving that purpose, and subsequently evaluate whether surveillance efforts are meeting the surveillance objectives (CDC, 2001; Meriwether 1996).

Depending on the objectives, a variety of methods can be used to conduct vector-borne public health surveillance (Hadler and Petersen, 2007). For example, to evaluate potential and emerging tickborne diseases, ongoing systematic efforts can be done to capture vector ticks, monitor their population size and determine infection rates. In addition, if appropriate serologic tests are available, serosurveys can be done to monitor the percentage of the population that has been infected with the disease agent. To determine the annual burden of human illness and its epidemiology, surveillance for human illness using provider and/or laboratory reporting to public health authorities, analysis of hospital discharge and death data, and for high incidence diseases population surveys can be done. To determine and monitor the prevalence of risk factors for tickborne disease (e.g., spending time outdoors, tick bites) and prevention practices (e.g., daily tick checks, wearing long light-colored pants tucked into socks, use of insect repellants), regular telephone and/or community surveys can be done.

Each method of surveillance has its particular limitations, however. Surveillance for ticks and tick infection rates is limited in part by the need to sample, the uneven distribution of vectors and infection rates geographically, and the need to confirm human risk by obtaining human infection data. Human disease reporting is limited by the need for laboratory and/or explicit symptom confirmation for diseases such as Lyme disease in which many other diseases may present with similar symptoms, and underreporting by healthcare providers who do not take the time needed to report. Reporting of laboratory findings alone, while less subject to underreporting than clinician reporting, is limited in part by the fact that positive tests may indicate infection long in the past or be falsely positive, necessitating the need to get clinical information to back up the laboratory report. In addition, they can take weeks to turn positive, so that persons in the early stages of infection may not have positive laboratory tests. Telephone and community surveys may have limited and non-representative response rates, and the results of community surveys are only clearly applicable to the communities in which they are done. In addition, each of these methods of surveillance has substantial costs to conduct and maintain.

*Human Disease Surveillance and Nationally Notifiable Diseases*

Constitutionally, local public health is a responsibility of state rather than federal government (Moulton et al., 2007). Correspondingly, surveillance for human disease using mandatory reporting of cases and laboratory findings to public health authorities is generally a state and local health department function rather than a federal one. State and local health departments have the legal authority, spelled out in statute in each state, to collect personally identifiable data on persons with selected diseases from laboratories and clinicians. Each state conducts surveillance for human disease according to its needs and resources. There is no standard list of diseases for which all states have reporting, and each has its own legislatively specified means for adding diseases to its state-specific list. The federal Centers for Disease Control and Prevention (CDC) conducts national surveillance for diseases reportable at the state level through collaboration with states via the Council of State and Territorial Epidemiologists (CSTE). Through resolutions passed by the majority of state representatives attending the annual CSTE meeting each June (a quorum is required, one vote per state present), a list of nationally notifiable diseases reportable to the CDC has been established, known as the National Notifiable Disease Surveillance System (NNDSS). For a disease to be included in the NNDSS, the purpose of national surveillance and a case definition to be used to count cases for national purposes must be agreed upon. Placement of a disease in the NNDSS does not obligate each state to conduct surveillance for it or to conduct surveillance in a standardized manner. The NNDSS is simply an agreement that states that conduct surveillance will de-identify and share their information with CDC using standard case definitions. Placement of a disease in the NNDSS also does not guarantee that resources are or will be available to each state to conduct surveillance. However, to the extent that CDC provides funding through cooperative agreements with states, CDC can require recipients to conduct surveillance for a specific disease and specify surveillance methods within the limits of funding provided.

*Principles of Surveillance Based on Case Reporting—Case Definitions*

There are at least four important principles of public health surveillance for human illness through disease reporting. First, surveillance for human disease based on clinician or laboratory reporting generally requires that a suspected case be confirmed. Cause-specific diagnoses based on a physician's best guess may be wrong, especially for persons with symptoms that can be caused by a number of different microbial agents or mechanisms other than infection (e.g., fever, malaise, skin rash, arthritis, headache, cough, diarrhea). Positive laboratory tests alone may reflect past disease (e.g., serologic tests for antibodies) or a carrier state without disease (e.g., bacterial colonization of the intestinal tract). Thus, case definitions are needed to define relevant symptoms in combination with relevant laboratory results that make it highly likely that a "case" really has the disease under surveillance, or, when laboratory confirmation is not possible, to define symptoms and findings that are characteristic of only of the disease under surveillance (e.g., erythema migrans for Lyme disease).

Second, because of the need for laboratory confirmation to make sure that only real cases of disease due to any given microbe are being counted, surveillance based on reporting is likely to underestimate the true magnitude of a disease. Cases for which it is technically difficult or too costly to confirm will not be counted, nor will cases that go unreported. Despite the legal requirements for reporting, some clinicians never get around to reporting patients they suspect of having a disease. To determine the true number of people with a given disease (e.g., Lyme disease), it may be necessary to conduct population and/or provider surveys.

Third, it is not critical for most surveillance purposes to count every possible case of a disease. For purposes of monitoring a disease over time to determine whether its epidemiology (which groups are most affected) is changing and its occurrence is stable, increasing or decreasing, it is only necessary to count cases in the same way and to invest the same effort over time. If one monitors a consistent part of the "iceberg" of disease, then changes in it will reflect what is happening to the whole iceberg.

Finally, consistency of the means of surveillance is important. It can be expected that there will be under-reporting and/or inability to follow-up every reported clinical case and laboratory finding because of resource restraints. If no funding is appropriated for surveillance, it may be impossible for a health department to conduct follow-up on thousands of laboratory reports to find out if a person had symptoms consistent with recent disease.

## Lyme Disease Surveillance and Case Definitions

Of the five tickborne diseases under national surveillance in the U.S., Lyme disease is by far the most common and has had the most public interest and dynamic surveillance history. Lyme disease was first recognized as a distinct entity in 1975 by epidemiologists investigating an apparent cluster of juvenile arthritis cases in Lyme, Connecticut. Informal national surveillance for human illness via annual surveys of states conducted by the CDC began in 1980 (CDC, 1981), and Lyme disease was formally added to the National Notifiable Disease Surveillance System in 1991 (CSTE, 1990). The causative infectious agent, *Borrelia burgdorferi*, was recognized in 1982, after which time laboratory tests were developed and gradually over several years began to be available for surveillance and clinical purposes.

### Features of Lyme Disease Relevant to Surveillance

Lyme disease has a number of clinical, laboratory and epidemiologic features that make conducting surveillance for human illness a challenge. These include: 1) erythema migrans (EM), an early stage disease manifestation and the most common one, a spreading skin lesion that begins as a papule or macule and over the course of days to weeks becomes a red, expanding lesion that must be diagnosed clinically because supportive laboratory tests are often negative, and only begins to be readily distinguishable from insect bite reactions or local skin infections when it gets to a substantial size and has a characteristic "target" pattern; 2) later clinical manifestations such as arthritis, neurologic involvement (lymphocytic meningitis, Bells' palsy, radiculoneuropathy) and cardiac complications (transient, high grade atrioventricular conduction defects sometimes accompanied by myocarditis) that are not unique to Lyme disease and need laboratory confirmation of *B. burgdorferi* infection; 3) confirmatory laboratory test methods which produce results that can be falsely positive and result in mistaken diagnosis of Lyme disease, especially in geographic areas where neither a competent tick vector (*Ixodes* ticks) nor *B. burgdoreri* are present; 4) positive serologic tests occurring after true infection that can remain positive indefinitely, making it essential that there be corroborating clinical data to back up laboratory findings (i.e., laboratory findings alone cannot be used for surveillance); 5) transmission from a tick that is small enough that attachment and feeding (i.e., "bites") often go unnoticed, making a history of having an antecedent tick bite an insensitive way to conduct surveillance; and 6) limited geographic areas in which infected, competent tick vectors are present, making it important for epidemiologic and public health purposes to distinguish between human disease in "endemic" areas and disease diagnosed in residents of geographic areas without a previous history of Lyme disease.

## Case Definitions of Lyme Disease for Public Health Surveillance

The objectives of formal national public health surveillance for human Lyme disease were agreed upon at the CSTE meeting in 1990 and have not changed since: (1) define the demographic, geographic, and seasonal distribution; (2) consistently monitor disease trends; (3) identify risk factors for transmission in areas where Lyme disease is newly emerging; and (4) develop strategies of prevention and control and evaluate the impact of prevention and control measures (CSTE, 1990, 2007). The recommended methods of surveillance for disease have also not changed: a combination of clinician and laboratory reporting of suspected cases with public health follow-up as needed to obtain detailed clinical information to confirm cases. The above clinical, laboratory and epidemiologic features of Lyme disease have been taken into consideration in the consensus case definitions that have been crafted over time by CSTE and CDC for surveillance to meet these public health surveillance objectives (CDC, 1990, 1997; CSTE, 2007). Importantly, as noted in the publication of each case definition, the surveillance definition for Lyme disease (and for other diseases under public health surveillance) was developed for national reporting of Lyme disease; it is NOT appropriate for clinical diagnosis, including determination of reimbursement by insurers.

To enable comparability between states and over time, public health epidemiologists have favored restriction of clinical manifestations that can be counted to those that are most likely to be Lyme disease rather than counting all possible cases. Thus, measurement of geographic distribution, the descriptive epidemiology and trends in Lyme occurrence within geographic areas have been emphasized over measuring the full magnitude of the problem.

To overcome the lack of specificity of small, evolving erythema migrans (EM) lesions, a lesion must be at least 5 centimeters in diameter to be counted. Annular erythematous lesions occurring within several hours of a tick bite represent hypersensitivity reactions and do not qualify as EM. For later musculoskeletal (joint), neurologic and cardiac manifestations to be counted, there must be laboratory confirmation. In addition, to count arthritis as being due to Lyme disease, the arthritis must be adequately characterized. Recurrent, brief attacks (weeks or months) of objective joint swelling in one or a few joints, sometimes followed by chronic arthritis in one or a few joints is typical of Lyme arthritis. However, manifestations not considered as criteria for diagnosis include chronic progressive arthritis not preceded by brief attacks and chronic symmetrical polyarthritis. Additionally, arthralgia, myalgia, or fibromyalgia syndromes alone are not criteria for musculoskeletal involvement. To count neurologic manifestations, any of the following, alone or in combination qualify in the absence of another explanation: lymphocytic meningitis; cranial neuritis, particularly facial palsy (may be bilateral); radiculoneuropathy; or, rarely, encephalomyelitis. Encephalomyelitis must be confirmed by demonstration of antibody production against *B. burgdorferi* in the cerebrospinal fluid (CSF), evidenced by a higher titer of antibody in CSF than in serum. Headache, fatigue, paresthesia, or mildly stiff neck alone are not criteria for neurologic involvement. Similar restrictions apply for cardiovascular manifestations. Acute onset of high-grade (2nd-degree or 3rd-degree) atrioventricular conduction defects that resolve in days to weeks and are sometimes associated with myocarditis can be counted. However, palpitations, bradycardia, bundle branch block, or myocarditis alone are not criteria for cardiovascular involvement.

To increase the probability that a case reported from a county in which Lyme disease has not previously been recognized is truly a case of Lyme disease, persons with suspected EM either should have been in a county in which Lyme disease is known to be endemic some time in the preceding 30 days or have laboratory confirmation. Endemic counties are those in which at least two laboratory confirmed cases meeting the clinical criteria defined above have been acquired and/or in which a known tick vector has been shown to be infected with *B. burgdorferi*. Of note, having a tick bite is not required for a case to be counted, as only about 20% of cases will report noticing a tick bite in the 3-30 days prior to the onset of EM (CDC, 1982).

There is also a definition for laboratory confirmation to assure the same standards for considering a test positive are used across states and, to the extent possible, over time.

### Modification of the Case Definition Over Time

The purpose of public health surveillance for Lyme disease has not changed over time. Thus with one exception (2007), there has not been a particular need to radically change the case definition. The focus has continued to be on specificity (counting only true cases) and on consistency in who is counted in order to monitor trends in geographic distribution and incidence within geographic areas over time.

The original case definition for national public health surveillance published in 1990 and used beginning in 1991 has been modified twice, in 1996 and in 2007 for use beginning the year after modification (CDC, 1990, 1997; CSTE, 1990, 1996, 1997). Most of the modifications have been to the laboratory criteria for confirming a diagnosis to incorporate new laboratory testing methods and to standardize methods for counting tests as positive for surveillance purposes. The latter has become particularly important as test methods for Lyme disease have proliferated and testing has become more common, and as states have been using laboratory reporting to supplement provider reporting to conduct surveillance for Lyme disease. In the 1990 definition, the laboratory criteria for a positive test were: 1) isolation of *Borrelia burgdorferi* from a clinical specimen, or 2) demonstration of diagnostic levels of IgM and IgG antibodies to the spirochete in serum or CSF, or 3) a significant change in IgM or IgG antibody response to *B. burgdorferi* in paired acute- and convalescent-phase serum samples. States were authorized to determine their own criteria for laboratory confirmation and diagnostic levels of antibody (CDC, 1990).

The main change in the case definition in 1996 was a new recommendation to use a two-test approach for laboratory confirmation, using a sensitive enzyme immunoassay or immunofluorescence antibody test followed by immunoblot confirmation (CDC, 1997; CSTE, 1996). In 2007, the laboratory criteria were modified slightly. The criterion: "demonstration of diagnostic levels of IgM and IgG antibodies in serum or CSF" was removed and a *requirement* made for "single-tier IgG immunoblot seropositivity interpreted using established criteria." (CSTE, 2007) This completed a shift from dependence on serologic tests using IFA or ELISA methods to only relying on immunoblot methods for confirmation, a positive immunoblot test providing firmer evidence of *B. burgdorferi* infection than positive tests using the other two methods.

There was another important revision contained in the 2007 case definition. In addition to having a category of "confirmed" cases, two new categories with less stringent criteria were added, "probable" and "suspect" cases. "Probable" cases were defined as "any other case of physician-diagnosed Lyme disease that has laboratory evidence of infection" (as defined above). This means that persons with laboratory criteria for infection who do not meet the strict clinical criteria specified in the confirmed case definition could be counted—for example, persons whose EM diameter is less than 5 centimeters and persons with any disease manifestation that a clinician diagnosed as Lyme disease. "Suspected" cases were defined as "a case of EM where there is no known exposure" (i.e., not having been in an endemic county in the 30 days before EM onset) and no laboratory evidence of infection, or "a case with laboratory evidence of infection but no clinical information available" (i.e., a person with only a positive laboratory report [as defined above]) (CSTE, 2007). The purpose of this change is to enable states to count more cases if they so chose and to better account for the surveillance burden of the huge number of laboratory reports, a burden that some states have been unable to meet (i.e., make efforts to obtain clinical information), resulting in potentially decreased confirmed case counts. Both confirmed and probable cases are designated as under national as well as state surveillance. The suspect case category is a category designed for optional use by states only. With these changes, it is expected that the national case counts will increase.

### Findings from National Surveillance

Taking the national surveillance findings at face value, national public health surveillance for Lyme disease has largely met the major public health surveillance objectives. The demographic, geographic and seasonal distribution of Lyme disease have been defined and trends from 1992 to 2006 have been measured (CDC, 2008). By age, the pattern is similar from year to year with all age groups being affected but incidence being bimodal with 5-9 year olds and 45-49 year olds providing the most cases. The sex distribution has been slowly changing over time, with the percentage of cases that are male gradually increasing, especially among 5-19 year olds and in the 10 states with the highest incidence. Clinically, EM has been present in nearly 70% of reported cases overall and over time, with a fairly wide variation by state, ranging from 87% in Minnesota to 51% in Delaware. Seasonally, new diagnoses of Lyme disease occur throughout the year, with peak occurrence of both early (EM) and later stage (arthritis, neurologic and cardiac) diagnoses during June through August when vector ticks most actively seek mammalian hosts and people spend the most time outdoors. Most importantly, national surveillance has documented the slowly expanding geographic distribution of Lyme disease and its initial intensification in areas as they become endemic, followed by reaching a fluctuating plateau in many endemic areas as, presumably, the ecologic dynamics of the tick, mice, deer and *B. burgdorferi* populations stabilize.

Figure A10-1 shows the annual number of reported cases to CDC from 1982 to 2008, including the period of informal national surveillance from 1982 to 1990.

There has been a steady upward trend in number of reported confirmed cases. Underlying this trend is an increasing number of states identifying and reporting Lyme disease (from 11 in 1982 to 21 in 1984 to all 50 by 1987) and increasing rates in most states and counties. Figure A10-2 shows maps of Lyme disease incidence by county in the U.S. in 1999 (the first time a county-level map was published by the CDC) and 2007. These illustrate the continually expanding geographic distribution and intensification in counties bordering well-established areas. In addition, using data from human surveillance, risk factor studies have been done (Ley et al., 1995; Orlosky et al., 1998; Cromley et al., 1998), a map of risk of acquiring Lyme disease was produced to guide vaccination recommendations when a

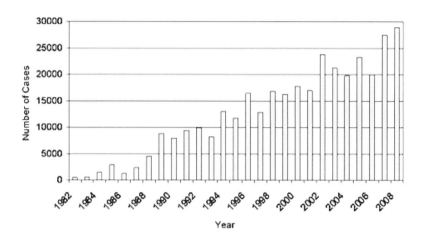

**FIGURE A10-1** Annual number of reported cases to CDC 1982 to 2008.

vaccine was transiently available (CDC, 1999), and prevention and control demonstration projects have been conducted in high Lyme disease incidence areas (Vazquez et al., 2008; Connally et al., 2009; Gould et al., 2008).

*Impact of Case Definition and Other Factors Affecting*
*Number of Reported Cases*

As previously mentioned, counting every single diagnosed case of human Lyme disease has not been the purpose of ongoing national public health surveillance. However, it is important to be able to define the extent to which current surveillance methods may underestimate the magnitude of the problem. With data from special studies conducted by states, often with CDC support, it is possible to crudely estimate the extent of undercounting of Lyme disease cases—or at least those with disease manifestations that are widely accepted as being due to *B. burgdorferi* infection. Studies done in Connecticut and Maryland in the early 1990s examined underreporting by physicians, and estimated that only 6-12% of EM cases were actually reported (Meek et al., 1996; Coyle et al., 1996). Laboratory reporting, which is particularly important for the 30% of reported cases that do not have EM, tends to be much more complete, but each report needs follow-up to obtain clinical data. States that attempt to follow up on positive laboratory

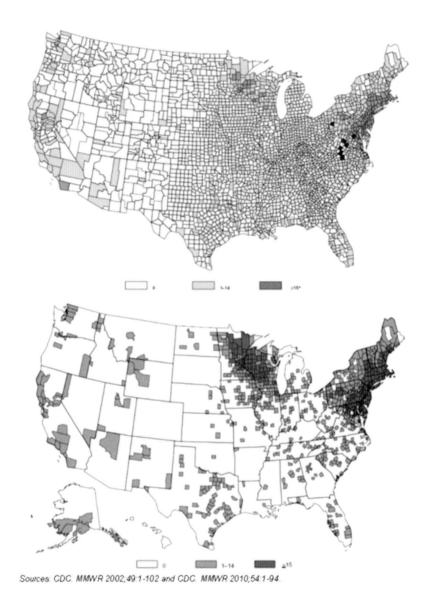

Sources: CDC. MMWR 2002;49:1-102 and CDC. MMWR 2010;54:1-94.

**FIGURE A10-2** Lyme disease incidence by county in the U.S. in 1999.

reports to obtain clinical information that could make a person with a positive laboratory test countable as a case, find that they have success in getting case information back from physicians on only about 40-50% of positive laboratory reports (Connecticut Department of Public Health and New York State Department of Health, personal communication). Assuming these findings apply to all states and are still pertinent, and that EM accounts for 70% of all reported cases, one can estimate that for every counted, reportable case, another 6-12 countable cases occur.

To the extent that the above factors, underreporting of EM and unsuccessful follow-up of positive laboratory reports, are stable, changes in numbers of cases reported and counted should be meaningful. However, to the extent that they are unstable, artifactual increases or decreases could occur. In recent years, several important and interrelated sources of instability of surveillance efforts have been identified, resulting in challenges to interpretation of trends within some states and nationally. Instability of effort has occurred when funding for surveillance has changed and as the work of surveillance has increased with increasing use of laboratory tests for Lyme disease. For example, between 1998 and 2002, Connecticut used CDC funding given to evaluate vaccine impact to support two full-time positions to initiate full scale laboratory result-based surveillance with multiple attempts at follow up of positive laboratory test results to obtain clinical information. This was done in part to be able to evaluate vaccine impact on laboratory test result-defined disease as well as on EM. As a consequence, the number of reported cases more than doubled (Ertel et al., 2006). After the vaccine was withdrawn and CDC switched emphasis from supporting enhanced surveillance to evaluate vaccine impact to other prevention efforts, Connecticut could no longer sustain nor needed such a labor-intensive level of surveillance and ceased laboratory surveillance beginning in 2003 in favor of Lyme disease prevention efforts. The result was a 70% decrease in cases from 4,631 in 2002 to 1,403 in 2003, although physician-reported cases were stable (Ertel et al., 2006).When reporting from laboratories that could submit data electronically was restarted in 2007 but with some lesser efforts at follow-up, the reported case count rose 71% from 1,788 in 2006 to 3,058 in 2007 (Ertel et al., 2008). In 2007, the Connecticut Department of Public Health had 16,799 positive laboratory reports. In New York State (excluding New York City), the number of unique persons with positive laboratory reports needing follow-up increased from 18,420 in 2005 to 38,503 in 2008 (New York State Health Department, personal communication).

These issues need to be taken into account when interpreting trends in national as well as state data. Thus, interpretation of national trends has balanced issues of changes in intensity of surveillance with data from states with stable surveillance. For example, from 2001 to 2002, there was a 40% increase in the number of reported cases of Lyme disease nationally. The interpretation was "Factors potentially contributing to the increase in reported cases include growing populations of deer that support the *Ixodes* tick vector, increased residential development of wooded areas, tick dispersal to new areas, improved disease recognition in areas where LD is endemic, and enhanced reporting" (CDC, 2004). When there was no substantial change in incidence from 2003-2005, in part because Connecticut dropped laboratory reporting and other states were also adjusting surveillance methods to resources, the interpretation was more measured: "Since Lyme disease became nationally notifiable in 1991, the annual number of reported cases has more than doubled. This increase likely is the result of several factors, including a true increase in disease incidence and enhanced case detection resulting from implementation of laboratory-based surveillance in several states. . . . To address this surveillance burden (laboratory reporting) and create more sustainable Lyme disease surveillance systems, some states (e.g., Connecticut) have modified components of their systems, leading to acute reductions in reported cases. However, no evidence exists to suggest a true decrease in Lyme disease incidence in these states" (CDC, 2007).

*Other Lyme Disease Surveillance Activities*

Although this report focuses on national public health surveillance for human Lyme disease, it should be noted that many states also conduct surveillance for vector tick density and percentage of *Ixodes* ticks infected with *B. burgdorferi*. This form of surveillance is used to complement human surveillance, to help define whether a county with reported cases for the first time is becoming endemic, and to help interpret fluctuating incidence in highly endemic areas. It has been well established that infected tick density can vary from year to year and that variations in infected tick density within a county or state correlate well with variation in human incidence (Stafford et al., 1998; Mather et al., 1996).

*Current Issues in Human Lyme Disease Surveillance:*
*Questions and Answers*

There are a number of Lyme disease human surveillance issues that have been raised recently by various persons and groups including state and local health departments conducting surveillance for Lyme disease. The following is a list of some of the issues with discussion in Issue and Response format.

**Issue:** Should we be making more of an effort through public health surveillance to fully measure the full magnitude of the Lyme disease problem annually, in part to call more attention to it and possibly to get more funding devoted to it?

**Response**: This would require a change in the objectives of public health surveillance and a change in the Lyme disease surveillance case definition to make it inclusive of any clinician-reported case of EM and any clinician-diagnosed case who has a positive laboratory test for *B. burgdorferi* infection. Such a change would require the consensus of the majority of the official state representatives (usually the State Epidemiologist) at the annual CSTE meeting. While CSTE decided not to change the objectives of surveillance the last time this was considered in 2007, they did partially address the issue of measuring more of the Lyme disease problem by creating new categories of Lyme disease case reports (CSTE, 2007). Beginning in 2008, any person with a positive laboratory test meeting the laboratory criteria who had a physician diagnosis of disease regardless of symptoms could be called a "probable" case. Thus, persons with non-classical manifestations of Lyme disease potentially could be counted as cases. In addition, persons with clinician-diagnosed EM that was less than 5 cm in diameter could be counted if they had a positive laboratory test. Further, persons with a qualifying positive laboratory test but no clinical information could be counted as a "suspect" case. Thus, all persons with qualifying positive laboratory reports can be counted in state-level surveillance. For national surveillance, however, only those with confirmed and probable status will be counted. It will take some years using this system before any additional changes are likely to be considered. Data from 2008 illustrates that it will take time for this system to become fully established. In 2008, there were a total of 28,921 confirmed and 6,277 probable cases reported nationally, a ratio of 0.22 probable cases per confirmed case (CDC, 2010). While 49 states (including Washington, DC) reported at least one confirmed case, only 36 states reported at least one probable case. Neither Pennsylvania nor Delaware, together accounting for 4,590 confirmed cases, reported any probable cases, although at least 1,000 probable cases might have been expected. Given inadequate staffing to initiate follow up or successfully follow up on laboratory reports, suspect cases are likely to provide many more additional reports than probable cases. In 2008, Connecticut reported 2,738 confirmed and 1,158 probable cases, but identified an additional 3,106 suspect cases in state surveillance (Connecticut Department of Public Health, personal communication).

**Issue**: How can we accurately determine the full magnitude of the human Lyme disease problem in the U.S.?

**Response**: A definition of what should be included in the full magnitude of the Lyme disease problem is needed. It potentially includes the following: 1) persons truly infected with *B. burgdorferi* who have widely agreed upon ("classic") symptoms and disease (currently being partially captured through confirmed case surveillance); 2) persons truly infected with *B. burgdorferi* who have non-classical Lyme disease symptoms that some would attribute to *B. burgdorferi* (e.g., persons with "chronic" Lyme disease, being partially addressed through "probable" case surveillance); 3) persons with a non-qualifying positive laboratory test who have been diagnosed as having Lyme disease (not all laboratories rely on immunoblot testing or a standard interpretation of the pattern found); and 4) persons without documented *B. burgdorferi* infection by any test or classic EM who are being treated for Lyme disease (includes persons with "seronegative Lyme disease"). In other words, the full impact of Lyme disease on the U.S. healthcare system potentially includes all persons who truly have Lyme disease and all persons getting treated for Lyme disease without standard laboratory confirmation, whether they have Lyme disease or not. There is no easy method to get at this. Given the limitations and challenges of public health surveillance in general and for Lyme disease in particular, conventional reporting of cases to public health departments will not give a complete answer no matter what the case definition, and it is unlikely that there will ever be a surveillance case definition for Lyme disease that is so inclusive. One could conduct a large population-based survey and ask respondents whether or not they have been treated for Lyme disease in the past year and the nature of that disease. However, this is not as easy as it sounds: the sample frame would have to be large, given that it is likely that the expected rate would be somewhere between 1 in a hundred and 1 in a thousand, given that the measured rate through national surveillance is most recently approximately 1.2 per 10,000 population (CDC, 2010). It might also need to be conducted in all states to determine state-specific rates and, subsequently, trends. Thus, a substantial financial investment would be needed to do this.

**Issue:** Can public health surveillance for human Lyme disease be used to determine whether there is chronic Lyme disease and the magnitude of the problem with it?

**Response:** Public health surveillance based on case reporting is dependent on having a case definition that can be applied to determine if a suspected case meets the criteria for being counted as a case. Clinically, many diseases can have similar symptoms. Clinicians faced with making a diagnosis of a patient with a given set of symptoms typically make a list of the possibilities (differential diagnoses) and then methodically do testing to determine what disease the patient likely has. It is similar with public health surveillance. At present, there is no standard case definition that could be used, as there is a lack of consensus even for whether there is "chronic Lyme disease." Until those involved in clinical research establish that there is such an entity and what a standard set of symptoms are, public health surveillance with all its limitations cannot be conducted.

**Issue:** Given current surveillance objectives and methods, how can we improve physician reporting and the percentage of laboratory reports on which we get clinical information?

**Response:** There is a hidden question in this issue. Given that clinician reporting of Lyme disease has been well established for a long time and that maintaining a constant level of surveillance is needed to accurately determine trends (a major public health objective of Lyme disease surveillance), do we want to improve physician reporting? Generally, we want to do whatever is necessary to keep it at more or less the same level. In order to maintain a constant level of surveillance, some states have established sentinel provider networks in which more active surveillance is done. Physicians in these networks are actively asked weekly to provide a list of all the persons they have seen with a new Lyme disease diagnosis. In some states, an epidemiologist will visit the practice to extract the necessary clinical information, limiting the work a physician has to do to report. The trends in the numbers of reports from these practices are compared to those from outside the network. As long as both show similar trend results, a state can reasonably assume that reporting levels are constant.

The laboratory question is a newer one. It is only recently that the number of positive laboratory reports in some high incidence states has overwhelmed the scarce public health resources to follow-up on them, threatening the ability to sustain laboratory surveillance for Lyme disease. One proposed solution that has worked well in New York State to address the problem created by the number of laboratory reports on unique individuals increasing from 18,420 in 2005 to 38,503 in 2008, has been to follow up on a random sample of reports (in New York, 1 in 5), then estimate the total number of cases based on the results of follow-up of the sample. In an unpublished validation, the sampling method has been shown to accurately predict what would have been obtained by following up all laboratory reports (New York State Health Department, personal communication). While sampling has not improved the percentage of laboratory reports successfully followed up (40-50% statewide, the percentage usually gotten by a single attempt by mail to contact the provider to complete a case report form), it takes a lot less work and may be a means that could be used by many states to achieve a sustainable, consistent level of Lyme disease laboratory based surveillance in the future. For sampling to be used for national surveillance purposes, it will ultimately be necessary for CSTE to endorse states reporting an estimated case count as a substitute for an exact one when reporting through the National Notifiable Disease Surveillance System.

**Issue:** Given the challenges of public health surveillance, can one fairly compare rates of reported Lyme disease between states? Within a single state over time?

**Response:** One cannot reliably compare rates of reported Lyme disease between states unless one knows whether or not they are making the same level of surveillance effort and what the density and infection rates of tick vectors are. Further, most states with high levels of endemic Lyme disease have very different rates from one part of the state to another. Thus, even the overall state incidence of Lyme disease does not reflect the different risk in different parts of the state (see Figure A10-2). The same principles apply to comparison of rates of Lyme disease within a state over time (Ertel, 2006 and 2008). If surveillance methods are stable, then data should accurately reflect changes in Lyme disease risk over time. However, overall state numbers and trends may not reflect risk and trends throughout the state. Some parts of the state may have plateaued and have some years when human disease incidence (and number of infected ticks) decrease while tick populations in other parts of the state and human illness are increasing.

**Issue:** A number of states and counties report cases of Lyme disease annually but are not known to have a competent tick vector or the presence of *B. burgdorferi* in tick populations. Do they really have Lyme disease? Are these really cases of Lyme disease?

**Response:** For purposes of national public health surveillance, a laboratory confirmed case meeting the clinical case definition will be counted from any state that chooses to count it, even if infection cannot be readily attributed to exposure where *B burgdorferi* and competent tick vectors are known to be well established (i.e., travel to an endemic area, as defined in the case definition). However, such a "case" in a state or county with no known competent tick vector or infected ticks could be a false case. Other diseases can cause similar symptoms and even immunoblot tests are not perfect. When such disease is diagnosed, it is incumbent on the state or county to attempt to look for the tick vector and find infected ticks before announcing that this is a new endemic area and counting persons who only could have been exposed locally. Definitive human risk in any given area is dependent on there being competent tick vectors and infected ticks. Of particular interest in this regard is the recognition of a new disease characterized by EM, Southern Tick-Associated Rash Illness (STARI) following the bite of the lone star tick (not a competent Lyme disease vector) which may be a more common cause of EM in some southern states than Lyme disease (Georgia Department of Human Resources, 2001; CDC, 2010). STARI was recognized during efforts to validate human risk for Lyme disease after EM was diagnosed in some southern states and counties without known *B. burgdorferi* infected *Ixodes* species.

### Public Health Surveillance for Other Tickborne Diseases in the U.S.

There are at least 6 other recognized tickborne diseases in the United States: Rocky Mountain Spotted Fever, Ehrlichiosis/anaplasmosis, babesiois,

Powassan virus meningoencephalitis, tickborne relapsing fever and STARI. Of these, four, Rocky Mountain Spotted Fever, Ehrlichiosis/anaplasmosis, Powassan virus encephalitis and babesiosis are included in the National Notifiable Disease Surveillance System. A presentation of the public health surveillance objectives for each and their past and current case definitions and history of public health surveillance are discussed below. None has had the public interest that has been generated by Lyme disease nor as complicated a clinical picture with different stages of illness. Thus far, there has been less concern about what surveillance efforts and case definitions for these diseases can and cannot do.

### Rocky Mountain Spotted Fever

Rocky Mountain Spotted Fever (RMSF) is an acute, severe and sometimes fatal tickborne illness transmitted in most parts of the country by the bite of *Dermacentor* species but in Arizona by *Rhiphicephalus sanguineus* (the brown dog tick). It has been under public health surveillance since at least 1944 (CDC, 1994). The main objective of public health surveillance is to provide information on the temporal, geographic, and demographic occurrence of Rocky Mountain Spotted Fever (and other spotted fever rickettsioses) to facilitate its prevention and control (CSTE, 2009). Recommended surveillance methods are both provider and laboratory reporting. Although under national public health surveillance for a long time, the case definition for national surveillance was first published in 1990 (CDC, 1990). At that time, a case was defined as follows:

"Clinical description—An illness most commonly characterized by acute onset and fever, usually accompanied by myalgia, headache, and petechial rash (on the palms and soles in two-thirds of the cases). To be counted as confirmed, a case needs to be laboratory confirmed. Four different laboratory criteria can independently be used to confirm a diagnosis: a) fourfold or greater rise in antibody titer to the spotted fever group antigen by immunofluorescent antibody (IFA), complement fixation (CF), latex agglutination (LA), microagglutination (MA), or indirect hemagglutination (IHA) test, or a single titer greater than or equal to 64 by IFA or greater than or equal to 16 by CF; or b) demonstration of positive immunofluorescence of skin lesion (biopsy) or organ tissue (autopsy); or c) Isolation of *Rickettsia rickettsii* from a clinical specimen. In addition to confirmed cases, a "probable" case is: "a clinically compatible case with supportive serology (fourfold rise in titer or a single titer greater than or equal to 320 by Proteus OX-19 or OX-2, or a single titer greater than or equal to 128 by LA, IHA, or MA test)."

Since 1990, the case definition has been revised several times, each time to make modifications based on newer laboratory test methods. In 1996, the laboratory confirmation criteria changed to include having a positive polymerase chain reaction assay to *R. rickettsii* as another independent confirmation criterion (CDC, 1997). In 2003, the 4 main confirmatory laboratory test results were reframed in an effort to make them clearer (CSTE, 2003).

In 2007, another revision was made to "clarify misleading or poorly defined laboratory statements, and to improve case classification for reporting" including adding a "suspected" case category (CSTE, 2007). The clinical description of disease was simplified to "any reported fever and one or more of the following: rash, headache, myalgia, anemia, thromobocytopenia, or any hepatic transaminase elevation," and the description of confirmatory laboratory tests was further clarified. A positive laboratory test became one of the following: a) serological evidence of a fourfold change in immunoglobulin G (IgG)-specific antibody titer reactive with *Rickettsia rickettsii* antigen by indirect immunofluorescence assay (IFA) between paired serum specimens (one taken in the first week of illness and a second 2-4 weeks later); b) detection of *R. rickettsii* DNA in a clinical specimen via amplification of a specific target by PCR assay; c) demonstration of spotted fever group antigen in a biopsy/autopsy specimen by IHC; or d) isolation of *R. rickettsii* from a clinical specimen in cell culture. Laboratory supportive evidence was defined as: has serologic evidence of elevated IgG or IgM antibody reactive with *R. rickettsii* antigen by IFA, enzyme-linked immunosorbent assay (ELISA), dot-ELISA, or latex agglutination. A confirmed case needed to have both clinical and laboratory confirmation, a probable case needed clinical confirmation in combination with laboratory supportive evidence, while a suspect case only needed laboratory evidence or recent or past infection (no clinical information needed).

The various iterations of surveillance definitions have been used to describe the geographic distribution within the U.S. and trends in occurrence over time. Most recently, without a substantial change in geographic distribution (mostly southeastern and south central U.S. with scattered cases throughout the country), the number of reported cases has increased 300% in the past decade with a trend toward stabilization in the 4 years since 2005 (CDC, 2010). In 2008, a total of 190 confirmed and 2,367 probable cases were reported.

*Erhlichiosis/Anaplasmosis*

Human ehrlichiosis was recognized as a distinct acute disease entity caused by an intracellular parasitic organism in the Rickettsiae family in the late 1980s, when human monocytic ehrlichiosis (HME) was described (CDC, 1988). Since then, three different species with their own ecology have been identified as causing ehrlichiosis and one has been reclassified as *Anaplasma*. Despite there being at least three known causes of ehrlichiosis, they have been grouped together for public health surveillance purposes. After recognition of a second type of ehrlichiosis that resulted in severe, acute disease with a predilection to affect granulocytes (human granulocytic ehrlichiosis, HGE) and which had an apparently different epidemiology than the previously described HME (Bakken et al., 1994; CDC, 1995), CSTE approved a standard case definition for voluntary reporting to CDC, recognizing that this was an emerging infection. However, it did not initially vote to include it in the Nationally Notifiable Disease Surveillance System, in part because it was reportable in only a minority of states (CSTE, 1996). At that time there were two known causes: *E. chaffeensis* causing HME, apparently transmitted by Lone Star (*Amblyomma americanum*) ticks, mainly affecting persons in the southeastern and south central U.S., and an *E. equi*-like agent causing HGE, suspected of being transmitted by *Ixodes* ticks and mainly affecting persons in the northeastern and north central states.

The provisional case definition included a clinical description of illness and laboratory criteria for diagnosis, a confirmed case being a person with a clinically compatible illness who met the laboratory criteria (CSTE, 1996). The clinical description was "A febrile illness most commonly characterized by acute onset, accompanied by headache, myalgia, rigors and/or malaise; clinical laboratory findings may include: intracytoplasmic microcolonies (morulae) in leukocytes of peripheral smear, cerebrospinal fluid or bone marrow aspirate or biopsy, cytopenias (especially thrombocytopenia and leukopenia), and elevated liver enzymes (especially alanine aminotransferase or aspartate aminotransferase)." Laboratory criteria included any of the following: "a) fourfold or greater change in antibody titer to *Ehrlichia* spp. antigen by immunofluorescence antibody (IFA) test in acute and convalescent specimens ideally taken four weeks or more apart. HME diagnosis requires *E. chaffeensis* antigen and HGE diagnosis currently requires *E. equi* or HGE-agent antigen; b) positive polymerase chain reaction (PCR) assay. Distinct primers are used for the diagnosis of HGE and HME; or c) intracytoplasmic morulae identified in blood, bone marrow or CSF leukocytes and an IFA antibody titer >=1:64." Probable cases were defined as persons with a compatible illness with a single IFA serologic titer >=1:64 or intracytoplasmic morulae identified in blood, bone marrow or CSF leukocytes.

In 1998, CSTE voted to formally add ehrlichiosis to the NNDSS effective January 1999 (CSTE, 1998). The purpose of public health surveillance was severalfold: 1) to define the epidemiology of ehrlichia infections in the United States; 2) to monitor incidence trends and changes in the geographic distribution of these infections over time; and 3) to identify risk factors for ehrlichia infections. The earlier recommended case definition was approved for national public health surveillance. In 2000, the case definition was revised to account for the recognition that *E. phagocytophilum* was the cause of HGE, to add a new human disease-causing species, *E. ewingii*, and to incorporate newer laboratory test methods (CSTE, 2000). In addition, the reporting classification was modified, "Three categories of confirmed or probable ehrlichiosis should be reported: 1) human ehrlichiosis caused by *E. chaffeensis* (HME), 2) human ehrlichiosis caused by *E. phagocytophilum* (HGE), and 3) human ehrlichiosis (other or unspecified agent), which includes cases that cannot be easily classified by available laboratory techniques, and cases caused by novel *Ehrlichia* species such as *E. ewingii*." In addition, the laboratory criteria became ehrlichia category-specific.

Additional changes to the case definition were made in 2007 in part to update taxonomic changes in the pathogens causing ehrlichiosis (CSTE, 2007). *E. phagocytophilum* was reclassified to *Anaplasma phagocytophilum,* the specific disease name changed from HGE to human granulocytic anaplasmosis (HGA) and the overall ehrlichiosis reporting classification was further expanded to 4 categories: 1) human ehrlichiosis caused by *Ehrlichia chaffeensis*, 2) human ehrlichiosis caused by *E. ewingii*, 3) human anaplasmosis caused by *Anaplasma phagocytophilum*, and 4) human ehrlichiosis/anaplasmosis—undetermined. Cases reported in the fourth sub-category can only be reported as "probable" because the cases are only weakly supported by ambiguous laboratory test results. Laboratory confirmatory and supportive (probable) criteria were modified to include *E. ewingii* and "undetermined" categories as follows: *E. ewingii*: "Because the organism has never been cultured, antigens are not available. Thus, *Ehrlichia ewingii* infections may only be diagnosed by molecular detection methods: *E ewingii* DNA detected in a clinical specimen via amplification of a specific target by polymerase chain reaction (PCR) assay." "Undetermined" infections "can only be reported as 'probable' because the cases are only weakly supported by ambiguous laboratory test results."

In 2008, a total of 2107 confirmed cases of human ehrlichiosis were reported, with disease caused by *A. phagocytophilum* (1,009 cases) and by *E. chaffeensis* (957 cases) accounting for 93% of all cases (CDC, 2010). The incidence of both major forms of ehrlichiosis (HGA, HME) has been steadily increasing since 1999, with a 4-5-fold increase since 2001. Surveillance has also confirmed the early findings on geographic distribution of HME and HGA and demonstrated that ehrlichiosis caused by *E. ewingii* has a similar geographic distribution as HME.

*Powassan Virus Encephalitis/Meningitis*

Powassan virus encephalitis/meningitis results from central nervous system infection with Powassan virus, a tickborne virus that causes rare cases of arboviral encephalitis in the upper Midwest and northeastern U.S. It was placed under national public health surveillance in 2002 to be included at the same time West Nile virus was added to the list of other domestic arboviral encephalitis viruses which had been under national public health surveillance since 1995, including California serogroup virus, equine encephalitis, St. Louis encephalitis, and western equine encephalitis (CSTE, 2001). At the time it was described as "an under-recognized tickborne disease." It was noted that laboratory testing was not widely available, but that 2 cases were diagnosed in New England during evaluation for West Nile virus infection and that there was a case-fatality rate of approximately 10%. The goals of surveillance were multiple: 1) assess the national public health impact of Powassan viral and other arboviral diseases of the CNS and monitor national trends, 2) identify high-risk population groups or geographic areas to target interventions and guide analytic studies, and 3) develop hypotheses leading to analytic studies about risk factors for infection and disease.

The original case definition was the same for all the arboviruses causing central nervous system infection and recognized that infection may result in clinical disease of variable severity and variable CNS involvement. There was no specific definition for Powassan virus infection. However, cases could be classified as "neuroinvasive" or "nonneuroinvasive" depending on symptoms and demonstration of CNS involvement and required laboratory confirmation in one of 4 ways: a) fourfold or greater change in virus-specific serum antibody titer; b) isolation of virus from or demonstration of specific viral antigen or genomic sequences in tissue, blood, cerebrospinal fluid (CSF), or other body fluid; c) virus-specific immunoglobulin M (IgM) antibodies demonstrated in CSF by antibody-capture enzyme immunoassay (EIA); or d) virus-specific IgM antibodies demonstrated in serum by antibody-capture EIA and confirmed by demonstration of virus-specific serum immunoglobulin G (IgG) antibodies in the same or a later specimen by another serologic assay (e.g., neutralization or hemagglutination inhibition).

From 2002-2008, a total of 13 cases of Powassan virus infection were reported with a peak of 7 cases in 2007. All were neuroinvasive, most from upstate New York with several from Maine, Minnesota and Wisconsin (CDC, 2010). In 2009, CSTE voted to continue surveillance for Powassan virus infection with the same objectives (CSTE, 2009). The one change to the case definition was to add a "probable" category. Confirmed cases continue to need clinical criteria for neuroinvasive (any of a variety of central nervous system symptoms plus pleocytosis on lumbar puncture) or non-neuroinvasive (at least fever) and laboratory confirmation. Probable cases need to have a compatible clinical illness plus a lesser degree of laboratory confirmation, either a) stable (less than or equal to a two-fold change) but elevated titer of virus-specific serum antibodies, or b) virus-specific serum IgM antibodies detected by antibody-capture EIA but with no available results of a confirmatory test for virus-specific serum IgG antibodies in the same or a later specimen.

*Babesiosis*

Babesiosis is a tickborne disease caused by several different species of malaria-like red blood cell infecting parasites of the genus *Babesia*. *B. microti* is the most common cause of babesiosis in the U.S., particularly in New England, East coast and Midwestern states, with *B. duncani* causing disease in California and Washington. Infection ranges from asymptomatic to a life-threatening illness resembling malaria, being most severe in immunosuppressed, asplenic and/or elderly persons. Prior to the 1980s, documented human illness was rare and largely acquired in islands off the coast of New England and New York. In addition to causing disease following tick bites, *Babesia* can be transmitted by blood transfusion from asymptomatically infected persons, with transfusion-associated disease first described in the U.S. in 1979.

During the 1980s, it was recognized that in some states, babesiosis was a growing problem. In some of those states, babesiosis was made reportable and increases in incidence and geographic range were documented. For example, New York made babesiosis reportable in 1986 following apparent increases in incidence on Long Island. In 1986, 18 cases were reported, all from Long Island. In 2008, 261 cases were reported: 96 from Long Island, 126 from 12 additional counties in New York state and 39 from New York City (New York State Department of Health, 1994 and 2008). In Connecticut, a cluster of 6 cases occurred in 1989 in New London County, near where Lyme disease was first recognized (CDC, 1989). Babesiosis was made reportable in 1991. In 2007, 156 cases were reported from all 8 counties (Connecticut Department of Public Health, 2007).

With the increasing incidence and spread of babesiois, the incidence of blood transfusion-associated disease increased (Stramer et al., 2009). Correspondingly, in 2010, CSTE voted to add babesiosis to the list of notifiable diseases under national public health surveillance (CSTE, 2010). The purpose of surveillance is to provide information on the temporal, geographic, and demographic occurrence of babesiosis, including transfusion-associated babesiosis, to facilitate its prevention and control. It is recommended that states conduct both healthcare provider and laboratory surveillance. The case definition has three categories of disease: confirmed, probable and suspect, with confirmed and probable being under national public health surveillance. The probable definition includes blood donors and recipients without symptoms associated with a transfusion case or a known infected donor, as long as the probable case has either supportive or confirmatory laboratory evidence of infection.

## Other Tickborne Illnesses, Coinfection

There are several other tickborne infections known to occur in the US that currently are not under national public health surveillance: STARI and tickborne relapsing fever. Neither disease is known to be common nor widespread enough for CSTE to seriously consider voting it to be part of the National Notifiable Disease Surveillance System. However, individual states in which they are present can choose to make them locally reportable.

Given that *Ixodes* ticks, especially in the northeast and north-central states, are vectors for Lyme disease, ehrlichiosis/anaplasmosis and babesiosis, it is possible for ticks to carry and transmit more than one agent. In fact, coinfections are not unusual and can result in more severe illness than infection with a single agent (Swanson et al., 2006). At present, there is no systematic effort at national surveillance for coinfection. However, the potential exists in any state to match persons reported with one infection to reports of those with either of the other infections. Thus far, no results of such matching to determine population levels of coinfection have been reported.

## References*

* All with Internet URLs accessed September 1-10, 2010.

Bakken J.S., J.S. Dumler, S.M. Chen, M.R. Eckman, L.L. Van Etta, and D.H. Walker. 1994. Human granulocytic ehrlichiosis in the upper midwest U.S. *J Am Med Assoc* 272:212–8.

CDC. 1981. Lyme disease—United States. 1980. *MMWR Morb Mortal Wkly Rep* 30:489-92,497.

CDC. 1982. Lyme disease. *MMWR Morb Mortal Wkly Rep* 31:367-368. Available at: http://www.cdc.gov/mmwr/preview/mmwrhtml/00015561.htm.

CDC. 1988. Epidemiologic notes and reports human ehrlichiosis – United States. *MMWR Morb Mortal Wkly Rep* 37:270,275-77. Available at http://www.cdc.gov/mmwr/preview/mmwrhtml/00000020.htm.

CDC. 1989. Epidemiologic notes and reports, babesiosis – Connecticut. *MMWR Morb Mortal Wkly Rep* 38:649-650. Available at http://www.cdc.gov/mmwr/preview/mmwrhtml/00001468.htm.

CDC. 1990. Case definitions for public health surveillance. *MMWR Morb Mortal Wkly Rep* 39(RR-13):1-43. Available at: http://www.cdc.gov/mmwr/preview/mmwrhtml/00025629.htm.

CDC. 1994. Summary of notifiable diseases – United States, 1993. *MMWR Morb Mortal Wkly Rep* 42:1-91. Available at http://www.cdc.gov/mmwr/PDF/wk/mm4253.pdf.

CDC. 1995. Human granulocytic ehrlichiosis – New York, 1995. *MMWR Morb Mortal Wkly Rep* 44:593-595. Available at http://www.cdc.gov/mmwr/PDF/wk/mm4432.pdf.

CSTE. 1996. Position statement 1996-17. Ehrlichiosis. Available at http://www.cste.org/ps/1996/1996-17.htm.

CDC. 1997. Case definitions for infectious conditions under public health surveillance. *MMWR Morb Mortal Wkly Rep* 46(RR-10):1-55. Available at: http://www.cdc.gov/mmwr/preview/mmwrhtml/00047449.htm.

CDC. 1999. Recommendations for the use of Lyme disease vaccine: recommendations of the Advisory Committee on Immunization Practices (ACIP). Appendix: methods used to create a national Lyme disease risk map. *MMWR Morb Mortal Wkly Rep* 48(RR-07):21-24. Available at: http://www.cdc.gov/mmwr/PDF/rr/rr4807.pdf.

CDC. 2001. Updated guidelines for evaluating public health surveillance systems: recommendations of the guidelines working group. *MMWR Morb Mortal Wkly Rep* 50(RR-13):1-36. Available at: http://www.cdc.gov/mmwr/PDF/rr/rr5013.pdf.

CDC. 2004. Lyme Disease — United States, 2001—2002 *MMWR Morb Mortal Wkly Rep* 53:365-369. Available at http://www.cdc.gov/mmwr/preview/mmwrhtml/mm5317a4.htm.

CDC. 2007. Lyme Disease — United States, 2003—2005. *MMWR Morb Mortal Wkly Rep* 56:573-76. Available at http://www.cdc.gov/mmwr/preview/mmwrhtml/mm5623a1.htm.

CDC. 2008. Surveillance for Lyme disease – United States, 1992-2006. *MMWR Morb Mortal Wkly Rep* 57(SS-10):1-9. Available at: http://www.cdc.gov/mmwr/preview/mmwrhtml/ss5710a1.htm.

CDC. 2010. Southern tick-associated rash illness. Available at http://www.cdc.gov/ncidod/dvbid/stari/.

CDC. 2010. Summary of notifiable diseases – United States, 2008. *MMWR Morb Mortal Wkly Rep* 54;1-94. Available at http://www.cdc.gov/mmwr/PDF/wk/mm5754.pdf.

Connally N.P., A.J. Durante, K.M. Yousey-Hindes, J.I. Meek, R.S. Nelson and R. Heimer. 2009. Peridomestic Lyme disease prevention: results of a population-based case-control study. *Am J PrevMed* 37(3):201-6.

Connecticut Department of Public Health. 2010. Reported cases of disease by county, 2007. Available at http://www.ct.gov/dph/lib/dph/infectious_diseases/pdf_forms_/ct_disease_cases_by_county_2007_fnl.pdf.

Coyle B.S., G.T. Strickland, Y.Y. Liang, C. Pena, R. McCarter, and E. Israel. 1996. The public health impact of Lyme disease in Maryland. *J Infect Dis* 173:1260-62.

Cromley, E.K., M.L. Cartter, R.D. Mrozinski, and S.H. Ertel. 1998. Residential setting as a risk factor for Lyme disease in a hyperendemic region. *Am J Epidemiol* 147:472-77.

CSTE. 1990. Position statement 1: National surveillance of Lyme disease and resources for Lyme disease and epidemiology. Available at: http://www.cste.org/ps/1990/1990-01.htm.

CSTE. 1996. Position statement 96-18: Revised case definitions for public health surveillance: infectious disease. Available at: http://www.cste.org/dnn/AnnualConference/PositionStatements/tabid/191/Default.aspx.

CSTE. 1998. Position statement 1998-ID-6. Adding Ehrlichiosis as a condition reportable to the National Public Health Surveillance System (NPHSS). Available at http://www.cste.org/ps/1998/1998-id-06.htm.

CSTE. 2000. Position statement 2000-ID-3. Changes in the case definition for human ehrlichiosis, and addition of a new ehrlichiosis category as a condition placed under surveillance according to the National Public Health Surveillance System (NPHSS). Available at http://www.cste.org/ps/2000/2000-id-03.htm.

CSTE. 2001. Position statement 2001-ID-06: Inclusion of West Nile encephalitis/meningitis and Powassan encephalitis/meningitis in the National Public Health Surveillance System (NPHSS), and revision of the national surveillance case definition of arboviral diseases of the central nervous system (CNS). Available at http://www.cste.org/ps/2001/2001-id-06.htm.

CSTE. 2003. Position statement 03-ID-08: Rocky Mountain spotted fever. Available at http://www.cste.org/PS/2003pdfs/2003finalpdf/03-ID-08Revised.pdf.

CSTE. 2007. Position statement 07-ID-11: Revised national surveillance case definition for Lyme disease. Available at: http://www.cste.org/PS/2007ps/2007psfinal/ID/07-ID-11.pdf.

CSTE. 2007. Position statement 2007-ID-05: Revision of the surveillance case definitions for Rocky Mountain spotted fever. Available at http://www.cste.org/PS/2007ps/2007psfinal/ID/07-ID-05.pdf.

CSTE. 2007. Position statement 2007-ID-03. Revision of the National Surveillance Case Definition for Ehrlichiosis (Ehrlichiosis/Anaplasmosis). Available at http://www.cste.org/PS/2007ps/2007psfinal/ID/07-ID-03.pdf.

CSTE. 2009. Position statement 2009-ID-16: Public health reporting and national notification for spotted fever rickettsiosis (including Rocky Mountain spotted fever). Available at http://www.cste.org/ps2009/09-ID-16.pdf.

CSTE. 2009. Position statement 09-ID-25: Public health reporting and national notification for Powassan virus disease. Available at http://www.cste.org/ps2009/09-ID-25.pdf.

CSTE. 2010. Position statement 2010-ID-27. Public health reporting and national surveillance for babesiosis. Available at http://www.cste.org/ps2010/10-ID-27.pdf.

Ertel S., B. Esponda, R. Nelson, and M.L. Cartter. 2006. Lyme disease- Connecticut, 2005. *Connecticut Epidemiologist* 26:13-14. Available at http://www.ct.gov/dph/lib/dph/infectious_diseases/pdf_forms_/vol26no4.pdf.

Ertel S. P. Gacek, R. Nelson, and M.L. Cartter. 2008. Lyme disease – Connecticut, 2007. *Connecticut Epidemiologist* 28:5-6. Available at http://www.ct.gov/dph/lib/dph/infectious_diseases/ctepinews/vol28no2.pdf.

Georgia Department of Human Resources, Division of Public Health, Epidemiology Branch. 2001. Tick bites and erythema migrans in Georgia: It Might NOT be Lyme disease! *Georgia Epidemiology Report* 17:1-3. Available at http://health.state.ga.us/pdfs/epi/gers/ger0801.pdf.

Gould H.L., R.S. Nelson, K.S. Griffith, E.B. Hayes, J. Piesman, P.S. Mead and M.L. Cartter. 2008. Knowledge, attitudes, and behaviors regarding Lyme disease prevention among Connecticut residents, 1999–2004. *Vector-borne and Zoonotic Diseases* 8:769-776.

Hadler, J.L. and L.R. Petersen. 2007. Surveillance for vector-borne diseases. In *Infectious Disease Surveillance*, edited by N.M. M'ikanatha, R. Lynfield, C.A. Van Beneden and H. de Valk. Oxford: Blackwell Publishing. Pp. 107-123.

Ley, C., E.M. Olshen, and A.L. Reingold. 1995. Case-control study of risk factors for incident Lyme disease in California. *Am J Epidemiol* 142:S39-S47.

Mather T.N., M.C. Nicholson, E.F. Donnelly, and B.T. Matyas. 1996 Entomologic index for human risk of Lyme disease. *Am J Epidemiol* 144:1066--9.

Meek J.I., C.L. Roberts, E.V. Smith, Jr, and M.L. Cartter. 1996. Underreporting of Lyme disease by Connecticut physicians, 1992. *J Public Health Manag Pract* 2:61-65.

Meriwether, R.A. 1996. Blueprint for a national public health surveillance system for the 21st century. *J Public Health Manag Pract* 2(4):16-23.

Moulton, A.D., R.A. Goodman and W.E. Permet. 2007. Perspective: law and great public health achievements. In *Law and Public Health Practice*, 2nd ed, edited by R.A. Goodman, R.E. Hoffman, W. Lopez, G.W. Matthews, M. Rothstein, and K.L. Foster. New York: Oxford University Press. P 13.

New York State Department of Health. 1994. Communicable disease in New York State, reported cases of selected diseases exclusive of New York City, 1984-1994. Available at http://www.nyhealth.gov/nysdoh/cdc/1994/sect5a.pdf

New York State Department of Health. 2008. Reported cases by disease and county, AIDS-dengue fever. Available at http://www.nyhealth.gov/statistics/diseases/communicable/2008/cases/1.htm.

Orloski, K., G. Campbell, C. Genese, J. Beckley, M. Schriefer, K. Spitalny, and D. Dennis. 1998. Emergence of Lyme disease in Hunterdon County, New Jersey, 1993: A case-control study of risk factors and evaluation of reporting patterns. *Am J Epidemiol* 147:391-7.

Stafford K.C., III, M.L. Cartter, L.A. Magnarelli, S. Ertel, and P.A. Mshar. 1998. Temporal correlations between tick abundance and prevalence of ticks infected with *Borrelia burdorferi* and increasing incidence of Lyme disease. *J Clin Microbiol* 36:1240-4.

Stramer S.L., F.B. Hollinger, L.M. Katz, S. Kleinman, P.S. Metzel, K.R. Gregory, and R.Y. Dodd. 2009. Emerging infectious disease agents and their potential threat to transfusion safety. *Transfusion* 49 Suppl 2:1S-29S.

Swanson S.J., D. Neitzel, K.D. Reed, and E.A. Belongia. 2006. Coinfections acquired from *Ixodes* ticks. *Clin Microbiol Rev* 19:708-27.

Vázquez M., C. Muehlenbein, M. Cartter, E.B. Hayes, S. Ertel and E.D. Shapiro. 2008. Effectiveness of personal protective measures to prevent Lyme disease. *Emerg Infect Dis* 14:210-216. Available at: http://www.cdc.gov/eid/content/14/2/210.htm.

# B

# Federal Funding of Tick-Borne Diseases

The Committee on Lyme disease and Other Tick-Borne Diseases surveyed federal agencies in the summer of 2010 to request information about the funding for tick-borne diseases to understand how the funding was distributed across agencies, across types of tick-borne diseases, and across study types. The following analysis is the result of the responses from the agencies, and while every effort was made to include all agencies, the Committee recognizes that some agencies may be missing and that it wasn't always possible to break out programs or dollar amounts. The analysis of this data was done by Andrea Bankoski, a graduate student at George Mason University, as an individually authored report to the Committee.

## TICK-BORNE DISEASE FUNDING

Figures B-1 and B-2, and Table B-1 report the funding for tick-borne disease studies[1] in the United States, which has totaled 369,61,539 from 2006 to 2010. Nine United States agencies[2] have allocated this funding

---

[1] Only studies with a monetary funding amount were used in the analysis.

[2] The data provided for this analysis included studies from the following organizations: NIH-NIAID (National Institute of Allergy and Infectious Diseases), CDC (Centers for Disease Control and Prevention), US Army Public Health Command (formerly US Army Center for Health Promotion & Preventive Medicine), NIH-NIAMS (National Institute of Arthritis and Musculoskeletal and Skin Diseases, NIH-NINDS (National Institute of Neurological Diseases and Stroke), NSF (National Science Foundation), USDA-ARS (Agricultural Research Service), EPA (Environmental Protection Agency), and the USDA-NWRC (National Wildlife Research Center).

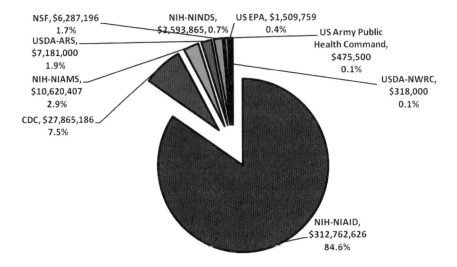

**FIGURE B-1** Total allocation of funding for tick-borne disease studies by agency/organization, 2006–2010.

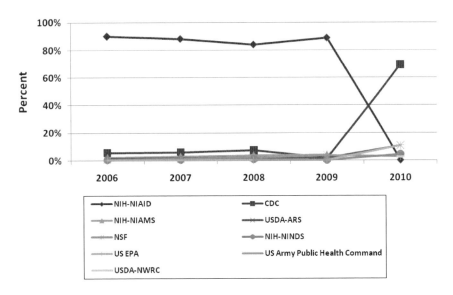

**FIGURE B-2** Annual proportion of agency/organization funding for tick-borne disease studies by year, 2006–2010.

**TABLE B-1** Annual Funding of Tick-Borne Disease Studies by Agency/Organization, 2006–2010

| Agency/Org (#) | 2006 | 2007 | 2008 | 2009 | 2010 | Average |
|---|---|---|---|---|---|---|
| NIH-NIAID (404) | $91,765,324 | $83,686,260 | $63,747,787 | $73,563,255 | — | **$62,552,525** |
| CDC (19) | $5,706,765 | $5,631,765 | $5,614,765 | $1,226,765 | $9,685,126 | $5,573,037 |
| NIH-NIAMS (15) | $2,051,376 | $2,579,209 | $2,758,608 | $3,231,214 | — | $2,655,102 |
| US-EPA (6) | — | — | — | — | $1,509,759 | **$1,509,759** |
| USDA-ARS (5) | $1,424,000 | $1,428,000 | $1,447,000 | $1,376,000 | $1,506,000 | $1,436,200 |
| NSF (5) | $390,196 | $1,093,733 | $1,436,180 | $2,990,954 | $376,133 | $1,256,439 |
| NIH-NINDS (4) | $662,366 | $458,834 | $654,163 | $220,625 | $597,877 | $518,776 |
| US Army PHC (1) | $237,750 | $237,750 | $243,500 | $232,000 | $237,750 | $237,750 |
| USDA-NWRC (2) | — | — | — | — | $318,000 | $318,000 |
| YEARLY TOTAL | $102,000,027 | $94,877,801 | $75,902,003 | $82,840,813 | $12,483,136 | **$73,620,756** |

to 45 studies. Tick-borne disease studies were grouped into six study type categories.

Figure B-1 shows the total allocation of funding by agency/organization for all studies between 2006 and 2010. The NIH-NIAID has funded the greatest amount of tick-borne disease studies—a total of 404 studies comprising 85% of the funding from all agencies and organizations. The CDC has funded 19 tick-borne disease studies from 2006 to 2010, 7% of the funding from all agencies and organizations. NIH-NIAMS has funded 15 tick-borne disease studies all between 2006 and 2009.The remaining agencies—USDA-ARS, NSF, NIH-NINDS, US Army Public Health Command, Environmental Protection Agency, and USDA-NWRS—have each funded six or less studies between 2006 and 2010.

Table B-1 shows the annual funding of tick-borne disease studies for each agency and organization from 2006 to 2010. Next to each agency name is the total number of studies funded for 2006 to 2010. Note that the annual total of funding had a significant drop ($12.4m) in 2010 since the provided data for analysis did not list any 2010 studies funded by the NIH-NIAID. The NIH-NIAID has allocated the most amount of funding, followed by the CDC and NIH-NIAMS. The US Army Public Health Command has funded just one study that spanned from 2008 to 2009, while the USDA-NWRC has granted funding only in 2010 for two studies that totaled $318,000.

The proportion of annual agency/organization funding for tick-borne disease studies by year is displayed in Figure B-2. All agencies and organizations allocated a steady proportion of funding until 2010. The NIH-NIAID contributed to the greatest proportion of funding for tick-borne disease studies until 2010. The CDC had the next greatest contribution to tick-borne disease funding until 2009, when they had a decline in their allocated funding; then, in 2010, the CDC increased their funding of tick-borne disease studies so significantly that it almost doubled their funding from previous years. In 2009, NIH-NIAMS and NSF had an increase in funding of tick-borne disease studies. In 2010, the NSF had a decrease in funding which was significantly lower than their funding from previous years, but was more closely aligned with the 2010 funding for the US EPA, USDA-ARS, USDA-NWRC, and NIH-NINDS.

### Tick-Borne Disease Funding by Study Type
### (Biological, Surveillance, Environmental)

Allocation of funding for tick-borne disease studies by study type is examined in this report. Tick-borne disease studies were grouped into six study type categories: Biological/Laboratory, Environmental, Surveillance (including human and animal surveillance), Treatment, Education/

Prevention, and Combination (the Combination study falls into at least two or more of the five other study type categories). Figure B-3 shows the total allocation of funding by study type for all studies between 2006 and 2010. Microbiological studies totaled $210m, which was 57% of the funding from all tick-borne disease studies. Prevention/Education studies were allocated $84.0m in funding (23%), followed by studies on a Combination of study types at $47.2m (13%), Treatment at $17.1m (4%), Environmental at $7.2m (2%), and Surveillance at $3.5m (1%).

Table B-2 shows the annual funding of tick-borne disease studies by study type from 2006 to 2010. Next to each agency name is the total number of studies funded for 2006 to 2010 (#). Note that the annual total of funding had a significant drop ($12.4m) in 2010 since the provided data for analysis did not list any 2010 studies funded by the NIH-NIAID. There were 304 Microbiological studies between 2006 and 2010 averaging $42m for annual funding, while Prevention/Education totaled 77 studies and averaged $16.8m for annual funding between 2006 and 2010. All other study types had between 10 to 39 studies and averaged between $711k and $9.4m for annual funding.

The proportion of annual funding for tick-borne diseases study types by year is displayed in Figure B-4. There was a steady allocation of funding for all study types until 2009 (last complete year for all agencies). Microbiological studies contributed to the greatest proportion of funding

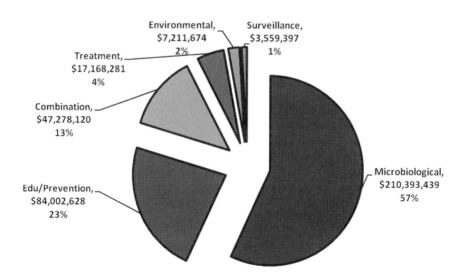

**FIGURE B-3** Total allocation of funding for tick-borne disease studies by study type, 2006–2010.

TABLE B-2 Annual Funding of Tick-Borne Disease Studies by Study Type, 2006–2010

| Study Type (#) | 2006 | 2007 | 2008 | 2009 | 2010 | Average |
|---|---|---|---|---|---|---|
| Microbiological (304) | $53,895,938 | $50,119,167 | $48,780,509 | $56,059,948 | $1,537,877 | $42,078,688 |
| Prevention/Edu (77) | $30,072,837 | $30,782,779 | $9,179,903 | $13,137,663 | $199,446 | $16,800,526 |
| Combination (39) | $11,989,868 | $9,348,166 | $11,696,074 | $4,229,879 | $10,014,133 | $9,455,624 |
| Treatment (16) | $3,975,791 | $3,433,126 | $4,820,748 | $4,938,616 | — | $3,433,656 |
| Environmental (14) | $1,030,142 | $995,563 | $453,989 | $3,206,541 | $1,525,439 | $1,442,335 |
| Surveillance (11) | $405,451 | $199,000 | $970,780 | $1,268,166 | $716,000 | $711,879 |
| YEARLY TOTAL | $102,000,027 | $94,877,801 | $75,907,003 | $82,340,813 | $12,483,136 | $73,620,756 |

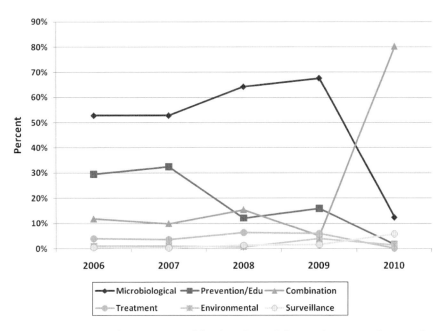

**FIGURE B-4** Annual proportion of funding for tick-borne disease study types by year, 2006–2010.

from 2006 to 2009. Combination studies had the greatest proportion of funding in 2010. There was a slight downward trend in funding of Prevention/Education studies from 2006 to 2010. Treatment, Environmental, and Surveillance, studies were all low in proportion to the other study types, but all three remained relatively stable from 2006 to 2010.

### Tick-Borne Disease by Study Topic (Pathogen, Tick, Host)

A further allocation of funding for tick-borne disease studies by study topic was examined. Tick-borne disease studies were grouped into five study topic categories—Pathogen, Tick, Host (including both humans and animals), Clinical Impact, and All Inclusive (the All Inclusive study falls into all four of other study topic categories).

Figure B-5 shows the total allocation of funding by study topic for all studies between 2006 and 2010. Pathogen studies have been allotted the greatest amount of funding at a total of $247m (67%). Clinical Impact studies were the next highest funding study topic with a total of $71.6m (20%). The other categories of study topics were Inclusive studies at $30.8m (8%), Tick studies at $11.9m (3%), and Host studies at $8.1m (2%).

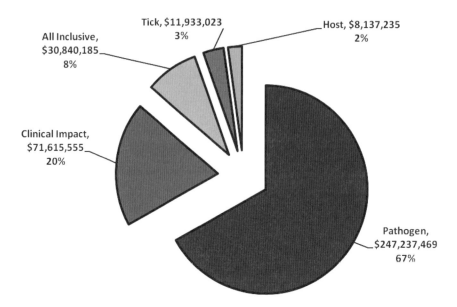

All Inclusive, $30,840,185 8%

Tick, $11,933,023 3%

Host, $8,137,235 2%

Clinical Impact, $71,615,555 20%

Pathogen, $247,237,469 67%

**FIGURE B-5** Total allocation of funding for tick-borne disease studies by study topic, 2006–2010.

Table B-3 shows the annual funding of tick-borne disease studies by study topic from 2006 to 2010. Next to each agency name is the total number of studies funded for 2006 to 2010 (#). Note that the annual total of funding had a significant drop ($12.4m) in 2010 since the provided data for analysis did not list any 2010 studies funded by the NIH-NIAID. There were 343 Pathogen studies between 2006 and 2010 averaging $49m for annual funding, while Clinical Impact studies totaled 64 and averaged $14.3m. Inclusive, Tick, and Host study topics had between 17 to 19 studies and averaged between $1.6m and $6.1m for average annual funding.

The proportion of annual funding for tick-borne diseases study topics by year is displayed in Figure B-6. The Pathogen studies contributed to the greatest proportion of funding until 2010 when Inclusive studies had a significant increase in funding. Clinical Impact studies slowly decreased in funding from 2006 to 2010 while Tick and Host studies remained low but stable in funding.

*Tick-Borne Disease by Tick Pathogen*

Allocation of funding for tick-borne disease studies by pathogen type was examined in this report. Tick-borne disease studies were grouped into

TABLE B-3 Annual Funding of Tick-Borne Disease Studies by Study Topic, 2006–2010

| Study Topic (#) | 2006 | 2007 | 2008 | 2009 | 2010 | Average |
|---|---|---|---|---|---|---|
| Pathogen (343) | $62,863,944 | $57,183,511 | $59,127,804 | $66,593,207 | $1,469,003 | $49,447,494 |
| Clinical Impact (64) | $28,775,092 | $27,390,105 | $6,225,497 | $9,224,861 | | $14,329,111 |
| Inclusive (17) | $7,215,128 | $6,943,735 | $7,001,369 | $611,953 | $9,068,000 | $6,168,037 |
| Tick (19) | $2,495,035 | $1,938,727 | $1,848,631 | $3,854,871 | $1,795,759 | $2,386,605 |
| Host (18) | $650,827 | $1,421,723 | $1,848,631 | $2,555,921 | $910,133 | $1,627,447 |
| YEARLY TOTAL | $102,000,026 | $94,877,801 | $75,902,003 | $82,840,813 | $12,483,136 | $73,620,756 |

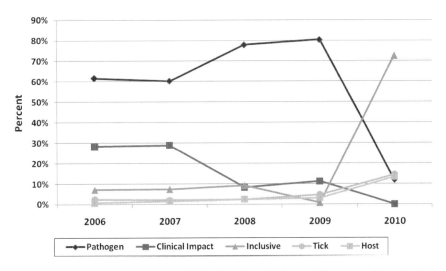

FIGURE B-6 Annual proportion of funding for tick-borne disease study topics by year, 2006–2010.

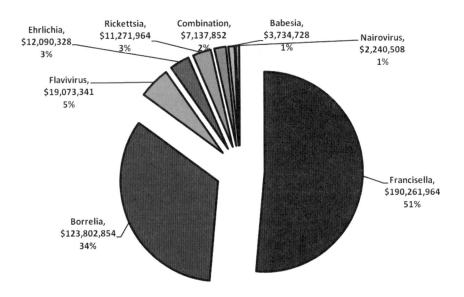

FIGURE B-7 Total allocation of funding for tick-borne disease studies by pathogen type, 2006–2010.

five types of tick-borne pathogens—*Borrelia*, *Rickettsia*, *Babesia*, *Ehrlichia*, and Combination (study focuses on at least two or more pathogens).

Figure B-7 shows the total allocation of funding by pathogen type for all studies between 2006 and 2010. Francisella studies have received the most funding at $190m (51%) followed by Borrelia studies at $123m (34%). Funding for Flavivirus totaled $19m (5%) and all other pathogens (Ehrlichia, Rickettsia, Combination, Babesia, and Nairovirus) were 3% or less of the total funding.

Table B-4 shows the annual funding of tick-borne disease studies by pathogen type from 2006 to 2010. Next to each agency name is the total number of studies funded for 2006 to 2010 (#). Note that the annual total of funding had a significant drop ($12.4m) in 2010 since the provided data for analysis did not list any 2010 studies funded by the NIH-NIAID. Francisella studies received the most funding, followed by Borrelia studies. A significant amount of Francisella and Borrelia studies were conducted (218 and 147) compared to other studies (all 26 or less).

The proportion of annual funding for tick-borne diseases pathogen studies by year is displayed in Figure B-8. The figure shows that Francisella studies received the highest proportion of funding from 2006 to 2009, followed by Borrelia studies. In 2010, Borrelia studies had a significant increase in funding taking the lead of the highest proportion of funding for tick-borne diseases, a likely artifact without the study allocation from NIH-NIAID for this year.

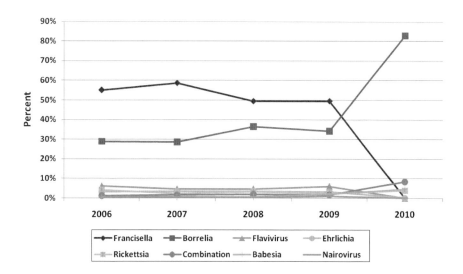

FIGURE B-8 Annual proportion of funding for tick-borne disease pathogen studies by year, 2006–2010.

**TABLE B-4** Annual Funding of Tick-Borne Disease Pathogen Studies by Year, 2006–2010

| Study Topic (#) | 2006 | 2007 | 2008 | 2009 | 2010 | Average |
|---|---|---|---|---|---|---|
| Francisella (218) | $56,234,585 | $55,565,617 | $37,493,378 | $40,968,384 | — | $38,052,393 |
| Borrelia (147) | $29,476,671 | $27,047,516 | $27,645,414 | $28,267,376 | $11,365,877 | $25,398,126 |
| Flavivirus (26) | $6,207,170 | $4,361,255 | $3,540,803 | $4,964,113 | — | $3,814,668 |
| Ehrlichia (18) | $3,384,192 | $3,282,096 | $2,650,076 | $2,748,964 | $25,000 | $2,418,066 |
| Rickettsia (18) | $4,136,723 | $2,299,654 | $2,503,017 | $1,840,737 | $491,833 | $2,254,393 |
| Combination (14) | $1,245,961 | $1,494,676 | $1,473,265 | $1,390,765 | $1,533,185 | $1,427,570 |
| Babesia (15) | $502,237 | $410,216 | $419,291 | $1,825,984 | $577,000 | $746,946 |
| Nairovirus (5) | $812,488 | $416,771 | $176,759 | $834,490 | — | $448,102 |
| YEARLY TOTAL | $102,000,027 | $94,877,801 | $75,907,003 | $82,840,813 | $12,483,136 | $73,620,756 |

# C

# Summary of Public Comment on Agenda

As part of its charge, the Institute of Medicine (IOM) Committee on Lyme Disease and Other Tick-Borne Diseases: the State of the Science was requested to include broad input from the public. To meet this goal, the committee held an open session on April 29, 2010, and four subsequent listening sessions. These sessions were structured to allow the public to briefly suggest topics of interest and speakers for the committee's workshop. The four sessions reached four geographic regions within the United States with high rates of Lyme disease and other tick-borne diseases. These sessions allowed participation from individuals who could not travel to the open session due to personal and financial hardships. Listening session participants came from Arizona, California, Connecticut, the District of Columbia, Florida, Georgia, Illinois, Iowa, Kansas, Kentucky, Maryland, Massachusetts, Michigan, Minnesota, Missouri, Nebraska, Nevada, New York, North Carolina, Oklahoma, Oregon, South Carolina, Tennessee, Texas, Washington, Wisconsin, and Native American tribes. During these sessions, the public were allowed to comment uninterrupted for up to 3 minutes, sharing personal experiences, suggesting topics to be considered by the committee, and offering the names of individuals whom they thought would be able to speak to the committee regarding Lyme disease and other tick-borne diseases. Views presented from the listening sessions do not represent conclusions from the committee.

## KEY POINTS FROM LISTENING SESSIONS

The first listening session targeted Georgia, North Carolina, and South Carolina and included participants from Florida, Georgia, Kentucky, Maryland, South Carolina, Tennessee, Virginia, and Wisconsin. Main topics gleaned from the listening session are

- Detecting and responding to tick-borne diseases remain challenging. Cases of STARI in the Southeast are poorly identified because there is no specific test; cases are hard to distinguish from Lyme disease and are often dismissed. Some *Borrelia* strains and species may not be detectible; there are more *Borrelia* strains in the South.
- There needs to be a regional Western blot using southern strains and species.
- Medical providers remain undereducated about tick-borne diseases. Health providers frequently dismiss patients and see positive cases as false—many are inadequately trained to diagnose tick-borne diseases. Providers also need to learn the vector biology of ticks and wildlife hosts. False positive cases of Lyme disease and other tick-borne diseases lack follow-up studies or evidence to confirm that it is a false case. The use of antibiotics, timing and fluctuating antibodies remain confusing to physicians. Varying criteria to diagnose Lyme disease lead to misinterpretation of lab reports.
- There is a need to fund independent, large-scale human studies conducted by new researchers in the Southeast.
- Cases of Lyme disease cannot be compared across the country because different methodologies are used to detect cases.
- Overall, the public lacks awareness of tick-borne diseases.

The second listening session targeted Arizona, California, and Texas and included participants from Arizona, California, Georgia, Iowa, Montana, New York, Oklahoma, Oregon, Texas, and Washington. The session highlighted the human face of tick-borne disease infections, definitions of cases and diagnoses, diagnostics, and physician education. Many felt that treatment guidelines did not always provide the relief to their ongoing symptoms. Assessments of clinical guidelines are outside the statement of task for this study.

Main topics gleaned from the listening session are

- There are varying strains of *Borrelia* species across geographic regions.
- Debates remain on the case definition versus clinical diagnosis of Lyme disease and other tick-borne diseases.

- Diagnostics on Lyme disease and other tick-borne disease have yet to be improved—specifically, the adequacy of current serology lab tests; current ELISA tests miss nearly half of those with Lyme disease; Western blot test may lead to false results; the timing of tests may conflict with antibiotics regimen.
- There is insufficient research on persistence and relapse of Lyme disease and other tick-borne diseases.

The third listening session targeted Michigan, Minnesota, and Wisconsin and included participants from Georgia, Illinois, Iowa, Kansas, Michigan, Minnesota, Missouri, Nebraska, Texas, and Wisconsin.

Main points outlined in session from Michigan, Minnesota, and Wisconsin include

- Existing diagnostic tests lack reliability, validity, sensitivity and specificity (serologic sensitivity)—the role of skin biopsy is unknown.
- Physicians frequently overlook co-infections that occur with the onset of Lyme disease.
- Healthcare providers need to be educated on the classic symptoms of Lyme disease.
- Research needs to examine the clinical significance of intracellular mechanisms (pathogenesis).
- Late neurological diseases may be triggered by Lyme disease and other tick-borne diseases.
- There is insufficient research on persistence and relapse of Lyme disease and other tick-borne diseases.
- Studies on behavioral change and non-pharmaceutical measures to treat Lyme disease (e.g., alternative and complementary therapy) are needed.

The final listening session was designed to engage the Native American tribes of Oklahoma and expanded to include the Native American population across the nation. The session included participants from Arizona, California, Connecticut, the District of Columbia, Florida, Iowa, Maryland, and Massachusetts.

Main points from the session include

- The *Borrelia* organism has changing morphology.
- There are alternative animal hosts for tick-borne diseases.
- Signs and symptoms associated with the *Borrelia* organism lack specificity.

- Existing diagnostics of the *Borrelia* organism remain inadequate. Resources are limited to develop a point-of-care test to improve clinical diagnosis in real time.
- State and local health departments should work with Native American tribes to develop behavioral, cultural, and educational efforts to prevent tick-borne diseases.
- There may be genetic differences in susceptibility to tick-borne diseases.

The committee greatly appreciates all who have participated during the listening sessions. Despite time limitations, the listening sessions strengthened the understanding of the current state of Lyme disease and other tick-borne diseases. The committee used information provided during the listening sessions to commission a paper on challenges to diagnostic development and the management of co-infection and past infections.

## SUMMARY OF PUBLIC COMMENTS PRIOR TO THE OCTOBER WORKSHOP

In reviewing the submissions to the Public Access file for the Committee on Lyme and Other Tick-Borne Diseases: The State of the Science, the following major themes were found among the submissions:

- the strong desire for the committee to know and understand what it is like for those living with Lyme disease and other tick-borne diseases in their day-to-day lives and the impact of being diagnosed or not having been diagnosed had on their physical and mental health, their economic situation, and their relationships in the community and with their health care providers, etc.
- the belief that the IDSA guidelines are immensely flawed and need to be rewritten and expanded. One commenter indicated the possibility of conflict of interest with IDSA and CDC, and which researchers get funded
- the need for improved diagnostics and testing. (There is a lot of frustration with the Western blot test and the CDC guidelines.)
- the strong push for more research and increased funding for Lyme disease especially in areas such as disease transmission, pathogenesis, new treatments and why old treatments fail, co-infection, persistence, and strain variability
- emphasis on physician and community education about Lyme disease and the need for physicians willing to treat for Lyme disease in areas that have not been recognized as endemic

- the possibility of and the need to look for alternative treatments and the use of different antibiotics other than doxyxyline and cefriaxone
- the lack of a national reporting standard and how different case definitins impact those in areas labeled "non-endemic"
- the need for more research into tick biology and the processes by which pathogens invade and multiple in the human host

Other comments raised the following issues:

- impact of vaccines and vaccine research adversely affecting the study of Lyme disease
- a possible link between Lyme disease and autism
- alternative modes of infection (e.g., bees and fungi)
- the need for environmental controls (e.g., decreasing the deer population in largely endemic areas)
- the need to look at special populations such as children, people with occupational risk of exposure, and low-income individuals
- genetic/immune factors that may cause the disease to vary from person-to-person
- a desire for an international standard for Lyme disease and the pathogens capable of transmitting Lyme disease in humans

In addition to these comments, the following individuals were suggested to give testimony to the committee because of their expertise in the area:

- Raphael Stricker (ILADS)
- Benjamin Luft (SUNY–Stony Brook)
- Steven Schutzer (University of Medicine and Dentistry, NJ)
- Steven Phillips
- Brian Fallon (Columbia University)
- David Cadavid (Biogen Idec)
- Allison Delong (Brown University)
- Kerry Clark (University of North Florida)
- Reinhard Strubinger (Ludwig-Maximilians-Universität)
- Elizabeth Maloney
- Dave Martz
- Eugene Davidson (Georgetown University Medical Center)
- Joseph Burrascano
- David Volkman (SUNY–Stony Brook)
- Steven Barthold (University of California Davis)
- Mario Phillip (Tulane University)
- Sam Donta

- Robert Lane (University of California Berkeley)
- Ellen Stromdahl (US Army Center for Health Promotion and Preventive Medicine)
- Judith Miklossy (University of British Columbia)
- Kenneth Leigner
- Eva Sapi (University of New Haven)
- Karen Newell (Texas A&M)
- Cheryl Koopman (Stanford University)
- Dan Cameron (International Lyme and Associated Disease Society)
- James Oliver (Georgia Southern University)
- John Aucott (Johns Hopkins)
- Joseph G. Jemsek (Washington, DC)
- Norton L. Fishman (Rockville, MD)

# D

# Workshop Agenda

**DAY ONE: OCTOBER 11, 2010**

8:00 am        Introduction
                    *Lonnie King, D.V.M., M.S., M.A.*
                    Chair, Committee on Lyme Disease and Other Tick-
                        Borne Diseases
                    Dean, College of Veterinary Medicine
                    The Ohio State University

8:15 am        A Systems Approach in Understanding Tick-Borne
                    Diseases: People, Animals, and the Ecosystem
                    *Richard Ostfeld, Ph.D.*
                    Disease Ecologist
                    Cary Institute of Ecosystem Studies

8:40 am        Discussion

**Surveillance, Spectrum, and Burden of Tick-Borne Diseases**

9:00 am        Moderator: *Gordon Schutze, M.D.*
                    Committee Member, Committee on Lyme Disease
                      and Other Tick-Borne Diseases
                    Professor and Vice-Chairman for Educational Affairs
                    Department of Pediatrics
                    Vice President, Baylor International Pediatric AIDS
                      Initiative
                    Baylor College of Medicine
                    Texas Children's Hospital

9:05 am          Landscape of Lyme Disease: Current Knowledge, Gaps,
                 and Research Needs
                     *Gary P. Wormser, M.D.*
                     Professor of Medicine
                     Chief, Division of Infectious Diseases
                     Vice-Chairman, Department of Medicine
                     New York Medical College

9:30 am          Spectrum of Lyme Disease: Approaches to Understanding
                 Multi-factorial and Multidimensional Diseases
                     *Benjamin J. Luft, M.D.*
                     Edmund D. Pellegrino Professor
                     Division of Infectious Diseases
                     State University of New York at Stony Brook

9:50 am          Discussion

10:10 am         Break

10:25 am         Clinical Manifestations, Co-infection, and Research
                 Needs of Human *Babesiosis*: The Increasing Health
                 Burden
                     *Peter Krause, M.D.*
                     Senior Research Scientist
                     Lecturer in Epidemiology, Microbial Diseases
                     Yale School of Public Health

10:40 am         Insights into *Ehrlichia* & *Anaplasma*: Surveillance,
                 Co-infection, and Research Needs
                     *J. Stephen Dumler, M.D.*
                     Professor, Department of Pathology
                     Division of Medical Microbiology
                     Johns Hopkins University School of Medicine

11:00 am         *Rickettsia* Diseases: Spectrum of Disease, Spatial
                 Clustering, At-Risk Populations, and Research Needs
                     *Jennifer McQuiston, D.V.M, M.S.*
                     National Center for Preparedness, Detection, and
                         Control of Infectious Diseases
                     Centers for Disease Control and Prevention

11:20 am         Discussion

| 11:40 am | Panel: Disease Surveillance & Co-infection<br>*J. Stephen Dumler, Peter Krause, Benjamin J. Luft,*<br>*Jennifer McQuiston, and Gary P. Wormser* |
|---|---|

| 12:15 pm | Summation: Unifying Knowledge Gaps and Needs<br>*Gordon Schutze* |
|---|---|

| 12:25 pm | **LUNCH (45 minutes)** |
|---|---|

**At-Risk Populations and Human Face of Tick-Borne Diseases**

| 1:10 pm | Moderator: *Lonnie King* |
|---|---|

| 1:15 pm | Panel: Genetic and Acquired Determinants of Host<br>Susceptibility and Vulnerable Populations<br>*David Weber, M.D.*<br>Professor of Medicine and Pediatrics, School of<br>    Medicine<br>Professor of Epidemiology, School of Public Health<br>University of North Carolina<br>*Peter Krause, M.D.*<br>Senior Research Scientist<br>Lecturer in Epidemiology Microbial Diseases<br>Yale School of Public Health |
|---|---|

| 1:40 pm | Discussion |
|---|---|

| 1:55 pm | The Human Face of Tick-Borne Disease Infections<br>*Pamela Weintraub*<br>Author, *Cure Unknown*<br>Features Editor, *Discover* Magazine |
|---|---|

| 2:15 pm | Discussion |
|---|---|

| 2:55 pm | Break |
|---|---|

**Diagnostics and Diagnosis**

| 3:05 pm | Moderators: *Lynn Gerber, M.D.*<br>Committee Member, Committee on Lyme Disease<br>    and Other Tick-Borne Diseases<br>Director, Center for the Study of Chronic Illness and<br>    Disability<br>College of Health and Human Services<br>George Mason University |
|---|---|

*David H. Walker, M.D.*
Committee Member, Committee on Lyme Disease and
    Other Tick-Borne Diseases
Professor and Chair
Department of Pathology
University of Texas Medical Branch at Galveston

3:10 pm          Diagnostics for Lyme Disease: Knowledge Gaps and
                 Needs
                 *Maria Aguero-Rosenfeld, M.D.*
                 Professor of Pathology
                 Director of Clinical Pathology and Microbiology
                     Laboratory
                 Bellevue Hospital Center

3:30 pm          Improved Diagnostics & Novel Approaches to Tick-
                 Borne Disease Infections
                 *Juan Olano, M.D.*
                 Associate Professor, Department of Pathology
                 Director, Residency Training Program
                 University of Texas Medical Branch Center

3:50 pm          Potential Bio-Marker Applications for Lyme Disease:
                 Aligning Multiple Symptoms with Biological Measures
                 *Afton Hassett, Psy.D.*
                 Associate Research Scientist, Department of
                     Anesthesiology
                 Chronic Pain & Fatigue Research Center
                 University of Michigan Medical School

4:10 pm          Discussion

4:40 pm          Panel: Challenges for Clinicians in Diagnosis and
                 Management of Chronic Illness Manifestations:
                 Knowledge Gaps
                 *Sam T. Donta, M.D.*
                 Infectious Disease Specialist
                 Falmouth Hospital, Massachusetts

> *Brian Fallon, M.D., M.P.H.*
> Director of the Center for Neuroinflammatory
> Disorders and Biobehavioral Medicine
> Director of the Lyme and Tick-Borne Diseases
> Research Center
> Columbia University Medical Center
>
> *Richard F. Jacobs, M.D., F.A.A.P.*
> Robert H. Fiser, Jr., M.D. Endowed Chair in Pediatrics
> Chairman, Department of Pediatrics
> University of Arkansas for Medical Sciences
> President, Arkansas Children's Hospital Research
> Institute
>
> *Matthew Liang, M.D., M.P.H.*
> Professor, Department of Health Policy and Management
> Harvard School of Public Health

5:20 pm          Discussion

5:45 pm          Summation
                 *Lynn Gerber and David Walker*

6:00 pm          Adjourn

### DAY TWO: OCTOBER 12, 2010

8:00 am          Introduction
                 *Lonnie King*

### Emerging Infections, Tick Biology, and Host-Vector Interactions

              Moderator: *Lonnie King*

8:05 am          Emerging and Re-Emerging Tick-Borne Infections
                 *Ulrike Munderloh, D.V.M., Ph.D.*
                 Associate Professor, Department of Entomology
                 University of Minnesota

8:25 am        Natural History of Ticks: Evolution, Adaptation and
               Biology
                    *Tom G. Schwan, Ph.D., M.S.*
                    Chief, Laboratory of Zoonotic Pathogens
                    Chief, Medical Entomology Section
                    National Institute of Allergy and Infectious Diseases

8:45 am        Wildlife and Domestic Hosts: Their Roles in
               Maintaining, Amplifying Pathogens, and their Changing
               Dynamics
                    *Howard Ginsberg, Ph.D.*
                    Research Ecologist
                    United States Geological Survey
                    Professor in Residence, Department of Plant Science
                    University of Rhode Island

9:05 am        Discussion

9:20 am        Comparative Medical Importance of a One Health
               Approach to Emerging Tick-borne Diseases
                    *Edward Breitschwerdt, D.V.M.*
                    Professor of Internal Medicine
                    College of Veterinary Medicine
                    North Carolina State University
                    Adjunct Professor of Medicine
                    Duke University Medical Center

9:40 am        Variation of *Borrelia* Subspecies: Implications for Human
               Disease
                    *James H. Oliver, Jr., Ph.D.*
                    Director, Institute of Arthropodology and
               Parasitology
                    Callaway Professor of Biology
                    Georgia Southern University

10:00 am       Discussion

10:20 am       Break

**Pathogenesis**

10:30 am        Moderator: *Guy Palmer, D.V.M., Ph.D.*
                Committee Member, Committee on Lyme Disease
                    and Other Tick-Borne Diseases
                Regents Professor of Pathology and Infectious
                    Diseases
                The Creighton Chair and Director, School for Global
                    Animal Health
                Washington State University

10:35 am        Pathogenesis of *Borrelia burgdorferi* Infection and
                Disease
                    *Janis Weis, Ph.D.*
                    Professor of Pathology, Department of Pathology
                    University of Utah

10:55 am        Duration of Spirochete Infection Following Antibiotic
                Treatment in Animals
                    *Linda Bockenstedt, M.D.*
                    Harold W. Jockers Professor of Medicine
                    Department of Rheumatology
                    Yale School of Medicine

11:15 am        Discussion

11:30 am        Antigenic Variation as a Mechanism for Persistent
                *Borrelia* Infection
                    *Steven Norris, Ph.D.*
                    Greer Professor
                    Vice Chair for Research
                    Pathology & Laboratory Medicine
                    University of Texas, Houston

11:50 am        Sequestration as a Mechanism for Persistent *Borrelia*
                Infection
                    *Stephen Barthold, D.V.M., Ph.D.*
                    Distinguished Professor
                    Department of Pathology, Microbiology and
                        Immunology
                    Center of Comparative Medicine
                    School of Veterinary Medicine
                    University of California, Davis

12:10 pm        Discussion

12:30 pm        **LUNCH (45 minutes)**

1:15 pm         Pathogenesis of *Ehrlichia* and *Anaplasma* Infection and
                Disease
                > **Nahed Ismail, M.D., M.Sc., Ph.D., S.M. (ASCP),**
                > **D. (ABMM)**
                > Associate Professor, Department of Pathology
                > Meharry Medical College

1:35 pm         Pathogenesis of *Rickettsia* Infection and Disease
                > **Gustavo Valbuena, M.D.**
                > Instructor, Department of Pathology
                > University of Texas Medical Branch

1:55 pm         Discussion

2:15 pm         Summation
                > **Guy Palmer**

                **Science, Society, and Disease**

2:20 pm         Moderator: **Lynn Gerber**

2:25 pm         The Social Construction of Lyme Disease
                > **Robert Aronowitz, M.D.**
                > Professor, Department of History and Sociology of
                >        Science
                > University of Pennsylvania

2:45 pm         Discussion

2:55 pm         Break

                **Prevention**

3:05 pm         Moderator: **Stephen M. Ostroff, M.D.**
                > Committee Member, Committee on Lyme Disease
                >        and Other Tick-Borne Diseases
                > Director, Bureau of Epidemiology
                > Pennsylvania Department of Health

| | |
|---|---|
| 3:10 pm | Current Vaccines for Tick-Borne Disease Infections and Vaccine Development |
| | *Jere McBride, Ph.D., M.S.* |
| | Associate Professor, Department of Pathology |
| | University of Texas Medical Branch |
| | |
| 3:30 pm | Developing Opportunities for Future Vaccines |
| | *Wendy Brown, Ph.D., M.P.H.* |
| | Regents Professor, Department of Veterinary |
| | Microbiology and Pathology |
| | Washington State University |
| | |
| 3:50 pm | Discussion |
| | |
| 4:10 pm | Education, Behavior Change, and Other Non-Pharmaceutical Measures Against Lyme and Other Tick-Borne Diseases |
| | *Paul Mead, M.D., M.P.H.* |
| | Medical Epidemiologist, Division of Vector-Borne |
| | Infectious Diseases |
| | National Center for Infectious Diseases |
| | Center for Disease Control and Prevention |
| | |
| 4:30 pm | Vector- and Host-Targeted Strategies for Prevention of Tick-Borne Diseases |
| | *José M.C. Ribeiro, M.D., Ph.D.* |
| | Chief, Vector Biology Section |
| | Laboratory of Malaria and Vector Research |
| | National Institute of Allergy and Infectious Diseases |
| | |
| 4:50 pm | Discussion |
| | |
| 5:10 pm | Summation |
| | *Steve Ostroff* |

## Closing

5:20 pm     Moderator: *Lonnie King*

5:25 pm     Panel: State of Science, General Research Gaps and
            Opportunities in Tick-Borne Diseases
            *John Aucott, M.D.*
            Founder, Lyme Disease Research Foundation of
                Maryland
            Physician, Park Medical Associates

            *Linda Bockenstedt, M.D.*
            Harold W. Jockers Professor of Medicine
            Department of Rheumatology
            Yale School of Medicine

            *J. Stephen Dumler, M.D.*
            Professor, Department of Pathology
            Division of Medical Microbiology
            Johns Hopkins University School of Medicine

            *Susan O'Connell, M.D.*
            Consultant Microbiologist
            Head of the Lyme Borreliosis Unit
            Southampton General Hospital

            *Gregg P. Skall, J.D.*
            Counsel, National Capital Lyme and Tick-borne
                Disease Association
            Member, Womble Carlyle Sandridge & Rice, PLLC

5:55 pm     Discussion

6:25 pm     Final Summation and Closing Remarks
            *Lonnie King*

6:35 pm     Adjourn

# E

# Public Comment Summary

During the workshop, a number of questions and comments were emailed to the panelists from online participants. Due to time limitations, many of the questions posed were not addressed. This appendix contains a list of questions asked during each session. The questions have been annotated, but they, along with any comments submitted during the workshop, can be found in their entirety in the committee's Public Access File.[1]

## SURVEILLANCE, SPECTRUM, AND BURDEN OF TICK-BORNE DISEASES

- Why is *Borrelia burgdorferi* the only recognized cause of Lyme disease in the United States?
- Are there standard criteria for a Lyme disease diagnosis?

---

[1] Written materials submitted to a study committee by external sources are listed in the project's Public Access File and can be made available to the public upon request. Contact the Public Access Records Office (PARO) for a copy of the list and to obtain copies of the materials. Copies of materials are free to government employees and educators. Please send an email or call PARO to make a request or an inquiry.

Public Access Records Office
The National Academies
Washington, DC 20001
Tel: 202.334.3543
FAX: 202.334.2158
E-mail: paro@nas.edu

- Is there a possibility of chronic Lyme disease, and if so, what data is there to support the existence of chronic or persistent Lyme disease? What symptoms could describe such a condition?
- In regards to RMSF case studies are other tick-borne infections—for example, *Bartonella*, *Babesia*, *Mycoplasma*—investigated as well? If not, is there an area where retrospective analysis could be helpful, particularly in fatal cases?
- Why is late-stage Lyme not considered a disability according to SSDI guidelines?
- Has anyone looked at the possibility of ongoing *Babesia* infection due to *Borrelia* coinfection?
- Is there a connection between acute or chronic Lyme disease and infection with *Bartonella* or a *Bartonella*-like organisms?
- If a patient has Lyme and *Babesia*, do you think it could complicate eradication of the diseases and warrant further antibiotics/antimalarials?
- What is the benefit of prophylactic antibiotic therapy, and how effective would such therapy be in preventing disease?
- What is being done to update the materials on tick-borne diseases taught to military personnel?
- Would data from alternative sources (for example, home health care workers) be of value to physicians and researchers in accurately recording cases and disease symptoms?
- How are researchers supposed to investigate a disease without proper funding when money is needed to begin the initial investigations (research paradox)?
- What efforts would you suggest to increase communication between researchers and physicians?

## AT-RISK POPULATIONS AND HUMAN
## FACE OF TICK-BORNE DISEASES

- Does Lyme disease have the potential to cause postural orthostatic tachycardia syndrome (POTS)?
- Has any research been done to investigate possible connections between Lyme disease and Alzheimer's disease?
- What genetic characteristics make one more susceptible to Lyme disease?
- Are there any strains of *Babesia* that, given current lab techniques, are only able to be clinically diagnosed?
- What services are available to help support families suffering from Lyme disease?

- What research is being done regarding the relationship between Lyme disease and movement disorders?

## DIAGNOSTICS AND DIAGNOSIS

- Why is IGM only useful in early disease?
- Why does IGM seem to cycle between positive and negative during treatment of other co-infections and returning Lyme symptoms? Why is this not clinically relevant to diagnostics?
- Should children be immediately screened for Lyme disease following a tick bite?
- What clinical markers are used to diagnosis "post Lyme"? Is the diagnosis made on the basis that any level of treatment means eradication of the pathogen?
- Should patients with post-treatment Lyme disease syndrome still test positive for *Borrelia* DNA? If not, what diagnosis would be given to a person who is post-treatment but still positive for *Borrelia*?
- How can you be certain that these patients are free of *Borrelia burgdorferi*, even when it is known that many people and animals have been sero-negative despite still having active disease?
- Using a SPECT scan of the brain, can you distinguish global hypoperfusion (brain damage) and cognitive dysfunction caused by tick-borne diseases versus that caused by long-term excessive medications?
- Do changes in the immune system alter the effectiveness of antibiotic treatment when recommended dosages are bacteriostatic not bactericidal?
- Is there any way to determine which stage of Lyme disease a patient with chronic Lyme disease is in whether through test results or the chronological progression of symptoms?
- When will the gap in testing knowledge be addressed? When will the weight of the evidence be acknowledged? When will this disease be robustly studied scientifically, without political or other interference?
- What factors effect the development of symptoms and diagnosis of Lyme disease?
- What tests are currently available besides the Western blot for Lyme disease patients and their physicians to more accurately determine the elimination of *Borrelia* after a course of antibiotic treatment?

## EMERGING INFECTIONS, TICK BIOLOGY,
## AND HOST–VECTOR INTERACTIONS

- How come people can have a negative Lyme disease result in the UK and yet have a positive Lyme disease test in the United States?
- Do ticks remain infectious after biting someone?
- Have you done any studies on biofilms as a way for *B. burgdorferi* to sequester itself?

## PATHOGENESIS

- How long must a tick be attached to transmit *Borrelia*?
- Can you explain tick regurgitation and pathogenic infection on improper removal or agitation?
- What research has been done to investigate intracellular *Borrelia* infection?
- Can ongoing infection be the result of residual primary infection after treatment?
- If no toxins [are] secreted from *B. burgdorferi*, why do patients experience a Jarish-Herxheimer reaction to treatment?
- How do the explanations of *Borrelia* antibodies affect interpretation of Elisa and Western blot testing?
- Is there a possibility of sexual transmission of Lyme disease? Are there any studies being done to support or disprove this?

## SCIENCE, SOCIETY, AND DISEASE

- For medical and psychological communities, what can be done to educate those who are in a position to encounter Lyme as a valid differential diagnoses? If mental health services have a Surgeon General Statement that translates to codes of ethics for the profession, is it possible that Lyme could be named as another such diversity group for which ethical consideration is merited? Currently, what propaganda is being downloaded to institutions of medicine and psychology, M.D.s, psychiatric and mental health services providers, educational personnel, etc., that promotes the well-being of those who suffer with Lyme?
- Can the CDC provide funding at the public grade school levels to educate staff and students on prevention techniques?
- What public health message should be relied to the public regarding Lyme disease?

## PREVENTION

- What tests are currently available, besides the Western blot for Lyme disease patients and their physicians to help them more accurately determine whether the patient is completely cured of the infection after a course of antibiotic treatment even though the patient may still exhibit symptoms?
- How can highly specific bands to *Borrelia* be used in current vaccine research and be excluded in diagnosis?
- Are there any factors such as body scent that attracts ticks to certain individuals?

# F

# Speaker Biosketches

**Maria Aguero-Rosenfeld, M.D.** is the director of the clinical pathology and microbiology laboratory at Bellevue Hospital Center and has worked on the laboratory diagnosis of tick-borne diseases for over 20 years. She has been a faculty member at New York Medical College since 1989 as a professor in the Departments of Pathology, Microbiology, and Medicine, and has been the director of clinical pathology at Westchester Medical Center since 2006.

Dr. Aguero-Rosenfeld obtained her M.D. from the University of Chile School of Medicine and completed residencies in internal medicine and clinical pathology, and a fellowship in medical microbiology, at the Hospital of the University of Pennsylvania.

**Robert A. Aronowitz, M.D.** is a professor and graduate chair of history and sociology of science, and professor of family medicine and community practice, at the University of Pennsylvania. At the University of Pennsylvania, Dr. Aronowitz was the founding director of the health and societies program. He also founded and co-directs the university's Robert Wood Johnson Foundation Health and Society Scholars Program. Dr. Aronowitz's first book, *Making Sense of Illness: Science, Society, and Disease* (Cambridge 1998), explores changing disease definitions and meanings in the 20th century. He is currently finishing a project on the history of health risks in American medicine and society.

Dr. Aronowitz received his M.D. from the Yale School of Medicine.

**John Aucott, M.D.** is the founder of the Lyme Disease Research Foundation of Maryland, a public nonprofit organization founded to promote research and education in Lyme disease. He is also the co-principal investigator for the prospective cohort study, SLICE, examining the impact of acute Lyme disease on long-term health outcomes and immune function. A graduate of the Johns Hopkins University School of Medicine, Dr. Aucott is a diplomate of the American Board of Internal Medicine with sub-specialty training in infectious disease and geographic medicine at University Hospitals of Cleveland. He served as the Section Head for General Internal Medicine and was the Residency Program Director at the Cleveland Veterans Affairs Medical Center while on the faculty at Case Western Reserve University School of Medicine from 1989–1996.

**Stephen Barthold, D.V.M., Ph.D.** is a Distinguished Professor of Veterinary and Medical Pathology at the University of California (UC) Davis, and director of the UC Davis Center for Comparative Medicine. His professional specialty is infectious diseases of laboratory rodents and biology of the laboratory mouse. In 1974, he was appointed assistant professor of comparative medicine at the Yale School of Medicine, with subsequent promotion to full professor in 1989. He earned diplomate status in the American College of Veterinary Pathologists in 1976, and he moved to UC, Davis, in 1997.

Dr. Barthold received his B.S. and D.V.M. from UC, Davis, in 1967 and 1969. He sought further training in experimental and comparative pathology at the University of Wisconsin, Madison, and received his M.S. and Ph.D. in 1973 and 1974, respectively.

**Linda K. Bockenstedt, M.D.** is the Harold W. Jockers Professor of Medicine in Rheumatology and director for Professional Development and Equity at Yale University School of Medicine. Dr. Bockenstedt's research interests are in infection-related rheumatic disease, with a focus on the tick-borne spirochetal infection Lyme disease. Her most recent studies employ state-of-the-art imaging techniques to examine tick-spirochete-mammalian host interactions, including optical tweezers to study spirochete outer membrane physical properties that promote evasion of phagocytosis, and multiphoton microscopy to image in real-time tick-borne spirochete invasion, dissemination, and persistence in mice.

Dr. Bockenstedt is a member of the Ad Hoc Lyme Disease Study Group and served on the panel that revised the clinical practice guidelines for the diagnosis and treatment of Lyme disease, human granulocytic anaplasmosis, and *babesiosis*, published in 2006 by the Infectious Diseases Society of America.

She is a graduate of Harvard College in 1977 and the Ohio State University College of Medicine in 1981, and completed residency training in internal medicine at Yale–New Haven Hospital in 1984.

**Edward B. Breitschwerdt, D.V.M.** is a professor of medicine and infectious diseases at North Carolina State University College of Veterinary Medicine. He is also an adjunct professor of medicine at Duke University Medical Center, and a diplomate, American College of Veterinary Internal Medicine (ACVIM). Dr. Breitschwerdt directs the Intracellular Pathogens Research Laboratory in the Center for Comparative Medicine and Translational Research at North Carolina State University. He also co-directs the Vector Borne Diseases Diagnostic Laboratory and is the director of the NCSU-CVM Biosafety Level 3 Laboratory.

Dr. Breitschwerdt's clinical interests include infectious diseases, immunology, and nephrology, and his research has emphasized vector-transmitted intracellular pathogens. Most recently, he has contributed to cutting-edge research in the areas of animal and human bartonellosis.

Dr. Breitschwerdt received his M.D. from the University of Georgia and completed an internship and residency in Internal Medicine at the University of Missouri between 1974 and 1977.

**Wendy Brown, Ph.D., M.P.H.** is a Regents Professor in the Department of Veterinary Microbiology and Pathology at Washington State University (WSU). Dr. Brown's major research interest has been in the area of vaccine development for globally important tick-borne infectious diseases. This includes understanding the host-pathogen interaction and identifying vaccine antigens that stimulate recall responses by T lymphocytes from immune animals.

At WSU, Dr. Brown initiated a new research program to identify candidate vaccine antigens within the protective outer membrane fraction of a tick-transmitted rickettsial pathogen of cattle, Anaplasma marginale.

**Sam T. Donta, M.D.** is retired from a long career as an infectious disease specialist. He worked at the University of Iowa where he became a professor of medicine and chief of infectious diseases before moving to the University of Connecticut where he was chief of infectious diseases for 11 years. Dr. Donta then moved to Boston University/Boston VA for 10 years before his retirement. His basic interests have been in microbial toxins, but he has also been involved in a number of clinical trials. For the last 20 years, he has been interested in Lyme disease, and he continues to practice and do research on the topic.

Dr. Donta received his B.S. from Allegheny College and his M.D. from Albert Einstein College of Medicine; he did an internship/residency in Internal Medicine at University of Pittsburgh Hospitals.

**J. Stephen Dumler, M.D.** is a professor in the Department of Pathology at the Johns Hopkins University School of Medicine. Dr. Dumler is a medical microbiologist and pathologist with extensive training in the cellular microbiology of infectious diseases, with a focus on rickettsial infections, tick-borne infections, and other vector-borne diseases. He played key roles in the discovery of human granulocytic anaplasmosis (HGA), identification of its etiologic agent, description of the disease, development of serological and molecular diagnostic methods, and investigation of the antimicrobial sensitivity of anaplasma phagocytophilum.

Dr. Dumler has also significantly contributed to the understanding of *Ehrlichia* and *anaplasma*. His work on these organisms includes initial discovery, phenotypic characterization, taxonomic classification, development of diagnostic tools that are the current laboratory standards, identification of the reservoirs and vector hosts of these pathogens, and characterization of the virulence factors and mechanisms of pathogenesis. His current work crosses from translational medicine to basic science, including the investigation of epigenetics of intracellular pathogen infections.

**Brian A. Fallon, M.D.** serves as director of the Lyme and Tick-borne Diseases Research Center at the Columbia University Medical Center, director of the Center for Neuroinflammatory Disorders and Biobehavioral Medicine, and professor of Clinical Psychiatry at Columbia University and the NYS Psychiatric Institute. As a clinical research scientist, Dr. Fallon has conducted NIH-supported research in the medical/neurologic domain on chronic Lyme encephalopathy and in the psychiatric domain on somatoform disorders and obsessive compulsive disorders. His primary research approaches have included structural and functional neuroimaging, spinal fluid and serologic assessments, and clinical treatment trials. His primary focus in Lyme disease over the last 10 years has been on identifying improved diagnostic tests and biomarkers of treatment response and on evaluating different treatments for patients with chronic symptoms that have persisted despite standard courses of antibiotic therapies for Lyme disease.

**Howard Ginsberg, Ph.D.** is a research ecologist with the U.S. Geological Survey, Biological Resources Discipline, at Patuxent Wildlife Research Center. He is unit leader of Patuxent's Coastal Field Station and Professor in Residence at the University of Rhode Island. His emphasis is on understanding transmission dynamics and factors that influence human exposure to vector-borne zoonotic pathogens. This knowledge is used to develop efficient approaches to surveillance and management of vector-borne diseases that protect public health while minimizing negative effects on sensitive natural systems.

Dr. Ginsberg received his Ph.D. in entomology from Cornell University in 1979.

**Afton Hassett, Psy.D.** is a licensed clinical psychologist and an associate research scientist in the Department of Anesthesiology, Division of Pain Medicine at the University of Michigan Medical School.

Currently, as a principal investigator at the Chronic Pain and Fatigue Research Center under the direction of Dr. Daniel Clauw, she conducts research exploring the role of psychological and affective factors in chronic pain conditions like fibromyalgia, rheumatoid arthritis, lupus, and Post Lyme Disease Syndrome. Although much of her research has targeted risk factors for poor symptomatic and neurobiological outcomes, she has been an advocate for identifying patient strengths and promoting resilience.

Dr. Hassett is a graduate of Colorado State University and received her doctorate from Alliant International University in San Diego, California, in 2000.

**Nahed Ismail, Ph.D., M.Sc.** is associate professor at the Department of Pathology, Meharry Medical College, and director of oral pathogen core at the Vanderbilt Institution of Clinical and Translational Research of the Vanderbilt-Meharry Alliance. Dr. Ismail studied several aspects of host-microbial interactions with particular emphasis on the immunopathogensis of infectious diseases caused by intracellular bacteria, and the immunoregulatory mechanisms that control the induction and effector functions of T lymphocytes during infection.

At the University of Texas Medical Branch, she established an independent research career in Ehrlichial and Rickettsial diseases with particular focus on protective immunity and immunopathogensis of this tick-borne emerging infectious disease. Her research on Rickettsial and Ehrlichial immunity, pathology, pathogenesis, and pathophysiology included important contributions to elucidating the protective or pathogenic immune mechanisms against *Rickettsiae* and *Ehrlichiae* that contribute to the development of mild or severe Ehrlichial and Rickettsial diseases.

She obtained a M.D. from Tanta University in Egypt in 1988, a M.Sc. in 1995 from the University of Toronto, and a Ph.D. from the University of Saskatchewan in Saskatoon, Canada, in 2000.

**Richard F. Jacobs, M.D.** is currently the Robert H. Fiser, Jr., Endowed Chair in Pediatrics and the chairman of the Department of Pediatrics at the University of Arkansas for Medical Sciences (UAMS), and the president of the Arkansas Children's Hospital Research Institute. His research interests include the clinical and translational research trials of neonatal-infant antiviral treatment of congenital and perinatal viral infections. He received his M. D. degree from UAMS in 1977 and completed his infectious diseases fellowship training in 1982 at the University of Washington in Seattle.

**Peter J. Krause, M.D.** is a senior research scientist in the Department of Epidemiology and Public Health at the Yale School of Medicine in New Haven, Connecticut. Dr. Krause carries out clinical, epidemiological, and translational research in the study of vector-borne disease. His primary focus has been on human babesiosis and two companion tick-borne infections, Lyme disease and human granulocytic anaplasmosis.

Dr. Krause and his colleagues were the first to identify the long-term persistence of babesial infection in people and the first to characterize persistent and relapsing babesiosis in immunocompromised hosts in a case series. They quantitated the risk of transmission of babesiosis and Lyme disease though blood transfusion, developed several antibody and molecular-based tests for the diagnosis of babesiosis, and carried out the first antibiotic trial for the treatment of human babesiosis. They also were the first to characterize the frequency and clinical outcome of tick-borne disease coinfection.

Dr. Krause received his B.A. with honors in biology from Williams College and his M.D. from Tufts University School of Medicine. He completed his pediatric internship and residency at Yale–New Haven Hospital and Stanford University Medical Center and his pediatric infectious diseases training at the University of California, Los Angeles.

**Matthew Liang, M.D., M.P.H.** is a professor of medicine at Harvard Medical School, professor of health policy and management at Harvard School of Public Health, and a primary care physician and rheumatologist. He is also the director of special projects of the Robert B. Brigham Arthritis and Musculoskeletal Diseases Clinical Research Center at the Brigham and Women's Hospital, and he is medical director of rehabilitation services.

His research interests include basic methodologic work in clinimetrics, clinical trials, the epidemiology of rheumatic disease and disability, outcomes research, and the identification of modifiable risk factors in high risk and disadvantaged populations. In Lyme disease, his group studied the cost-effectiveness of the Lyme vaccine, studied long-term outcomes of Lyme disease, identified barriers to tick removal and avoidance, and conducted a clinical trial of over 30,000 travelers demonstrating the effectiveness of a novel health educational intervention in preventing Lyme and other tick-borne illnesses.

He is a graduate of Johns Hopkins University in philosophy and chemistry, Harvard Medical School, and the Harvard School of Public Health where he studied tropical public health and epidemiology.

**Benjamin J. Luft, M.D.** is an Edmund D. Pellegrino Professor in the Department of Infectious Diseases at State University of New York (SUNY) at Stony Brook.

From 1994–2006, he was chairman of the Department of Medicine and Director of Infectious Diseases. His research into the molecular biological structure of antigens of *Borrelia* species is for developing sensitive and specific diagnostic tests, as well as the development of a vaccine, which is undergoing testing in Europe. Dr. Luft led the NIH AIDS Clinical Trials Group effort on toxoplasmosis from 1986–1996. He has developed new antibiotics and diagnostic approaches to *Toxoplasma gondii*.

Dr. Luft obtained his B.A. from SUNY at Stony Brook in 1973 and his M.D. from Albert Einstein College of Medicine in 1976. He received his infectious disease training at Stanford University School of Medicine.

**Jere W. McBride, Ph.D., M.S.** is associate professor in the Departments of Pathology and Microbiology and Immunology at the University of Texas Medical Branch at Galveston. In addition to his academic appointments, he is a scientist in the Sealy Center for Vaccine Development, and a member of the Center for Biofense and Emerging Infectious Diseases and the Institute of Human Infections and Immunity. He is has research projects to study pathobiology, immunity and vaccine and diagnostic development related to human and veterinary ehrlichioses.

His current research interests include identification and molecular characterization of protective immunodeterminants of *Ehrlichia*, investigation of pathogenic mechanisms and host-pathogen interactions involving secreted effector proteins of *Ehrlichia*, understanding the molecular mechanisms involved in the adaptation of *Ehrlichia* to mammalian and arthropod hosts, and translational research directed at the development of diagnostics and vaccines for the ehrlichioses.

He received his doctorate in comparative pathology from the University of California at Davis in 1997, followed by postdoctoral fellowship at the University of Texas Medical Branch from 1998–2000, where his studies focused on vaccine development for the ehrlichioses.

**Captain Jennifer McQuiston, D.V.M., M.S.** serves as the epidemiology activity leader in the Rickettsial Zoonoses Branch in the Division of Vectorborne Diseases (DVBD) at the National Center for Emerging and Zoonotic Infectious Diseases in the Centers for Disease Control and Prevention (CDC).

Dr. McQuiston joined CDC in 1998 as an epidemic intelligence service officer, conducting research and the investigation of outbreaks related to zoonotic diseases. She has worked extensively on rickettsial diseases such as Rocky Mountain spotted fever, ehrlichiosis, anaplasmosis, Q fever, typhus, and cat scratch disease.

She attended Virginia-Maryland Regional College of Veterinary Medicine, where she received a D.V.M. in 1997 and an M.S. in Molecular

Biology in 1998. She is a diplomate of the American College of Veterinary Preventive Medicine.

**Paul Mead, M.D., M.P.H.** is chief of the epidemiology and surveillance activity in the Bacterial Diseases Branch of the Division of Vector-borne Diseases at the Centers of Disease Control and Prevention (CDC). His current responsibilities include surveillance, research, and prevention activities for Lyme disease, plague, tularemia, and tick-borne relapsing fever. Dr. Mead is board certified in Infectious Diseases by the American Board of Internal Medicine.

Dr. Mead received his M.D. from the University of Colorado and completed Internal Medicine Residency at Dartmouth Hitchcock Medical Center, followed by an Infectious Diseases Fellowship at the University of California, San Francisco. In 1994, Dr. Mead received a M.P.H. from the University of California, Berkeley.

**Ulrike (Uli) G. Munderloh, D.V.M, Ph.D.** is an associate professor in the Department of Entomology at the University of Minnesota. At the University of Minnesota, Dr. Munderloh examines the host-vector-pathogen interface of *Anaplasma* and *Rickettsia* species, using cell and molecular biology tools to study the functional genomics of this highly evolved relationship between bacteria, ticks, and humans.

Dr. Munderloh received her academic education in Munich and graduated from the school of veterinary medicine in 1975. She received a doctorate in the area of tropical veterinary medicine from the Institute of Comparative Tropical Medicine and Parasitology, Ludwig-Maximilians-Universität, Munich, in 1977.

**Steven J. Norris, Ph.D.** is currently the Robert Greer Professor in Biomedical Sciences and vice chair of pathology and laboratory medicine at the University of Texas Medical School at Houston. Dr. Norris began his faculty career at the University of Texas Medical School at Houston in 1982 and continued studies on the physiology and in vitro culture of *Treponema pallidum*, the spirochete that causes syphilis. His group is currently screening a transposon insertion library in *B. burgdorferi* in an attempt to identify every gene important in Lyme disease pathogenesis. He is a Fellow of the American Academy of Microbiology and has served as the chair of the American Society for Microbiology Division of General Medical Microbiology and of the Gordon Research Conference on the Biology of Spirochetes.

Dr. Norris received a B.A. in psychobiology at the University of California, Los Angeles (UCLA), then gradually evolved toward microbiology while obtaining an M.S. in biochemistry and molecular biology at UC Santa Barbara, and a Ph.D. in microbiology and immunology at UCLA in 1980.

**Susan O'Connell, M.D.** is head of the Lyme Borreliosis Unit (LBU) at the Health Protection Agency's Microbiology Laboratory at Southampton University Hospitals Trust, Southampton UK. The LBU provides laboratory diagnostic and clinical advisory service on Lyme disease and other tick-borne infections for the UK. She graduated in medicine from Dublin and trained in general medicine and family practice in the UK before specializing in microbiology and infectious diseases. She has worked at the LBU since 1990 and was a leading participant in the European Union Concerted Action on Lyme Borreliosis (EUCALB) initiative, in addition to other international collaborations. Current activities include an epidemiologic overview of European Lyme borreliosis for the European Centre for Disease Control, review of the EUCALB clinical case definitions, and development of European guidelines for the prevention, diagnosis, and management of Lyme borreliosis and other tick-borne infections.

She has a major commitment nationally to the prevention and early recognition of Lyme borreliosis, and she works closely with a wide range of health-care workers, occupational groups, recreational groups, and the media to promote awareness and risk reduction measures.

**James H. Oliver, Jr., Ph.D.** is director of the James H. Oliver, Jr. Institute of Arthropodology and Parasitology, and Callaway Professor of Biology Emeritus at Georgia Southern University. His current research focuses on more than 300 cultured *Borrelia* isolates and 5 tick vector species from the southeastern United States.

Dr. Oliver's fields of specialization include medical entomology, acarology, and genetics focusing on defining tick-host-pathogen interrelationships including tick phenology and ecology, vector competency, transmission of microorganisms, isolation and *in vitro* cultivation of pathogens, their infectivity and pathogenesis, and vertebrate hosts as reservoirs of pathogens, among other topics. His emphasis is on producing fundamental knowledge that can be applied to prevention and intervention of arthropod pests and vectors of pathogens important in livestock, agriculture, and biomedicine.

Dr. Oliver has obtained a B.S. in biology, a M.S. in zoology, and a Ph.D. in entomology.

**Richard S. Ostfeld, Ph.D.** is a senior scientist at the Cary Institute of Ecosystem Studies, a not-for-profit research institution in Millbrook, New York, dedicated to providing the science behind environmental solutions. He is also adjunct professor at Rutgers University and the University of

Connecticut. His research focuses on ecological determinants of human risk of exposure to infectious diseases, emphasizing Lyme and other tick-borne diseases as well as West Nile Virus.

He obtained his B.A. from the University of California, Santa Cruz, and his Ph.D. from the University of California, Berkeley.

**Juan Olano, M.D.** is an associate professor in the Department of Pathology and director of the residency training program at the University of Texas Medical Branch.

His research interests are focused on obligate intracellular bacteria, namely, *Rickettsiae* and *Ehrlichiae*. His current research focuses on development of aerosolized animal models for *rickettsiae*, development of ultrasensitive diagnostic methods for rickettsial infections, and pathogenesis of rickettsial infections as it relates to molecular mechanisms of increased microvascular permeability.

Dr. Olano received his M.D. from the University of Cauca in Colombia in 1987.

**José M. C. Ribeiro, M.D., Ph.D.** is chief of the Vector Biology Section of the Laboratory of Malaria and Vector Research at the National Institute of Allergy and Infectious Diseases (NIAID) at the National Institutes of Health. His research focus is on the role of vector saliva in feeding and parasite transmission by arthropods and in the ecology of vector-borne diseases. He joined the Department of Entomology of the University of Arizona in 1990 as full professor, and in 1996, he moved to NIAID as head of the Section of Vector Biology.

Dr. Ribeiro graduated from the State University of Rio de Janeiro and obtained his Ph.D. at the Biophysics Institute of the Federal University of Rio de Janeiro.

**Tom G. Schwan, Ph.D., M.S.** is chief of the Laboratory of Zoonotic Pathogens and the Medical Entomology Section of the National Institute of Allergy and Infectious Diseases. In recent years, his work has narrowed its focus to the biology of soft (argasid) ticks, the interaction of spirochetes in their tick vectors, improving serological tests for identifying human infections with spirochetes, and identifying geographic areas where tick-borne relapsing fever poses a risk for humans.

He received his undergraduate training in biology at California State University, Hayward, where he also did his M.A. research on the fleas parasitizing grassland rodents. Dr. Schwan then studied at the University of California, Berkeley, to earn his Ph.D. in parasitology and medical entomology, while he also worked on fleas and the surveillance of plague with the Vector Control Section of the California State Department of Health.

**Gregg Skall, J.D.** is a member of the law firm Womble Carlyle Sandridge & Rice, PLLC. He serves as counsel to the National Capital Lyme & Tick-Borne Disease Association, a pro bono client of Womble Carlyle Sandridge & Rice, PLLC.

He received his B.A. in 1966 at the Ohio State University and his J.D. in 1969 at the University of Cincinnati College of Law.

**Gustavo Valbuena, M.D.** is an instructor in the Department of Pathology at the University of Texas. He is a physician-scientist with training in anatomical, clinical, and experimental pathology. His expertise includes pathogenesis, immunology, and the development of animal models and *in vitro* systems for the study of rickettsial diseases. The research interests of his laboratory currently focus on four areas that are funded by the National Institutes of Health. These areas are the role of the endothelium in the regulation of the anti-rickettsial immune response, the identification of rickettsial antigens recognized by T cells and B cells (the first step in the development of an anti-rickettsial vaccine), the optimization of a humanized mouse model of rickettsial infections, and the development of a mouse model of scrub typhus.

He obtained his M.D. from Javeriana University in Bogota, Colombia, and subsequently completed residency training in pathology at the University of Texas Medical Branch (UTMB) in Galveston, Texas. Dr. Valbuena also received a Ph.D. in experimental pathology from UTMB.

**David Jay Weber, M.D., M.P.H.** is currently a professor of medicine and pediatrics in the University of North Carolina (UNC) School of Medicine, and a Professor of Epidemiology in the UNC School of Public Health. He also serves as the medical director of the Departments of Hospital Epidemiology (Infection Control), Occupational Health, and Environmental Health and Safety for the UNC Health Care System. He is an associate director of the North Carolina Statewide Infection Control Program and serves as director of the Regulatory Core for the UNC Clinical Translational Research Award. He is board-certified in internal medicine, infectious disease, critical care medicine, and preventive medicine.

His research interests include the epidemiology of healthcare-associated infections, new and emerging infectious diseases (Pfisteria, nontuberculous mycobacteria, SAR-coV, norovirus, community-associated MRSA), control of drug resistant pathogens, immunization practices (especially of healthcare workers), zoonotic diseases, and epidemiology of tuberculosis.

He received his B.A. from Wesleyan University in 1973, his M.D. from the University of California, San Diego, in 1977, his M.P.H. from Harvard

University in 1985. He completed his medicine residency and infectious disease fellowship at the Massachusetts General Hospital in 1985.

**Pamela Weintraub** is the features editor at *Discover* magazine and the author of *Cure Unknown: Inside the Lyme Epidemic*, a personal memoir and journalistic investigation into the medical history, patient experience, and brutal political war over Lyme disease and the winner of the American Medical Writer Association book award, 2009. Weintraub has worked as a journalist covering health and biomedicine for national media since 1981 and is the author of 16 prior books on topics from the infant brain to bioterrorism to emergency medicine.

**Janis J. Weis, Ph.D.** is a professor in the Department of Pathology at the University of Utah School of Medicine in Salt Lake City. Her laboratory studies the host–pathogen interactions associated with *Borrelia burgdorferi* infection and the pathogenesis of Lyme arthritis. The overall goals of her research are to understand the bacterial triggers required for arthritis development and the signaling pathways involved in disease progression. Dr. Weis maintains an active research laboratory at the University of Utah studying the mechanism and genetic regulation of Lyme arthritis development.

Dr. Weis received a B.A. in microbiology from the University of Kansas and a Ph.D. in microbiology from the University of Minnesota. She received post-doctoral training in Immunology at Brigham and Women's Hospital/Harvard Medical School from 1982–1986, where she studied structure/function aspects of innate host defense and viral infection.

**Gary P. Wormser, M.D.** is chief of the Division of Infectious Diseases and vice chairperson of the Department of Medicine at New York Medical College. He is professor of medicine and pharmacology. At Westchester Medical Center, Dr. Wormser is chief of the section of infectious diseases, director and founder of the Infectious Diseases Fellowship Program, and director and founder of the Lyme Disease Diagnostic Center. Dr. Wormser's principal research interests are Lyme disease, babesiosis, and human granulocytic anaplasmosis.

Dr. Wormser received his B.A. from the University of Pennsylvania and his M.D. from the Johns Hopkins University School of Medicine.